Review and
Self-Assessment
to Accompany

EMERGENCY MEDICINE

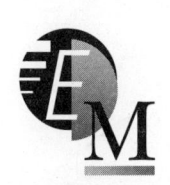

John M. Howell, MD, FACEP
Associate Professor and Chairman
Department of Emergency Medicine
Georgetown University Hospital
Washington, DC

Judith Linden, MD, FACEP
Assistant Professor and Associate Residency
Director of Emergency Medicine
Department of Emergency Medicine
Boston Medical Center
Boston, Massachusetts

Donald Barton, MD
Clinical Assistant Professor and Associate
Director
Department of Emergency Medicine
Mount Sinai Services
Elmhurst Hospital Center
Elmhurst, New York

Sheree Givre, MD
Clinical Assistant Professor and
Associate Director
Department of Emergency Medicine
Mount Sinai School of Medicine
Associate Director of Emergency Department
Elmhurst Hospital Center
Elmhurst, New York

W.B. SAUNDERS COMPANY
A Division of Harcourt Brace & Company
Philadelphia • London • Toronto • Montreal • Sydney • Tokyo

W.B. SAUNDERS COMPANY
A Division of Harcourt Brace & Company

The Curtis Center
Independence Square West
Philadelphia, Pennsylvania 19106

Library of Congress Cataloging-in-Publication Data

Review and self assessment to accompany Emergency medicine / [edited by] John M. Howell . . . [et al.].—1st ed.

p.   cm.

ISBN 0–7216–5821–0

1. Emergency medicine—Examinations, questions, etc.   2. Emergency medicine—Outlines, syllabi, etc.   I. Howell, John M., M.D. [DNLM: 1. Emergencies outlines.   2. Emergency Medical Services outlines.   WB 105 E537 1998 Suppl. 1999]

RC86.7.E5792   1998 Suppl.

616.02′5′076—dc21

DNLM/DLC   98-19199

REVIEW AND SELF-ASSESSMENT TO ACCOMPANY EMERGENCY MEDICINE   ISBN 0–7216–5821–0

Copyright © 1999 by W.B. Saunders Company.

All rights reserved. No part of this publication may be reproduced or transmitted in any form or by any means, electronic or mechanical, including photocopy, recording, or any information storage and retrieval system, without permission in writing from the publisher.

Printed in the United States of America.

Last digit is the print number: 9   8   7   6   5   4   3   2   1

I would like to give special recognition to my new husband, Stephen Marcus, whose support and encouragement were invaluable during the completion of this study guide and my many other projects.

Judy Linden

To my daughter Eliana, you're my joy and inspiration in life.

Sheree Givre

CONTRIBUTORS

Robert A. Aldoroty, PhD, MD
Assistant Professor, Mount Sinai School of Medicine, New York, New York
Abdominal and Urogenital Trauma and Pelvic Trauma: Abdominal and Urogenital Trauma

Paul A. Andrulonis, MD
Resident, University of Pennsylvania School of Medicine, and Department of Emergency Medicine, Hospital of the University of Pennsylvania, Philadelphia, Pennsylvania
Disorders of the Ears, Nose, and Sinuses

Carol Leah Barsky, MD
Assistant Clinical Professor of Medicine, College of Physicians and Surgeons, Columbia University; Director, Emergency Medicine Education, and Associate Residency Program Director, St. Luke's–Roosevelt Hospital Center, New York, New York
Upper Extremity: Shoulder, Humerus, Elbow, Forearm, Wrist, and Hand; Lower Extremity: Leg, Knee, Ankle, and Foot; Pediatric Orthopedic Emergencies, Joint and Bone Inflammation and Infection, Hip Injuries, and Disorders of the Spine

Donald Barton, MD
Clinical Assistant Professor and Associate Director, Department of Emergency Medicine, Mount Sinai Services, Elmhurst Hospital Center, Elmhurst, New York
Sepsis; Autoimmune Disorders; Breast Disorders; Administrative and Medicolegal Aspects of Emergency Medicine, Organ Procurement, and Wellness and Ethics

Kevin Baumlin, MD
Assistant Professor of Emergency Medicine, Department of Emergency Medicine, Mount Sinai School of Medicine; Assistant Residency Director, Emergency Medicine Residency, Mount Sinai Hospital, New York, New York
Cerebrovascular Emergencies and Cranial Nerve Disorders

Tareg Bey, MD
Clinical Instructor, University of Arizona Health Sciences Center, University of Arizona, Division of Emergency Medicine, Tucson, Arizona
Approach to Delirium and Psychiatric Illness, Thought Disorder, and Suicide; Substance Abuse, Addiction, and Withdrawal; Trauma in Special Populations: Pediatric and Pregnant Patients

Adrienne Birnbaum, MD
Assistant Professor and Residency Director, Department of Emergency Medicine, Albert Einstein College of Medicine Jacobi Medical Center and Montefiore Medical Center, Bronx, New York
Head Trauma

John C. Brancato, MD
Assistant Professor of Pediatrics, University of Connecticut School of Medicine, Farmington; Attending Physician, Division of Pediatric Emergency Medicine, Connecticut Children's Medical Center, Hartford, Connecticut
Congenital Heart Disease; Fluid and Electrolyte Management

Jeremy Brown, MD
Instructor in Medicine, Harvard Medical School; Attending Physician, Division of Emergency Medicine, Beth Israel Deaconess Medical Center, Boston, Massachusetts
Maxillofacial Trauma and Neck Trauma

Paul Buckley, MD, PhD
Emergency Medicine Resident, St. Luke's–Roosevelt Hospital Center, New York, New York
Upper Extremity: Shoulder, Humerus, Elbow, Forearm, Wrist, and Hand; Lower Extremity: Leg, Knee, Ankle, and Foot; Pediatric Orthopedic Emergencies, Joint and Bone Inflammation and Infection, Hip Injuries, and Disorders of the Spine

Richard Caggiano, MD
Attending Physician, Director of Emergency Services, Pullman Memorial Hospital, Pullman, Washington
Approach to Chest Pain, Myocardial Ischemia, and Congestive Heart Failure

Yvette Calderon, MD, FACEP
Assistant Professor and Site Residency Director, Albert Einstein College of Medicine; Assistant Director of Operations, Assistant Director of Quality Assurance, Hyperbaric Medicine and Snakebite Consultant, Jacobi Medical Center, Bronx, New York
Approach to Multiple Trauma and Spinal Trauma

Melissa E. Clarke, MD, FACEP
Assistant Professor, Howard University College of Medicine; Attending Physician, Emergency Medicine, Howard University Hospital, Washington, DC
Diseases of the Arteries and Veins and Aortic Emergencies; Pericarditis, Myocarditis, and Endocarditis

Kathryn Craig, MD
Lecturer/Research Fellow, University of Michigan Medical Center, Section of Emergency Medicine, Ann Arbor, Michigan; Resident, St. Luke's–Roosevelt Hospital, Department of Emergency Medicine, New York, New York
Upper Extremity: Shoulder, Humerus, Elbow, Forearm, Wrist, and Hand; Pediatric Orthopedic Emergencies, Joint and Bone Inflammation and Infection, Hip Injuries, and Disorders of the Spine

Fernando Daniels III, MD, FACEP
Assistant Professor, EMS Director, Howard University, College of Medicine; Attending Physician, Emergency Medicine, Howard University Hospital, Washington, DC
Diseases of the Arteries and Veins and Aortic Emergencies

Robert Dart, MD
Assistant Professor, Department of Emergency Medicine, Boston Medical Center, Boston, Massachusetts
Adult Medical Resuscitation; Airway Management

Elizabeth M. Datner, MD
Assistant Professor, University of Pennsylvania School of Medicine and Department of Emergency Medicine, Hospital of the University of Pennsylvania, Philadelphia, Pennsylvania
Disorders of the Ears, Nose, and Sinuses

Charles DiMaggio, PA-C, MPH
Assistant Adjunct Professor, Department of Allied Health Sciences, Nassau Community College, Garden City; Chief Physician Assistant, Emergency Department, Mount Sinai Services, Elmhurst Hospital Center, Elmhurst, New York
Parasitic and Exotic Illnesses (Malaria, Dengue Fever, and Trypanosomiasis) and Syphilis and Leptospirosis: Parasitic Diseases (Malaria, Dengue Fever, and Trypanosomiasis)

Gail D'Onofrio, MD
Associate Professor of Emergency Medicine, Research Director, Section of Emergency Medicine, Yale University School of Medicine, New Haven, Connecticut
Arrhythmias, Hypertension, and Syncope

David H. Dorfman, MD
Assistant Professor of Pediatrics, Boston University School of Medicine; Active Staff, Boston Medical Center, Boston, Massachusetts
Pediatric Resuscitation; Fluid and Electrolyte Management

Sophia Dyer, MD
Fellow in Medical Toxicology, Instructor in Pediatrics, Harvard Medical School, Childrens Hospital, Boston, Massachusetts
Adult Medical Resuscitation; Airway Management

Phillip Fairweather, MD
Clinical Assistant Professor, Department of Emergency Medicine, Mount Sinai School of Medicine, New York; Associate Residency Director, Mount Sinai Emergency Medicine Residency, Elmhurst Hospital Center, Elmhurst, New York
Cerebrovascular Emergencies and Cranial Nerve Disorders; Renal Failure, Hematuria, Renal Insufficiency, and Urinary Tract Infection

Jane Federman, MD
Clinical Assistant Professor, College of Physicians and Surgeons of Columbia University; Attending Emergency Medicine Faculty, St. Luke's–Roosevelt Hospital Center, New York, New York
Injury Prevention, Sexual Assault, and Domestic Violence

Douglas W. Fields, MD
Resident, Emergency Medicine, Mount Sinai Medical Center, New York, New York
Noninfectious Disorders of the Male Genital Tract; Renal and Ureteral Calculi

Luanne Freer, MD, FACEP
Assistant Clinical Professor of Emergency Medicine, George Washington University School of Medicine, Washington, DC; Assistant Professor, Department of Surgery, Division of Emergency Medicine, University of Maryland, Baltimore, Maryland; Medical Director, Air Idaho Rescue, Eastern Idaho Regional Medical Center, Idaho Falls, Idaho; Associate Medical Director, Yellowstone National Park, Wyoming
Altitude Illness, Heat- and Cold-Related Illness, and Lightning and Electric Injury

Jeff Galvin, MD
Attending Physician, Department of Emergency Medicine, 1SW Hospital, Langley Air Force Base, Hampton, Virginia
Wound Management, Burns, and Blast Injuries

Marian L. Gambrell, MD
Clinical Professor of Emergency Medicine, Columbia University, Columbia Presbyterian College of Physicians and Surgeons; Attending Physician of Emergency Medicine, St. Luke's–Roosevelt Hospital Center, New York, New York
Gastrointestinal Hemorrhage and Appendicitis

Syndee J. Givre, MD
Resident, Department of Ophthalmology, Mount Sinai Medical Center, New York, New York
Traumatic and Nontraumatic Eye Disorders

Richard J. Hamilton, MD
Assistant Professor of Emergency Medicine and Program Director, Medical Toxicology Fellowship, MCP Hahnemann University; Clinical Director, Emergency Center, Medical College of Pennsylvania Hospital, Philadelphia, Pennsylvania
Approach to the Poisoned Patient, Acetaminophen, Salicylates and NSAIDs, and Iron; Anticholinergics, Antidepressants, Cardiac Drug Ingestions, Theophylline, and Beta-Agonists; Ethanol, Toxic Alcohols, Benzodiazepines, and Anticonvulsants; Cocaine and Stimulants, Hallucinogens, Mushrooms and Toxic Vegetations, Opioids, Pesticides, Phenothiazines, and Other Neuroleptics; Caustic Ingestions, Hydrocarbon Ingestions, Physical and Chemical Irritants and Asphyxiants, Methemoglobinemia, and Lead

Debra Heitmann, MD
Clinical Instructor, University of Massachusetts Medical School; Attending Physician, Department of Emergency Medicine, University of Massachusetts Memorial Medical Center, Worcester, Massachusetts
Abdominal and Urogenital Trauma and Pelvic Trauma: Abdominal and Urogenital Trauma

Lynne Holden, MD
Assistant Professor, Albert Einstein Medical College; Assistant Residency Director, Emergency Medicine, and Associate Site Director, Montefiore Medical Center, Bronx, New York
Approach to the Patient with Abdominal Pain and Diarrhea; Disorders of the Esophagus, Liver, Pancreas, and Gallbladder

Judd E. Hollander, MD
Associate Professor, Department of Emergency Medicine, University of Pennsylvania School of Medicine; Clinical Research Director, Department of Emergency Medicine, Hospital of the University of Pennsylvania, Philadelphia, Pennsylvania
Cricothyroidotomy and Percutaneous Transtracheal Ventilation and Peritoneal Lavage; Lumbar Puncture and Gastrostomy Tubes; Percutaneous Central Venous Catheterization and Pericardiocentesis; Joint Aspiration, Major Joint Reduction, and Intraosseous Infusion

Erik Holt, MD
Resident, University of Pittsburgh Affiliated Residency in Emergency Medicine, Pittsburgh, Pennsylvania
Bites, Stings, and Rabies; Diving Injuries and Illness; and Radiation

CONTRIBUTORS

David K. Hoshizaki, MD
Assistant Clinical Professor, Division of Emergency Medicine, University of Alberta, Edmonton, Alberta, Canada
Rashes, Dermatitis, and Skin Lesions

Carl K. Hsu, MD
Clinical Assistant, Albert Einstein College of Medicine; Attending Physician, Department of Emergency Medicine, Beth Israel Medical Center, New York, New York
Pregnancy, Labor, and Delivery; Approach to Pelvic Pain and Infectious and Noninfectious Disorders

Oliver Hung, MD
Toxicology Fellow, New York City Poison Control Center, New York, New York
Approach to the Poisoned Patient, Acetaminophen, Salicylates and NSAIDs, and Iron; Anticholinergics, Antidepressants, Cardiac Drug Ingestions, Theophylline, and Beta-Agonists; Ethanol, Toxic Alcohols, Benzodiazepines, and Anticonvulsants; Cocaine and Stimulants, Hallucinogens, Mushrooms and Toxic Vegetations, Opioids, Pesticides, Phenothiazines, and Other Neuroleptics; Caustic Ingestions, Hydrocarbon Ingestions, Physical and Chemical Irritants and Asphyxiants, Methemoglobinemia, and Lead

Andy Jagoda, MD
Associate Professor, Department of Emergency Medicine, Associate Residency Director, Mount Sinai Emergency Medicine Residency, Mount Sinai Medical Center, New York, New York
Seizures and Headaches

Thea James, MD
Assistant Professor, Emergency Medicine, Boston University School of Medicine; Attending Physician, Boston Medical Center, Boston, Massachusetts
Hemoglobinopathies; Disorders of Hemostasis

Daniel M. Joyce, MD
Assistant Professor, Department of Emergency Medicine, State University of New York, Syracuse, New York
Approach to Pelvic Pain and Infectious and Noninfectious Disorders; Breast Disorders

Steven C. Larson, MD
Assistant Professor of Emergency Medicine, University of Pennsylvania School of Medicine, Hospital of the University of Pennsylvania, Philadelphia, Pennsylvania
Disorders of the Oropharynx and Throat

David L. Levine, MD
Assistant Professor, Emergency Medicine, Rush Medical College; Associate Director, Adult Emergency Services, Cook County Hospital, Chicago, Illinois
Rashes, Dermatitis, and Skin Lesions; Infections and Infestations, Skin Cancer, and Cutaneous Manifestations of Illness

Frank LoVecchio, DO
Assistant Clinical Professor and Director, Clinical Correlations, Midwestern University/Arizona College of Osteopathic Medicine, Glendale; Emergency Medicine Faculty, Maricopa Medical Center, Phoenix, Arizona
CNS Infections (Meningitis and Encephalitis); Mycobacterial and Tick-Borne Infections; Parasitic and Exotic Illnesses (Malaria, Dengue Fever, and Trypanosomiasis) and Syphilis and Leptospirosis: Syphilis and Leptospirosis

Robby Mahadeo, MD
Assistant Professor, Mount Sinai School of Medicine; Associate Director, Pediatric Emergency Medicine, Mount Sinai Medical Center, New York, New York
The Infant with Apnea by History; Febrile Child

John Mahoney, MD
Assistant Professor of Emergency Medicine, University of Pittsburgh School of Medicine, Pittsburgh, Pennsylvania
Bites, Stings, and Rabies; Diving Injuries and Illness; and Radiation

Ron Medzon, MD
Clinical Instructor, Department of Emergency Medicine, Boston University School of Medicine; Attending Physician, Emergency Department, Boston Medical Center, Boston, Massachusetts
Endocrine Disorders

Elizabeth L. Mitchell, MD
Assistant Professor of Emergency Medicine, Boston University School of Medicine and Boston Medical Center, Boston, Massachusetts
Extremity Trauma

Lisa B. Namerow, MD
Assistant Professor of Pediatrics and Psychiatry, University of Connecticut School of Medicine, Farmington; Division Chief, Child and Adolescent Psychiatry, and Training Director, Child and Adolescent Psychiatry, Institute of Living/Hartford Hospital, Connecticut Children's Medical Center, Hartford, Connecticut
Approach to Delirium and Psychiatric Illness, Thought Disorder, and Suicide; Substance Abuse, Addiction, and Withdrawal

Lewis Nelson, MD
Assistant Professor of Clinical Surgery/Emergency Medicine, New York University School of Medicine; Director, Fellowship in Medical Toxicology, New York City Poison Control Center, New York, New York
Pulmonary Embolism and Chronic Obstructive Pulmonary Disease

William O'Callahan, MD
Attending Physician, University of Massachusetts Memorial Hospital, Worcester, Massachusetts
Dental Emergencies

Neill S. Oster, MD
Assistant Professor of Emergency Medicine, Mount Sinai School of Medicine, Department of Emergency Medicine, New York; Director, Disaster Emergency Medical Services, and Assistant Residency Director, Mount Sinai Services, Elmhurst Hospital Center, Elmhurst, New York
Approach to a Disaster, EMS Systems Organization and Operation, Patient Transfer, and Air Medical Transport; Administrative and Medicolegal Aspects of Emergency Medicine, Organ Procurement, and Wellness and Ethics: Wellness and Ethics

Mary Palmer, MD
Toxicology Fellow, New York City Poison Control Center, New York, New York
Approach to the Poisoned Patient, Acetaminophen, Salicylates and NSAIDs, and Iron; Anticholinergics, Antidepressants, Cardiac Drug Ingestions, Theophylline, and Beta-Agonists; Ethanol, Toxic Alcohols, Benzodiazepines, and Anticonvulsants; Cocaine and Stimulants, Hallucinogens, Mushrooms and Toxic Vegetations, Opioids, Pesticides, Phenothiazines, and Other

Neuroleptics; Caustic Ingestions, Hydrocarbon Ingestions, Physical and Chemical Irritants and Asphyxiants, Methemoglobinemia, and Lead

Ernst Paul, Jr, MD
Clinical Assistant Professor, Department of Emergency Medicine, Mount Sinai School of Medicine, Elmhurst Hospital Center, Elmhurst, New York
Adult Respiratory Failure; Gastrointestinal Obstruction and Anorectal Disorders; Renal Failure, Hematuria, Renal Insufficiency, and Urinary Tract Infection

Rama B. Rao, MD
Faculty, Department of Surgery/Emergency Medicine, Bellevue Hospital Center/NYU Medical Center, New York, New York
Approach to the Poisoned Patient, Acetaminophen, Salicylates and NSAIDs, and Iron; Anticholinergics, Antidepressants, Cardiac Drug Ingestions, Theophylline, and Beta-Agonists; Ethanol, Toxic Alcohols, Benzodiazepines, and Anticonvulsants; Cocaine and Stimulants, Hallucinogens, Mushrooms and Toxic Vegetations, Opioids, Pesticides, Phenothiazines, and Other Neuroleptics; Caustic Ingestions, Hydrocarbon Ingestions, Physical and Chemical Irritants and Asphyxiants, Methemoglobinemia, and Lead

Niels K. Rathlev, MD
Associate Clinical Professor and Vice-Chairman, Boston University School of Medicine; Clinical Director, Boston Medical Center, Boston, Massachusetts
Maxillofacial Trauma and Neck Trauma

Luis Rodriguez, MD
Assistant Professor of Pediatrics, Mount Sinai School of Medicine, New York; Assistant Attending Physician, Mount Sinai Services, Elmhurst Hospital Center, Elmhurst, New York
Asthma, Pneumonia, Pleurisy, Empyema, and Disorders of the Pleura and Mediastinum

Todd C. Rothenhaus, MD
Assistant Professor, Department of Emergency Medicine, Boston University School of Medicine; Attending Physician, Emergency Department, Boston Medical Center, Boston, Massachusetts
Endocrine Disorders

Simon Roy, MD
Assistant Professor of Emergency Medicine, Boston University School of Medicine and Boston Medical Center, Boston, Massachusetts
Chest Trauma; Emergency Department Thoracotomy and Tube Thoracostomy

Mary Ryan, MD
Attending Physician, Lincoln Medical and Mental Health Center, Bronx, New York
Gastrointestinal Obstruction and Anorectal Disorders; Neuromuscular Disorders; Abdominal and Urogenital Trauma and Pelvic Trauma: Pelvic Trauma

Mark J. Sagarin, MD
Resident in Emergency Medicine, Harvard Medical School, Brigham and Women's Hospital and Massachusetts General Hospital, Boston, Massachusetts
Oncologic Emergencies, Red Blood Cell Disorders, and White Blood Cell Disorders; Disorders of Hemostasis

Sandra Sallustio, MD, PhD
Chief Resident, Department of Emergency Medicine, Mount Sinai Medical Center, New York, New York
Renal Failure, Hematuria, Renal Insufficiency, and Urinary Tract Infection

Peter Shearer, MD
Clinical Instructor, Mount Sinai School of Medicine, New York; Assistant Attending Physician, Department of Emergency Medicine, Elmhurst Hospital, Elmhurst, and Mount Sinai Hospital, New York, New York
Arrhythmias, Hypertension, and Syncope

Adam J. Singer, MD
Associate Professor, Research Director, Department of Emergency Medicine, State University of New York, Stony Brook, New York
Cricothyroidotomy and Percutaneous Transtracheal Ventilation and Peritoneal Lavage; Lumbar Puncture and Gastrostomy Tubes; Percutaneous Central Venous Catheterization and Pericardiocentesis; Joint Aspiration, Major Joint Reduction, and Intraosseous Infusion

Fred F. Tilden, MD
Assistant Professor, University of Connecticut School of Medicine, Farmington; Emergency Physician, Hartford Hospital, Hartford, Connecticut
Hypersensitivity and Related Disorders; Pain Management and Sedation

Barry J. Tils, MD
Emergency Department Staff, Newton-Wellesley Hospital, Newton, Massachusetts
Approach to Chest Pain, Myocardial Ischemia, and Congestive Heart Failure

Joseph Turban, MD
Attending Physician, Department of Emergency Medicine, Wahiawa General Hospital, Wahiawa, Hawaii
Approach to Altered Mental Status and Coma, Dizziness, and Vertigo

Andrew Ulrich, MD
Assistant Professor, Department of Emergency Medicine, Boston University School of Medicine; Residency Director, Department of Emergency Medicine, Boston Medical Center, Boston, Massachusetts
Wound Management, Burns, and Blast Injuries

Robert J. Vissers, MD
Assistant Professor, Emergency Medicine, and Assistant Residency Director, University of North Carolina, Chapel Hill, Chapel Hill, North Carolina
Oncologic Emergencies, Red Blood Cell Disorders, and White Blood Cell Disorders; Disorders of Hemostasis

Anthony J. Weekes, MD
Assistant Residency Director, Department of Emergency Medicine, Columbia–Presbyterian College of Physicians and Surgeons, St. Luke's–Roosevelt Hospital, New York, New York
Gastrointestinal Hemorrhage and Appendicitis

Ping Wong, MD
Department of Emergency Medicine, Elmhurst Hospital Center, Elmhurst, New York
Autoimmune Disorders

Richard J. Wong, MD
Clinical Assistant Professor, Department of Emergency Medicine, Mount Sinai School of Medicine, Elmhurst Hospital Center, New York
Approach to the Patient with HIV Infection and AIDS

PREFACE

Review and Self-Assessment to Accompany Emergency Medicine is a comprehensive study guide in Emergency Medicine. Intended for use by students, residents, and practicing physicians, it is designed in an easy-to-use question and answer format. While it is an ideal tool for use when preparing for the yearly in-service and American Board of Emergency Medicine (ABEM) certification examination, it may also be used by the practicing physician to more easily target topics for additional reading.

The study guide is divided into chapters consisting of 20 to 40 questions by topic. We recommend setting aside 30 to 60 minutes to answer the questions, then review the one-paragraph explanations. As the participant identifies areas of strength and weakness, we recommend further reading directed to targeted areas. Most answers are referenced to the Howell *Emergency Medicine* textbook chapter, and many include recent references for additional reading.

JOHN M. HOWELL
JUDITH LINDEN
DONALD BARTON
SHEREE GIVRE

ACKNOWLEDGMENTS

This study guide is dedicated to the students and residents at Boston Medical Center/Boston University School of Medicine and Elmhurst Hospital/Mount Sinai School of Medicine, who renew our sense of enthusiasm and curiosity, inspiring us to continually strive for academic excellence.

We would like to thank the contributors, who made this study guide possible through their hard work and timely completion. Finally, we would like to thank Dolores Meloni and all of the editors at W.B. Saunders for their helpful input and support in completing this study guide.

NOTICE

Emergency Medicine is an ever-changing field. Standard safety precautions must be followed, but as new research and clinical experience broaden our knowledge, changes in treatment and drug therapy become necessary or appropriate. Readers are advised to check the product information currently provided by the manufacturer of each drug to be administered to verify the recommended dose, the method and duration of administration, and the contraindications. It is the responsibility of the treating physician, relying on experience and knowledge of the patient, to determine dosages and the best treatment for the patient. Neither the publisher nor the editor assumes any responsibility for any injury and/or damage to persons or property.

THE PUBLISHER

Contents

Glossary of Abbreviations xxi

Section One
Resuscitation

1 Adult Medical Resuscitation 3
Robert Dart, MD and
Sophia Dyer, MD

2 Pediatric Resuscitation 6
David H. Dorfman, MD

3 The Infant with Apnea by History 11
Robby Mahadeo, MD

4 Adult Respiratory Failure 13
Ernst Paul, Jr, MD

5 Airway Management 15
Robert Dart, MD and
Sophia Dyer, MD

Section Two
Heart and Vascular System

6 Approach to Chest Pain, Myocardial Ischemia, and Congestive Heart Failure 21
Richard Caggiano, MD and
Barry J. Tils, MD

7 Arrhythmias, Hypertension, and Syncope 32
Peter Shearer, MD and
Gail D'Onofrio, MD

8 Diseases of the Arteries and Veins and Aortic Emergencies 45
Melissa E. Clarke, MD, FACEP and
Fernando Daniels III, MD, FACEP

9 Pericarditis, Myocarditis, and Endocarditis 51
Melissa E. Clarke, MD, FACEP

10 Congenital Heart Disease 56
John C. Brancato, MD

Section Three
Pulmonary Disorders

11 Pulmonary Embolism and Chronic Obstructive Pulmonary Disease .. 61
Lewis Nelson, MD

12 Asthma, Pneumonia, Pleurisy, Empyema, and Disorders of the Pleura and Mediastinum 67
Luis Rodriguez, MD

Section Four
Gastrointestinal Disorders

13 Approach to the Patient with Abdominal Pain and Diarrhea 75
Lynne Holden, MD

14 Disorders of the Esophagus, Liver, Pancreas, and Gallbladder 78
Lynne Holden, MD

15 Gastrointestinal Hemorrhage and Appendicitis 82
Anthony J. Weekes, MD and
Marian L. Gambrell, MD

16 Gastrointestinal Obstruction and Anorectal Disorders 88
Ernst Paul, Jr, MD and
Mary Ryan, MD

Section Five
Serious Infections

17 Febrile Child 95
Robby Mahadeo, MD

18 Approach to the Patient with HIV Infection and AIDS 99
Richard J. Wong, MD

19 Sepsis 102
Donald Barton, MD

20 CNS Infections (Meningitis and Encephalitis) 105
Frank LoVecchio, DO

21 Mycobacterial and Tick-Borne Infections 107
Frank LoVecchio, DO

22 Parasitic and Exotic Illnesses (Malaria, Dengue Fever, and Trypanosomiasis) and Syphilis and Leptospirosis 112
Charles DiMaggio, PA-C, MPH and Frank LoVecchio, DO

Section Six
Immune Disorders

23 Autoimmune Disorders 117
Ping Wong, MD and
Donald Barton, MD

24 Hypersensitivity and Related Disorders 123
Fred F. Tilden, MD

Section Seven
Endocrine and Fluid and Electrolyte Disorders

25 Fluid and Electrolyte Management 129
David H. Dorfman, MD and
John C. Brancato, MD

26 Endocrine Disorders 135
Ron Medzon, MD and
Todd C. Rothenhaus, MD

Section Eight
Head and Neck Disorders

27 Traumatic and Nontraumatic Eye Disorders 145
Syndee J. Givre, MD

28 Disorders of the Ears, Nose, and Sinuses 151
Paul A. Andrulonis, MD and
Elizabeth M. Datner, MD

29 Disorders of the Oropharynx and Throat 157
Steven C. Larson, MD

30 Dental Emergencies 163
William O'Callahan, MD

Section Nine
Oncology and Blood Disorders

31 Oncologic Emergencies, Red Blood Cell Disorders, and White Blood Cell Disorders 173
Mark J. Sagarin, MD and
Robert J. Vissers, MD

32 Hemoglobinopathies 180
Thea James, MD

33 Disorders of Hemostasis 184
Thea James, MD, Mark Sagarin, MD,
and Robert J. Vissers, MD

Section Ten
Neurologic Disorders

34 Approach to Altered Mental Status and Coma, Dizziness, and Vertigo 191
Joseph Turban, MD

35 Cerebrovascular Emergencies and Cranial Nerve Disorders 197
Kevin Baumlin, MD and
Phillip Fairweather, MD

36 Neuromuscular Disorders 200
Mary Ryan, MD

37 Seizures and Headaches 203
Andy Jagoda, MD

Section Eleven
Renal, Urinary, and Male Genitourinary System Disorders

38 Renal Failure, Hematuria, Renal Insufficiency, and Urinary Tract Infection 211
Ernst Paul, Jr, MD,
Phillip Fairweather, MD, and
Sandra Sallustio, MD, PhD

39 Noninfectious Disorders of the Male Genital Tract; Renal and Ureteral Calculi 217
Douglas W. Fields, MD

Section Twelve
Dermatologic Disorders

40 Rashes, Dermatitis, and Skin Lesions 223
David K. Hoshizaki, MD and
David L. Levine, MD

41 Infections and Infestations, Skin Cancer, and Cutaneous Manifestations of Illness 227
David L. Levine, MD

Section Thirteen
Behavioral Disorders and Substance Abuse

42 Approach to Delirium and Psychiatric Illness, Thought Disorder, and Suicide 233
Lisa B. Namerow, MD and
Tareg Bey, MD

43 Substance Abuse, Addiction, and Withdrawal 238
Lisa B. Namerow, MD and
Tareg Bey, MD

Section Fourteen
Trauma

44 Approach to Multiple Trauma and Spinal Trauma 243
Yvette Calderon, MD

45 Head Trauma 247
Adrienne Birnbaum, MD

46 Maxillofacial Trauma and Neck Trauma 251
Niels K. Rathlev, MD and
Jeremy Brown, MD

47 Chest Trauma 257
Simon Roy, MD

48 Abdominal and Urogenital Trauma and Pelvic Trauma 261
Robert A. Aldoroty, PhD, MD,
Debra Heitmann, MD, and
Mary Ryan, MD

49 Extremity Trauma 269
Elizabeth L. Mitchell, MD

50 Trauma in Special Populations: Pediatric and Pregnant Patients 271
Tareg Bey, MD

51 Wound Management, Burns, and Blast Injuries 277
Andrew Ulrich, MD and
Jeff Galvin, MD

Section Fifteen
Musculoskeletal Injuries

52 Upper Extremity: Shoulder, Humerus, Elbow, Forearm, Wrist, and Hand 285
Carol Leah Barsky, MD,
Paul Buckley, MD, PhD, and
Kathryn Craig, MD

53 Lower Extremity: Leg, Knee, Ankle, and Foot 290
Carol Leah Barsky, MD and
Paul Buckley MD, PhD

54 Pediatric Orthopedic Emergencies, Joint and Bone Inflammation and Infection, Hip Injuries, and Disorders of the Spine 293
Carol Leah Barsky, MD,
Paul Buckley, MD, PhD, and
Kathryn Craig, MD

Section Sixteen
Obstetric and Gynecologic Disorders

55 Pregnancy, Labor, and Delivery 301
Carl K. Hsu, MD

56 Approach to Pelvic Pain and Infectious and Noninfectious Disorders 307
Daniel M. Joyce, MD and
Carl K. Hsu, MD

57 Breast Disorders 313
Donald Barton, MD and
Daniel M. Joyce, MD

Section Seventeen
Toxicologic Emergencies

58 Approach to the Poisoned Patient, Acetaminophen, Salicylates and NSAIDs, and Iron 317
Richard J. Hamilton, MD,
Oliver Hung, MD,
Mary Palmer, MD, and
Rama B. Rao, MD

59 Anticholinergics, Antidepressants, Cardiac Drug Ingestions, Theophylline, and Beta-Agonists 321
Richard J. Hamilton, MD,
Oliver Hung, MD,
Mary Palmer, MD, and
Rama B. Rao, MD

60 Ethanol, Toxic Alcohols, Benzodiazepines, and Anticonvulsants 325
Richard J. Hamilton, MD,
Oliver Hung, MD,
Mary Palmer, MD, and
Rama B. Rao, MD

61 Cocaine and Stimulants, Hallucinogens, Mushrooms and Toxic Vegetations, Opioids, Pesticides, Phenothiazines, and Other Neuroleptics 329
Richard J. Hamilton, MD,
Oliver Hung, MD,
Mary Palmer, MD, and
Rama B. Rao, MD

62 Caustic Ingestions, Hydrocarbon Ingestions, Physical and Chemical Irritants and Asphyxiants, Methemoglobinemia, and Lead 332
Richard J. Hamilton, MD,
Oliver Hung, MD,
Mary Palmer, MD, and
Rama B. Rao, MD

Section Eighteen
Environmental Emergencies

63 Bites, Stings, and Rabies; Diving Injuries and Illness; and Radiation 339
John Mahoney, MD and
Erik Holt, MD

64 Altitude Illness, Heat- and Cold-Related Illness, and Lightning and Electric Injury 347
Luanne Freer, MD

Section Nineteen
Administration, Emergency Medical Services, and Disaster

65 Pain Management and Sedation 355
Fred F. Tilden, MD

66 Injury Prevention, Sexual Assault, and Domestic Violence 357
Jane Federman, MD

67 Approach to a Disaster, EMS Systems Organization and Operation, Patient Transfer, and Air Medical Transport 363
Neill S. Oster, MD

68 Administrative and Medicolegal Aspects of Emergency Medicine, Organ Procurement, and Wellness and Ethics 367
Donald Barton, MD and
Neill S. Oster, MD

Section Twenty
Procedures

69 Emergency Department Thoracotomy and Tube Thoracostomy 379
Simon Roy, MD

70 Cricothyroidotomy and Percutaneous Transtracheal Ventilation and Peritoneal Lavage 383
Judd E. Hollander, MD and Adam J. Singer, MD

71 Lumbar Puncture and Gastrostomy Tubes 385
Judd E. Hollander, MD and Adam J. Singer, MD

72 Percutaneous Central Venous Catheterization and Pericardiocentesis 387
Adam J. Singer, MD and Judd E. Hollander, MD

73 Joint Aspiration, Major Joint Reduction, and Intraosseous Infusion 389
Adam J. Singer, MD and Judd E. Hollander, MD

Index 391

GLOSSARY OF ABBREVIATIONS

A–a	alveolar–arterial
ABCs	airway, breathing, circulation
ABGs	arterial blood gases
ACE	angiotensin-converting enzyme
ACLS	advanced cardiac life support
ACTH	adrenocorticotropic hormone
AIDS	acquired immunodeficiency syndrome
ALT	alanine aminotransferase
AMI	acute myocardial infarction
AMP	adenosine monophosphate
AP	anteroposterior
ARDS	adult respiratory distress syndrome
AST	aspartate aminotransferase
AV	atrioventricular
BiPAP	bilevel positive airway pressure
BP	blood pressure
BUN	blood urea nitrogen
CBC	complete blood count
CHF	congestive heart failure
CK-MB	creatine kinase-MB
CNS	central nervous system
COPD	chronic obstructive pulmonary disease
CPAP	continuous positive airway pressure
CPR	cardiopulmonary resuscitation
CT	computed tomography
DC	direct current
DMSA	2,3-dimercaptosuccinic acid
DNR	do not resuscitate
DVT	deep vein thrombosis
ECG	electrocardiogram
ED	emergency department
EDTA	ethylenediaminetetraacetic acid
ELISA	enzyme-linked immunosorbent assay
EMS	emergency medical service
EMT	emergency medical technician
ESR	erythrocyte sedimentation rate
FEV_1	forced expiratory volume in 1 second
FIO_2	fraction of inspired air
HIDA	hepato-iminodiacetic acid
HIV	human immunodeficiency virus
ICU	intensive care unit
Ig	immunoglobulin
IM	intramuscular
INR	International Normalized Ratio
IO	intraosseous
IPG	impedance plethysmography
IV	intravenous
LV	left ventricular
MEN	multiple endocrine neoplasia
MI	myocardial infarction
MRI	magnetic resonance imaging
NADH	nicotinamide adenine dinucleotide phosphate
NADPH	nicotinamide adenine dinucleotide phosphate, reduced form
NPO	nothing by mouth
NSAIDs	nonsteroidal anti-inflammatory drugs
OR	operating room
PA	posteroanterior
$Paco_2$	partial pressure of carbon dioxide, arterial
Pao_2	partial pressure of oxygen, arterial
Pco_2	partial pressure of carbon dioxide
PEEP	positive end-expiratory pressure
PO	by mouth
Po_2	partial pressure of oxygen
PT	prothrombin time
PTT	partial prothromboplastin time
QD	four times a day
qhs	every hour of sleep
RBC	red blood cell
RPR	rapid plasma reagin
RR	respiratory rate
RV	right ventricular
SIDS	sudden infant death syndrome
SQ	subcutaneous
SVT	supraventricular tachycardia
TCA	tricyclic antidepressant
TPA	tissue plasminogen activator
$\dot{V}/\dot{Q}$	ventilation/perfusion
VDRL	Venereal Disease Research Laboratory
VF	ventricular fibrillation
VT	ventricular tachycardia
WBC	white blood cell

SECTION ONE

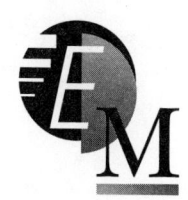

Resuscitation

1 Adult Medical Resuscitation

ROBERT DART, MD   SOPHIA DYER, MD

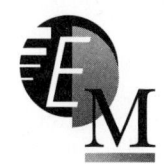

1. The best predictor of survival in the setting of cardiac arrest is:
   a. Elapsed time prior to initiation of resuscitation
   b. Initial rhythm
   c. Premorbid disease
   d. Blood gas results
   e. Age

2. Links in the prehospital chain of survival include all of the following except:
   a. Early ACLS
   b. Early basic CPR
   c. Early defibrillation
   d. Distance to the hospital

3. The probability of successful defibrillation declines by what percentage per minute?
   a. 2% to 10% per minute
   b. 25% to 50% per minute
   c. 70% per minute
   d. 90% to 95% per minute

4. All of the following statements are true about procainamide except:
   a. May be used in the setting of refractory VT
   b. Rate of infusion is 0.30 mg per minute
   c. Total maximum dose is 17 mg per kg
   b. Infusion should be stopped if the QRS complex widens by 50% over baseline
   e. Infusion should be stopped if PR or QT intervals lengthen by 50%

5. Sodium bicarbonate is potentially useful in cardiac arrest in all of the following settings except:
   a. Known or suspected hyperkalemia
   b. Tricyclic antidepressant overdose
   c. Preexisting acidosis
   d. Hypoxic lactic acidosis

6. Reversible causes of pulseless electrical activity include all of the following except:
   a. Severe myocardial ischemia with depletion of high-energy phosphate bonds
   b. Hypovolemia
   c. Tension pneumothorax
   d. Pulmonary embolism
   e. Pericardial tamponade

7. Potentially treatable causes of a wide complex pulseless rhythm include all of the following except:
   a. Hypothermia
   b. Hyperkalemia
   c. Tricyclic antidepressant overdose
   d. Digitalis
   e. Myocardial injury

8. Appropriate therapy for slow, wide, complex pulseless rhythms includes all of the following except:
   a. Lidocaine
   b. Norepinephrine
   c. Dopamine
   d. Volume expansion
   e. Airway management

9. Standard therapy for asystole includes all of the following except:
   a. CPR
   b. Epinephrine
   c. Atropine
   d. Hyperventilation
   e. Routine use of defibrillation

10. In the treatment of bradycardia or asystole, the maximum dose of IV atropine is:
    a. 1 to 2 mg/kg
    b. 2 to 3 mg/kg
    c. 0.03 mg/kg
    d. 0.01 mg/kg
    e. None of the above

11. Atropine should be used with caution or avoided in the following situation:
    a. New-onset complete heart block
    b. Mobitz type II AV block with an associated bundle branch block
    c. Mobitz type I AV block

d. Asystole
e. None of the above

12. The rate of recurrence of paroxysmal SVT after treatment with adenosine is:
    a. 10% to 20%
    b. 20% to 45%
    c. 50% to 60%
    d. None of the above

13. The first intervention in a patient with a witnessed VF arrest is:
    a. Airway management
    b. CPR
    c. Defibrillation
    d. Administration of epinephrine
    e. None of the above

14. Design features of automatic external defibrillators that allow safe and effective use by first responders with limited medical training include:
    a. Computer analysis of the rhythms
    b. Adhesive pads for both sensing and shocking
    c. Limited number of shocks can be delivered
    d. All of the above

15. Historical and ECG findings that increase the likelihood that a wide complex tachycardia is VT include all of the following except:
    a. History of prior MI
    b. rSR′ pattern in V1
    c. QRS duration greater than 0.16 seconds
    d. AV dissociation
    e. Positive concordance in the frontal leads

16. The most common underlying cause of CHF is:
    a. Valvular heart disease
    b. Hypertension
    c. Coronary artery disease
    d. Nonischemic cardiomyopathies

17. A 20-year-old male without underlying lung disease presents unconscious with decreased respirations after a heroin overdose. Expected blood gas findings will include:
    a. Normal CO_2; normal A–a gradient
    b. Elevated CO_2; elevated A–a gradient
    c. Normal CO_2; elevated A–a gradient
    d. Elevated CO_2; normal A–a gradient
    e. None of the above

Answers

1.a. Although ventricular fibrillation has the best prognosis as a presenting rhythm in patients with cardiac arrest, the time elapsed from arrest to start of resuscitation has the most critical impact on survival. (*Emergency Medicine, Chapter 2, pp 14–26*)

2.d. Distance to the hospital is not considered one of the American Hospital Association's "chain of survival" prehospital links. These links are early access to EMS, early basic CPR, early defibrillation, and early advanced life support. (*Emergency Medicine, Chapter 2, pp 14–26*)

3.a. VF/VT is the primary dysrhythmia in 80% of all atraumatic out-of-hospital cardiac arrests. The probability of successful defibrillation declines by 2% to 10% per minute. The probability of successful defibrillation at time zero is 80%. (*Emergency Medicine, Chapter 2, pp 14–26*)

4.b. Procainamide can be given at a rate of 20 to 30 mg per minute to a maximum cumulative dose of 17 mg/kg. Hypotension, termination of VT, and 50% widening of the QRS complex are other reasons to discontinue therapy with procainamide. Procainamide is second-line therapy for refractory VT, after lidocaine and bretylium (5 mg/kg). Procainamide is also useful in wide complex tachycardia (VT versus SVT) and in arrhythmias secondary to WPW. (*Emergency Medicine, Chapter 2, pp 14–26*)

5.d. Sodium bicarbonate administration is helpful in tricyclic antidepressant overdose because tricyclic antidepressant binding to serum proteins is altered by PTT. As the pH increases (becoming less acidic), more drug becomes protein bound. Because only the unbound drug is active, raising the pH decreases the proportion of active drug. Raising the pH in hyperkalemia causes K+ to move intracellularly as hydrogen ions move out of the intracellular space and into the serum. Sodium bicarbonate is not considered helpful in the patient with hypoxic lactic acidosis from prolonged cardiac arrest, where the preferred treatment is optimizing ventilation and restoration of circulation. (*Emergency Medicine, Chapter 2, pp 14–26*)

6.a. Reversible causes for pulseless electrical activity (electromechanical dissociation) include hypovolemia, tension pneumothorax, pericardial effusion, and massive pulmonary embolism. Once the heart is depleted of high-energy phosphate stores, pulseless electrical activity is no longer reversible. (*Emergency Medicine, Chapter 2, pp 14–26*)

7.e. Slow, wide complex pulseless rhythms can be associated with potentially treatable causes such as hypothermia, hyperkalemia, tricyclic antidepressant overdose, and calcium channel and beta-blocker overdose, as well as digitalis overdose. (*Emergency Medicine, Chapter 2, pp 14–26*)

8.a. Therapy for slow, wide complex pulseless rhythms may include volume expansion, atropine, dopamine, norepinephrine, transcutaneous pacing as well as intubation and hyperventilation with 100% O_2. Lidocaine is not indicated in slow, wide complex rhythms because it may suppress a ventricular escape rhythm (resulting in asystole). (*Emergency Medicine, Chapter 2, pp 14–26*)

9. e. CPR, early intubation, and pharmacologic treatment are all standard interventions for asystole. Routine defibrillation is not helpful and is possibly detrimental. Whenever asystole is the presumed rhythm it should be confirmed in another lead to rule out fine ventricular fibrillation. *(Emergency Medicine, Chapter 2, pp 14–26)*

10. c. In the treatment of bradydysrhythmias, the maximal IV dose of atropine is 0.03 to 0.04 mg/kg. Doses of 0.5 to 1 mg IV may be repeated every 3 to 5 minutes until you reach the maximum cumulative dose (approximately 3 mg for the average adult). Doses of less than 0.5 mg (in adults) may be vagotonic and decrease heart rate. *(Emergency Medicine, Chapter 2, pp 14–26)*

11. b. Mobitz type II AV block is typically associated with a block below the level of the AV node. In some circumstances, atropine leads to both an increase in the atrial rate and an increase in the grade of AV block, which could lead to a slower ventricular response. For example, with an atrial rate of 80 and a 2:1 block, the ventricular rate would be 40. An increase of the atrial rate to 90 with an increase in the grade of block to 3:1 would decrease the ventricular rate to 30. Placement of an external pacer is therefore the treatment of choice in this circumstance. *(Emergency Medicine, Chapter 2, pp 14–26)*

12. c. The recurrence rate of paroxysmal SVT after treatment with adenosine is 50% to 60%. This recurrence rate is higher than with verapamil. Verapamil is considered a second-line agent at a dose of 1.5 to 5 mg IV. *(Emergency Medicine, Chapter 2, pp 14–26)*

13. c. Time to defibrillation is the most important factor in determining survival after a VF arrest; therefore, rapid defibrillation is the number one priority once VF is identified. *(Emergency Medicine, Chapter 2, pp 14–26)*

14. d. A number of features are built into automatic external defibrillators that allow safe and easy use by individuals with limited medical training. Pad application is simplified by allowing sensing and shocking to take place with the same pads. Rhythm analysis is performed by the defibrillator. The number of repeated shocks is limited to avoid recurrent defibrillation of an inappropriate rhythm. *(Emergency Medicine, Chapter 2, pp 14–26)*

15. b. History of a previous MI, QRS duration more than 0.16 seconds, AV dissociation, and positive concordance in the frontal leads all increase the probability that a wide complex tachycardia is ventricular in origin. An rSR′ pattern in V1 increases the likelihood that the rhythm is supraventricular.[1,2]

16. c. The most common underlying cause of CHF is ischemic heart disease, followed by hypertension. Clinicians should consider coronary ischemia as a possible precipitant in any patient with new-onset or worsening CHF. *(Emergency Medicine, Chapter 2, pp 14–26)*

17. d. Hypoxemia from hypoventilation alone is caused by an increased partial pressure of CO_2 within the alveoli, which leads to a reduction in the partial pressure of O_2 within the alveoli. Patients with hypoxemia from hyperventilation alone do not have an elevated A–a gradient. A secondary cause other than hypoventilation alone should be considered in patients with an elevated CO_2 as well as a widened A–a gradient. *(Emergency Medicine, Chapter 2, pp 14–26)*

REFERENCES

1. Brugada P, Brugada J, Mont L, et al: A new approach to the differential diagnosis of a regular tachycardia with a wide QRS complex. Circulation 1991; 83(5):1649–1659.
2. Podrid P: How is SVT with aberrancy distinguished from VT? Choices Cardiol 1991; 5(suppl 3):18–25.

BIBLIOGRAPHY

Blum FC: Adult medical resuscitation. *In* Howell JM, Altieri M, Jagoda AS, et al (eds): Emergency Medicine. Philadelphia, WB Saunders, 1998, pp 14–26.

Goodenberger DM: Adult respiratory failure. *In* Howell JM, Altieri M, Jagoda AS, et al (eds): Emergency Medicine. Philadelphia, WB Saunders, 1998, pp 3–13.

2 Pediatric Resuscitation

DAVID H. DORFMAN, MD

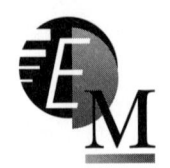

1. Premature infants are at particular risk of developing hypothermia because of each of the following reasons except:
   a. Infants have a larger surface area relative to their mass.
   b. Acidosis and hypoglycemia lead to decreased heat generation.
   c. They have little subcutaneous fat.
   d. If not dried sufficiently after birth, they will lose more heat through evaporation.
   e. Asphyxia increases heat production by causing an adrenergic surge.

2. A child's airway differs from that of an adult in all of the following except:
   a. A child has a larger tongue relative to the size of the oral cavity.
   b. A child's epiglottis is relatively shorter and thicker than that of an adult.
   c. Tonsils are more prominent in children.
   d. The larynx is positioned more anteriorly in the airway.
   e. The young child's larger head may necessitate placing a roll under the shoulders in order to align the airway for visualization during intubation.

3. All of the following statements about pediatric arrest are false except:
   a. Most cardiac arrests in pediatrics are secondary to respiratory arrest.
   b. Asystole in children is often responsive to defibrillation because of the greater automaticity of their hearts' conduction systems.
   c. Atropine is often helpful in treating asystole in children because of their active parasympathetic tone.
   d. Calcium, important for cardiac contractility, should be given to pediatric patients with asystole that is unresponsive to airway management and epinephrine.
   e. Asystole from drowning is particularly resistant to therapy, and interventions should be kept to a minimum in these victims.

4. To choose the correct size endotracheal tube for children, you may do any of the following except:
   a. Use a Broselow tape.
   b. Use the formula $(16 + \text{age in years}) \div 4$.
   c. Use the formula $4 + (\text{age in years} \div 4)$.
   d. Choose a tube with an outside diameter equal to that of the child's index finger.
   e. Choose a tube with an outside diameter equal to that of the child's little finger.

5. A full-term infant is born with thick meconium. The baby is depressed at birth without respiratory effort. The appropriate order of steps in resuscitation are:
   a. Intubate the child immediately and begin positive pressure ventilation while monitoring heart rate.
   b. Try to stimulate the child to elicit spontaneous respirations. After 30 to 45 seconds, if heart rate is below 100 begin positive pressure ventilation.
   c. Suction the infant's oral pharynx and nose at the perineum. Intubate the child's trachea and suction out the meconium while simultaneously monitoring heart rate. After clearing the trachea, stimulate the infant and proceed with the usual steps in neonatal resuscitation.
   d. Stimulate the infant until there are spontaneous respirations and heart rate greater than 100. Then proceed to intubate and clear the airway.
   e. Suction the child's pharynx at the perineum. Then intubate the trachea and continue positive pressure ventilation for 6 to 12 hours until it is clear the child will not have respiratory distress.

6. A 6-month-old infant presents to the ED in full arrest. Which of the following steps should be taken in the resuscitation?
   a. Proceed with CPR until a "quick look" can be obtained. Defibrillate if VF is seen. Start with 2 J/kg.
   b. Proceed with CPR. Intubate with a 4.0-mm endotracheal tube. Allow 90 seconds to obtain an intravenous line. If unsuccessful, proceed to a central line or saphenous vein cutdown.
   c. Proceed with CPR. Intubate with a 4.0-mm endotra-

cheal tube. Give 90 seconds of trying to obtain a peripheral IV line, place an IO line in the proximal tibia. Give 0.1 mg/kg of epinephrine via the endotracheal tube while awaiting venous access.
d. Proceed with CPR. Intubate with a 4.0-mm endotracheal tube. Once an IV line is placed, give epinephrine 0.01 mg/kg. A broad-spectrum antibiotic such as ceftriaxone should be given because sepsis is a common cause of SIDS.
e. Proceed with CPR. Once the infant has been intubated with a 4.0-mm endotracheal tube, give 0.01 mg/kg of epinephrine via endotracheal tube. After an IV or IO line is in place, epinephrine may be given again.

7. A full-term infant is born depressed, without spontaneous respirations. Appropriate measures in the resuscitation are as follows:
a. Measure the heart rate, and if less than 60, start chest compressions. Then intubate the child and begin positive pressure ventilation.
b. Wait 1 minute to obtain an accurate Apgar score. Then begin resuscitation as indicated by the Apgar.
c. Intubate the child and begin positive pressure ventilation. Measure the heart rate, and if less than 60 or between 60 and 80 and not increasing, start chest compressions.
d. Position the infant on its back and suction the infant's mouth. Stimulate the child by vigorously rubbing child's back. If within 10 to 15 seconds the infant is not breathing, start positive pressure ventilation with a bag valve mask. After 15 to 30 seconds, reassess for spontaneous respirations and heart rate.
e. Vigorously stimulate the child for 30 seconds, and if not spontaneously breathing, intubate the infant and provide positive pressure ventilation. If the heart rate is greater than 100 and the child is breathing well after 30 seconds, extubate the child and reassess.

8. A 4-year-old boy is found at the bottom of a swimming pool. He is quickly pulled out. He is not breathing but has a heart rate of 80. CPR is quickly initiated and the child responds with coughing and quickly resumes spontaneous respirations. The child is responsive but combative. He is breathing at 40 with bilateral crackles and has central cyanosis despite receiving O_2 via a nonrebreather mask. The child is intubated in the field. Upon arrival to the ED, the child remains intubated but is bucking the ventilator. The following would be the most appropriate sedatives and muscle relaxants for this child:
a. None. Children may have severe allergic reactions to a wide variety of medications and giving medications may just put the child at greater risk.
b. Succinylcholine, 1 to 2 mg/kg IV. The child should be paralyzed to gain control of his breathing. Succinylcholine has the advantage of being very short acting, so if the child is accidentally extubated, he can be ventilated with a bag valve mask until the drug wears off.
c. Vecuronium, 0.1 to 0.3 mg/kg IV. Nondepolarizing agents do not cause fasciculations and do not have a significant risk for malignant hyperthermia.
d. Versed and fentanyl for sedation and analgesia. If paralysis is necessary, vecuronium may be used.
e. Ketamine, 1.5 mg/kg IV.

9. Which of the following statements about cardiac arrest in children is correct?
a. Cardiac arrest is, unfortunately, a common event.
b. Cardiac arrest is effectively treated in most cases as long as CPR is initiated quickly.
c. Cardiac arrest is associated with far better outcomes among survivors than in adults.
d. Drowning victims who have a cardiac arrest have especially poor outcomes.
e. Cardiac arrest is most common in children under 1 year of age and during adolescence.

10. Which of the following pairs represents the most common arrhythmia in children and the proper treatment of this arrhythmia?
a. SVT—verapamil
b. Asystole—epinephrine
c. Ventricular tachycardia—cardioversion
d. SVT—adenosine
e. First-degree heart block—atropine

11. Appropriate order of vascular access attempts for a 3-year-old child in cardiopulmonary arrest is:
a. Femoral line, peripheral IV, radial artery line, IO line
b. Radial artery line, IO line, peripheral IV, femoral line
c. Peripheral IV, femoral line, IO line, radial artery line
d. IO line, peripheral IV, radial artery line, femoral line
e. Peripheral IV, IO line, femoral line, radial artery line

Answers

1.e. Infants and premature infants, especially, are at increased risk to develop hypothermia. Hypothermia may hinder resuscitation by causing acidosis and hypoglycemia. Infants have far greater surface areas relative to their mass. Newborns need to be dried and kept warm at birth. This can be accomplished by bundling them in warm blankets on their mothers' chests if they are healthy, or in the case of premature infants or less healthy newborns, putting them under warming lights for resuscitation. Premature babies have very little subcutaneous fat, which puts them at even greater risk. Their skin does not insulate well. Also, with little subcutaneous fat and little glycogen stores, hypoglycemia is more likely. For all these reasons, positioning, warming, and drying are the initial steps in neonatal resuscitation. (*Emergency Medicine, Chapter 3, pp 27–35*)

2.b. The larynx in children is more anteriorly placed. In addition, the epiglottis is relatively larger and thinner. Children have large tongues and their tonsils may be quite big. For these reasons, oral airways are placed with a different technique than that used for adults. In children, oral airways are placed by opening the mouth, depressing the tongue with a tongue depressor, and putting the airway straight back. They are not twisted over as in adults. The relatively large head of young children may cause flexion of the neck when infants are placed on their backs. When intubating newborns, a towel roll placed under the shoulders helps alleviate this problem and align the airway for easier visualization. *(Emergency Medicine, Chapter 3, pp 27–35)*

3.a. Cardiac arrest in children is most frequently caused by respiratory arrest and hypoxia. Asystole is not responsive to defibrillation, which is reserved for treating pulseless VT and VF. Airway measures and epinephrine are first-line therapies in treating asystole in children. Atropine may be used, but it is uncertain whether it is useful in treating asystole. Calcium should be given only in instances of marked hyperkalemia with ECG changes, documented hypocalcemia, hypermagnesemia, and calcium channel blocker overdose. Cardiac arrest in children has very poor clinical outcome. Victims of ice-water submersion are the one subset of pediatric patients in whom good neurologic outcomes have been reported after prolonged asystole. One commonly stated dictum is that patients who appear dead after prolonged exposure to cold temperatures should not be considered dead until they are warm and dead. *(Emergency Medicine, Chapter 3, pp 27–35)*

4.d. Finding the correct size equipment can pose difficulty in pediatric resuscitations. The Broselow tape serves to remove most of the guesswork and includes medication doses as well as equipment sizes. The tape is accurate to within 15% of the actual weight for patients weighing less than 25 kg. The formulas (16 + age in years) ÷ 4 and 4 + (age in years ÷ 4) are equivalent, work very well, and with a little practice are easy to remember and use. A 3.5-mm endotracheal tube is appropriate for most full-term newborns. Premature infants weighing approximately 1 kg or less take a 2.5-mm tube, and a 3.0-mm tube is appropriate for infants weighing 1 to 2 kg. The child's little finger may be used to estimate the appropriate size of the endotracheal tube. The external diameter of the tube corresponds with the diameter of the fifth finger. When preparing to intubate, have on hand tubes one size larger and one size smaller than you envision using. *(Emergency Medicine, Chapter 3, pp 27–35)*

5.c. Children born with thick meconium require that their airway be cleared before proceeding with the usual steps of newborn resuscitation. This is best accomplished by suctioning the child's oral pharynx and nose just after the head is delivered. The delivery should then be completed and the child brought to the warmer immediately without stimulating him or her. The infant is then quickly intubated and the airway suctioned via the endotracheal tube. Meconium aspirators connect directly to the endotracheal tube and allow easy suctioning. The endotracheal tube is then removed as suction is applied. If thick meconium is aspirated, another intubation may be required to further clear the airway. However, there is a fine balance between continuing to clear the airway and proceeding to the next step in resuscitation. Monitor the heart rate of the infant throughout these initial steps. If bradycardia is significant, it is time to stop clearing the airway. Instead stimulate the child to initiate spontaneous respirations. Give positive pressure breaths if necessary. If at delivery the infant is crying or already breathing and only thin meconium is present, the trachea need not be suctioned. *(Emergency Medicine, Chapter 3, pp 27–35)*

6.c. A 6-month-old is in full arrest. The proper order of actions in resuscitation is first to continue CPR, then intubate. Cardiac arrhythmias such as VF are exceedingly rare in children who do not have underlying congenital heart disease, metabolic illness, toxic ingestion, or myocarditis. Cardiac arrest is overwhelmingly caused by respiratory arrest in children. Intravenous access should be attempted while monitoring is obtained. The dose of epinephrine given via ET tube is 10 times the initial IV dose (0.1 mg/kg). If 90 seconds pass and an IV line is not secured, an IO line should be placed. The medial aspect of the proximal tibia is the easiest site for IO placement. Once the line is secured, epinephrine is given again (0.01 mg/kg if it is the first dose, 0.1 mg/kg if a dose of epinephrine has been given via endotracheal tube). If asystole is confirmed, continue with epinephrine every 3 to 5 minutes. Atropine (0.02 mg/kg; minimum 0.1 mg) may be given, although its efficacy has not been shown in treating asystole. If there is documented metabolic acidosis, sodium bicarbonate (1 to 2 mEq/kg) may be helpful. Outcomes in asystolic arrests are very poor, and it is important to know when to call the code and declare the child dead if there is no response. *(Emergency Medicine, Chapter 3, pp 27–35)*

7.d. The first steps in neonatal resuscitation are quickly warming, drying, positioning, and suctioning the airway. The infant is then stimulated if it is not moving vigorously and breathing effectively. Appropriate stimulation includes rubbing the infant's back or flicking your finger at or slapping the infant's feet. Many newborns will respond to this with spontaneous respirations and require no further resuscitative measures. If the child is still not breathing well on its own, initiate positive pressure ventilation via bag valve mask while monitoring the heart rate. After 20 to 30 seconds, if the child is making appropriate respiratory effort, reassess the infant. If the child responds by breathing well with a good heart rate (>100) continue to watch the child, paying close attention to respiratory status, heart rate, and color. If the child has central cyanosis after respirations and the heart rate is above 100, supply high-concentration oxygen. This can be accomplished by oxygen tubing, mask, or bag valve mask. If the child does not respond to the above measures, intubate and continue resuscitation. *(Emergency Medicine, Chapter 3, pp 27–35)*

8.d. This child required intubation for persistent hypoxia despite receiving 100% oxygen via a non-rebreather mask. On arrival to the ED, the child is intubated but combative. The child's behavior may be caused by persistent hypoxia or fear and discomfort. The placement of the endotracheal tube needs to be confirmed. This should be assessed by listening, CO_2 detector, or direct visualization. Then the child's breathing must be assessed by listening, pulse oximetry, and/or arterial blood gas. The child requiring medication for airway control should receive sedation and analgesia. It would be cruel to paralyze the child in this vignette without appropriate sedation. Versed and fentanyl are reasonable choices for this child. Ketamine can cause production of copious secretions. In this child, without the use of atropine or another antisialagogue, ketamine may worsen the already compromised respiratory status. Ketamine is also associated with upsetting hallucinations and dreams, which can be lessened or eliminated by using it in conjunction with a benzodiazepine. **(Emergency Medicine, Chapter 3, pp 27–35)**

9.e. Cardiac arrest in pediatric patients has an extremely poor outcome in the majority of cases. Most cardiac arrests in children are the outcome of severe illness or injury, leading to hypoxia, acidosis, and respiratory arrest, or in adolescence, caused by trauma. Emphasis is therefore placed on airway management and optimizing oxygen delivery. Many children with cardiac arrest present in asystole, and only about 10% of children with asystole survive. Most of the survivors have very poor neurologic outcomes. Patients with isolated respiratory arrests have a much better prognosis, with about 50% survival. Cold-water drowning is one area where there has been some success with prolonged resuscitations after cardiac arrest. **(Emergency Medicine, Chapter 3, pp 27–35)**

10.d. Supraventricular tachycardia is far and away the most common arrhythmia in children. In older children, it presents with the sensation of rapid heart rate. In infants and younger children, SVT may present with poor feeding, diaphoresis, fussiness, tachypnea, and hepatomegaly. If the arrhythmia is prolonged or associated with poor cardiac output, physical signs may include weak peripheral pulses, delayed capillary refill, and decreased sensorium. In most cases of SVT, the onset is paroxysmal and the rate is faster than 230 beats per second. In approximately 95% of patients, the QRS complex is identical to that seen in normal sinus rhythm. Most infants with very rapid sinus rhythms have dehydration, fever, or some historical finding to help explain the tachycardia. Most infants with SVT are otherwise well.

The first determination to make in the child with SVT is whether there is significant vascular compromise. For the child in shock, obtain vascular access immediately. After 90 seconds or three unsuccessful attempts at a peripheral IV line, an IO line should be placed in the proximal tibia. While this is being done, if ice is available, a rubber glove filled with crushed ice may be placed on the child's face. This initiates the diving reflex and is often successful in converting SVT to sinus rhythm. Once vascular access is established, adenosine (0.1 mg/kg; maximum 0.25 mg/kg up to 12 mg) is given by rapid push. If adenosine fails and the child is unstable, the next step is cardioversion (0.5 to 1.5 J/kg). If there is a delay in obtaining vascular access or if adenosine is not available, cardioversion is indicated for the unstable child. In the stable child, if adenosine does not cause conversion, intravenous digitalis may be used. Verapamil is a dangerous drug to use to treat SVT in young children. It has been associated with vascular collapse. The other rhythms listed as potential answers are all uncommon in children. **(Emergency Medicine, Chapter 3, pp 27–35)**

11.e. Three attempts or 90 seconds are devoted to obtaining a peripheral IV. In children 6 years or less, if the physician is unsuccessful after this short duration, an IO line is placed. This recommendation was developed after research showed that while treating children in arrest or shock, vascular access was frequently delayed or not obtained at all. Additionally, cutdowns were shown to be enormously time consuming, taking an average of 24 minutes to complete.[1] Intraosseous lines in contrast are very easy to do and are easily learned. One study showed an 80% success rate in children under 1 year of age, with 85% being completed within 1 minute.[2] Intraosseous needles can be placed in a number of sites, but the easiest and recommended site is the medial aspect of the proximal tibia. Any medication, crystalloid fluid, or blood product can be given through an IO line. The dose of medications used is the same as with peripheral IV lines. Research has shown that the duration of action and the peak drug level is unchanged when using IO lines. Even adenosine, which has an extremely short half-life (10 seconds), is effective when given via IO and does not require a change of dose. The only common contraindications of IO placement are bone fracture and vascular interruption. If an unsuccessful IO attempt is made at one site, another site should be used.

For children older than 6 years, the current recommendation is to proceed to percutaneous femoral line or saphenous vein cutdown if one is not successful obtaining a peripheral intravenous line. The reason for this is that as children get older IO placement becomes more difficult. The bone cortex becomes thicker and more difficult to penetrate, and delivery of fluid may be slowed somewhat as the bone marrow becomes less vascular. Also, with older children, femoral lines and saphenous cutdowns are easier simply because the children are larger. Despite this recommendation, IO lines are effective and can be used in older children and adults. The medial aspect of the lower leg, just above the medial malleolus, is a favored site in older children because the cortex is thinner there than at the proximal tibia. Femoral veins are the preferred site for central lines, as there is a lower complication rate compared with other sites. Also, during code situations there is often more room near that part of the patient compared to the head and neck, where airway issues and chest compressions may take precedence. *(Emergency Medicine, Chapter 3, pp 27–35)*

REFERENCES

1. Rosetti VA, Thompson BM, Miller J, et al: Intraosseus infusion: An alternative route of pediatric vascular access. Ann Emerg Med 14:885–888, 1985.

2. Glaeser PW, Hellmich TR, Szewczuga D, et al: Five-year experience in pre-hospital intraosseous infusion in children and adults. Ann Emerg Med 22:1119–1124, 1993.

BIBLIOGRAPHY

Patterson M: Pediatric resuscitation. *In* Howell JM, Altieri M, Jagoda AS, et al (eds): Emergency Medicine. Philadelphia, WB Saunders, 1998, pp 27–35.

3 The Infant with Apnea by History

ROBBY MAHADEO, MD

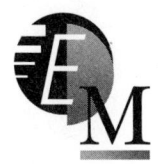

1. Which risk factors are associated with apnea?
   a. Respiratory syncytial virus bronchiolitis
   b. Prematurity
   c. Gastroesophageal reflux–associated laryngospasm
   d. Concurrent emesis or choking episodes
   e. All of the above

2. Which of the following statements regarding the physical examination of a child with a history of apnea is false?
   a. A rapid cardiopulmonary assessment is necessary.
   b. The skin should be assessed for pallor, cyanosis, and jaundice.
   c. Retinal hemorrhages are a common finding after resuscitation attempts by the parents.
   d. The nares should be assessed for patency and rhinorrhea.
   e. The oropharynx should be evaluated for congenital malformations or trauma.

3. An infant with a first episode of apnea who has normal vital signs and a physical examination in the ED requires all of the following studies except:
   a. CBC
   b. Electrolytes
   c. Chest radiograph
   d. ECG
   e. Head CT scan

4. Management options in the treatment of an apneic infant include all of the following except:
   a. Intravenous antibiotics
   b. Nebulized racemic epinephrine
   c. Intravenous calcium chloride
   d. Intravenous morphine
   e. Intravenous lorazepam

5. Which of the following is included in the differential diagnosis of apnea?
   a. Pertussis
   b. Disorders of fatty acid metabolism
   c. Infant botulism
   d. Prolonged QT syndrome
   e. All of the above

Answers

1.e. Concurrent respiratory infection is perhaps the most common risk factor associated with apneic episodes in infants. There is a well-described association between respiratory syncytial virus bronchiolitis and apnea, particularly in infants born prematurely or in the first 2 months of life. Another common association observed is that of gastroesophageal reflux–associated laryngospasm, so that a history of concurrent emesis or choking temporally related to a recent feeding is significant. *(Emergency Medicine, Chapter 51, pp 489–492)*

2.c. After a rapid cardiopulmonary assessment and appropriate treatment if indicated, a general survey should be done. The skin should be carefully evaluated for pallor, cyanosis, and jaundice. The nares should be carefully examined for patency and rhinorrhea, and the oropharynx should be evaluated for foreign bodies or obstruction. Concomitant retinal hemorrhages are pathognomonic of "shaken baby syndrome," mandating a careful fundoscopic examination. *(Emergency Medicine, Chapter 51, pp 489–492)*

3.e. Even asymptomatic infants require a minimum evaluation, including a CBC; electrolytes (including glucose); a chest radiograph to evaluate for occult aspiration, anatomic variants, or cardiopulmonary disease; and an ECG to screen for a prolonged QT interval or for evidence of recent myocardial injury. *(Emergency Medicine, Chapter 51, pp 489–492)*

4.d. Suspected infection would require that appropriate antibiotic therapy be initiated. A clinical diagnosis of viral croup with stridor would require nebulized racemic epinephrine. Hypocalcemia (<8 mg/dL) can be corrected with IV calcium chloride. Intravenous lorazepam is used to treat seizures, especially in the presence of respiratory depression. Intravenous morphine can precipitate respiratory depression and is not a treatment for apnea. *(Emergency Medicine, Chapter 51, pp 489–492)*

5.e. The differential diagnosis of apnea is extensive. It includes infections, metabolic disturbances, cardiac dysrhythmias, gastroesophageal reflux with laryngospasm, anatomic airway abnormalities, and idiopathic apnea of infancy. *(Emergency Medicine, Chapter 51, pp 489–492)*

BIBLIOGRAPHY

Keller SR: The infant with apnea by history. *In* Howell JM, Altieri M, Jagoda AS, et al (eds): Emergency Medicine. Philadelphia, WB Saunders, 1998, pp 489–492.

4 Adult Respiratory Failure

ERNST PAUL, Jr, MD

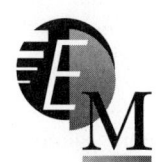

1. Which of the following statements about the physical examination of the patient in respiratory distress is true?
   a. In pulmonary edema, a systolic ejection murmur radiating to the carotids is a significant finding.
   b. In COPD, diaphragmatic fatigue is heralded by respiratory alternans or paradoxical abdominal breathing.
   c. The asthmatic in respiratory distress with few wheezes or a silent chest will likely need intubation.
   d. Upper airway obstruction is suggested by the inability to ventilate with a bag valve mask device.
   e. All the above are true.

2. Which statement concerning the usefulness of an ABG in evaluating a patient for respiratory failure is true?
   a. It can help differentiate asthma from respiratory failure caused by CNS depression.
   b. The presence of hypercapnia suggests increasing respiratory muscle fatigue and impending respiratory failure.
   c. The P_{CO_2} is the only useful value in evaluating decompensated COPD.
   d. An increased A–a oxygen gradient is specific to pulmonary edema.
   e. A P_{O_2} greater than 80 suggests that ventilation is adequate.

3. The typical prehospital management of a patient in respiratory failure includes all of the following except:
   a. Administering furosemide to the patient with pulmonary edema
   b. Treating asthma with nebulized albuterol
   c. Treating COPD with nebulized ipratropium bromide (Atrovent)
   d. Withholding oxygen in COPD to avoid CO_2 retention
   e. Giving epinephrine to a patient with angioedema

4. In the mechanically ventilated patient, which parameter may be adjusted to help prevent auto-PEEP?
   a. Tidal volume (V_T)
   b. F_{IO_2}
   c. Inspiratory flow rate
   d. PEEP
   e. RR

5. All of the following are true regarding mechanical ventilation in respiratory distress except:
   a. BiPAP may be an acceptable alternative to intubation in certain patients.
   b. The decision to initiate mechanical ventilation should be based on spirometry.
   c. Orotracheal intubation is the route of choice for airway management in most respiratory conditions.
   d. Permissive hypercapnia can be used to manage respiratory failure caused by asthma.
   e. Nasotracheal intubation is usually contraindicated with severe facial trauma.

Answers

1.e. In pulmonary edema, a systolic ejection murmur radiating to the carotids with a characteristic single S1 suggests critical aortic stenosis. This is important to recognize, because the use of nitrates in these patients will decrease preload and thus further decrease left ventricular output and systemic perfusion in an already compromised output state. In COPD, respiratory alternans (alternating accessory muscle and diaphragm breathing) and abdominal paradox (inward movement of the abdomen with inspiration) are signs of diaphragmatic fatigue, suggesting the need for mechanical support. Mechanical support is also indicated in the asthmatic patient with few wheezes and/or a silent chest, suggesting inadequate air movement and impending respiratory failure. In the patient with an appropriate history who is properly positioned for optimal airway management, the inability to ventilate via bag valve mask suggests critical airway obstruction and the need for airway management to alleviate the obstruction. *(Emergency Medicine, Chapter 1, pp 3–13)*

2.b. The ability to differentiate asthma from acute CNS depression (caused by a cerebrovascular accident or drug overdose) is mainly established by history and physical examination. Asthmatics usually present with a history of recurrent attacks, often caused by particular stressors, whereas respiratory failure caused by CNS depression is sudden in onset and associated with depressed mental status, often caused by a particular event (e.g., overdose). In COPD, worsening CO_2 retention on ABG testing is important to recognize, but clinical evaluation and change in the pH is more helpful in determining decompensation. Acute hypercapnia is highly suggestive of respiratory muscle fatigue and the need for close monitoring and intubation. An increase in the A–a gradient is not specific to pulmonary edema and can also occur in atelectasis, pulmonary embolism, and pneumonia. The adequacy of ventilation is determined using the P_{CO_2}, not the P_{O_2}, because CO_2 is freely diffusible in the lung and therefore more accurately reflects the rate of gas exchange, whereas P_{O_2} can be affected by intrapulmonary and intracardiac shunting of blood (e.g., $\dot{V}/\dot{Q}$ mismatching). *(Emergency Medicine, Chapter 1, pp 3–13)*

3.d. Respiratory compromise caused by pulmonary edema can be managed in the prehospital setting by giving IV furosemide (Lasix). Lasix causes an initial venodilation (decreasing the central venous pressure) and a later diuresis, which lasts up to 6 hours. Sublingual nitroglycerin decreases cardiac preload and systolic cardiac wall tension. The early management of asthma includes nebulized albuterol. Subcutaneous epinephrine and terbutaline are helpful in the asthmatic patient in extremis. Allergic angioedema can also be managed with subcutaneous epinephrine (0.3–0.5 mg of 1:1000 solution). Ultimately, failure of these measures is managed by securing the airway by endotracheal intubation. Oxygen must never be withheld in any patient in respiratory distress, including patients with COPD. Progressive hypoxemia is far more dangerous than hypercapnea. Patients with COPD should receive low-flow oxygen to maintain an O_2 saturation of 90%, as well as nebulized albuterol and ipratropium bromide. *(Emergency Medicine, Chapter 1, pp 3–13)*

4.c. Auto-PEEP, the process of progressive air trapping, with resultant hyperinflation of small air spaces, is caused by insufficient expiratory time. This phenomenon is mostly seen in the intubated asthmatic. The respiratory time is most effectively controlled by manipulating the inspiratory flow rate. The inspiratory flow rate predicts the time required for inspiration and, in conjunction with the respiratory rate, will determine the time available for expiration (the I:E ratio). Auto-PEEP should be avoided because it causes increased intrathoracic pressures that can lead to hypotension (caused by decreased venous return) and a pneumothorax (caused by barotrauma). Although the respiratory rate determines the cycle time for a single respiration, varying it alone will not result in auto-PEEP unless the rate is set too high to complete an entire cycle given the inspiratory flow rate and the patient's lung compliance. Tidal volume, fraction of inspired O_2, and PEEP have no direct correlation to auto-PEEP. *(Emergency Medicine, Chapter 1, pp 3–13)*

5.b. Clinical assessment of the patient's respiratory pattern, degree of distress, sense of tiring, and mental status is more important than spirometry in determining the need for mechanical support. Mechanical ventilation remains the most assured means of securing an unstable airway. Because of its intrinsic invasiveness and the technical expertise required, less aggressive procedures have regained popularity. This includes BiPAP, which delivers pressurized ventilation to assist the patient's own respirations. When successful, this method may obviate the need for intubation. Nonetheless, orotracheal intubation remains the method of choice in airway management. Nasotracheal intubation is less favorable because of the smaller endotracheal tube required; the need for a cooperative, spontaneously breathing patient; and the risk of complications (nasal bleeding or infection). Because of the risk of injury to the cribriform plate, nasotracheal intubation should not be attempted in the patient with facial trauma. After intubation of an asthmatic patient, higher P_{CO_2} ranges (therefore lower pH) may be acceptable in order to decrease the risk of barotrauma. This "permissive hypercapnia" is achieved by adjusting the respiratory rate and the inspiratory flow rate to provide adequate time for expiration and thus prevent auto-PEEP. *(Emergency Medicine, Chapter 1, pp 3–13)*

BIBLIOGRAPHY

Goodenberger DM: Adult respiratory failure. *In* Howell JM, Altieri M, Jagoda AS, et al (eds): Emergency Medicine. Philadelphia, WB Saunders, 1998, pp 3–13.

5 Airway Management

ROBERT DART, MD   SOPHIA DYER, MD

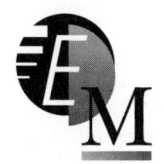

1. In the event of airway obstruction and mandibular fracture, the jaw thrust maneuver is contraindicated.
   True or False

2. The use of which of the following devices is most appropriate when suctioning large particulate matter?
   a. Tonsil tip
   b. Dental tip
   c. Catheter tip
   d. None of the above
   e. All of the above

3. Landmarks used in determining the correct size for an oropharyngeal airway are:
   a. Angle of jaw to lip
   b. Thyroid cartilage to angle of jaw
   c. Tip of ear to nose
   d. Tip of ear to angle of jaw
   e. None of the above

4. Indications for the use of esophageal obturator airway or esophageal gastric tube airway include all of the following except:
   a. Inability to endotracheally intubate
   b. Comatose patient
   c. Possibility of upper airway obstruction
   d. Unavailability of endotracheal intubation
   e. Apnea

5. The rate of inadvertent tracheal intubation with the esophageal obturator airway or esophageal gastric tube airway is:
   a. 0.5% to 1%
   b. 50% to 60%
   c. 5% to 15%
   d. 20% to 25%

6. Contraindications to the pharyngotracheal lumen airway include all of the following except:
   a. Upper airway obstruction
   b. Suspected cervical spine injury
   c. Semiconscious or conscious patient
   d. Esophageal disease or caustic ingestion
   e. Age younger than 16 years and/or height less than 5 feet

7. The correct formula for determining endotracheal tube size in the pediatric patient is:
   a. Internal diameter = (4 ÷ age in months) + 4
   b. Internal diameter = (age in years ÷ 10) × 4
   c. Internal diameter = (age in years ÷ 4) + 4
   d. Internal diameter = (4 ÷ age in years) + 4

8. In children, the distance from the alveolar ridge to the midtrachea can be calculated using the following formula:
   a. (Age in years ÷ 2) + 20
   b. (Age in years ÷ 4) + 4
   c. (Age in years ÷ 4) + 12
   d. (Age in years ÷ 2) + 12

9. The appropriate size for a nasotracheal tube is:
   a. 0.5 mm larger than for orotracheal intubation
   b. 0.5 mm smaller than for orotracheal intubation
   c. 1 mm larger than for orotracheal intubation
   d. 1 mm smaller than for orotracheal intubation
   e. None of the above

10. Potential side effects of thiopental in the setting of endotracheal intubation include all of the following except:
    a. Hypotension
    b. Bronchospasm
    c. Chest wall rigidity
    d. Decrease in intracranial pressure
    e. Porphyria exacerbations

11. Succinylcholine is metabolized by:
    a. Liver
    b. Plasma
    c. Kidney
    d. Liver and plasma

12. Histamine release is an effect of which of the following?
    a. Vecuronium
    b. Pancuronium
    c. Rocuronium
    d. None of the above

13. Which of the nondepolarizing agents is primarily metabolized by plasma enzymes?

a. Atracurium
b. Succinylcholine
c. Pancuronium
d. Vecuronium

14. Pediatric endotracheal tubes are uncuffed up to size 6:
    a. Because cuffs are always needed up to age 8 years
    b. Because of the normal anatomic narrowing at the level of the cricoid cartilage
    c. Because the cuff makes the tube more difficult to manage in a small airway
    d. All of the above
    e. None of the above

15. Contraindications to blind nasotracheal intubation include all of the following except:
    a. Apnea
    b. Midface trauma
    c. Intracranial hemorrhage
    d. Coagulopathy

16. Which of the following statements about disposable colorimetric end-tidal CO_2 detectors is false?
    a. They use photochemical reactions to detect the presence of CO_2.
    b. Their sensitivity is up to 100%.
    c. They can be used in pediatric as well as adult patients.
    d. They have no false-negative readings.

17. Which of the following statements about intermittent mandatory ventilation is true?
    a. It ensures a defined number of breaths.
    b. The tidal volume and rate are preset.
    c. Spontaneous breaths are not assisted.
    d. All of the above are true.
    e. None of the above are true.

18. PEEP can:
    a. Reverse hypoxic pulmonary vasoconstriction
    b. Reduce intrapulmonary shunting
    c. Reduce the right ventricular ejection fraction
    d. a and b
    e. a and c

19. Tidal volume on a ventilated patient should be set at:
    a. 5 to 6 mL/kg
    b. 7 to 8 mL/kg
    c. 2 to 5 mL/kg
    d. 10 to 12 mL/kg

20. The effects of CPAP are often beneficial in which of the following conditions?
    a. COPD
    b. Restrictive lung disease
    c. Acute respiratory failure from any cause
    d. a and b
    e. b and c

21. The following statements about colorimetric readings are true except:
    a. A purple color is associated with CO_2 less than 4 mm Hg.
    b. A yellow color is associated with CO_2 greater than 15 mm Hg.
    c. Ambient CO_2 levels in the esophagus are less than 4 mm Hg.
    d. Purple generally indicates esophageal intubation.
    e. All of the above are true.

Answers

1. False. The jaw thrust maneuver is not contraindicated in the event of a mandibular fracture. It could be a temporizing measure until the airway is secured. Airway narrowing from the tongue resting on the posterior pharyngeal wall is the most common cause of obstruction in the obtunded or unconscious patient. Because the tongue is connected to the mandible, moving the mandible anteriorly will elevate the tongue off the posterior pharynx and will thereby relieve the airway obstruction. To accomplish the jaw thrust maneuver, the operator should place his or her fingers around the angle of the jaw and lift anteriorly. The thumbs can then be used to position the face mask. Because the attachments of the tongue remain intact when the mandible is fractured, the maneuver remains effective. *(Emergency Medicine, Chapter 4, pp 39–53)*

2.b. The dental tip suction device has the largest opening and is therefore the most effective device when suctioning particulate matter. Catheter tips (with small diameters) are useful for suctioning endotracheal tubes. The tonsil tip is the device of choice when suctioning secretions and blood. Its multiple openings allow suctioning to continue even when one of these openings is obstructed. *(Emergency Medicine, Chapter 4, pp 39–54)*

3.a. The appropriate size of an oropharyngeal airway can be approximated by measuring from the lip to the angle of the jaw. *((Emergency Medicine, Chapter 4, pp 39–53)*

4.c. The use of the esophageal obturator airway or esophageal gastric tube airway is contraindicated in the setting of upper airway obstruction because it may further impact the obstructing object into the airway. Other contraindications include age less than 16 years, conscious or semiconscious patient, known or suspected caustic ingestion, or esophageal disease. Complications include inadvertent tracheal intubation in 10% of attempts, esophageal rupture, aspiration, and hemorrhage. Before removing the esophageal obturator airway or esophageal gastric tube airway in the ED, the patient should be intubated tracheally, the cuff should be inflated, and suction should be readily available because aspiration is common. *(Emergency Medicine, Chapter 4, pp 39–53)*

5.c. Along with esophageal injury and rupture (from inflation of the cuff), inadvertent tracheal intubation is a potential complication of esophageal obturator airway or esophageal gastric tube airway. Ten percent of attempts at esophageal obturator airway or esophageal gastric tube airway insertion result in intubation of the trachea. The operator should check for chest rise before cuff inflation to identify inadvertent tracheal intubation and to avoid tracheal injury from cuff inflation. *(Emergency Medicine, Chapter 4, pp 39–53)*

6.b. Because insertion of the pharyngotracheal lumen does not require neck movement, it is not contraindicated in patients with suspected cervical spine fractures. *(Emergency Medicine, Chapter 4, pp 39–53)*

7.c. The correct calculation is internal diameter = (age in years ÷ 4) + 4. In addition, a rough estimate can be obtained by estimating the width of the fingernail of the fifth digit. *(Emergency Medicine, Chapter 4, pp 39–53)*

8.d. In children older than 2 years, the distance from the alveolar ridge to the midportion of the trachea can be approximated by (age in years ÷ 2) + 12. This allows for movement of the patient's head without risking extubation or right main stem bronchus intubation. In adults, the tube should be positioned at the 21-cm mark at the corner of the mouth for females and the 23-cm mark for males. *(Emergency Medicine, Chapter 4, pp 39–53)*

9.b. The correct size tube for nasotracheal intubation is 0.5 mm smaller than the tube size to be used if performing an orotracheal intubation. It is best to place the patient in the sniffing position and treat each nostril with topical anesthetic and an agent for vasoconstriction (e.g., Neo-Synephrine). The right naris is preferred. By ensuring that the bevel of the tube is facing the septum, the clinician can avoid excessive bleeding from Kiesselbach's plexus. If the left naris must be used, the tube should be inserted with the curvature of the tube opposite the natural curvature of the airway, and then the tube is rotated into the AP plane until it approximates the same curvature as the airway. *(Emergency Medicine, Chapter 4, pp 39–53)*

10.c. Thiopental may be used as a sedative agent before endotracheal intubation to avoid increased intracranial pressure in patients with head injuries. The onset of action is very rapid (<1 minute) and the duration of action is also brief (5 to 10 minutes). It is highly metabolized by liver enzymes, so a prolonged duration of action could be expected in patients with hepatic disease. Potential side effects include hypotension and bronchospasm, which must be considered before its use. Chest wall rigidity is associated with rapid administration of higher doses of fentanyl. *(Emergency Medicine, Chapter 4, pp 39–53)*

11.d. Succinylcholine is a depolarizing neuromuscular blocking paralytic agent for rapid-sequence intubation. It is metabolized by liver and plasma enzymes. Its major side effect is muscle fasciculations that secondarily can lead to elevated potassium levels. Patients with chronic denervating injuries, such as chronic spinal cord injuries, older (not acute) burns, and crush injuries, are particularly at risk for clinically significant hyperkalemia. Succinylcholine may also cause increased intracranial and intraocular pressure during fasciculations. Fasciculations can be minimized by pretreating with a nondepolarizing agent. Succinylcholine's onset of action is about 1 minute, and the duration of action is typically about 5 to 10 minutes. Duration of action may be prolonged in patients with hepatic insufficiency or pseudocholinesterase deficiency. *(Emergency Medicine, Chapter 4, pp 39–53)*

12.b. Both atracurium and pancuronium cause histamine release and, therefore, may cause hypotension. *(Emergency Medicine, Chapter 4, pp 39–53)*

13.a. Atracurium is the only nondepolarizing agent that is metabolized by plasma enzymes. Succinylcholine is a depolarizing paralytic agent. The others listed are nondepolarizing paralytic agents. Atracurium may be useful in this regard if the patient has hepatic and/or renal failure. *(Emergency Medicine, Chapter 4, pp 39–53)*

14.b. Pediatric endotracheal tubes are uncuffed because the anatomic narrowing at the level of the cricoid cartilage provides sufficient seal to minimize air leak around the tube without an inflatable cuff. Using the appropriate tube size is critical because tubes that are too small relative to the diameter of the airway can have a significant retrograde air leak around the tube. *(Emergency Medicine, Chapter 4, pp 39–53)*

15.c. Correct placement of the endotracheal tube using the blind nasotracheal technique requires that the clinician adjust positioning based on the flow of air through the tube, which requires that the patient is spontaneously breathing. Nosebleeds are a complication of nasotracheal intubation, and the risk of this increases in patients with underlying coagulopathy. Patients with significant midface trauma will have distorted anatomy and are at higher risk of having bleeding induced by tube placement. In addition, the possibility of a cribriform plate fracture places these patients at higher risk for inadvertent intracranial tube placement as well as for infectious complications. *(Emergency Medicine, Chapter 4, pp 39–53)*

16.d. False-negative results with colorimetric end-tidal CO_2 can occur when the patient is pulseless. During pulseless rhythms, total body CO_2 production is markedly decreased. Because of this, the concentration of CO_2 in expired air may be below the threshold of these detectors. Colorimetric CO_2 detectors are available in pediatric and adult sizes. Sensitivity is between 88% and 100%. *(Emergency Medicine, Chapter 5, pp 55–60)*

17.d. Intermittent mandatory ventilation ensures a defined number of breaths per minute at a preset tidal volume. It is well tolerated by patients and is typically not associated with barotrauma. Occasionally, with intermittent mandatory ventilation, a process of "stacking" of spontaneous ventilations on top of mechanical ventilations occurs. Synchronized intermittent mandatory ventilation was developed to reduce this complication. *(Emergency Medicine, Chapter 5, pp 55–60)*

18.d. Statements a and b are correct. By reducing hypoxemia, PEEP also reduces hypoxic pulmonary vasoconstriction. Because pulmonary vascular resistance is decreased, the right ventricular ejection fraction is increased. In addition, PEEP reduces intrapulmonary shunting and allows a reduction of F_{IO_2}. *(Emergency Medicine, Chapter 5, pp 55–60)*

19.d. The tidal volume should be 10 to 12 mL/kg. *(Emergency Medicine, Chapter 5, pp 55–60)*

20.d. The CPAP full face mask can be used in the patient with respiratory insufficiency caused by COPD or chronic restrictive lung disease. CPAP provides positive airway pressure with a full face mask, as opposed to BiPAP, which is only a nasal mask. *(Emergency Medicine, Chapter 5, pp 55–60)*

21.e. The ambient CO_2 level in the esophagus is 4 mm Hg; therefore, purple color, which indicates CO_2 below 4 mm Hg, would indicate esophageal intubation. In the patient with a prolonged loss of circulation, the colorimetric reading may be purple even in the setting of tracheal intubation. *(Emergency Medicine, Chapter 5, pp 55–60)*

BIBLIOGRAPHY

Anderson DM: Airway management. *In* Howell JM, Altieri M, Jagoda AS, et al (eds): Emergency Medicine. Philadelphia, WB Saunders, 1998, pp 39–53.

Verdile VP: Capnography, ventilator management, and alternative ventilation techniques. *In* Howell JM, Altieri M, Jagoda AS, et al (eds): Emergency Medicine. Philadelphia, WB Saunders, 1998, pp 55–60.

SECTION TWO

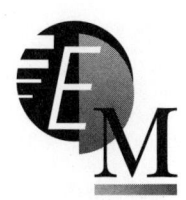

Heart and Vascular System

6 Approach to Chest Pain, Myocardial Ischemia, and Congestive Heart Failure

RICHARD CAGGIANO, MD   BARRY J. TILS, MD

Chest Pain

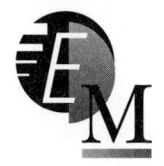

1. Risk factors for AMI include all of the following except:
   a. Cocaine use
   b. Male sex
   c. Diabetes
   d. Hypertension
   e. Family history of an elderly grandfather with a recent myocardial infarction

2. Which is least helpful in distinguishing which patient with stable angina has become unstable?
   a. Increasing frequency of chest pain
   b. Longer duration of chest pain
   c. The overall severity of the chest pain
   d. Chest pain that no longer requires provocation
   e. Lack of any response to nitroglycerin

3. All of the following statements are true for both unstable angina and AMI except:
   a. Risk factors include diabetes mellitus and hyperlipidemia.
   b. They can occur at rest and with exertion.
   c. Symptoms may not be relieved quickly with nitroglycerin.
   d. Elevation of cardiac enzymes aids in diagnosis.
   e. Initial ECG may be normal.

4. Variant, or Prinzmetal's, angina not associated with a fixed coronary artery lesion is seldom associated with which of the following?
   a. Psychological stress
   b. Exposure to the cold
   c. Effort
   d. Sleep
   e. Hyperventilation

5. All of the following statements are true of cocaine-associated chest pain except:
   a. It is frequently atypical.
   b. It can be treated with oxygen, nitrates, and beta-adrenergic blockers.
   c. It can occur in patients without other risk factors for coronary artery disease.
   d. It can occur several days after using cocaine.
   e. Hypertension and tachycardia are commonly associated findings.

6. All of the following predispose to altered cardiac pain perception and silent cardiac ischemia except:
   a. Advanced age
   b. Prior myocardial infarction
   c. Diabetes
   d. Prior thoracic or pericardial surgery
   e. Multiple sclerosis

7. A 62-year-old woman with a history of stable angina and hypertension presents with 4 hours of substernal chest pain associated with nausea and vomiting. Her BP is 160/100, pulse 80, RR 20. She is in moderate distress with no rales or wheezing. Her ECG shows 2 mm of ST-T depression in V_1 through V_3 not present on a recent ECG. She presently is on nitroglycerin parenterally for chest pain and hydrochlorothiazide for hypertension. All of the following would be appropriate considerations for treatment except:
   a. Nifedipine, 20 mg PO
   b. Sublingual nitroglycerin, 1/150, every 5 minutes for chest pain
   c. Aspirin, 160 mg PO, chewable
   d. IV heparin bolus followed by a continuous infusion
   e. Atenolol, 5 mg IV, followed by the oral route if her heart rate is 60 or greater

8. All of the following statements are true of hypertrophic cardiomyopathy except:
   a. Ten percent of patients have chest pain similar to myocardial ischemia.
   b. There may be a family history, but often the disorder is idiopathic.
   c. Hypertrophic cardiomyopathy accounts for a large percent of sudden cardiac death in otherwise young and healthy people.
   d. The patient usually has characteristic ECG findings that are highly suggestive of hypertrophic cardiomyopathy.
   e. It is best diagnosed with cardiac ultrasound.

22 HEART AND VASCULAR SYSTEM

9. Which of the following symptoms of aortic stenosis may warrant urgent surgical correction?
   a. Dyspnea on exertion
   b. Syncope with minimal exertion
   c. Occasional palpitations
   d. Chest pain with exertion
   e. Decreased exercise tolerance

10. In patients with chest pain, physical findings that may be associated with aortic stenosis include all of the following except:
    a. A brisk carotid upstroke
    b. Paradoxical splitting of the second heart sound
    c. A narrowed pulse pressure
    d. LV hypertrophy on ECG
    e. A systolic murmur that diminishes with the Valsalva maneuver

11. Which of the following is least characteristic of the pain associated with pericarditis?
    a. It often worsens with leaning forward.
    b. Chest pain usually worsens with swallowing or inspiration.
    c. It may radiate to the neck and acromial region.
    d. It is usually described as sharp and stabbing.
    e. It may develop 1 week to several weeks after an MI.

12. The most appropriate therapy for the chest pain associated with Dressler's syndrome (post-MI syndrome) is:
    a. Oxygen
    b. Magnesium sulfate
    c. Beta-adrenergic blockers
    d. Aspirin
    e. Heparin

13. Findings associated with the ECG during the early stage of acute pericarditis include all of the following except:
    a. Depression of the PR segment
    b. Low-voltage QRS complexes on ECG
    c. Sinus tachycardia
    d. Diffuse ST-segment elevations
    e. Diffuse T-wave inversion

14. Which one of the following noncardiac diagnoses must be differentiated urgently?
    a. Boerhaave's syndrome
    b. Cervicoprecordial angina
    c. Nutcracker esophagus
    d. Precordial catch syndrome
    e. Cholelithiasis

15. Chest pain accompanied by which of the following symptoms is most specific for esophageal reflux disease?
    a. Belching
    b. Acid regurgitation
    c. Nocturnal cough
    d. Dyspepsia
    e. Nausea

16. All of the following conditions may be associated with chest pain that worsens with deep inspiration except:
    a. Pericarditis
    b. Myocardial infarction
    c. Boerhaave's syndrome
    d. Aortic stenosis
    e. Tietze's syndrome

17. All of the following may be acutely worsened by thrombolytic therapy if mistaken for an MI except:
    a. Aortic dissection
    b. Peptic ulcer disease
    c. Pulmonary embolus
    d. Pericarditis
    e. Pancreatitis

18. A 60-year-old woman presents with severe substernal chest pain radiating to her back. Her BP is 200/100 in the right arm and 150/70 in the left arm. Her ECG reveals diffuse ST-segment depression. Of the following, the most appropriate initial therapy would be:
    a. Esmolol
    b. Aspirin
    c. Nitroglycerin
    d. Heparin
    e. Nipride

19. Which one of the following patients could be appropriately discharged home from the ED?
    a. A 40-year-old woman without cardiac risk factors who had nonpleuritic chest pain for 1 hour and a normal ECG
    b. A 50-year-old man with hypertension who has epigastric discomfort and nonspecific ECG changes
    c. A 45-year-old woman with a syncopal episode and an ECG with flipped T waves in leads V_4, V_5, V_6, I, and aV_L
    d. A 20-year-old smoker who had 1 hour of severe chest pain after smoking crack cocaine and has a normal ECG
    e. A 30-year-old woman with pleuritic chest pain and a normal ECG who is otherwise healthy

20. Which of the following is true regarding the ECG in the evaluation of chest pain?
    a. Variant (Prinzmetal's) angina can cause ST-segment elevation.
    b. Q waves may indicate myocardial necrosis.
    c. Twenty-five percent to 50% of the initial ECGs during AMI reveal ST-segment elevation.
    d. Peaked T waves may precede ST elevation in AMI.
    e. All of the above are true.

21. In children, all of the following could predispose them to acute cardiac ischemia except:
    a. Congenital heart disease
    b. Marfan's syndrome
    c. Use of cocaine
    d. Kawasaki syndrome
    e. Anatomic coronary artery aberrations

22. The most common cause of chest pain in children is:
    a. Chest wall pain
    b. Pericarditis
    c. Pleurisy

d. Reactive airway disease
e. Pneumothorax

23. Commonly described cardiovascular complications of Kawasaki syndrome include all of the following except:
    a. Valvular insufficiency
    b. Pericardial effusions
    c. Aortic dissection
    d. Coronary artery aneurysm
    e. CHF

24. In children with sickle cell disease, common findings associated with chest pain crises include all of the following except:
    a. Fever
    b. ECG changes consistent with ischemia
    c. Pulmonary friction rub
    d. Pulmonary infiltrates
    e. Leukocytosis

Answers

1.e. All of the rest are well-established risk factors for atherosclerosis and myocardial infarction. Cocaine may precipitate a myocardial infarction, with or without underlying coronary artery disease. Cigarette smoking, advancing age, hypercholesterolemia, and a family history of premature atherosclerosis are additional risk factors. (*Emergency Medicine, Chapter 17, pp 129–141*)

2.e. Stable angina is usually predictable in its frequency, duration, and severity as well as in the factors that provoke it. It is usually short lived and relieved with rest or nitroglycerin. Although it is usually milder than the pain or discomfort of an AMI, this is not always a distinguishing feature in regard to unstable angina. Chest pain that is not relieved with nitroglycerin is least useful, because this may result from a noncardiac cause. (*Emergency Medicine, Chapter 17, pp 129–141*)

3.d. It may be difficult to distinguish unstable angina from AMI, depending on the clinical setting. They are associated with similar risk factors (history of diabetes, hyperlipidemia, hypertension, and cigarette use) and may occur at rest or with exertion. Unstable angina may be associated with a changing pattern from baseline stable angina, with chest pain at rest or less exertion, or pain not relieved as quickly with nitroglycerin. In both AMI and unstable angina, early ECGs may be normal. Although measurements of cardiac enzymes are useful in the diagnosis of myocardial infarction, they are not helpful in confirming or excluding unstable angina. (*Emergency Medicine, Chapter 17, pp 129–141*)

4.c. Variant, or Prinzmetal's, angina may or may not be associated with atherosclerotic coronary artery disease. When there are no coronary artery lesions, it usually occurs in the early morning hours at rest or with psychological stress, cold exposure, or hyperventilation or in response to alpha-adrenergic agents. It often lasts longer than classic angina, but it is usually relieved by nitrates and calcium channel blockers. When an ECG is obtained during the chest pain it will often demonstrate ST-segment elevations, which return to baseline when the symptoms resolve. (*Emergency Medicine, Chapter 17, pp 129–141*)

5.b. Patients using cocaine can develop chest pain and MI immediately or days afterward. The pain is frequently atypical, and patients may have some, all, or no risk factors for atherosclerosis. Rest, oxygen, nitrates, benzodiazepines, and calcium channel blockers may be used as therapy. Beta-adrenergic blockers are contraindicated because they may cause unopposed alpha-adrenergic stimulation, leading to worsening vasoconstriction, hypertension, and ischemia. (*Emergency Medicine, Chapter 17, pp 129–141*)

6.b. Elderly patients, diabetics with neuropathy, patients who had prior cardiothoracic surgery, and patients with degenerative neurologic diseases such as amyotrophic lateral sclerosis and multiple sclerosis are all more likely to have atypical presentations with myocardial ischemia, including a truly silent MI. These patients may present with dyspnea without chest pain, syncope, or new dysrhythmias. Prior MI does not necessarily predict an atypical or silent presentation of future cardiac ischemia. (*Emergency Medicine, Chapter 17, pp 129–141*)

7.a. This patient is most likely having a subendocardial or non–Q-wave infarction. Thrombolytic therapy is not indicated in this set of patients with MI. Aspirin, nitrates, heparin, and beta-blockers have all been shown to be beneficial in reducing pain, extension, reinfarction, and thus early mortality. This has not been the case for calcium channel blockers used in the first 24 hours of management. Angiotensin-converting enzyme inhibitors may also be beneficial when initiated within the first 24 to 48 hours of infarction. (*Emergency Medicine, Chapter 17, pp 129–141*)

8.d. Hypertrophic cardiomyopathy is an idiopathic, asymmetric hypertrophy of subvalvular myocardium, characterized by symptoms of shortness of breath, palpitations, and syncope and even sudden death. In some series, it was the most common reason for sudden unexpected cardiac death in adolescents and young adults. Although there may be characteristic ECG findings in some patients, such as large Q waves, especially in the anterior septal region, none are diagnostic, and the ECG is often normal. Cardiac ultrasound is the most useful diagnostic tool and can be used for family screening in genetically linked cases. Chest pain is often atypical when present but may be similar to myocardial ischemia in 10% of cases. (*Emergency Medicine, Chapter 17, pp 129–141*)

9.b. Symptoms from aortic stenosis depend on the reduction in valve area and coexisting cardiac diseases, such as coronary atherosclerosis. All of the listed symptoms may be present with aortic stenosis, but syncope with minimal exertion implies a critical narrowing resulting in an inability to maintain cardiac output with exertion. Congestive heart failure is also an ominous finding. Limited exercise tolerance, palpitations, chest pain, and dyspnea on exertion may be present with less critical stenosis. *(Emergency Medicine, Chapter 17, pp 129–141)*

10.a. Angina pectoris develops in aortic stenosis as a result of increased myocardial oxygen requirements (hypertrophied myocardium) and decreased myocardial blood flow (from accompanying coronary artery disease as well as compression of coronary vessels by the increased myocardial mass). Findings in aortic stenosis include a gradual carotid upstroke with a delayed peak (pulsus parvus et tardus), paradoxical splitting of the second heart sound (caused by delayed closure of the stenotic valve), narrowed pulse pressure, and a murmur that diminishes with the Valsalva maneuver.

11.a. Pericarditis is caused by inflammation of the pericardium and produces a sharp, usually well-localized somatic chest pain, which may radiate to the neck, shoulder, or interscapular area. The pain usually worsens with inspiration, swallowing, or coughing but improves with leaning forward. Pericarditis may develop 1 week to 1 month after cardiac injury from trauma, surgery, or infarction (Dressler's syndrome). *(Emergency Medicine, Chapter 17, pp 129–141)*

12.d. Dressler's syndrome, or post-MI syndrome, is characterized by fever and pleuropericardial chest pain occurring from a week to several months after an AMI. The syndrome usually responds quickly to salicylates, but glucocorticoids may be used in refractory cases. Anticoagulants are contraindicated because they can create hemorrhagic pericardial effusions.

13.e. In the early stage of pericarditis, global ST-segment elevation with upward concavity is the characteristic finding. PR segment depression is also seen. Diffuse T-wave inversions characterize the second stage of pericarditis and usually follow the resolution of the ST-segment changes. Low voltage can be seen during both stages. Each stage may take several weeks to resolve.

14.a. Boerhaave's syndrome (esophageal perforation caused by forceful vomiting) is fatal if not diagnosed within 24 hours. The tear most commonly occurs in the distal posterior lateral aspect of the esophagus in a middle-aged male alcoholic. It begins with severe left-sided chest pain and shortness of breath and progresses to mediastinitis with septic shock. The history along with subcutaneous air, pneumomediastinum, pneumothorax, or a new left pleural effusion suggests the diagnosis. The other four conditions are usually self-limited and non–life-threatening gastrointestinal or musculoskeletal disorders. Cholelithiasis may lead to acute cholecystitis with sepsis, but it is biliary colic that may mimic acute cardiac ischemia.

15.b. Burning chest pain and regurgitation (the unexpected presence of gastric contents in the back of the throat) are more specific for esophageal reflux disease than the other symptoms associated with reflux—belching, dyspepsia, indigestion, and nocturnal cough.

16.d. The angina seen in aortic stenosis is usually exertional and is often associated with exertional dyspnea and syncope. The chest pain of pericarditis is often worsened with the supine position, breathing, and swallowing. Boerhaave's syndrome (esophageal rupture) usually occurs on the left side and is accompanied by fever and shortness of breath. Tietze's syndrome can cause inflammation and swelling of one or more upper costal cartilages, resulting in pleuritic and palpable chest pain. Up to 19% of patients with MI describe sharp or respirophasic chest pain. *(Emergency Medicine, Chapter 17, pp 129–141)*

17.c. Thrombolytic therapy may or may not be indicated for an acute pulmonary embolus, but it should not be harmful. Pericarditis may progress to tamponade from bleeding; aortic dissection, to hemorrhagic shock. A peptic ulcer that is active may bleed profusely, and pancreatitis could become hemorrhagic.

18.a. Given the clinical findings in this case, the patient should be assumed to be suffering from an aortic dissection until proved otherwise. The goal of therapy in aortic dissection is to reduce myocardial, heart rate, and systemic arterial pressure, therefore decreasing shear stress (dP/dT). Beta-adrenergic blocking agents are very effective in acute aortic dissection unless signs of CHF are present. Nipride can be used to lower BP but should only be used in conjunction with beta-blockers to avoid reflex tachycardia. Anticoagulants should not be used because they interfere with clot formation and may result in death. *(Emergency Medicine, Chapter 17, pp 129–141)*

19.e. Pleuritic chest pain as a sole presenting complaint is very unlikely to be caused by myocardial ischemia; however, chest pain associated with cocaine use even days later may be caused by myocardial ischemia or infarction. Syncope is usually not caused by ischemic heart disease or cardiac dysrhythmia if the patient has no known heart disease and a *normal* ECG. Nonpleuritic chest pain, even in patients who have no cardiac risk factors or a normal or nonspecific ECG, must be considered ischemic, unless the physical examination or additional testing points toward another diagnosis.

20.e. Variant, or Prinzmetal's, angina is a condition caused by coronary artery vasospasm that may occur at rest or on exertion. Reversible ST-segment elevation may occur. In general, abnormal Q waves are indicative of myocardial muscle infarction or necrosis. Peaked T waves occur very early in the course of an AMI and may precede ST-segment elevation. The initial ED

ECG shows ST-segment elevation in only 25% to 50% of patients with MI. *(Emergency Medicine, Chapter 17, pp 129–141)*

21.b. Ischemic cardiac chest pain is distinctly uncommon in children. It may occur as a result of vascular abnormalities of the coronary arteries, which could be congenital or acquired from a vasculitic disease, such as Kawasaki syndrome. This can result in coronary artery aneurysms in 20% of these patients if untreated. Cocaine use in adolescents, severe hyperlipidemia, and a number of congenital heart abnormalities, such as tetralogy of Fallot, patent ductus arteriosus, and aortic valve stenosis, may all result in myocardial ischemia. Marfan's syndrome predisposes to aortic aneurysms and mitral valve prolapse but not directly to myocardial ischemia or infarction.

22.a. Chest wall pain is the most common cause of chest discomfort in children. Asthma-associated chest pain and pleurisy caused by infection are also commonly seen, although usually with other accompanying symptoms. Pericarditis is less common but may accompany or follow a viral infection. Pneumothorax must always be considered, especially in tall, thin male adolescent cigarette smokers. Cardiac ischemia in children is uncommon unless there are cardiac abnormalities or distinct cardiac risk factors are identified. *(Emergency Medicine, Chapter 17, pp 129–141)*

23.c. Kawasaki syndrome, or mucocutaneous lymph node syndrome, is an acute multisystem disease of unknown etiology. The peak incidence is in children 18 to 24 months of age, with 80% of cases occurring in children younger than 4 years of age. Cardiovascular manifestations make up the major complications of Kawasaki syndrome. They include coronary aneurysms, valvular insufficiency, CHF, myocarditis, MI, dysrhythmias, and pericardial effusions. *(Emergency Medicine, Chapter 17, pp 129–141)*

24.b. The primary cause of the morbidity and mortality of sickle cell disease is the recurrence of vaso-occlusive episodes. When these episodes occur in the lungs, chest pain may occur and is often associated with fever, leukocytosis, pulmonary infiltrates or effusions, or a pulmonary friction rub. Vaso-occlusive events rarely occur in the heart, probably because of the relatively rapid blood flow through the myocardial circulation.

Myocardial Ischemia

1. All of the following statements are true concerning prehospital 12-lead ECG diagnosis and field-initiated thrombolytic therapy except:
   a. The diagnosis of AMI is made an average of 47 ± 21 minutes earlier.
   b. Patients who receive thrombolytic therapy within 70 minutes of symptom onset had a mortality of only 1.2%.
   c. Only a small number of patients would be eligible for prehospital thrombolytic therapy.
   d. Prehospital-initiated thrombolytic therapy decreases the time from symptom onset to treatment.
   e. Overall mortality from AMI is reduced with prehospital initiated thrombolysis by 7%.

2. In cardiogenic shock, the appropriate use of dobutamine is best described in which of the following statements?
   a. When systolic BP is less than 90 mm Hg, a dobutamine infusion will increase BP.
   b. After the systolic BP is greater than 90 mm Hg following a dopamine infusion, dobutamine can be initiated for inotropic support, if peripheral hypoperfusion still exists.
   c. Its inotropic effect is more pronounced than that of isoproterenol.
   d. It should be used before a trial of IV normal saline in patients with cardiogenic shock.
   e. At higher doses (10 to 20 µg/kg per minute) it is less dysrhythmogenic than isoproterenol.

3. A 70-year-old woman presents to the ED with 2 hours of substernal chest pain. She is agitated and has a systolic pressure of 80 mm Hg. Her lung fields are clear on examination. An ECG reveals an acute inferolateral myocardial infarction. All of the following statements are true except:
   a. Intravenous crystalloid should be given.
   b. Thrombolytics may be indicated.
   c. The patient is in cardiogenic shock.
   d. Primary angioplasty may be appropriate.
   e. Dopamine should be used initially to stabilize the BP.

4. All of the following statements are true concerning the ECG in patients with AMI except:
   a. The initial ECG is nondiagnostic in 50% of patients.
   b. At least 1 mm of ST-T elevation in two contiguous leads should be present for the diagnosis of an acute transmural infarction.
   c. An AMI cannot be diagnosed electrocardiographically with a left bundle branch block.
   d. An accelerated idioventricular rhythm may be seen following reperfusion, but is not associated with an increased risk of VF.

e. Reperfusion therapy should be considered with a new left bundle branch block in a clinical setting consistent with the diagnosis of AMI.

5. True statements regarding new left bundle branch block in the setting of an AMI of the anterior wall include all of the following except:
   a. Left bundle branch block is a risk factor for a higher mortality rate.
   b. Patients with left bundle branch block are more likely to develop CHF.
   c. Left bundle branch block is a relative contraindication to the use of thrombolytic agents.
   d. Patients with left bundle branch block are more likely to develop third-degree AV block.
   e. Left bundle branch block identifies patients more likely to develop VF.

6. A 58-year-old man presents to the ED with 2 hours of crushing substernal chest pain. He has a history of hypertension but denies other medical problems. Vital signs reveal a BP of 210/120 in both arms, heart rate of 90, and RR of 20. Physical examination reveals no evidence of jugular venous distention, a normal lung and cardiac examination, and no peripheral edema. ECG reveals sinus rhythm at 90 and 3 to 4 mm ST-segment elevation in leads I, aV$_L$, and V$_2$ to V$_6$. Appropriate next steps in the management of this patient include all of the following except:
   a. Metoprolol, 5 mg IV
   b. Oxygen, 2 L by nasal cannula
   c. Tissue plasminogen activator, 100 mg over 90 minutes
   d. Aspirin, 160 mg chewed
   e. Nitroglycerin, 0.4 mg sublingual

7. All of the following should be considered adjunctive therapies for AMI except:
   a. Calcium channel antagonist
   b. Aspirin
   c. Beta-blockers
   d. Heparin
   e. ACE inhibitors

8. The use of IV lidocaine in the setting of an AMI is indicated as initial therapy for which one of the following cardiac rhythms?
   a. Torsades de pointes
   b. Sinus rhythm, to prevent VF from developing
   c. Accelerated idioventricular rhythm during reperfusion therapy
   d. Unstable VT
   e. Frequent episodes of nonsustained VT

9. All of the following statements about serum markers for AMI are true except:
   a. Creatine kinase-MB (CK-MB) is 48% sensitive for AMI at 6 hours following symptom onset.
   b. Myoglobin can be elevated 1 to 2 hours following symptom onset but is nonspecific.
   c. Troponin T is specific for AMI and is elevated in approximately one third of patients with unstable angina.
   d. CK-MB subforms are 95.7% sensitive for AMI at 6 hours following symptom onset with the same specificity as CK-MB.
   e. Troponin T may be elevated for as long as 1 to 2 days after the onset of an AMI.

10. Of the following serum markers used to diagnose AMI, which one will be present in the serum the earliest?
    a. CK-MB
    b. Myoglobin
    c. Cardiac troponin T
    d. Cardiac troponin I
    e. Lactate dehydrogenase

11. All of the following statements are true concerning AMI in the United States except:
    a. Of the patients who die from AMI, about 50% die within 1 hour of symptom onset.
    b. Coronary artery disease is no longer the leading cause of death in the United States.
    c. About 45% of all AMIs occur in people under the age of 65.
    d. The majority of deaths from AMI are caused by dysrhythmias.
    e. The death rate from AMI has declined by more than 50% in the last 40 years.

Answers

1.e. Overall mortality has not been reduced in studies looking at prehospital diagnoses and treatment of AMI. Thrombolytic therapy does occur closer to symptom onset, but at the expense of overdiagnosing AMI. Only a few patients actually receive prehospital thrombolytics in the field. Early recognition of AMI, rapid transport, and prehospital transfer of critical information can improve door-to-drug time at the receiving hospital. *(Emergency Medicine, Chapter 19, pp 147–154)*

2.b. Dobutamine is predominately a beta$_1$-agonist with very minimal beta$_2$ peripheral vasodilating effects; therefore, it is less chronotropic and dysrhythmogenic but only at lower infusion rates (1 to 10 μg/kg per minute) than its cousin isoproterenol. It is an inotropic agent best used in patients with CHF not responsive to Lasix and nitrates or with signs of hypoperfusion despite a systolic BP greater than 90 mm Hg. In patients with cardiogenic shock with a systolic BP less than 90 mm Hg, it is best to begin with dopamine to improve coronary perfusion by raising the systolic to 90 mg Hg before initiating dobutamine. In all patients with cardiogenic shock, adequate volume status and optimal preload must be ensured. *(Emergency Medicine, Chapter 19, pp 147–154)*

3.e. Hypotension in the setting of AMI may result from several etiologies. Cardiogenic shock is typically characterized by hypotension (systolic BP less than 90 mm Hg), a decreased cardiac output, and elevated LV filling pressures. Patients with LV infarction have clinical evidence of pulmonary edema and low cardiac output, e.g., altered mental status, acidosis, and low urine output. Twenty percent of patients in cardiogenic shock develop peripheral hypoperfusion without pulmonary congestion. Patients with hypotension in the setting of AMI may be hypovolemic and may respond to boluses of IV fluids. Dopamine in this setting should not be used until after a trial of volume replacement. Hypotension in the setting of MI is not a contraindication to thrombolytic therapy. Primary angioplasty in the patient with cardiogenic shock may be an effective approach to therapy at some centers. *(Emergency Medicine, Chapter 19, pp 147–154)*

4.c. The initial ECG is diagnostic 50% of the time in AMI; therefore, it is wise to repeat the ECG for continued symptoms. A new left bundle branch block or ST-T elevation of at least 1 mm in contiguous leads represents ECG criteria for reperfusion therapy. Following reperfusion, an accelerated idioventricular rhythm may appear. This is usually benign and transient. An AMI can be diagnosed with a left bundle branch block present, especially when compared to a prior ECG with more pronounced ST-T segment elevation greater than 4 mm or significant ST-T depression greater than 1 mm. *(Emergency Medicine, Chapter 19, pp 147–154)*

5.c. The development of left bundle branch block during AMI usually indicates an extensive anterior wall infarct. The development of left bundle branch block during AMI has been shown to identify patients who are more likely to develop high-degree heart block, CHF, and VF. In addition, these patients have a higher mortality rate. In patients with a history consistent with AMI, the presence of new left bundle branch block may be an indication for reperfusion therapy. Left bundle branch block is not a contraindication to thrombolysis. *(Emergency Medicine, Chapter 19, pp 147–154)*

6.c. Appropriate management in the patient with AMI includes oxygen therapy, which increases oxygen delivery to ischemic myocardium; beta-adrenergic blockers, which can help reduce ischemia, protect against dysrhythmias, and in this case, reduce BP; aspirin therapy, which has been shown to reduce mortality and reinfarction; and nitroglycerin, which reduces preload on the heart and can help relieve pain by improving coronary blood flow. Thrombolytics in this case are contraindicated because the patient's systolic BP is greater than 200 mm Hg and the diastolic BP is greater than 120 mm Hg. Many clinicians would give thrombolytics if a sustained reduction in BP has been achieved. Other absolute contraindications include active peptic ulcer disease with internal bleeding, intracranial or intraspinal surgery or trauma within 2 months, intracranial neoplasm, or a known bleeding diathesis. *(Emergency Medicine, Chapter 19, pp 147–154)*

7.a. In addition to reperfusion therapy, aspirin should be given immediately. Aspirin has been associated with 23% reduction in the 35-day mortality. Beta-blockade, if no contraindications exist, reduces mortality in the first week by 15% when given in the first hours of infarction. Heparin is used with or without tissue plasminogen activator or with percutaneous transluminal coronary angioplasty to prevent reocclusion. Heparin also prevents cardiac thrombus formation and systemic embolization in large infarcts as well as venous thrombosis with pulmonary embolization. ACE inhibitors given within 24 hours after reperfusion or stabilization showed a 7% reduction in 5-week mortality. Calcium channel blockers have not been shown to reduce mortality and have some adverse effects that may complicate management of AMI, especially when combined with beta-blockade therapy. Although nitroglycerin can be used in AMI cautiously, it does not improve mortality and may reduce the reperfusion rate by enhancing the liver's metabolism of tissue plasminogen activator. *(Emergency Medicine, Chapter 19, pp 147–154)*

8.e. During AMI, lidocaine can be used as initial therapy for stable VT or frequent short runs of VT. Routine use of lidocaine to prevent VF in AMI does not improve mortality and is not recommended. Unstable VT is treated initially with an unsynchronized electric shock of 200 J, repeating at 300 J and 360 J if necessary. Torsades de pointes is initially treated with magnesium, 1 to 2 mg IV bolus. Lidocaine is not effective. Accelerated idioventricular rhythm may occur during reperfusion therapy and is often brief, requiring no treatment. It does not increase the risk of VF. *(Emergency Medicine, Chapter 19, pp 147–154)*

9.e. All of the statements are true except that the troponins may be elevated for 5.5 to 10 days (longer than 1 to 2 days). This would allow for the late diagnosis of AMI when CPK-MB, its isoforms, and myoglobin are all normal. A reasonable strategy would be to obtain a myoglobin level for a sensitive early assay and a troponin assay to confirm an elevated myoglobin, to detect a late MI or severe unstable angina. *(Emergency Medicine, Chapter 19, pp 147–154)*

10.b. During AMI, myoglobin is a serum marker for myocardial necrosis, which can be elevated as early as 1 to 2 hours after symptom onset. It has poor specificity and remains elevated for only 12 to 24 hours. CK-MB is not elevated until 3 or more hours after symptom onset and returns to normal by 48 to 72 hours. Cardiac troponin T and I levels become elevated in 3 to 4 hours and can remain elevated for as long as 5.5 to 10 days. Lactate dehydrogenase rises later, within 24 to 48 hours, and can remain elevated for 7 to 14 days.

11.b. Coronary artery disease remains the leading cause of death in the United States despite the fact that the death rate from AMI has declined by 54% over the past 40 years. The majority of these deaths are due to ventricular dysrhythmias. Of the 500,000 people who die from AMI each year in the United States, about 50% die within 1 hour of symptom onset. Forty-five percent of all AMIs occur in people younger than age 65.

Congestive Heart Failure

1. Prehospital personnel should consider endotracheal intubation in patients with acute CHF and the following signs and symptoms except:
   a. Altered mental status
   b. Poor respiratory effort with cyanosis
   c. AMI
   d. Extreme respiratory distress, with a respiratory rate greater than 30 breaths/minute
   e. Cardiogenic shock

2. Adverse effects to sublingual nitroglycerin include all of the following except:
   a. Sinus bradycardia
   b. Coronary artery steal
   c. Hypotension
   d. Sinus tachycardia
   e. Headache

3. For the patient presenting with acute CHF who is hemodynamically stable, all of the following may be appropriate initial therapies except:
   a. Sublingual nitroglycerin
   b. Endotracheal intubation
   c. Furosemide
   d. Propranolol
   e. Supplemental oxygen

4. Immediate angioplasty is most likely to be considered in which one of the following circumstances?
   a. Acute transmural MI 24 hours after the onset of chest pain
   b. Unstable angina not responsive to outpatient medical therapy
   c. Uncomplicated subendocardiac MI 3 hours after the onset of chest pain
   d. Reinfarction 2 weeks after MI
   e. Acute transmural MI with cardiogenic shock

5. Acceptable approaches to the definitive treatment of respiratory failure in CHF include all of the following except:
   a. CPAP or BiPAP
   b. Blind nasotracheal intubation
   c. Fiberoptic nasotracheal intubation
   d. Bag valve mask ventilation
   e. Rapid-sequence intubation

6. Of the following, which are contraindicated during rapid-sequence intubation of the patient in cardiogenic shock?
   a. Midazolam
   b. Thiopental
   c. Succinylcholine
   d. Bag valve mask ventilation prior to intubation
   e. Placing the patient supine

7. Accompanying signs of cardiogenic shock include all of the following except:
   a. Systolic BP less than 90 mg Hg
   b. Jugular venous distention
   c. An S4 gallop
   d. Cold moist skin
   e. Bilateral rales

8. Which statement is most true about the therapeutic effect of dobutamine in CHF?
   a. Cardiac output is increased; ventricular filling pressures are decreased.
   b. Cardiac output is increased, as is peripheral vascular resistance.
   c. The increase in cardiac output results in an increase in the patient's BP.
   d. Cardiac output is unchanged; ventricular filling pressures are decreased.
   e. Tachyarrhythmias are common at doses of 2.5 to 15 μg/kg per minute.

9. Reduction of preload or afterload is an important mechanism of all of the following medications except:
   a. Morphine, 4 mg IV
   b. Furosemide, 40 mg IV
   c. Nitroglycerin, 30 μg/min
   d. Dobutamine, 10 μg/kg per minute
   e. Dopamine, 15 μg/kg per minute

10. The hemodynamic profile of a patient with cardiogenic shock without pulmonary congestion is best described by which of the following?
    a. Low cardiac output, high peripheral resistance, high LV filling pressure
    b. Low cardiac output, low peripheral resistance, low LV filling pressure
    c. Low cardiac output, low peripheral resistance, low RV filling pressure
    d. Low cardiac output, high peripheral resistance, low RV filling pressure
    e. Low cardiac output, high peripheral resistance, high RV filling pressure

11. Clinical findings in patients with acute left-sided heart failure may include all of the following except:
    a. Diaphoresis
    b. Peripheral edema
    c. Confusion
    d. Elevated pulmonary capillary wedge pressure
    e. Interstitial edema on chest radiograph

12. High-output heart failure (i.e., heart failure in the setting of elevated cardiac output) may be seen in patients with all of the following except:
    a. Dilated cardiomyopathy

b. Hyperthyroidism
c. Anemia
d. Arteriovenous fistulas
e. Pregnancy

13. In the patient with underlying heart disease, acute CHF may be precipitated by which of the following conditions?
    a. Dysrhythmias
    b. Pregnancy
    c. Physical exercise
    d. Pulmonary embolus
    e. All of the above

14. Risk factors for the development of cardiogenic shock after MI include all of the following except:
    a. History of cigarette use
    b. Advanced age
    c. Large infarct size
    d. History of previous MI
    e. History of diabetes mellitus

15. Which of the following best estimates the long-term mortality in patients with CHF from cardiac causes?
    a. 50% mortality within 4 years
    b. 10% mortality within 4 years
    c. 5% mortality per year
    d. 80% mortality in 1 year
    e. 80% mortality in 4 years

16. True statements concerning the mortality associated with CHF include all of the following except:
    a. Ten percent of patients die of ventricular arrhythmias.
    b. Worsening CHF causes more frequent arrhythmias.
    c. Fifty percent of patients with severe symptoms die within 1 year.
    d. Electrolyte disturbances contribute to increased mortality.
    e. Mortality is increased in patients with AMI and evidence of peripheral hypoperfusion.

17. All of the following can be used to describe CHF except:
    a. High or low output
    b. Primary or secondary
    c. Acute or chronic
    d. Dilated or restrictive
    e. Right or left sided

18. In infants, which of the following is least likely to be a cause of heart failure?
    a. Wolff-Parkinson-White syndrome
    b. Endocarditis
    c. Tetralogy of Fallot
    d. Pulmonic stenosis
    e. Hypoplastic left heart syndrome

19. The most common cause of CHF in children is:
    a. MI
    b. Congenital heart disease
    c. Pericarditis
    d. SVT
    e. Viral myocarditis

20. Common findings in infants with CHF include all of the following except:
    a. Periorbital edema
    b. Hepatomegaly
    c. Wheezing
    d. Pedal edema
    e. Feeding difficulties

Answers

1.c. Respiratory failure should be the primary reason for endotracheal intubation of the severely ill patient with CHF. Alteration in mental status, cyanosis, measured hypoxemia, and inadequate respiratory effort due to respiratory muscle fatigue are all indications that ventilation needs to be mechanically supported. In cardiogenic shock, mechanical ventilation will reduce the work of breathing and correct hypoxemia. The physician must be prepared for worsening hypoperfusion in some cases because of a reduction in venous return from positive intrathoracic pressure and an increased functional residual volume. MI by itself is not an indication to intubate. *(Emergency Medicine, Chapter 20, pp 155–160)*

2.b. Nitroglycerin results in preload reduction because of an increase in venous capacitance. Afterload is reduced to a lesser extent. Together this could lead to hypotension with or without sinus tachycardia. In some patients, an increase in vagal tone can lead to bradycardia or even heart block. In either case, hypotension can be reversed with IV fluids. Atropine may be necessary if the bradycardia contributes to the hypotension. Coronary artery dilation occurs especially in diseased segments, improving perfusion to the most ischemic areas. Headache is common with acute and chronic nitroglycerin therapy. *(Emergency Medicine, Chapter 20, pp 155–160)*

3.d. The most important goal in treating patients with acute CHF is to initiate therapy early. Supplemental oxygen is appropriate, as is the administration of nitrates and furosemide, both of which can reduce myocardial preload. In patients who are in extremis, endotracheal intubation may be necessary. Beta-blockers such as propranolol should generally be avoided initially because they can reduce myocardial contractility and worsen CHF. *(Emergency Medicine, Chapter 19, pp 149–154)*

4.e. Primary emergency angioplasty is usually reserved for patients with extensive transmural infarctions, resulting in cardiogenic shock or severe pulmonary edema. It is also an option for patients who have absolute contraindications to thrombolytic therapy or complications from thrombolytic therapy leading to its discontinuance or failure to reperfuse. It must be available without delay. Results approaching 95% reperfusion are obtained in experienced hands. The risk of reocclusion is relatively low with heparin therapy.

The procedure should be performed as close to the onset of infarction as possible, but not later than 24 hours. Emergent angioplasty has not been adequately studied for acute unstable angina or nontransmural infarctions. (*Emergency Medicine, Chapter 20, pp 155–160*)

5.d. All of these approaches are acceptable except for bag valve mask ventilation. This is only a temporary measure, is often inadequate, and frequently causes gastric distention with the risk of aspiration. The nasotracheal approach allows the patient to remain upright but carries a significant risk of airway trauma and epistaxis, particularly with the use of thrombolytic or anticoagulation therapy. In addition, hypoxemia is often worsened during the procedure and the success rate is lower than a controlled rapid-sequence intubation using a rapidly acting sedative with few hemodynamic side effects. CPAP and BiPAP are alternatives to intubation in a patient who is alert and cooperative, allowing time to pharmacologically treat the CHF while reducing hypoxemia and the work of breathing. (*Emergency Medicine, Chapter 20, pp 155–160*)

6.b. Endotracheal intubation may be necessary in the patient with respiratory compromise in cardiogenic shock. Bag valve mask ventilation, although not an effective definitive form of therapy in patients with pulmonary edema, may be a temporizing measure before rapid-sequence intubation oxygenation. Although the supine position may restrict a patient's ability to ventilate on his or her own, it is usually necessary for orotracheal intubation and can be done safely before intubation. As an induction agent, thiopental may cause severe hypotension and is contraindicated in patients who are hemodynamically unstable. Succinylcholine is not contraindicated, and midazolam can be used in small doses without adversely affecting the BP. (*Emergency Medicine, Chapter 20, pp 155–160*)

7.c. In cardiogenic shock, cardiac muscle dysfunction causes decreased ventricular function and inadequate cardiac output. The LV filling pressure is high, and an S3 gallop is present along with pulmonary edema. Jugular venous distention is present when the right ventricular filling pressures are high as a result of direct muscle dysfunction or pulmonary hypertension, most frequently from chronic LV failure. An RV infarction therefore can result in cardiogenic shock without CHF. This carries a better prognosis than LV infarction with shock and will respond to IV crystalloid therapy. An S4 gallop is common in older adults because stiffening causes the ventricle to vibrate with each atrial contraction. It is therefore not a helpful finding in patients with either MI or CHF. (*Emergency Medicine, Chapter 20, pp 155–160*)

8.a. Dobutamine stimulates principally beta-receptors, increasing cardiac inotropy while decreasing peripheral resistance. At doses of 2.5 to 15 μg/kg per minute, dobutamine increases cardiac output directly by improving cardiac muscle performance and indirectly by reducing systemic venous resistance. There is little change in BP because of the reduction in peripheral vascular resistance. Dobutamine is used to treat CHF that is unresponsive or only partially responsive to nitrates and diuretics or when hypoperfusion persists despite a BP above 90 mm systolic. (*Emergency Medicine, Chapter 20, pp 155–160*)

9.e. Morphine in doses up to 8 to 10 mg decreases afterload and produces a sedative effect. Furosemide in doses greater than 20 mg IV reduces preload within minutes of administration, whereas the peak diuretic effect is delayed 30 to 60 minutes. Nitroglycerin is a potent preload reducer and, in higher doses, reduces afterload as well. Dobutamine exerts its effect by increasing cardiac output as well as decreasing afterload. In low doses (1 to 10 μg/kg per minute), dopamine increases renal and mesenteric blood flow by stimulating dopaminergic receptors. At doses of 10 to 20 μg/kg per minute, dopamine becomes more of an alpha- and beta-adrenergic agent, increasing myocardial contractility through $beta_1$-adrenergic stimulation. (*Emergency Medicine, Chapter 20, pp 155–160*)

10.e. Twenty percent of patients with cardiogenic shock from myocardial infarction have a hemodynamic profile of hypoperfusion, high peripheral resistance, and low or normal LV filling pressures. There is no pulmonary congestion. In these patients, decreased cardiac output causes increased vasoconstriction and increased systemic vascular resistance. Increasing intravascular volume increases the filling of the RV (which is volume dependent), therefore increasing cardiac output. Peripheral resistance will fall and hypoperfusion can be corrected. These patients require careful hemodynamic monitoring to optimize cardiac output. (*Emergency Medicine, Chapter 20, pp 155–160*)

11.b. Acute left-sided heart failure produces clinical manifestations that reflect both elevated left heart pressures and decreased cardiac output and diminished peripheral blood flow. Peripheral arterial vasoconstriction in the setting of a low cardiac output may produce diaphoresis. Diminished forward blood flow may also cause altered mental status, low urine output, and fatigue. The elevated left-sided heart pressures will produce pulmonary vascular congestion and edema and be reflected by an elevation of the pulmonary capillary wedge pressure. Peripheral edema is generally seen in patients with right-sided heart failure, chronic left-sided heart failure, or biventricular failure. (*Emergency Medicine, Chapter 20, pp 155–160*)

12.a. Heart failure may be seen in the setting of both low and high cardiac output. Common causes of low-output heart failure include hypertension, myocardial ischemia, valvular disease, and dilated cardiomyopathy. Common causes of high-output heart failure include pregnancy, beriberi, Paget's disease, arteriovenous fistulas, hyperthyroidism, and anemia. (*Emergency Medicine, Chapter 20, pp 155–160*)

13.e. Any condition that places an additional burden on a chronically overloaded and compensated myocardium may precipitate an episode of acute CHF. Increased metabolic demands in conditions such as infections, thyrotoxicosis, pregnancy, and exercise may precipitate heart failure. Dysrhythmias may precipitate heart failure in chronically diseased as well as normal hearts. Pulmonary emboli may cause an elevation of pulmonary arterial pressure, which can cause or worsen ventricular failure. *(Emergency Medicine, Chapter 20, pp 155–160)*

14.a. Cardiogenic shock may develop during the first few hours of an AMI or may develop later, up to a week after in some cases. Risk factors for the development of shock after MI include advanced age, decreased LV function at presentation, large infarct size, history of diabetes mellitus, and previous MI. Cigarette use, although an independent risk factor for coronary artery disease, does not predispose the patient with an AMI to develop cardiogenic shock. *(Emergency Medicine, Chapter 20, pp 155–160)*

15.a. Although CHF initially responds to medical therapy with a relatively low immediate mortality, long-term prognosis is poor. Nearly half the deaths are due to cardiac dysrhythmias. CHF may become chronic and progressive, leading to multiorgan system failure, with mortality approaching 50% by 3 to 4 years. *(Emergency Medicine, Chapter 20, pp 155–160)*

16.a. Approximately 50% of patients with CHF die within 1 year of the onset of severe symptoms. Between 30% and 40% of patients with CHF die suddenly of ventricular arrhythmias. The incidence of ventricular arrhythmias increases with worsening heart failure and may be prevented by treating electrolyte disturbances (hypokalemia and hypomagnesemia). In patients with AMI, mortality is 10% in patients with isolated pulmonary congestion, but it increases to 55% in patients with both pulmonary congestion and peripheral hypoperfusion.

17.d. Heart failure occurs when the heart cannot pump adequate blood to meet the body's metabolic needs. Pulmonary or systemic venous congestion will occur depending on which ventricle is failing. Primary cardiac causes include valvular heart disease, myocarditis, myocardial infarction, or hypertrophy from systemic hypertension. Secondary noncardiac causes include severe prolonged anemia, large or multiple AV fistulas, thyrotoxicosis, and advanced renal failure. Systolic dysfunction results from a failure in contractility. Diastolic dysfunction results from a failure in ventricular relaxation due to poor compliance. Heart failure may be acute from a new MI or chronic as a result of prior infarction and progressive pump failure. High-output failure occurs when high peripheral demand exceeds the heart's ability to match this, in spite of higher than baseline cardiac output. Progressive worsening of myocardial contractility will develop unless the underlying process is corrected. Both dilated and restricted cardiomyopathy may result in CHF but are not terms used to describe CHF. *(Emergency Medicine, Chapter 20, pp 155–160)*

18.b. In infants, congenital cardiac abnormalities and supraventricular tachydysrhythmias from an accessory pathway are the most likely causes of CHF. Congenital cardiac disorders include tetralogy of Fallot, hypoplastic heart, valvular stenosis, coarctation of the aorta, and anomalous pulmonary venous return. In adolescents, acquired causes such as thyrotoxicosis, endocarditis, or myocarditis become more common. Myocardial ischemia is distinctly uncommon in children and adolescents. If an adolescent has an MI, illicit drug use (cocaine or methamphetamine) should be suspected. *(Emergency Medicine, Chapter 20, pp 155–160)*

19.b. Overall, the most common cause of CHF in the pediatric patient is congenital heart disease. This includes patent ductus arteriosus (premature neonates), hypoplastic left ventricle, coarctation of the aorta, transposition of the great arteries, and ventricular septal defects. Acquired heart disease leading to CHF is more common in older children, and the cause is usually myocarditis. Myocardial ischemia is rare in the pediatric patient. *(Emergency Medicine, Chapter 20, pp 155–160)*

20.d. In children, clinical manifestations of CHF are age related. In older children and adolescents, signs and symptoms of CHF are similar to those in adults. In infants, clinical signs of CHF may be more subtle. Edema, if present, is usually seen around the eyes and over the flanks. Pretibial and pedal edema is not common. Other findings in infants include tachypnea, feeding difficulties, poor weight gain, excessive perspiration, hepatomegaly, and wheezing. *(Emergency Medicine, Chapter 20, pp 155–160)*

BIBLIOGRAPHY

Baxter MS: Acute myocardial ischemia. *In* Howell JM, Altieri M, Jagoda AS, et al (eds): Emergency Medicine. Philadelphia, WB Saunders, 1998, pp 147–154.

Dhindsa HS, Howell JM: Acute congestive heart failure. *In* Howell JM, Altieri M, Jagoda AS, et al (eds): Emergency Medicine. Philadelphia, WB Saunders, 1998, pp 155–160.

Howell JM, Hedges JR: Approach to chest pain. *In* Howell JM, Altieri M, Jagoda AS, et al (eds): Emergency Medicine. Philadelphia, WB Saunders, 1998, pp 129–141.

Sgarbossa EB, Pinski SL, Barbagelata A, et al: Electrocardiographic diagnosis of evolving myocardial infarction in the presence of left bundle branch block. N Engl J Med 1996; 334(8):481–487.

7. Arrhythmias, Hypertension, and Syncope

PETER SHEARER, MD   GAIL D'ONOFRIO, MD

Arrhythmias

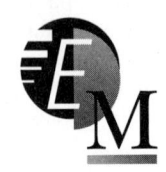

1. A 55-year-old woman presents during an AMI. One hour after receiving thrombolytic therapy, she develops a wide complex rhythm in the 80s (Fig. 7–1). Her BP is 110/70. You would treat this arrhythmia with:
   a. Digoxin
   b. Verapamil
   c. Lidocaine
   d. Procainamide
   e. None of the above

2. Criteria for admitting a patient with new-onset atrial fibrillation include all of the following except:
   a. Unknown onset time
   b. Moderate aortic insufficiency
   c. Presence of heart failure
   d. Onset less than 72 hours ago
   e. Older age

3. All of the following are part of the Brugada criteria for distinguishing VT from SVT in a wide complex tachycardia except:
   a. Presence of AV dissociation
   b. Absence of RS complex in leads V_1 to V_6
   c. QRS complex >0.14
   d. Onset of R wave to nadir of S wave >100 msec in any chest lead
   e. Presence of fusion beats

4. A 55-year-old man complains of intermittent chest pain. He is hemodynamically stable and denies chest pain or shortness of breath. His ECG findings are shown in Figure 7–2. Proper treatment includes:
   a. Admitting him for possible coronary ischemia and monitoring his rhythm; consider external pacer placement
   b. Reassuring him and sending him home
   c. Checking his electrolytes and discharging to home if normal
   d. Placing him on a transcutaneous pacemaker at a rate of 70 beats/min
   e. Permanent pacemaker insertion

5. Adenosine's side effects or metabolism may be altered in all of the following situations except:
   a. Patients taking phenytoin
   b. Patients with a history of asthma
   c. Patients taking theophylline
   d. Patients taking dipyridamole
   e. Patients taking carbamazepine

6. A patient with a pacemaker presents with shortness of breath. His ECG reveals pacemaker spikes before some P waves, before some of the QRS complexes, and occasionally before both. There are also intrinsic beats that are not paced at all. His pacemaker is most likely a(n):
   a. AAI
   b. DDI
   c. VVI
   d. DDD
   e. Unable to tell from information given

7. A patient presents 2 weeks after implantation of a pacemaker. He complains of fatigue and dyspnea on exertion. His ECG reveals a second-degree AV block, Mobitz type II. He takes propranolol. There are frequent pacer spikes at various intervals before and after the QRS complexes without capture. All of the following may have produced this except:
   a. Dislodgment of lead from the myocardium
   b. Beta-blocker overdose
   c. Increased pacing threshold
   d. Hyperkalemia
   e. Lead fracture

8. An 18-year-old male presents to the ED with acute onset of palpitations while watching an action movie. He denies chest pain or shortness of breath. He had a similar episode 4 years ago that resolved spontaneously. The ECG reveals a narrow complex tachycardia at 160. He is given adenosine 6 mg IV with resolution. His subsequent ECG is shown in Figure 7–3. What is his diagnosis?
   a. Atrial flutter—resolved
   b. AV nodal reentrant tachycardia
   c. Wolff-Parkinson-White syndrome with orthodromic conduction
   d. Wolff-Parkinson-White syndrome with antidromic conduction
   e. Paroxysmal atrial tachycardia

ARRHYTHMIAS, HYPERTENSION, AND SYNCOPE 33

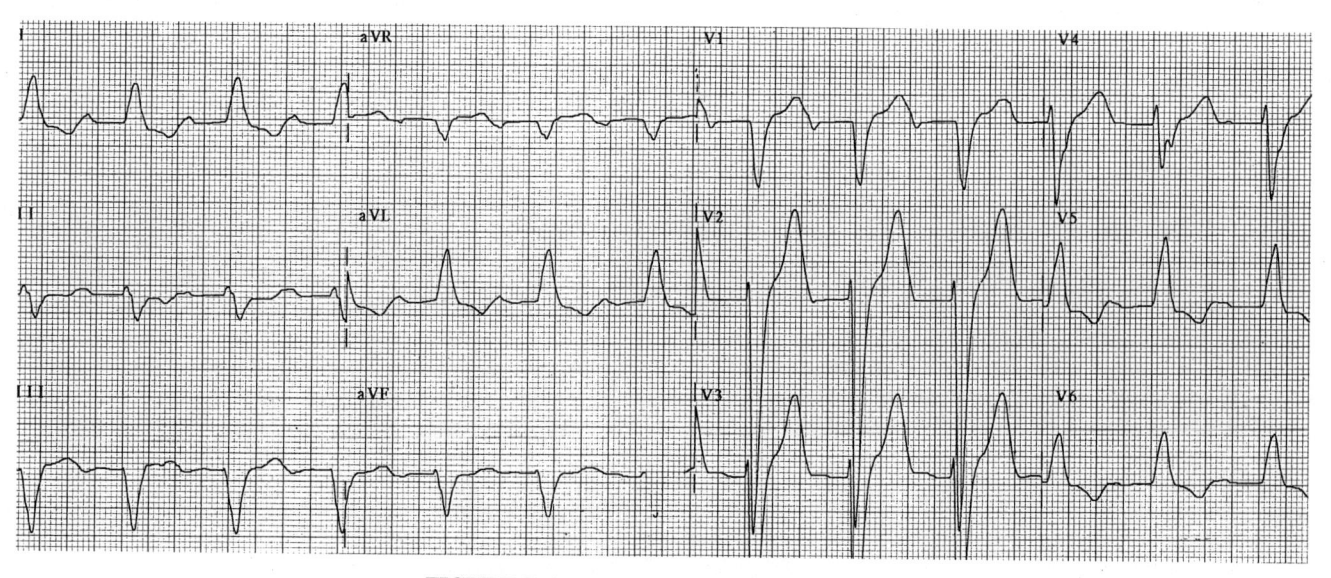

FIGURE 7–1. (Courtesy of Dr. Sheilah Bernard.)

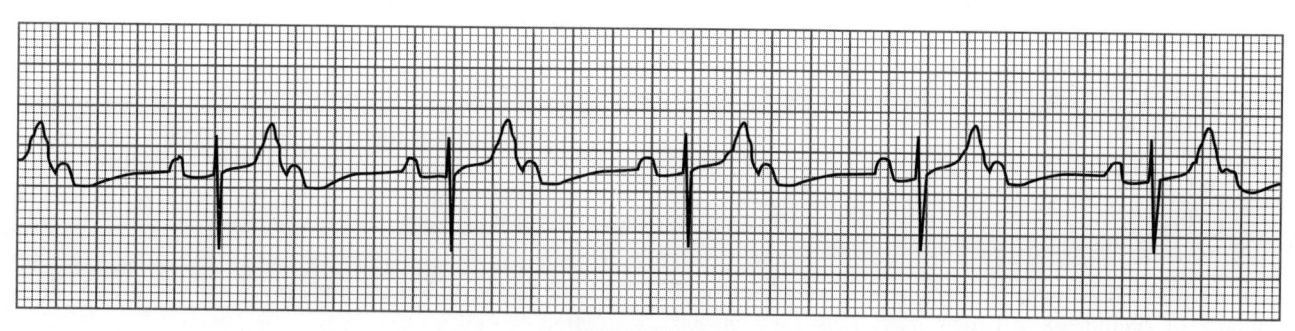

FIGURE 7–2.

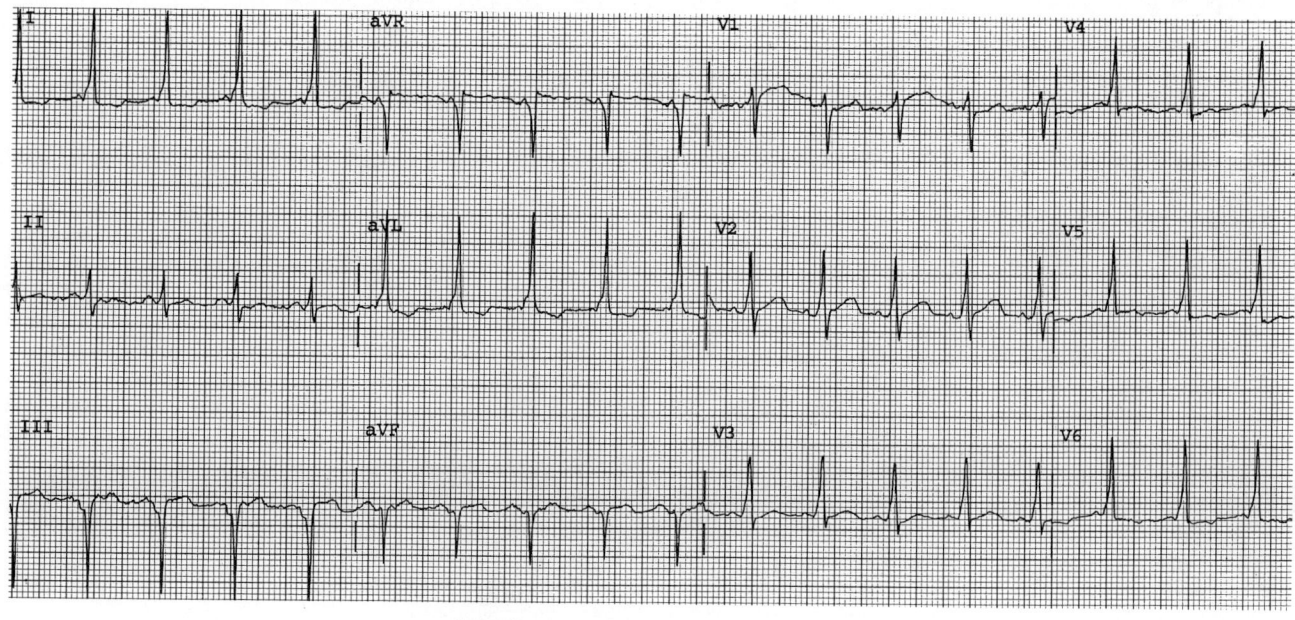

FIGURE 7–3. (Courtesy of Dr. Sheilah Bernard.)

9. All of the following are appropriate for treating cocaine-induced hypertension and arrhythmias except:
   a. Lidocaine
   b. Diazepam
   c. Metoprolol
   d. Nitroglycerin
   e. Nitroprusside

10. A 22-year-old college student who has been taking phenelzine for depression presents with a chief complaint of a headache. She is agitated and has BP 220/110, heart rate 115. Further history reveals that she has been taking an over-the-counter cold medication. The drug of choice for treating her hypertension is:
    a. Metoprolol
    b. Phentolamine
    c. Nifedipine
    d. Enalapril
    e. Clonidine

11. A 62-year-old woman with a history of previous coronary artery bypass graft complains of her typical substernal chest pain. She requires IV nitroglycerin, heparin, and an aspirin to make her pain-free. The nurse points out that the patient has frequent runs of bigeminy and trigeminy and would like to treat this before the patient develops an unstable rhythm. The drug of choice is:
    a. Lidocaine
    b. Metoprolol
    c. Verapamil
    d. Amiodarone
    e. None of the above

12. A 64-year-old woman presents with a complaint of 2 hours of feeling an irregular heart rate. She has no significant past medical history and she is on no medications. You find her to be in atrial fibrillation at a rate of 75. She is hemodynamically stable and would like to go home to return tomorrow for elective cardioversion. At this point you:
    a. Admit her to the CCU to rule out MI and give heparin
    b. Load her with digoxin to chemically cardiovert her before discharge
    c. Send her home on warfarin to return tomorrow to see a cardiologist
    d. Admit her to telemetry to monitor her while attempting chemical cardioversion
    e. Admit her for IV heparin and warfarin, to be cardioverted at a later date

13. For patients who present with new onset of a wide complex, regular tachycardia and who are hemodynamically stable, which of the following cannot be used:
    a. Lidocaine
    b. Procainamide
    c. Verapamil
    d. Adenosine
    e. All of the above can be used

14. A 28-year-old woman presents with 2 hours of palpitations and is found to have atrial fibrillation at a rate of 130. She is hemodynamically stable and you decide to chemically cardiovert her with quinidine. The order in which you give the drugs is:
    a. Quinidine only
    b. Heparin first, then quinidine
    c. Beta-blocker for rate control and then quinidine
    d. Heparin, then beta-blocker, then quinidine
    e. None of the above: quinidine should not be used for cardioversion

15. All of the following are associated with atrial fibrillation except:
    a. A 5 to 7 times increased risk of stroke
    b. Thyrotoxicosis
    c. Pulmonary embolism
    d. Aortic stenosis
    e. Rheumatic mitral valve disease

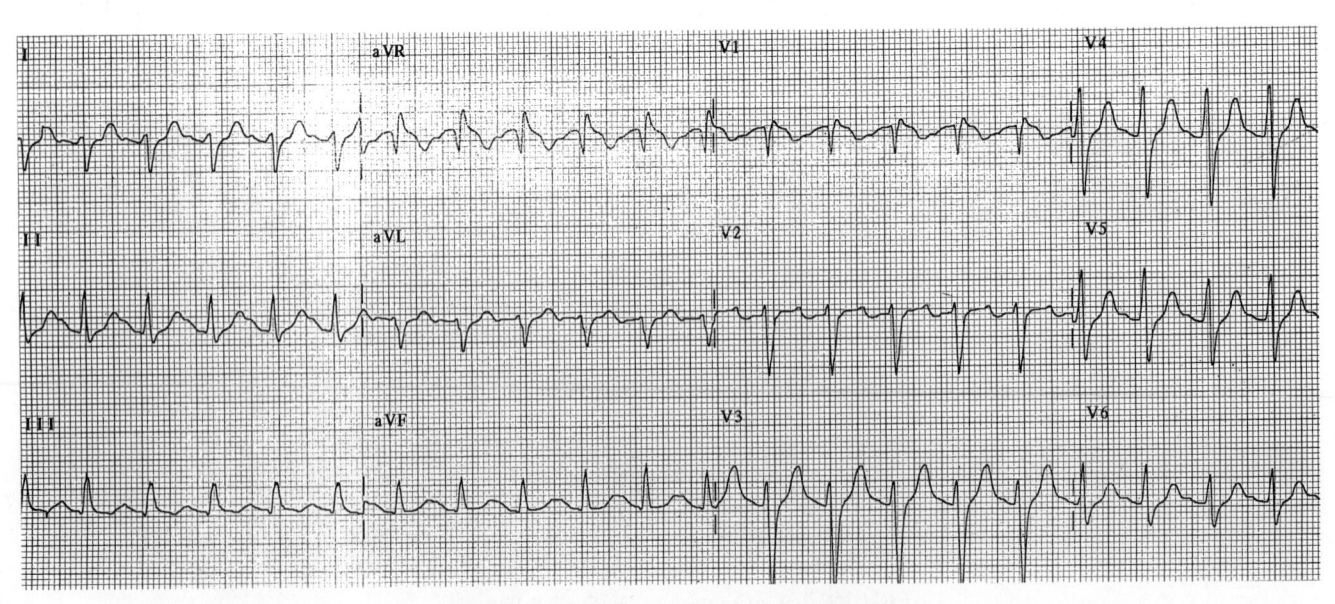

FIGURE 7–4. (Courtesy of Dr. Sheilah Bernard.)

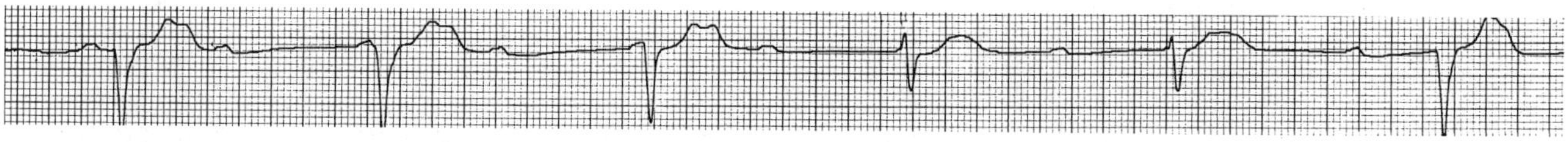

FIGURE 7–5. (Courtesy of Dr. Sheilah Bernard.)

16. An 18-year-old girl is found comatose by her probation officer. On arousal she becomes extremely combative. After arrival to the ED her BP is110/65, heart rate 115. Her ECG is shown in Figure 7–4. What is the first medication to be given?
    a. Lidocaine
    b. Procainamide
    c. Sodium bicarbonate
    d. A benzodiazepine
    e. None of the above

17. A 28-year-old man presents with lightheadedness and near-syncope that began while at home at rest. He reports no current medications or past history except for a viral illness and rash 2 months prior after a hunting trip. His BP is 105/70, heart rate 40. The ECG is shown in Figure 7–5. Treatment for this includes all of the following except:
    a. Antimicrobials
    b. Transcutaneous pacing, as needed
    c. Admission for intensive monitoring
    d. Lidocaine
    e. Infectious disease consultation

18. In a patient with second-degree heart block and 2:1 conduction, which of the following is helpful in distinguishing type I (Wenckebach) from type II ?
    a. The width of the QRS
    b. The administration of a beta-blocker
    c. The length of the QT
    d. Prolongation of consecutive PR intervals
    e. None of the above

19. A 74-year-old man presents to the ED with 48 hours of nausea, weakness, and confusion. He has a history of CHF and is taking digoxin and warfarin. His wife reports that his doctor recently started him on a "water pill" for fluid in his lungs. All of the following are typical of this patient's presentation with digoxin toxicity except:
    a. Visual perception of halos around lights
    b. Hyperkalemia
    c. Ventricular dysrhythmias
    d. Minimally elevated or "normal" digoxin levels
    e. Hypomagnesemia

20. All of the following dysrhythmias are common complications of MI except:
    a. Atrial fibrillation
    b. Atrial flutter
    c. Sinus bradycardia
    d. VT
    e. VF

21. A 22-year-old man presents to you complaining of a fluttering in his chest. He denies chest pain or shortness of breath but reports a past medical history of Wolff-Parkinson-White syndrome. He has a BP of 124/72. His ECG reveals a wide complex tachycardia. Which of the following medications would you not give?
    a. Diltiazem
    b. Lidocaine
    c. Adenosine
    d. Procainamide

22. The best therapy for asymptomatic bradycardia after MI is:
    a. Atropine
    b. Transvenous, temporary pacing
    c. Observation with transcutaneous pacer on standby
    d. Isoproterenol
    e. Nothing

23. A 55-year-old man presents with a complaint of feeling weak for "a few days." You find him to have a rhythm of atrial fibrillation at a rate of 140. He has no other cardiac history. The best treatment plan is:
    a. Admission for initiation of anticoagulation with subsequent discharge and cardioversion after 4 to 6 weeks
    b. Rate control in the ED and outpatient anticoagulation
    c. Begin digoxin and plan for cardioversion in the ED
    d. Rate control in the ED and admission to rule out MI
    e. None of the above

24. A call from EMS comes over the radio. They are with a 72-year-old man who reports new onset of palpitations at rest with slight sternal chest pressure. He has a history of an MI. His BP is 130/80 and his ECG reveals a wide complex tachycardia, at a regular rate of 170. The paramedics have already tried adenosine 12 mg IV twice without any change in rhythm. Which of the following would you give next?
    a. Adenosine, 24 mg IV
    b. Lidocaine, 1 mg/kg IV
    c. Diltiazem, 20 mg IV
    d. Verapamil, 5 mg IV
    e. None of the above

25. A 20-year-old man presents with feeling lightheaded. His BP is 100/70, heart rate 200. His ECG is shown in Figure 7–6. Your drug of choice is:
    a. Verapamil
    b. Metoprolol
    c. Digoxin
    d. Procainamide
    e. Adenosine

26. A 72-year-old man is sent from a local nursing home for evaluation of tachycardia. He has a past history of a stroke and dementia and is on no cardiac medications.

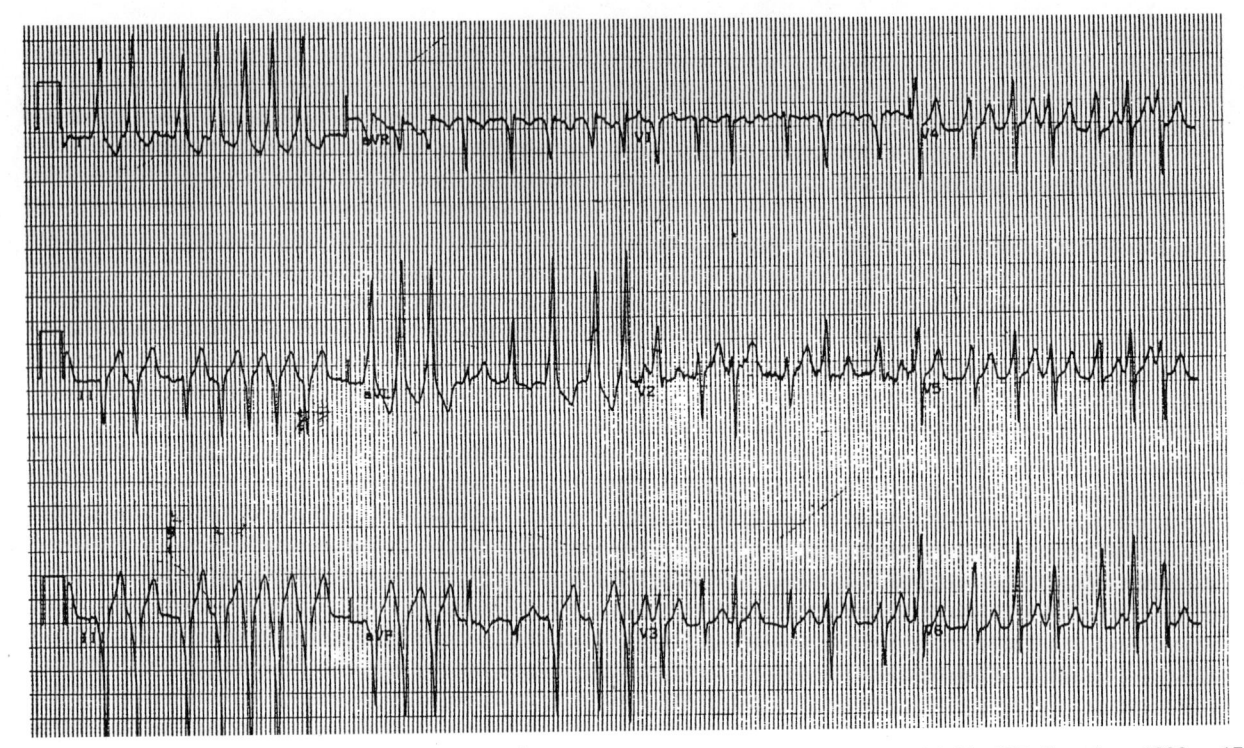

FIGURE 7–6. (From Howell JM, Altieri M, Jagoda AS, et al [eds]: Emergency Medicine. Philadelphia, WB Saunders, 1998, p 176.)

His vital signs are BP 110/65, HR 124, oral temperature 38°C. His ECG shows a sinus tachycardia of 128. What is the first choice for treating his tachycardia?
  a. Adenosine
  b. Verapamil
  c. Isoproterenol
  d. Digoxin
  e. None of the above

27. A 24-year-old woman with no past medical history presents complaining of skipped heartbeats. She has a normal ECG with occasional premature ventricular beats that are associated with her sensation of "skipped beats." How would you manage this patient?
  a. Admission for monitoring
  b. Admission for evaluation of possible ischemia
  c. Discharge home with a beta-blocker
  d. Treat with lidocaine and admit
  e. Check serum electrolytes, outpatient Holter monitor, and discharge with instructions to eliminate caffeine and smoking

Answers

1.e. This is an example of accelerated idioventricular rhythm, and it is seen in up to 30% of anterior MIs and in 40% to 50% of patients during thrombolytic therapy. This is caused by an abnormal focus within the ventricle that takes over pacemaker function. With a slower rate than VT, it is easier to identify fusion beats and retrograde conduction to the atria. In a hemodynamically stable patient, especially during an MI, this rhythm should not be treated: suppressing the ectopic focus may not leave an available pacemaker, leading to asystole or VF. *(Emergency Medicine, Chapter 21, pp 161–192)*

2.d. Sometimes it is possible to identify the time within which atrial fibrillation occurred by the sensation of palpitations. It is only after 72 hours of fibrillation that the risk for thrombus formation begins and anticoagulation is necessary. If the onset has been less than 72 hours, chemical or electrical cardioversion can be planned urgently. If the duration of the atrial fibrillation has been more than 72 hours, or if the duration is unknown, the patient should be admitted for heparinization. Some patients tolerate atrial fibrillation very well. Patients with aortic insufficiency depend upon the preload of the left ventricle to maintain an adequate ejection fraction. In atrial fibrillation, this is impaired because of the loss of the atrial kick and the lost diastolic filling time secondary to the rapid heart rate. Patients that either have a history of heart failure or develop it with the onset of atrial fibrillation should be admitted, because they are not stable. *(Emergency Medicine, Chapter 21, pp 161–192)*

3.c. The differentiation between VT and SVT with aberrancy is very difficult. Some factors, such as fusion beats, history of dilated cardiomyopathy, and past VT, are all very suggestive of VT. The Brugada approach is a stepwise algorithm to diagnosing VT in wide complex tachycardia by ECG criteria. Steps include 1) the absence of an RS complex in all precordial leads; 2) RS interval (measured from beginning of the R to the deepest point of the S wave) >100 msec; 3) AV dissociation; 4) criteria for VT in leads V_1, V_2, and V_6. If any of the above steps are positive, VT is diagnosed.¹ *(Emergency Medicine, Chapter 21, pp 161–192)*

4.a. The rhythm strip is an example of first- and second-degree AV block. Because it has 2:1 conduction, one cannot measure successive PR intervals to determine if they lengthen prior to the dropped beat; it could be Mobitz I (Wenckebach) or Mobitz II. The narrow shape of the QRS complex, however, is more likely to be Mobitz I. Because Mobitz II is an unstable rhythm that threatens to degenerate into complete heart block, this must be observed until proven otherwise. This patient needs admission. Transcutaneous pacer therapy is needed only if his rhythm becomes unstable. *(Emergency Medicine, Chapter 21, pp 161–192)*

5.a. Phenytoin is not of concern; however, adenosine should not be used in combination with carbamazepine because it may produce a higher degree of AV block. Adenosine can precipitate bronchoconstriction and so should be used with caution in patients predisposed to asthma. Methylxanthines (i.e., theophylline) antagonize the effects of adenosine and thus larger doses may be needed. Dipyridamole is an older antiplatelet drug, not frequently used, that may potentiate the effects of adenosine. *(Emergency Medicine, Chapter 21, pp 161–192)*

6.d. The first letter refers to the chamber paced; the second letter refers to the chamber sensed; the third letter refers to the pacemaker mode. In this example, the pacemaker can pace both the atria and ventricles (D for "dual"). The pacemaker can sense both natural P waves and QRS complexes (D for "dual") and inhibits its firing in both of these chambers (D for "dual"). The pacemaker must be a DDD pacemaker.² *(Emergency Medicine, Chapter 21, pp 161–192)*

7.b. This scenario is one of failure to capture. After a new pacer wire is placed and programmed, the healing of the myocardium produces a small scar that may require a higher threshold of energy to capture. Hyperkalemia can also change the polarization of the myocardium, increasing the energy requirement to produce depolarization and contraction. Some new leads can also become dislodged from the myocardium. Leads can fracture, causing malfunction in pacing, sensing, or both. Many people with pacemakers are on beta-blockers to keep their intrinsic heart rate slow, allowing the pacemaker to set the rhythm. Excessive beta-blockade does not lead to failure to capture. *(Emergency Medicine, Chapter 21, pp 161–192)*

8.c. The ECG contains two signs of Wolff-Parkinson-White syndrome: The first is a short PR interval, which is the result of fast conduction down the bypass tract. The second is the delta wave, best seen in leads V_2, V_3, and V_4, which represents preexcitation of the ventricle by early conduction down the bypass tract. A patient with an underlying Wolff-Parkinson-White syndrome bypass tract such as this can enter a reentrant tachycardia by one of two mechanisms. In this case, the impulse is conducted down the AV node and retrograde through the accessory pathway. Since the signal still reaches the ventricle via the AV node and His-Purkinje system, the QRS has a narrow complex (orthodromic conduction). In approximately 10% of cases conduction is down the accessory pathway and retrograde though the AV node, giving a wide complex tachycardia (antidromic conduction). *(Emergency Medicine, Chapter 21, pp 161–192)*

9.c. The peripheral vasoconstrictive effects of cocaine are related to both alpha- and beta-adrenergic agonist effects. Use of a beta-blocking agent may slow the patient's tachycardia, but by blocking peripheral beta₂ receptors responsible for vasodilatation, the overall effect is to create unopposed alpha stimulation, leading to worsening hypertension. Studies with both dogs and humans have shown that beta-blockers do not help and can worsen cocaine-related cardiac effects, whereas benzodiazepines such as diazepam do decrease events and mortality. The cardiac effects of cocaine are mediated through sodium channels, but the channels are probably different for those where lidocaine has its effect, making it safe for concomitant use. *(Emergency Medicine, Chapter 21, pp 161–192)*

10.b. Phenelzine is a monoamine oxidase inhibitor used to treat depression. It blocks the breakdown of norepinephrine, dopamine, and serotonin. Ingestion of certain foods high in tyramine content (cheese, aged meats, some alcohols, pickled fish, and others) by patients on monoamine oxidase inhibitors may precipitate a tyramine reaction, because tyramine is bioconverted to norepinephrine and dopamine. Similarly, ingestion of other sympathomimetic agents (i.e., pseudoephedrine found in over-the-counter cold remedies) will increase the synaptic availability of norepinephrine and dopamine, potentially precipitating a hypertensive urgency or emergency. Because the main effects leading to hypertension are alpha-receptor mediated, an alpha-blocker such as phentolamine is one of the first choices for treating the hypertension. Because the hypertension may be followed by hypotension, longer-acting drugs such as clonidine or enalapril are not recommended. Metoprolol may cause unopposed alpha-adrenergic effects and worsen the hypertension. *(Emergency Medicine, Chapter 21, pp 161–192)*

11.e. It was well demonstrated that in post-MI patients prophylaxis for VT and VF may increase the risk of sudden death. In a patient with known coronary artery disease such as this one, ventricular ectopy *does* reflect the underlying electrical instability of the heart and an increased risk of VF, but it is still not clear if treatment for these "warning arrhythmias" prevents sudden cardiac death. *(Emergency Medicine, Chapter 21, pp 161–192)*

12.d. Not all patients with new-onset atrial fibrillation need to be admitted, just as they do not all need anticoagulation. Rate control is often achieved with IV beta-blockers, calcium channel blockers, or digoxin. Note that digoxin is used for rate control—it does not achieve cardioversion. Patients with new-onset atrial fibrillation with rapid ventricular response of less than 2 days can be cardioverted (chemically or electrically) without anticoagulation, but if the onset of the atrial fibrillation is greater than 2 days or if it is unknown, they should be anticoagulated and cardioverted after 4 to 6 weeks. If they are easily rate controlled and hemodynamically stable, this can be done on an outpatient basis. The exception is the patient (as in this case) who presents with new-onset atrial fibrillation that has a naturally slow ventricular response. In these patients, the slow response suggests a sinus or AV node dysfunction (i.e., the "tachy-brady syndrome"), and attempted cardioversion can lead to symptomatic bradyarrhythmias or even asystole. They need admission for closer observation and planning for long-term therapy such as a pacemaker. *(Emergency Medicine, Chapter 21, pp 161–192)*

13.c. The difficulty here is in distinguishing VT from SVT with aberrancy. Often the diagnosis cannot be made definitively before beginning treatment. Since the rhythm could be Wolff-Parkinson-White syndrome with anterograde conduction down the accessory pathway (the bundle of Kent) and retrograde conduction up the AV node, verapamil will only block the AV node conduction and allow increased conduction through the bypass tract, possibly precipitating VT or VF. Procainamide has antiarrhythmic effects in both the atrium and ventricle and is safe for either SVT or VT. Lidocaine, the first line in pharmacologic therapy for VT, is usually safe for use with SVT, though it rarely increases conduction down a bypass tract. Adenosine, the treatment of choice for SVT, is now also being used experimentally to treat VT, and although its definitive use in this area has yet to be determined, it is not absolutely contraindicated as is verapamil. *(Emergency Medicine, Chapter 21, pp 161–192)*

14.c. As has been previously stated, there is no need for anticoagulation for atrial fibrillation that has less than a 72-hour duration. When using quinidine for cardioversion, there is often an increase in the heart rate when the drug is taking effect, which can precipitate a tachyarrhythmia. For this reason, patients are usually rate controlled (i.e., with a beta-blocker) prior to cardioversion with quinidine. *(Emergency Medicine, Chapter 21, pp 161–192)*

15.d. Atrial fibrillation is associated with an overall fivefold to sevenfold increased risk of stroke, although this risk is even greater in patients who have underlying valvular abnormalities. Mitral valve disease can lead to atrial fibrillation, but the same is not true for aortic stenosis. Other factors that can produce atrial fibrillation include thyrotoxicosis and pulmonary embolism. *(Emergency Medicine, Chapter 21, pp 161–192)*

16.c. The patient in this scenario most likely has a tricyclic antidepressant overdose with a change in mental status and tachycardia typical of the anticholinergic effects of tricyclics, and a widening QRS due to the quinidine-like effects. The widened QRS indicates cardiac toxicity; a QRS duration of greater than .16 increases the risk of deterioration to VT. The ECG also demonstrates rightward axis deviation of the terminal .04 msec of the QRS complex (the terminal .04 msec of the QRS complex is down in lead 1 and upright in lead aV_R). The treatment of choice is sodium bicarbonate, because the alkalization helps unbind the tricyclic from cardiac tissue, and the sodium competes with the tricyclic for sodium channels that mediate the toxic effects. Neither lidocaine nor procainamide is indicated for a wide complex tachycardia with a sinus node origin. *(Emergency Medicine, Chapter 21, pp 161–192)*

17.d. The patient has complete heart block. There is AV dissociation and the ventricular rate is slower than the atrial rate (the opposite is seen with VT). In this case, the history suggests that the dysrhythmia is due to Lyme disease. The disease results from the spirochete *Borrelia burgdorferi*, transmitted by the deer tick. Early manifestations include a viral-like illness and the rash of erythema migrans. Late manifestations include cardiac and/or neurologic effects that develop weeks to months later. The cardiac effects include AV blocks (as in this patient) and myocarditis. The treatment includes treating the underlying disease with either high-dose penicillin or ceftriaxone and treatment for the dysrhythmia with temporary pacing and cardiac monitoring. Lidocaine is contraindicated because it will suppress the escape rhythm, leading to asystole. *(Emergency Medicine, Chapter 21, pp 161–192)*

18.a. In second-degree AV block with 2:1 conduction, every other beat is a blocked beat. There must be at least 3:1 conduction (i.e., two conducted P waves followed by a third nonconducted P wave) in order to determine progressive PR lengthening. In type I block, the site of block is usually at the AV node, producing a normal QRS duration. In type II the site is usually below the AV node, which is why this dysrhythmia is subject to deterioration to third-degree AV block. Thus, the QRS can be used to suggest the site of origin of the block. Also, carotid sinus massage tends to make type I block worse (i.e., worsening AV node block) while transiently improving type II. *(Emergency Medicine, Chapter 21, pp 161–192)*

19.b. This is a patient with chronic digoxin toxicity. There are some marked differences between acute and chronic digoxin toxicity. With acute ingestion of large quantities of digoxin the rapid poisoning of the sodium-potassium pump leads to a rapid increase in serum potassium. Most chronic overdoses occur when a patient with a fixed dose begins using or changes the dose of a diuretic or develops renal insufficiency. Further, diuretic-induced hypokalemia worsens the symptoms of digoxin toxicity. Those with chronic toxicity tend to be older, with more subtle gastrointestinal and CNS symptoms. Also, the dysrhythmias of chronic toxicity tend to be of (but are not limited to) ventricular origin, whereas in acute toxicity the gastrointestinal symptoms are dramatic and the dysrhythmias are more often supraventricular with AV block. *(Emergency Medicine, Chapter 21, pp 161–192)*

20.b. Atrial fibrillation presents 10% to 20% of the time; sinus bradycardia, 16% to 25%; and VT, up to 40% in the setting of a MI. In comparison, atrial flutter is a rare occurrence. *(Emergency Medicine, Chapter 21, pp 161–192)*

21.a. In 70% of cases of Wolff-Parkinson-White syndrome that have developed into a reentrant tachycardia, the rapid conduction to the ventricle is down the AV node, thus producing a narrow complex, so slowing AV nodal conduction with a beta-blocker, calcium channel blocker, or even digoxin can be safe. When there is a wide complex with the reentrant tachycardia, the conduction to the ventricle is via the bypass tract. Any medication slowing the AV conduction (retrograde in these cases) will not affect the bypass tract and will leave the ventricle open to receiving impulses only from the bypass tract, leading to a faster rate and risk of deterioration to VT or VF. Diltiazem would do this, essentially leaving the rapidly conducting bypass tract as the only form of conduction. *(Emergency Medicine, Chapter 21, pp 161–192)*

22.c. As with an asymptomatic accelerated idioventricular rhythm, sinus bradycardia most often presents in patients with acute infarction of the inferior or posterior wall and is often transient and asymptomatic. If the patient is symptomatic with worsening ischemia, CNS changes, or CHF, then atropine or temporary pacing is necessary. In the asymptomatic patient, observation with a standby transcutaneous pacemaker until the rhythm resolves is acceptable treatment. *(Emergency Medicine, Chapter 21, pp 161–192)*

23.a. Patients who meet admission criteria include those with hemodynamic instability; those with significant underlying cardiac disease; and those with duration less than 2 days in whom cardioversion is an option but who have a slow ventricular response. This patient should be admitted for heparinization in anticipation of anticoagulation for 4 to 6 weeks prior to cardioversion. *(Emergency Medicine, Chapter 21, pp 161–192)*

24.b. It would be best if a 12-lead ECG were available, but that is not always the case. Beginning treatment of a wide complex, stable tachycardia with adenosine is acceptable; even VT can be treated this way as long as emergent defibrillation is available. In a case where the rhythm is not responsive to adenosine, the rhythm should be assumed to be VT and treated as such with lidocaine. Higher adenosine doses are unlikely to be effective. *(Emergency Medicine, Chapter 21, pp 161–192)*

25.d. This ECG most likely represents atrial fibrillation with a preexcitation pattern, such as Wolff-Parkinson-White syndrome with conduction intermittently down the bypass tract. Note the intermittent delta waves. Rate control with agents that increase AV nodal blockade could precipitate a fatal arrhythmia. Procainamide prolongs the refractory period of the accessory pathway, slowing ventricular rate. Lidocaine and possibly adenosine may also lead to a faster ventricular rate, VF, and cardiac arrest. *(Emergency Medicine, Chapter 21, pp 161–192)*

26.e. For patients with sinus tachycardia, the key is to treat the underlying etiology of the tachycardia. In this case it is the fever and possibly dehydration. Treating the rhythm alone might not be successful and may lead to a more complicated heart block once the fever resolves. *(Emergency Medicine, Chapter 21, pp 161–192)*

27.e. Premature ventricular beats are very common in young healthy people. In the past, it was thought that exercise-induced premature ventricular contractions in young, otherwise healthy people indicated underlying cardiac abnormalities, but this has since been proven false. If there is no underlying cause for electrolyte abnormality (diarrhea, diuretic medication), there is little yield to their testing. Outpatient Holter monitoring can be set up to document the frequency of the events, but continued hospital monitoring is not necessary. If the premature ventricular contractions are unifocal and are not present in runs of two or more, they are safe and not predictive of adverse events. Patients should be instructed to cut down on excessive cardiac stimulants (caffeine, smoking). *(Emergency Medicine, Chapter 21, pp 161–192)*

Hypertension

1. Which of the following is the best choice of drug regimen to lower the blood pressure in a patient with an aortic dissection?
   a. Hydralazine
   b. Sodium nitroprusside
   c. Labetalol followed by sodium nitroprusside
   d. Sodium nitroprusside followed by labetalol
   e. IV nitroglycerin

2. All of the following may be used for the treatment of hypertensive urgencies except:
   a. Oral nifedipine

b. Oral metoprolol
c. Oral clonidine
d. Oral labetalol
e. ACE inhibitors

3. A 35-year-old woman in the third trimester of pregnancy had been developing headaches. Prior to presentation she had a tonic-clonic seizure. Her BP is 180/94. Treatment may include all of the following except:
   a. Nitroprusside
   b. Enalapril
   c. Magnesium
   d. Hydralazine
   e. Emergent delivery

4. The goals of lowering BP in hypertensive encephalopathy include:
   a. Lowering the systolic BP below 160
   b. Lowering the diastolic BP below 95 mm Hg over 2 to 3 hours
   c. Lowering the diastolic BP below 95 mm Hg over 12 hours
   d. Lowering mean arterial pressure by no more than 25% to 30% over 2 to 3 hours
   e. Lowering mean arterial pressure by no more than 25% to 30% over 12 hours

5. A 52-year-old man presents to your department requesting a BP check. He has no other complaints. He has a regular heart rate of 82 and BP of 220/125. His fundoscopic examination, ECG, and neurologic examination are all normal. The urinalysis, however, shows 2+ hematuria and 2+ proteinuria, and his serum creatinine is 1.9 mg/dL. Your best treatment plan is:
   a. Begin oral therapy with goal of a diastolic BP of 90 to 100 in 2 to 3 days
   b. IV therapy to lower mean arterial pressure by 25% in the first 24 hours
   c. Reduction of systolic BP by 25% within the next 2 to 3 hours
   d. Reduction of mean arterial pressure by 25% within the next 2 to 3 hours
   e. Reduction of diastolic BP to 90 to 100 in the next 2 to 3 hours

6. All of the following pairs of hypertensive crisis and antihypertensive treatment are correct except:
   a. Cocaine-induced hypertension—benzodiazepines
   b. CHF—nitroglycerin
   c. Ischemic cerebrovascular accident—nitroprusside
   d. Aortic dissection—nitroprusside followed by esmolol
   e. Subarachnoid hemorrhage—nimodipine

Answers

1.c. The goal of lowering BP in thoracic aortic dissection is to reduce the sheer forces created by that pressure along the area of the dissection. Acute vasodilatation with hydralazine, nitroglycerin, or nitroprusside may worsen these sheer forces by causing an increased heart rate. Labetalol alone is adequate, but if further BP control is needed, nitroprusside should be added after starting labetalol or some other beta-blocker. (*Emergency Medicine, Chapter 24, pp 207–215*)

2.a. Though most urgencies do not need acute lowering of BP, often the physician prefers to see an initial lowering of BP before discharging the patient from the ED. To this end, many physicians have given oral, chewed, or even sublingual nifedipine that often produces a lowering of BP within 5 to 10 minutes, with a maximal effect at 20 to 30 minutes. Use of short-acting nifedipine may cause precipitous drops in BP, which can cause a stroke or MI, particularly in patients with a fixed cardiac outflow obstruction (i.e., aortic stenosis). Therefore, the use of nifedipine for hypertensive emergencies is contraindicated. All other medications listed will lower the BP—some, such as clonidine, faster than the others—without the same risks as nifedipine. (*Emergency Medicine, Chapter 24, pp 207–215*)

3.b. This patient has eclampsia, which is defined as hypertension in pregnancy with seizures. Preeclampsia is a milder form of hypertension in pregnancy and presents with edema, hyperreflexia, proteinuria, headache, and sometimes epigastric pain. Severe preeclampsia occasionally presents with coma or mental status changes. The ultimate treatment is delivery of the fetus, but the hypertension can be treated with any of the other above drugs. The ACE inhibitors can cross the placenta and may depress angiotensin II levels in the fetus. Magnesium is the drug of choice and can be given in doses of a 4 to 6 g bolus followed by 1 to 2 g/hr infusion, with care to decrease the rate or stop the infusion once the hypertension is controlled, or the patient will lose her deep tendon reflexes (toxic levels of magnesium). Nitroprusside can be used only for the short term because it can produce toxic thiocyanide levels.[3] (*Emergency Medicine, Chapter 24, pp 207–215*)

4.d. There are no set numbers after which patients develop hypertensive emergencies or urgencies, although diastolic pressure above 130 mm Hg is considered a high risk for patients with chronic hypertension. The designation as an emergency or urgency is dependent upon the signs and symptoms of end-organ damage. Although the goal of therapy is to expeditiously lower BP, a precipitous decrease in BP can precipitate myocardial ischemia or a cerebrovascular accident. Thus, the goals of therapy are not based upon absolute numbers but on the degree of initial BP lowering. The initial goal is a decrease in the mean arterial pressure by 25% to 30%, but if the presenting signs and symptoms of the emergency resolve before that level is reached, that can be used as an end point in therapy as well. (*Emergency Medicine, Chapter 24, pp 207–215*)

5.d. The patient has signs of early acute renal failure revealed by both the urinalysis (protein and blood) and his serum creatinine elevation. He therefore has a hypertensive emergency and requires emergent therapy even though he has few complaints. As BP is lowered, the mean arterial pressure is the best parameter to watch. BP should be decreased rapidly and cautiously over a 2- to 3-hour period, except in cases where hypertension is associated with cerebrovascular accident or if there are worsening neurologic symptoms after lowering BP. *(Emergency Medicine, Chapter 24, pp 207–215)*

6.d. Nitroprusside alone, although it rapidly lowers BP, causes a hyperdynamic cardiac response that will increase the arterial shear forces across the dissection. A beta-blocker, such as esmolol or labetalol, is needed to blunt this response and *must* be given prior to starting the nitroprusside. *(Emergency Medicine, Chapter 24, pp 207–215)*

Syncope

1. The 1-year mortality for a patient with cardiogenic syncope is:
   a. 18% to 30%
   b. 12%
   c. 6%
   d. Greater than 50%

2. The etiology of syncope is most frequently diagnosed through history and physical examination rather than using ancillary tests.
   True or False

3. A 55-year-old man with no past medical history or medications has just finished a long day of shopping and walking in the sun during which he skipped lunch. At 4 p.m. after sitting on a bench he stood up and had a witnessed syncopal event with transient loss of consciousness for 60 seconds. Which of the following is least likely to reveal the etiology of his syncope?
   a. Orthostatic vital signs
   b. Hematocrit
   c. Electrolytes and glucose
   d. Electrocardiogram
   e. Stool for occult blood

4. An athletic 40-year-old man is brought to your ED after fainting on the soccer field within 5 minutes of beginning to exercise. He had no preceding symptoms and was running downfield when this happened. It is the fourth such episode in the past month. The most likely diagnosis for the etiology of this man's event is:
   a. Aortic outflow tract obstruction
   b. Dehydration
   c. Carotid sinus syndrome
   d. Vasodepressor syncope
   e. A tachydysrhythmia

5. A 22-year-old dancer presents with syncope after rehearsal. She is thin and well appearing. There are no cardiac murmurs. She insists that her "sugar" is just low because she forgot to eat breakfast. Her vital signs are BP 110/70, heart rate 88, oxygen saturation 98%. What else should be done in her evaluation?
   a. Electrolytes
   b. Hematocrit
   c. ECG
   d. Orthostatic vital signs
   e. All of the above

6. A 78-year-old man had been seated while trying to urinate. On standing he felt lightheaded and then "everything went black." His wife found him getting up from the floor. He denies chest pain or palpitations. He takes terazosin for prostate hypertrophy. His ECG and his physical examination are unremarkable. At this time your diagnosis is:
   a. Vasodepressor syncope ("micturition syncope")
   b. Dysrhythmia
   c. Medicine related (hypotension)
   d. Myocardial ischemia
   e. Cannot be determined without further testing

7. A 10-year-old boy has a syncopal event while playing outside. No seizure activity is noted. He is not noted to be cyanotic. His ECG and physical examination are normal. The ECG in this case can be used to exclude cardiac arrhythmias.
   True or False

8. A 72-year-old woman presents with complaints of three episodes of dizziness and passing out. She is taking medication to control her atrial fibrillation. Her initial ECG shows a sinus rhythm of 72 with a QT interval of 0.52. While in your department she develops a rhythm on the monitor and becomes lightheaded. The rhythm is shown in Figure 7–7.
   a. VT
   b. Coarse VF
   c. Polymorphic VT
   d. Hyperkalemia
   e. Hypokalemia

Answers

1.a. The 1-year mortality of syncope from a cardiac etiology is 18% to 33%. The 1-year mortality for syncope of a

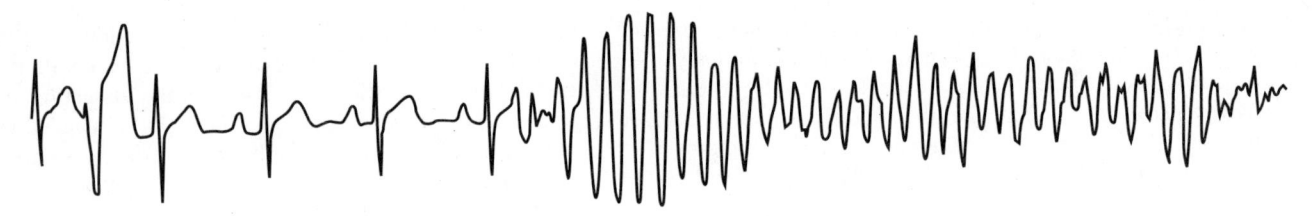

FIGURE 7-7.

noncardiogenic etiology is 12%, and that for those patients with an unknown etiology of their syncope is 6%. *(Emergency Medicine, Chapter 18, pp 142–146)*

2. True. History and physical examination alone can be used to diagnose 55% to 85% of cases of syncope. Past medical history (including detailed cardiac and neurologic history), drug use (prescription, over-the-counter, and illicit), other symptoms (including nausea, vomiting, diarrhea, or blood loss from gastrointestinal or gynecologic sources), preceding events (position changes, Valsalva maneuvers, dystonic stimuli), and symptoms (lightheadedness, vertigo, palpitations) are all historical facts that may be useful. *(Emergency Medicine, Chapter 18, pp 142–146)*

3.c. Although all the above should be done in the evaluation of a syncopal event, hypoglycemia is not likely to have caused a syncopal event that resolved spontaneously. It may cause seizures or weakness but not a transient loss of consciousness that completely resolves in such a short period. *(Emergency Medicine, Chapter 18, pp 142–146)*

4.a. This patient has not been exercising long enough to have become dehydrated. He has no direct stimulus pushing upon his carotid sinus. There is no stimulus to cause a vasodepressor event. Aortic outflow tract obstruction must be considered, especially in young people with syncope on exercise. The exercise creates a demand for increased cardiac output that the heart cannot meet because of the fixed obstruction. This leads to decreased cerebral perfusion as a greater proportion of the fixed output is used by the extremities. *(Emergency Medicine, Chapter 18, pp 142–146)*

5.e. Prior to any testing, a history of vaginal bleeding and eating disorders (i.e., self-induced emesis, irregular menses) must be elicited, and the patient should be observed for signs of anorexia (fingernail changes, low body weight). Regardless, electrolytes and ECG must be done when there is a suspicion of an eating disorder because the patient may have hypokalemia, a metabolic alkalosis, or volume depletion. *(Emergency Medicine, Chapter 18, pp 142–146)*

6.e. Though all of the above are potential causes for the syncopal event and need to be investigated, the diagnosis cannot be made at this time; further testing must be done. A normal ECG does not exclude arrhythmia, and the absence of chest pain or shortness of breath does not exclude ischemia. Especially in the elderly, vasodepressor syncope is a diagnosis of exclusion. *(Emergency Medicine, Chapter 18, pp 142–146)*

7. True. Children with an arrhythmia causing syncope most likely have supraventricular arrhythmias. Potentially dangerous conduction defects can be picked up from the baseline ECG such as prolonged QT syndrome, PR lengthening or other AV blocks, or a preexcitation pattern. Thus, the physical examination, ECG, a chest radiograph looking for cardiomegaly, and appropriate follow-up are enough for the ED evaluation. Without abnormalities in any of these the patient is not at an increased risk for sudden cardiac death, as opposed to an adult who may still be at risk even with a normal ECG. *(Emergency Medicine, Chapter 18, pp 142–146)*

8.c. Polymorphic VT is also referred to as torsades de pointes. It is a VT with a shifting QRS axis that goes from negative to positive although the arrhythmia arises from a single focus. It can be a complication of the congenital QT syndrome in children, it can result as a complication of medications in adults, or it may be related to ischemia and MI. Typical medications are those that prolong the QT and include type Ia antiarrhythmics (quinidine, procainamide, disopyramide) or class III drugs (sotalol, amiodarone). The QT is usually considered prolonged if it is greater than 0.44 sec (the QT must be corrected for the rate). It can also occur with drug combinations, particularly terfenadine (now off the market) with erythromycin or ketoconazole. Most episodes of torsades are spontaneously self-limited, but they can often lead to VT, as in this ECG. Main therapies include IV magnesium sulfate or overdrive pacing and removal of the underlying cause. *(Emergency Medicine, Chapter 18, pp 142–146)*

REFERENCES

1. Brugada P, Brugada J, Mont L, et al: A new approach to the differentiation of a regular tachycardia with a wide QRS complex. Circulation 1991; 83:1649–1659.
2. Kusimoto FM, Goldschlager N: Cardiac pacing. N Engl J Med 1996; 334(2):89–98.
3. Cunningham GF, MacDonald PC, Gant GF, et al: Hypertensive disorders of pregnancy. *In* Williams Obstetrics. Norwalk, CT, Appleton & Lange, 1993, pp 763–817.

BIBLIOGRAPHY

Linden J: Hypertension. *In* Howell JM, Altieri M, Jagoda AS, et al (eds): Emergency Medicine. Philadelphia, WB Saunders, 1998, pp 207–215.

MacMahon S, Collins R, Peto R, et al: Effects of prophylactic lidocaine in suspected myocardial infarction. JAMA 1988; 260(13):1910–1916.

Pelucio M, Jacoby RM: Dysrhythmias. *In* Howell JM, Altieri M, Jagoda AS, et al (eds): Emergency Medicine. Philadelphia, WB Saunders, 1998, pp 161–192.

Pigman EC: Approach to syncope. *In* Howell JM, Altieri M, Jagoda AS, et al (eds): Emergency Medicine. Philadelphia, WB Saunders, 1998, pp 142–146.

8 Diseases of the Arteries and Veins and Aortic Emergencies

MELISSA E. CLARKE, MD, FACEP   FERNANDO DANIELS III, MD, FACEP

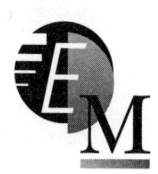

1. Urgent surgical intervention is suggested in the patient who presents with acute leg pain and which of the following signs?
   a. Ankle/brachial index of greater than 0.9
   b. Unilateral leg swelling
   c. Ankle BP less than 90 mm Hg
   d. Cool distal extremity
   e. All of the above

2. Tissue plasminogen activator may be considered a treatment in all of the following clinical scenarios except:
   a. A 25-year-old nonpregnant woman with 24 hours of symptoms of leg swelling found to have a large proximal extremity deep venous thrombosis
   b. A 60-year-old woman with a large proximal deep venous thrombosis and cerulea dolens
   c. A 65-year-old man with a large milky-white leg, severe leg edema, a large proximal deep venous thrombosis, and absent distal pulses
   d. A 40-year-old woman with an isolated calf deep venous thrombosis and a remote history of pulmonary embolus
   e. All of the above would warrant the use of tissue plasminogen activator

3. Risk factors for deep venous thrombosis include all except:
   a. Stroke
   b. Pregnancy
   c. CHF
   d. IV contrast
   e. All of the above are risk factors

4. Which of the following conditions is matched with an inappropriate therapy?
   a. Arterial claudication—elevation, support hose
   b. Superficial thrombophlebitis—NSAIDs, warm compresses
   c. Deep venous thrombosis—inferior vena cava interruption
   d. Varicose veins—vein sclerotherapy
   e. Arterial embolus with absent distal pulses—embolectomy

5. All of the following are true regarding the management of deep venous thrombosis except:
   a. Timely anticoagulation of patients with high likelihood of deep venous thrombosis helps prevent embolization.
   b. Heparin can be safely discontinued in a patient with high clinical suspicion of deep venous thrombosis with a negative ultrasound result.
   c. Isolated calf deep venous thrombosis may be treated on an outpatient basis without anticoagulation.
   d. In patients undergoing anticoagulation for deep venous thrombosis, the target INR is 2 to 3.
   e. Patients with isolated leg swelling and suspected deep venous thrombosis can be transported nonemergently to the ED if no signs or symptoms of pulmonary embolus are present.

6. All of the following are true in the evaluation of lower-extremity deep venous thrombosis except:
   a. Ultrasound is the superior diagnostic modality for pelvic deep venous thrombosis.
   b. Clot can be directly visualized on ultrasound.
   c. MRI and venography are rarely used in the diagnosis of deep venous thrombosis because of cost.
   d. Ultrasound is useful in identifying clot above the level of the popliteal fossa.
   e. Homans' sign is seen in a minority of patients with deep venous thrombosis.

7. All of the following studies are useful in the diagnosis of deep venous thrombosis except:
   a. Impedance plethysmography
   b. D-dimer serum levels
   c. CT scan
   d. MRI
   e. Contrast venogram

8. Which of the following is not related to the probability that deep venous thrombosis will occur?
   a. Existence of concomitant infection
   b. Degree of blood stasis
   c. Local vessel injury

d. Systemic hypercoagulability
e. Capacity for fibrinolysis

9. All of the following are characteristics of phlegmasia cerulea dolens except:
   a. Association with large proximal deep venous thrombosis
   b. Association with atrial fibrillation
   c. Severe leg edema
   d. Results in arterial occlusion
   e. Requires urgent anticoagulation

10. For patients with symptoms suggesting thoracic aortic aneurysm or dissection, a good history and heightened clinical suspicion shortens transport times and may improve outcomes. All of the following should be done in the prehospital setting except:
    a. Maintain adequate oxygenation.
    b. Apply a cardiac monitor and monitor breathing.
    c. Treat shock by starting two large-bore IVs.
    d. Do bilateral BP and transport patient as soon as possible.
    e. Obtain historical information and notify the receiving hospital of an incoming patient.

11. Nearly 50% of patients with thoracic aortic dissection are asymptomatic. Which of the following signs or symptoms may suggest dissection?
    a. Focal neurologic deficits
    b. BP difference between right and left arms of 20 mm Hg or greater
    c. Dysphagia and hoarseness
    d. Stridor and wheezing
    e. All of the above

12. All of the following are predisposing factors for thoracic aortic dissection before age 40 years except:
    a. Ehlers-Danlos syndrome
    b. Turner's syndrome
    c. Pregnancy
    d. Coarctation of aorta
    e. Arteriosclerosis

13. Although the onset of pain from abdominal aortic aneurysm is generally abrupt, associated physical findings may be subtle. All of the following are true except:
    a. The presence of a pulsatile abdominal mass is diagnostic but is found in less than half of the cases.
    b. Careful palpation of the abdomen is contraindicated because of increased risk of aortic rupture.
    c. Lateral propagation of the aortic pulse wave is found more often than a pulsatile mass.
    d. Almost half of abdominal aortic aneurysms are missed on initial presentation.
    e. Symptoms may be misinterpreted as renal colic.

14. Diagnostic findings on chest radiography of thoracic aortic dissection include all of the following except:
    a. Widened mediastinum
    b. Pleural effusion
    c. Enlarged cardiac silhouette from acute tamponade
    d. Aortic shadow beyond its calcified wall
    e. Tracheal deviation

15. Which of the following diagnostic modalities offers the clinician the most useful information, in a timely manner, when thoracic aortic dissection is suspected?
    a. CT
    b. MRI
    c. Transthoracic echocardiography
    d. Transesophageal echocardiography
    e. Aortogram

16. All of the following are true concerning the use of abdominal CT for the diagnosis of abdominal aortic aneurysm except:
    a. It detects leakage and permits concomitant kidney evaluation.
    b. It is not limited by obesity or bowel gas.
    c. It detects branch vessel and adjacent organ involvement.
    d. It defines cranial-caudal extent and extension into the suprarenal aorta.
    e. CT technique for diagnosing abdominal aortic aneurysm does not require the administration of IV contrast.

17. A patient presents to the ED with acute onset of chest pain radiating between his shoulder blades. Diagnostic studies reveal a dissection propagating distally from the left subclavian artery extending below the diaphragm. How is this classified using the Stanford system?
    a. Type I
    b. Type II
    c. Type A
    d. Type B
    e. Type C

18. All of the following are true concerning abdominal aortic aneurysm except:
    a. In stable asymptomatic patients, diagnostic evaluation takes precedence.
    b. Follow-up with a vascular surgeon is warranted if the aneurysm exceeds 3 cm in width.
    c. Patients having abdominal aortic aneurysm more than 6 cm in diameter require serial ultrasound.
    d. Patients with abdominal aortic aneurysm caused by inflammatory process or with evidence of distal emboli require emergent operative repair regardless of aneurysm size.
    e. Comorbid conditions require stabilization before surgical repair, if possible.

19. All of the following statements concerning abdominal aortic aneurysm are true except:
    a. Males are affected 7 times more commonly than females.
    b. Black males have the highest incidence of any age group.
    c. Abdominal aortic aneurysm occurs in 3% of the adult population.
    d. Abdominal aortic aneurysm has an 11% incidence in males older than 65 years.
    e. Three fourths of patients are older than age 60 years.

20. All of the following statements concerning thoracic aorta dissection are true except:
    a. It is two to three times more common in males than females.
    b. It is more common in blacks.
    c. The majority of the cases occur between ages 50 and 70 years.
    d. In women younger than age 40, pregnancy is a risk factor.
    e. Thoracic dissection is caused by atherosclerosis.

Answers

1.b. Acute leg pain associated with an absence of distal pulses, a cool distal extremity, ankle/brachial index less than 0.9, or an ankle BP of 50 mm Hg or less is highly suggestive of arterial embolism with acute arterial insufficiency and suggests the need for urgent surgical interventions. *(Emergency Medicine, Chapter 23, p 205)*

2.d. Tissue plasminogen activator should be considered in consultation for any patient with a large proximal deep venous thrombosis, especially if the patient is young, the thrombosis is recent, or the patient has alba or cerulea dolens *(Emergency Medicine, Chapter 23, pp 205–206)*. Isolated calf deep venous thromboses rarely embolize and, if treated, usually require only heparin anticoagulation. *(Emergency Medicine, Chapter 23, p 205)*

3.e. All of these are considered risk factors for deep venous thrombosis *(Emergency Medicine, Table 23–2)*. CHF, pregnancy, and stroke increase the likelihood of stasis, whereas IV contrast and chemotherapy damage local vessels.

4.a. Proximal deep venous thrombosis is treated with inferior vena cava interruption when anticoagulation is contraindicated. Superficial thrombophlebitis is treated with NSAIDs and warm compresses. Antimicrobials can be added if a septic cause is suspected. Varicose veins are treated with support hose and elevation. Sclerotherapy is indicated if refractory. Arterial claudication is managed with aspirin or pentoxifylline (Trental), but if there is evidence of embolus with acute ischemia, surgery is required. Elevation may actually worsen the pain of claudication. *(Emergency Medicine, Chapter 23, p 205)*

5.b. Heparin should be started for all patients with high suspicion of deep venous thrombosis to prevent embolization, with a target INR of 2 to 3. A negative ultrasound should be followed by MRI or venography in a patient with high likelihood of deep venous thrombosis. If suspected deep venous thrombosis is isolated to the calf, with no evidence for pulmonary embolus, patients can be treated as outpatients with serial ultrasound to check for clot propagation because these rarely embolize *(Emergency Medicine, Chapter 23, p 205)*. Patients do not require urgent transport for evaluation if symptoms suggest only deep venous thrombosis. *(Emergency Medicine, Chapter 23, p 203)*

6.a. Ultrasound has replaced venography in the diagnosis of deep venous thrombosis because it is readily available, can identify clot propagation, and does not have the side effects or cost of venography. Its drawback is that it is not effective in identifying pelvic clots. Magnetic resonance imaging is superior in detecting pelvic deep venous thrombosis, but it is also expensive and not always available. Homans' sign is seen only in 20% of patients with deep venous thrombosis. *(Emergency Medicine, Chapter 23, p 204)*

7.c. Along with ultrasound, impedence plethysmography, venogram, and MRI are all diagnostic modalities for detecting deep venous thrombosis, with MRI being the most sensitive for pelvic or iliac clots and Baker's cyst. The serum D-dimer test will be elevated in cases of deep venous thrombosis and is helpful in conjunction with imaging studies, but it is often not available in the ED and not specific for deep venous thrombosis. *(Emergency Medicine, Chapter 23, p 204)*

8.a. All risk factors associated with the occurrence of deep venous thrombosis can be grouped into four categories—the degree of blood stasis, systemic hypercoagulability, local vessel injury (Virchow's triad), and capacity for fibrinolysis. Existence of infection is not associated with increased probability for deep venous thrombosis formation. *(Emergency Medicine, Chapter 23, p 206)*

9.b. Phlegmasia cerulea dolens is caused by a large proximal deep venous thrombosis with the sequelae of severe leg edema, causing increased compartment pressures, arterial occlusion, and an ischemic, blue leg (cerulea dolens). The leg may also appear milky-white (alba dolens). It is a vascular emergency requiring urgent anticoagulation. Unlike arterial embolism, it is not associated with atrial fibrillation. *(Emergency Medicine, Chapter 23, p 203)*

10.d. For patients with symptoms suggesting thoracic aortic aneurysm or dissection, prehospital personnel must monitor breathing, maintain adequate oxygenation, treat shock (e.g., two large-bore IVs), apply a cardiac monitor, obtain historical information that expedites treatment on ED arrival, and transport as quickly as possible. Although it is usually difficult or impossible to establish these diagnoses in the field, heightened clinical suspicion shortens transport may be times and may improve outcomes. Operative management may be essential to optimal outcome, and all of the above measures may help to expedite diagnosis and definitive treatment. A BP difference between each arm of 20 mm Hg or greater supports the diagnosis of either thoracic aortic dissection or aneurysm. Stabilization and transport take precedence over attempts at rendering a diagnosis in the field; hence, the routine use of bilateral BP measurements by paramedics is not recommended. *(Emergency Medicine, Chapter 22, p 193)*

11.e. Ninety percent of patients with thoracic aortic dissection develop abrupt, excruciating pain. Severity is greatest at onset and may be localized to the anterior chest, neck, jaw, or back, depending on whether the ascending portion, arch, or descending aorta is involved. Migratory pain indicates either proximal or distal extension of the dissection. The patient may appear ashen, diaphoretic, and apprehensive. Vomiting and nausea occur frequently. Other symptoms depend on the structures being compressed by the aortic dissection. Stridor and wheezing may result from tracheal compression. Dysphagia may be caused by esophageal compression, and hoarseness, by laryngeal nerve compression. Associated neurologic deficits occur in 20% of patients, caused by dissection into the carotids or subclavian branches, and syncope occurs in 5% of patients. Occasionally, symptoms are indistinguishable from AMI. It is imperative that the two disorders are distinguished because thrombolytic therapy, which is beneficial in the setting of AMI, is life-threatening in dissection. AMI is approximately 1000 times more common than acute aortic dissection. *(Emergency Medicine, Chapter 22, p 194)*

12.e. Acute dissection results from a degenerative process of the arterial media in the setting of elevated BP, not from atherosclerosis. *(Emergency Medicine, Chapter 22, p 200)*

13.b. Although the onset of pain from abdominal aortic aneurysm is generally abrupt, associated physical findings may be subtle. Vital signs may be normal if there is retroperitoneal containment of the hematoma. The presence of a pulsatile abdominal mass is diagnostic, but it is found in fewer than half of cases and more commonly seen with aneurysmal rupture. Misdiagnosis is fairly common because the classic triad of back pain associated with hypotension and a pulsatile abdominal mass is present in only 30% to 50% of such patients who present to the ED. An abdominal bruit or lateral propagation of aortic pulse wave offers more subtle clues to the diagnosis of abdominal aortic aneurysm and is found more often than a pulsatile mass. There is no evidence that aortic rupture is precipitated by careful palpation of the abdomen. *(Emergency Medicine, Chapter 22, p 196)*

14.c. If thoracic aortic dissection is suspected, chest radiography should be performed because 80% to 90% of these patients have diagnostic findings such as a widened mediastinum, left-sided pleural effusion, extension of the aortic shadow beyond its calcified wall (greater than 6 mm), a localized mass on the arch, tracheal deviation, or changes in the aorta compared with old films. The cardiac silhouette often remains unchanged in tamponade that develops acutely. *(Emergency Medicine, Chapter 22, p 196)*

15.d. Echocardiography is extremely useful, especially when transthoracic, suprasternal, subcostal, and transesophageal techniques are used in combination Ultrasound visualizes the intimal membrane, the true and false lumens, the intimal tear, the extent of dissection, wall motion abnormalities caused by myocardial ischemia, aortic valvular insufficiency, side branch involvement, and pericardial or pleural effusions. The study is performed at bedside in 5 to 15 minutes, and a positive result obviates further evaluation. The main limitation of the study is poor visualization of the ascending aorta because of tracheal interposition, although false-negative results are rare when it is performed by an experienced echocardiographer. CT reliably diagnoses aortic dissection, with both sensitivity and specificity above 95%. CT does not require arterial cannulation and offers the additional advantage over aortography of consistently demonstrating a thrombosed false lumen or intimal flap. Disadvantages compared with aortography include limited information on aortic valvular and side branch involvement. MRI is noninvasive, requires no contrast material, and does not expose the patient to radiation. The procedure is very sensitive and specific in demonstrating the type and extent of dissection, intimal tears, true and false lumens, and aortic insufficiency. However, MRI is incompatible with life-support equipment and is time-consuming. MRI seems most appropriate for patients who are stable, cannot be given contrast material, or need follow-up after starting treatment. Aortography has a sensitivity of 90% and is considered the gold standard. Aortography will reveal the extent of dissection and involvement of branch vessels and helps the surgeon plan for operative intervention. Disadvantages include a large dye load and false-positive results. Given the relative strengths and weaknesses of each study, it is prudent to consult a radiologist and thoracic surgeon early, consider bedside ultrasonography (i.e., transesophageal echocardiography) first, and use a second test if echocardiographic results are unclear or inconsistent with clinical data. *(Emergency Medicine, Chapter 22, p 197)*

16.e. In stable patients in whom further radiologic investigation is warranted, CT is 100% sensitive for abdominal aortic aneurysm and offers certain advantages compared with ultrasound: defining aortic size, rostral-caudal extent, involvement of visceral arteries, and extension into the suprarenal aorta. CT visualizes the retroperitoneum, is not limited by obesity or bowel gas, detects leakage, and permits concomitant kidney evaluation. Newer technology with spiral CT images the abdomen in three dimensions, enhancing the detection of branch vessel and adjacent organ involvement. The major disadvantages are technician availability, cost, longer study time, the need for IV contrast, and the time spent out of the department *(Emergency Medicine, Chapter 22, p 197)*

17.d. Decisions concerning surgery for thoracic aortic dissection are predicated, in part, on anatomic classification by either the DeBakey or Stanford system (Fig.

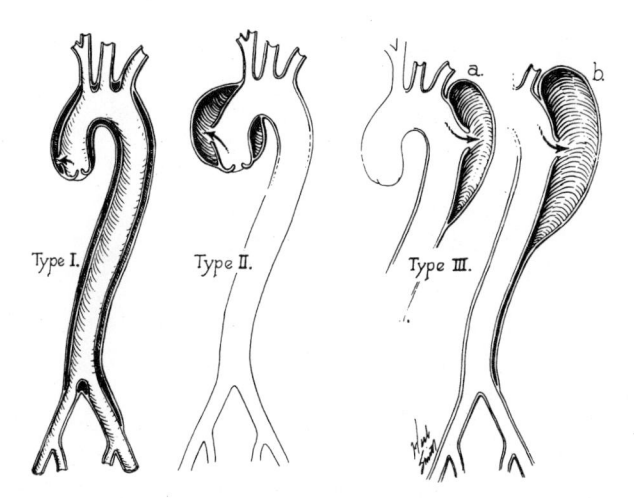

FIGURE 8–1. DeBakey's classification of dissecting aortic aneurysms: type I, type II, and type III. (From DeBakey ME, Henly WS, Cooley DA, et al: Surgical management of dissecting aneurysms of the aorta. J Thorac Cardiovasc Surg 1965;49:130.)

8–1). The DeBakey system classifies dissection into three categories: type I occurs 65% of the time and involves the ascending aorta, arch, and descending aorta; type II occurs 10% of the time and is limited to the ascending aorta; type III occurs 25% of the time and propagates distally from the left subclavian artery. Type IIIa does not extend below the diaphragm, and type IIIB does. The Stanford system is simpler and classifies dissections into two categories: type A involves the ascending aorta and type B does not. Type A dissections are more common, are associated with a higher mortality, and are usually treated operatively (except if stroke is present). Type B dissections are often treated medically, with strict BP control, but may require urgent operative intervention for organ/limb ischemia or progression. *(Emergency Medicine, Chapter 22, p 198)*

18.c. In abdominal aortic aneurysms, stability of the patient dictates the urgency of consultation. In stable, asymptomatic patients, diagnostic evaluation takes precedence, and consideration should be given to consulting radiology to determine whether ultrasound, CT, or MRI is most appropriate. Follow-up with a vascular surgeon is warranted if the abdominal aorta exceeds 3 cm in width or if any segment is greater than 1.5 times the diameter of an adjacent section. Patients having abdominal aortic aneurysms less than 4 cm in diameter require serial ultrasound twice a year. If the diameter increases by more than 0.5 cm over 6 months, exceeds 4 to 5 cm, or is more than twice the width of native aorta, surgical repair is warranted. The 5-year risk of rupture is 3% to 12% for aneurysms between 4 and 5 cm and 25% to 41% for aneurysms greater than 5.0 cm. *(Emergency Medicine, Chapter 22, p 197)*

19.b. Ruptured abdominal aortic aneurysm is the 13th leading cause of death in the United States, with an estimated 15,000 deaths per year. Abdominal aortic aneurysm occurs in 2% to 4% of the adult population, with 11% incidence in males older than 65 years. Despite increased survival after diagnosis, the incidence and crude mortality seem to be increasing. More than three fourths of patients with abdominal aortic aneurysms are older than 60 years. Risk factors include atherosclerosis and family history. Males are affected 7 times more commonly than females, with white males having the highest incidence of any group. *(Emergency Medicine, Chapter 22, pp 193–202)*

20.e. Thoracic aortic dissection occurs in 5 to 10 individuals per million, is more common in blacks, and is 2 to 3 times more common in males than females. The majority of cases occur between 50 and 70 years of age. Hypertension appears to be the main risk factor, with trauma and structural abnormalities contributing. Although atherosclerosis is often present in patients with dissections, it is not causative. Dissections in persons younger than 40 years are associated with Ehlers-Danlos syndrome, Marfan's syndrome, Turner's syndrome, pregnancy, and aortic coarctation. *(Emergency Medicine, Chapter 22, pp 193–202)*

BIBLIOGRAPHY

Cigarroa JE, Isselbacher EM, DeSanctis RW, Zagle KA: Diagnostic imaging in the evaluation of suspected aortic dissection. N Engl J Med 1993;328(1):35–43.

Howell JM: Acquired diseases of the arteries and veins. *In* Howell JM, Altieri M, Jagoda AS, et al (eds): Emergency Medicine. Philadelphia, WB Saunders, 1998, pp 203–206.

Nienbar CA, Von Kodolitisch Y, Nicolas V, et al. The diagnosis of thoracic aortic dissection on noninvasive imaging procedures. N Engl J Med 1993;328(1):2–9.

O'Connor RE: Aortic aneurysms and dissections. *In* Howell JM, Altieri M, Jagoda AS, et al (eds): Emergency Medicine. Philadelphia, WB Saunders, 1998, pp 193–202.

9 Pericarditis, Myocarditis, and Endocarditis

MELISSA E. CLARKE, MD, FACEP

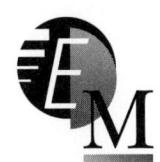

1. All of the following statements regarding acute cardiac tamponade are true except:
   a. Beck's triad includes a decrease in systolic blood pressure, neck vein distention, and muffled heart sounds.
   b. Nitroglycerin can be used as a temporizing agent to relieve the ischemic chest discomfort associated with cardiac tamponade because it increases arteriolar dilation and cardiac perfusion.
   c. Life-threatening hypotension caused by cardiac tamponade is treated by emergent pericardiocentesis.
   d. A 12-mm Hg or greater fall in arterial pressure during inspiration, although not specific for tamponade, can serve as an early warning sign.
   e. ICU admission is required for patients with hemodynamically stable cardiac tamponade.

2. All of the following ECG changes are characteristic of acute pericarditis except:
   a. Slightly taller, peaked, and symmetric T waves in the early phase
   b. ST segment deviation toward the injured epicardial surface
   c. Diminished magnitude of the P, QRS, and T wave deflections as well as possible electrical alternans
   d. Reciprocal ST segment changes similar to those present with AMI
   e. Concave upward ST segment elevation in stage 2

3. The ECGs of chronic pericarditis and myxedema are similar in all aspects except:
   a. Low-amplitude QRS wave
   b. Diminished T waves
   c. Sinus tachycardia
   d. Inverted T waves
   e. None of the above

4. The most common etiologic agent associated with myocarditis is:
   a. Lyme disease
   b. *Staphylococcus aureus*
   c. HIV
   d. Coxsackie B virus
   e. *Haemophilus influenzae*

5. All of the following statements are true regarding dilated cardiomyopathy from acute myocarditis except:
   a. A majority of patients with Coxsackie B virus as an etiologic agent develop cardiomyopathy.
   b. Delayed cellular response leading to cardiomyopathy is caused by a disorder in immune regulation.
   c. Patients with prior myocarditis have cardiomyopathy at a greater rate than control subjects.
   d. Death from dilated cardiomyopathy is caused by sequelae of the massively dilated heart, CHF, or dysrhythmia.
   e. None of the above are true.

6. Appropriate initial management of acute myocarditis presenting with hypotension and respiratory distress includes:
   a. Fluid challenges and broad-spectrum antimicrobials
   b. Airway management, diuretics, and inotropic agents
   c. MRI or CT scan in order to demonstrate a myocardial thickening
   d. Echocardiography
   e. ECG

7. The following drugs are all known to be causative agents in pericarditis except:
   a. Penicillin
   b. Isoniazid
   c. Prednisone
   d. Phenytoin
   e. Methyldopa

8. All of the following historical features are seen in acute pericarditis except:
   a. Retrosternal chest pain improved by lying flat and worsened with sitting up
   b. A preceding upper respiratory infection
   c. Odynophagia
   d. An association with certain medications such as procainamide and hydralazine
   e. Radiation of pain to the trapezoidal ridge

9. Which statement is the most accurate regarding the management of acute pericarditis?

a. All patients with an effusion require observation to monitor for possible additional fluid accumulation.
b. All patients diagnosed with acute pericarditis should receive a 1-week taper of corticosteroids.
c. All patients diagnosed with acute pericarditis require ICU admission.
d. All patients with purulent pericarditis require pericardial window.
e. Antimicrobials are the best single management for acute pericarditis.

10. The following statements are true regarding pericardial friction rub except:
    a. The rub is best heard during expiration with the patient sitting up and leaning forward.
    b. In the presence of pericardial effusion, the rub becomes more prominent.
    c. The classic rub is triphasic, with a component before, during, and after systole.
    d. The rub is intermittent and may not be present in every patient.
    e. The sound of the rub has a sandpaper-like quality.

11. Which of the following conditions is most appropriately matched to its correct presentation?
    a. Acute pericarditis with effusion—pericardial "knock"
    b. Dressler's syndrome—pleuritic chest pain 1 day postinfarction
    c. Malignant pericarditis—facial swelling and a superior vena cava syndrome
    d. Cardiac tamponade—hypertension and distended neck veins
    e. Constrictive pericarditis—signs of left heart failure

12. All of the following are accepted treatments for pericarditis except:
    a. NSAIDs
    b. Steroids
    c. Interferon therapy
    d. Azathioprine
    e. Acetaminophen

13. All of the following statements regarding pericarditis in renal failure are true except:
    a. Pericarditis usually resolves with increased hemodialysis and anti-inflammatory agents.
    b. Tamponade is a rare complication in uremic pericarditis.
    c. Hemorrhagic effusion is the most common type of effusion seen in uremic pericarditis.
    d. Pain may precede objective evidence of pericarditis by weeks.
    e. Severe azotemia may be a cause of pericarditis in patients without previous dialysis.

14. Presenting symptoms of myocarditis include:
    a. CHF
    b. Dysrhythmias
    c. Conduction disturbances
    d. Tachycardia
    e. All of the above

15. Constrictive pericarditis is associated with:
    a. Radiation therapy
    b. Renal failure
    c. Trauma
    d. Tuberculosis
    e. All of the above

16. All of the following cardiac lesions predispose patients to an episode of endocarditis except:
    a. Mitral valve prolapse with regurgitation
    b. Known calcific degenerative valvular disease
    c. Idiopathic subaortic stenosis
    d. Prosthetic valves
    e. Bicuspid aortic valve

17. All of the following are helpful signs in the diagnosis of patients with endocarditis except:
    a. Hypertension
    b. Hematuria
    c. Splenomegaly
    d. Osler's nodes
    e. Roth's spots

18. The following are true in the management of endocarditis except:
    a. Auscultating a murmur of valvular insufficiency in the setting of acute CHF requires prompt consultation with a cardiothoracic surgeon.
    b. Three to five sets of blood cultures 1 hour apart are important in making a diagnosis.
    c. Patients without septic shock or acute heart failure can be managed in a non-ICU setting.
    d. Patients with low probability for endocarditis with three negative blood cultures can be discharged with timely follow-up if stable.
    e. Because of the rapidly progressive nature of endocarditis, antimicrobials should be given immediately after the first two sets of blood cultures are obtained.

19. Patients who most benefit from surgical intervention include those with:
    a. Valvular insufficiency
    b. Annular or myocardial abscess
    c. Aortic endocarditis
    d. Prosthetic endocarditis
    e. All of the above

20. Which of the following is true in the pathophysiology of endocarditis?
    a. On a normal heart valve, only a small inoculum of bacteria is necessary for infection.
    b. Circulating immune complexes correlate with a higher rate of complicating arthritis, splenomegaly, and glomerulonephritis.
    c. Rupture of the chordae tendineae is an immune-complex mediated complication of endocarditis.
    d. Subacute endocarditis frequently results in metastatic infection.
    e. *H. influenzae* and *Streptococcus viridans* have the same frequency as causal agents of subacute endocarditis.

21. The most common skin finding in endocarditis is:
    a. Roth's spots
    b. Osler's nodes
    c. Janeway lesions
    d. Petechiae
    e. Splinter hemorrhages

Answers

1.b. Cardiac tamponade is characterized clinically by a decrease in systolic BP, neck vein distention reflective of an increased venous pressure, and muffled heart sounds—a constellation of signs known as Beck's triad. Pulsus paradoxus, present early in tamponade, is defined as a 12-mm Hg or greater fall in arterial pressure with inspiration. It is caused by the rapid equalization of pressures between ventricles and the pericardium as fluid accumulates. Pulsus paradoxus may also be seen in severe asthma, COPD, pulmonary embolism, and RV infarction. Giving nitroglycerin to a patient will decrease venous return, thereby decreasing preload and cardiac output and worsening hypotension. Nitroglycerin is contraindicated in patients with cardiac tamponade. *(Emergency Medicine, Chapter 25, pp 217–224)*

2.d. Four stages of ECG changes in pericarditis have been described. In the earliest stage, the T waves become tall and peaked, and there is diffuse ST elevation, with or without PR depression. The ST segment deviates toward the injured epicardial surface and has a concave upward appearance. ST segment changes that are convex, upward, or reciprocal in other leads are more consistent with myocardial ischemia. During stage 2, the ST junction returns to baseline, while PR depression may persist. During stage 3, T waves become inverted, and during stage 4, the ECG returns to normal. The pericardial effusion acts to short-circuit the electrical impulses, resulting in diminished magnitude of the wave deflections. *(Emergency Medicine, Chapter 25, pp 217–224)*

3.c. All of the above are true about the ECG of myxedema and chronic pericarditis except the heart rate. Myxedema usually presents with sinus bradycardia, whereas chronic and acute pericarditis usually are accompanied by sinus tachycardia. *(Emergency Medicine, Chapter 25, pp 217–224)*

4.d. All of the above etiologic agents are seen with myocarditis. Coxsackie B virus is the causative agent in more than 50% of all cases, although other viruses, bacteria, fungi, protozoa, rickettsiae, and spirochetes have been documented.[1,2]

5.a. The conclusion that myocarditis can progress to cardiomyopathy is supported by the observation that patients with previous myocarditis have cardiomyopathy at a greater rate than do control subjects. The mechanism is thought to be autoimmune, with a clinically latent period between the two stages of up to years, during which cumulative myocardial damage occurs.[3] Once cardiomyopathy has developed, mortality is estimated to be greater than 50% at 2 years, usually from CHF or dysrhythmias. Coxsackievirus cases progress at a greater rate; however, only a minority of patients with myocarditis ever have complications. Most recover without sequelae.[4] *(Emergency Medicine, Chapter 25, pp 217–224)*

6.b. Patients with hypotension and respiratory distress caused by myocarditis need definitive airway management. The hypotension usually results from poor cardiac output, and giving fluid challenges might actually worsen cardiac status, especially if the examination is consistent with adequate hydration. Inotropic agents, along with diuretics, improve cardiac output. Optimal management would include ICU admission and invasive hemodynamic monitoring. Bedside echocardiography would best demonstrate myocardial thickening but would not be important in the initial management. Although purulent pericarditis is seen in pediatric cases, it is much less common than viral or autoimmune causes. *(Emergency Medicine, Chapter 25, pp 217–224)*

7.c. All of the drugs listed except prednisone have been linked etiologically to acute pericarditis. Prednisone is actually a treatment for pericarditis refractory to NSAIDs. For the complete list of associated agents, see Table 25–4 in *Emergency Medicine, Chapter 25, p 222.*

8.a. The chest pain typical of acute pericarditis is sharp, retrosternal, relieved by sitting up, and aggravated by motions of the chest wall, including lying flat, deep breathing, and turning. Painful swallowing is another typical symptom reported. Pericarditis of viral etiology is often preceded by a viral respiratory infection within 2 weeks of presentation. Procainamide and hydralazine are two of the medications known to cause pericarditis.[3] *(Emergency Medicine, Chapter 25, pp 217–224)*

9.a. The management of acute pericarditis is determined by the presence of effusion as determined by echocardiography. Patients with effusion require monitoring in an ICU setting for accumulation of fluid leading to the rare complication of tamponade. Pericarditis without effusion is initially treated with NSAIDs. Steroids are used in refractory cases. Patients without effusion can be treated as outpatients, as long as pain management is adequate. Patients diagnosed with purulent pericarditis require ICU admission and appropriate antimicrobials after pericardiocentesis. In cases where pericardial fluid reaccumulates, partial surgical resection may be required to prevent progression to constrictive pericarditis. *(Emergency Medicine, Chapter 25, pp 217–224)*

10.b. Pericardial friction rub, pathognomonic of acute pericarditis, is best auscultated over the left lower sternal border with the patient sitting up and leaning forward, thus bringing the heart closest to the chest wall. Although not heard in all patients, when heard it has three classic components. The presence of effusion, which separates the parietal from the visceral pericardium, may actually eliminate the friction rub. *(Emergency Medicine, Chapter 25, pp 217–224)*

11.c. A pericardial knock, caused by the filling of a noncompliant ventricle, is seen in constrictive pericarditis. Dressler's syndrome (postinfarction pericarditis) occurs a *few days to 6 weeks* after infarct and presents with pleuritic chest pain, fever, or pneumonitis. Malignant pericarditis is most often caused by invasion by primary or metastatic tumors (most often breast, melanoma, lymphoma, leukemia, or lung). If pericarditis is caused by extension of a lung tumor, facial swelling and a superior vena cava syndrome may be present because of vascular obstruction. Cardiac tamponade is characterized by a *decrease* in systolic BP, pulsus paradoxus, neck vein distention, and muffled heart sounds. Constrictive pericarditis more often presents with signs of *right* heart failure—ascites, hepatomegaly, dyspnea, fatigue, and peripheral edema. *(Emergency Medicine, Chapter 25, pp 217–224)*

12.e. Although acetaminophen may help in fever reduction, it has no anti-inflammatory properties to assist in resolution of the acute inflammation. Agents used in addition to the mainstay of therapy—NSAIDs—include steroids, interferon, colchicine, and azathioprine. *(Emergency Medicine, Chapter 25, pp 217–224)*

13.b. Three types of pericarditis are associated with renal failure: uremic, dialysis-related, and constrictive. Effusions are common, are usually bloody, and occasionally progress to tamponade. Pain may precede objective evidence of pericarditis by weeks, and altered mental status may be the only presenting sign. *(Emergency Medicine, Chapter 25, pp 217–224)*

14.e. All of the above are seen with myocarditis. An unexplained increase in heart size on physical exam or chest radiograph is also seen. *(Emergency Medicine, Chapter 25, pp 217–224)*

15.e. Constrictive pericarditis results when the pericardium forms diffuse fibrous adhesions to the epicardium in response to a previous insult. The most common causes are neoplasm, previous irradiation, renal disease, previous thoracic trauma, infections, and collagen vascular disease. *(Emergency Medicine, Chapter 25, pp 217–224)*

16.c. Risk factors for endocarditis include any cardiac lesions involving damaged valves. These include previous valve surgery, known calcific degenerative valvular disease, mitral valve prolapse, bicuspid aortic valve, history of rheumatic fever, and a previous episode of endocarditis. *(Emergency Medicine, Chapter 26, p 225)*

17.a. Clinical manifestations of endocarditis result from embolization of septic fragments from vegetations to remote sites: the kidney (hematuria), the spleen (splenomegaly), and the skin (Osler's nodes—tender erythematous nodes on distal extremities—and Roth's spots—embolic retinal lesions *(Emergency Medicine, Chapter 26, p 226)*. Blood pressure tends to be low given the propensity for septic or cardiogenic shock.

18.e. Patients with valvular insufficiency and severe heart failure require prompt surgery to restore valvular competence and remove septic foci. Three to five sets of blood cultures are required a least 1 hour apart to identify the offending organism before treatment. Patients with septic shock or acute heart failure are admitted to an ICU setting. All others go to a regular hospital floor for IV antimicrobials and further study. Those who are unlikely to have acute endocarditis can be discharged after three blood cultures if stable. *(Emergency Medicine, Chapter 26, pp 225–227)*

19.e. Patients with prominent valvular insufficiency and severe heart failure, abscesses, or aortic or prosthetic endocarditis most benefit from surgical intervention. *(Emergency Medicine, Chapter 26, p 226)*

20.b. The presence of circulating immune complexes correlates with extracardiac manifestations such as arthritis, glomerulonephritis, and splenomegaly. Large inocula of bacteria are required to infect a normal heart valve. This colonization can result in a local bacterial infection that can invade contiguous structures such as the chordae tendineae, leading to rupture. Subacute endocarditis evolves slowly and rarely causes metastatic infection. *S. viridans* is one of the leading pathogens in subacute bacterial endocarditis, whereas *H. influenzae* is a less common cause. *(Emergency Medicine, Chapter 26, pp 227–228)*

21.d. Petechiae are the most common skin finding in endocarditis. Other findings, which are not commonly seen, include Roth's spots (embolic retinal lesions), splinter hemorrhages, Janeway lesions (hemorrhagic lesion on palms and soles) and Osler's nodes (tender, raised lesions on pads of fingers and toes). *(Emergency Medicine, Chapter 26, p 226)*

REFERENCES

1. Cohen IS, Anderson DW, Mirmani R, et al: Congestive cardiomyopathy in association with the acquired immunodeficiency syndrome. N Engl J Med 1986; 315:628
2. McAlister HG, Klementowicz J, Andrews C, et al: Lyme carditis: An important cause of reversible heart block. Ann Intern Med 1989; 110:339–345.
3. Leslie K, Blay R, Haisch C, et al: Clinical and experimental aspects of viral myocarditis. Clin Microbiol Rev 1989; 2:191–203.
4. Kereiakea DJ, Parmely WW: Myocarditis and cardiomyopathy. Am Heart J 1984; 108:1318–1326.

BIBLIOGRAPHY

Debehnke DJ: Cardiac related acute infectious disease. *In* Gibler WB, Aufderheide TP (eds): Emergency Cardiac Care. St. Louis, Mosby–Year Book, 1994, p 464.

Dhindsa HS, Howell JM: Endocarditis. *In* Howell JM, Altieri M, Jagoda AS, et al (eds): Emergency Medicine. Philadelphia, WB Saunders, 1998, pp 225–228.

O'Keefe KP, Sanson TG: Pericarditis, myocarditis, and pericardial tamponade. *In* Howell JM, Altieri M, Jagoda AS, et al (eds): Emergency Medicine. Philadelphia, WB Saunders, 1998, pp 217–224.

10 Congenital Heart Disease

JOHN C. BRANCATO, MD

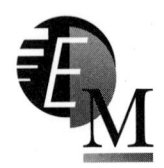

1. A 5-day-old female who was well in the immediate postnatal period is brought in by her parents because of cyanosis. On physical exam, the infant is quiet, warm, and well perfused with a low O_2 saturation and no murmur. Initial management should include all of the following except:
   a. ECG
   b. Chest radiograph
   c. ABG
   d. Lumbar puncture
   e. 100% oxygen challenge

2. If this same infant has no response to oxygen and no evidence of overwhelming lung disease, the most important subsequent therapy is:
   a. Dopamine infusion at 10 μg/kg per minute
   b. Epinephrine, 0.1 mg/kg of 1:10,000
   c. Digoxin, 40 μg/kg
   d. Prostaglandin E infusion at 0.1 μg/kg per minute
   e. Furosemide, 0.5 mg/kg

3. Tetralogy of Fallot is composed of all of the following except:
   a. Atrial septal defect
   b. Ventricular septal defect
   c. Overriding aorta
   d. Pulmonic stenosis
   e. RV hypertrophy

4. A 5-week-old male is brought to the ED because of fussiness and slightly decreased oral intake. In triage, he is noted to be tachycardic, with a rate of 250 beats/min. The most useful initial therapy is probably:
   a. Normal saline bolus, 20 mL/kg
   b. D_5 half-normal saline bolus, 20 mL/kg
   c. Ice bag applied to the face
   d. Verapamil, 0.1 mg/kg
   e. Immediate broad-spectrum antimicrobials

5. If the initial therapy is unsuccessful or if the patient is unstable, the next step is cardioversion at a dose of:
   a. 1 J/kg
   b. 10 J/kg
   c. 20 J/kg
   d. 50 J/kg
   e. 100 J/kg

6. A patient known to have tetralogy of Fallot arrives at the ED and is agitated, crying, and cyanotic. Appropriate management steps include all of the following except:
   a. Placing the patient in knee-to-chest position
   b. Administration of oxygen
   c. Giving an IM dose of morphine sulfate
   d. Vagal maneuvers
   e. Giving a bolus of IV crystalloid

7. Findings on history and physical examination consistent with a diagnosis of Kawasaki's disease include all of the following except:
   a. Nonpurulent conjunctival injection
   b. Cervical lymphadenopathy
   c. Peeling palms and soles
   d. Strawberry tongue
   e. Splinter hemorrhages

8. The classic Blalock-Taussig shunt connects:
   a. Descending aorta to left pulmonary artery
   b. Superior vena cava to right pulmonary artery
   c. Superior vena cava to left atrium
   d. Right atrium to left pulmonary artery
   e. Subclavian to pulmonary artery

9. Children with Down's syndrome and congenital heart disease most commonly have a ventricular septal defect or which of the following?
   a. Coarctation of the aorta
   b. Endocardial cushion defect
   c. Pulmonic stenosis
   d. Transposition of the great arteries
   e. Atrial septal defect

10. A 2-month-old infant presents with a 10- to 12-day history of poor feeding, intermittent tachycardia, and sweating. On examination, she is somewhat fussy with nasal flaring and mild retractions and is tachycardic to 180 beats/min. She has a few scattered rhonchi, no rales,

and a III/VI systolic murmur at the left lower sternal border. Her liver edge is down 3 to 4 cm, and her cardiac silhouette is enlarged on chest radiography. The most likely diagnosis is:
  a. Anomalous left coronary artery
  b. Myocarditis
  c. Myocardial infarction
  d. Supraventricular tachycardia
  e. Ventricular septal defect

Answers

1.d. Cyanosis presenting in the neonatal period has a broad differential diagnosis, including sepsis, metabolic causes such as adrenogenital syndrome and hypoglycemia, CNS depression, respiratory distress syndrome, and meconium aspiration pneumonia. In this patient who was previously acyanotic and is otherwise not in distress, congenital heart disease with ductal-dependent flow is most likely. Therefore, while keeping infection in the differential diagnosis, it is most appropriate to perform tests that will confirm the diagnosis of heart disease and help distinguish the specific lesion. The ECG may indicate which side of the heart is affected by demonstrating right or left axis deviation and ventricular hypertrophy. Chest radiographs are particularly useful to show increased or decreased pulmonary blood flow and often cardiac silhouettes suggestive of specific diagnoses, such as the "coeur en sabot" or "wooden shoe" heart of tetralogy of Fallot. ABG is used to clarify the acid-base status and confirm normal ventilatory function. The 100% oxygen challenge or hyperoxia test is the easiest way of distinguishing cyanotic heart disease from pulmonary disease. When administered 100% oxygen, those neonates with cyanotic lesions will generally not raise their PaO_2 above 150 mm Hg. *(Emergency Medicine, Chapter 27, pp 229–237)*

2.d. If the patient has failed the hyperoxia test and echocardiography is not immediately available, a prostaglandin infusion should be started to help maintain flow through the patent ductus arteriosus. A practitioner skilled at neonatal intubation should be available because the drug is associated with a greater than 10% risk of apnea. Vasoactive drugs and diuretics are not indicated in the absence of any evidence of failure or volume overload. *(Emergency Medicine, Chapter 27, pp 229–237)*

3.a. Tetralogy of Fallot classically consists of (1) right ventricular outflow tract/pulmonic obstruction; (2) ventricular septal defect; (3) dextroposition of the aorta with septal override; and (4) right ventricular hypertrophy. *(Emergency Medicine, Chapter 27, pp 229–237)*

4.c. Tachycardia in the neonate must be determined to be of sinus, other supraventricular, or ventricular origin. Because the normal heart rate of a newborn may easily reach 180 beats/min with mild exertion and 220 to 230 beats/min with crying, differentiation may be difficult. A rate greater than 230 beats/min with a regular R-R interval and an abnormal P-wave axis suggests SVT. Atrial flutter is characterized by an atrial rate of 250 to 400 and saw-toothed flutter waves but may have a ventricular response rate of 100 to 320 beats/min if there is variable conduction. Ventricular tachycardia with a rate of 120 to 240 is much less common in infants. Although significant sinus tachycardia caused by hypovolemia is best treated with IV fluids, a patient presumed to have SVT but who is otherwise stable may respond to vagal stimulation with an ice bag held on the face. If that fails, adenosine is the preferred therapy at a dose of 0.1 mg/kg, which may be increased to 0.2 mg/kg/dose (no more than 12 mg). The patient should have continuous ECG monitoring throughout the procedure. Digoxin may be used subsequently as maintenance therapy because it slows conduction within the AV node. Verapamil should *not* be used in infants because it may produce profound hypotension and cardiac arrest. *(Emergency Medicine, Chapter 27, pp 229–237)*

5.a. If a patient with SVT fails conservative therapies (vagal maneuvers, adenosine) or presents after the onset of CHF, synchronized DC cardioversion is recommended at an initial dose of 0.5 to 1.0 J/kg. *(Emergency Medicine, Chapter 27, pp 229–237)*

6.d. The degree of cyanosis experienced by patients with tetralogy of Fallot is related to the amount of RV obstruction and flow across the ventricular septal defect. The already compromised pulmonary blood flow is further reduced by pulmonary artery constriction in the setting of vigorous crying and hyperventilation, and blood is further shunted across the ventricular septal defect, resulting in worsening cyanosis progressing to severe hypoxia and metabolic acidosis. Infants who have only mild cyanosis at rest are at greater risk, not having developed mechanisms such as polycythemia to tolerate the decrease in oxygen saturation. Initial measures include maneuvers such as placing the infant on the abdomen in the knee-to-chest position, thereby raising the systemic vascular resistance and decreasing the right-to-left shunt. The administration of supplemental oxygen and a dose of morphine to depress the respiratory center slows the "thoracic pump," resulting in decreased systemic venous return, less blood arriving at the RV, and less shunting across the ventricular septal defect. *(Emergency Medicine, Chapter 27, pp 229–237)*

7.e. Kawasaki's disease or mucocutaneous lymph node syndrome is the leading cause of acquired heart disease in U.S. children. The etiology is uncertain. Bacterial toxins may be involved in the pathogenesis. Diagnosis is made on the following criteria: fever for at least 5 days, illness not explained by other disease process, and the presence of four of the following five conditions:
  1. Bilateral nonpurulent conjunctival injection
  2. Changes of the oropharyngeal mucosa, including infected pharynx; infected and/or dry, fissured lips; strawberry tongue

3. Changes of the peripheral extremities, such as edema and/or erythema of the hands or feet, desquamation
4. Rash, primarily truncal, polymorphous but nonvesicular
5. Cervical lymphadenopathy

Cardiac involvement is the most important manifestation of the disease. Ten percent to 40% of untreated children have evidence of coronary vasculitis within the first few weeks as evidenced by dilatation or aneurysm on 2-D echocardiography. *(Emergency Medicine, Chapter 27, pp 229–237)*

8.e. One of a number of shunt procedures used to alleviate the effects of RV outflow tract obstruction, the classic Blalock-Taussig shunt is a direct anastomosis of the subclavian artery to a branch pulmonary artery. It has largely been replaced by the modified Blalock-Taussig shunt, in which a Gore-Tex conduit is anastomosed between the subclavian and branch pulmonary arteries. Other shunt procedures include the descending aorta to left pulmonary artery (Potts shunt), the superior vena cava to the right pulmonary artery (Glenn anastomosis), and the right atrium to left pulmonary artery (Fontan procedure). *(Emergency Medicine, Chapter 27, pp 229–237)*

9.b. Children with Down's syndrome have a 50% chance of congenital heart disease. The most common defect is either a ventricular septal defect or an endocardial cushion defect, also known as atrio-ventricular septal defects—a group of contiguous atrial and ventricular septal defects with markedly abnormal AV valves. The most severe form is represented by a single AV valve or AV canal. *(Emergency Medicine, Chapter 27, pp 229–237)*

10.e. Although myocarditis remains in the differential diagnosis of this patient's disease, a lack of viral or infectious symptoms make it less likely. Ventricular septal defects account for approximately 25% of congenital heart disease. Although the left-to-right shunt through a ventricular septal defect may be small in the neonatal period, this flow increases with the normal fall in pulmonary vascular resistance during the first few weeks of life. This patient, with signs and symptoms of congestive failure in early infancy, likely has a large shunt with excessive pulmonary flow and pulmonary hypertension. *(Emergency Medicine, Chapter 27, pp 229–237)*

BIBLIOGRAPHY

Greene A: Pediatric cardiac disease. *In* Howell JM, Altieri M, Jagoda AS, et al (eds): Emergency Medicine. Philadelphia, WB Saunders, 1998, pp 229–237.

SECTION THREE

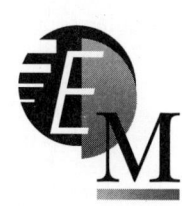

Pulmonary Disorders

11 Pulmonary Embolism and Chronic Obstructive Pulmonary Disease

LEWIS NELSON, MD

Pulmonary Embolism

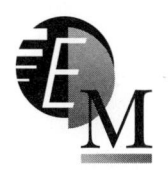

1. Patients who present with each of the following are at increased risk for pulmonary embolism except for those:
   a. With recent trans-Atlantic airplane travel
   b. With malignancies
   c. With a recent extremity injury
   d. Using NSAIDs
   e. With protein S deficiency

2. Patients with the following complaints should heighten the provider's clinical suspicion for pulmonary embolism except for those with:
   a. Angina-like chest pain
   b. Atypical chest pain
   c. Headache
   d. Hemoptysis
   e. Anxiety-doom sensation

3. Which of the following is true about pulmonary embolism?
   a. The incidence of pulmonary embolism is overestimated because of referral bias.
   b. Pulmonary embolism is easily ruled out by clinical criteria alone.
   c. Almost all patients present with hypotension and tachycardia.
   d. Pulmonary embolism may be asymptomatic in as many as 40% of patients with deep venous thrombosis.
   e. Risk factors are present in nearly all patients with pulmonary embolism.

4. The relationship between deep venous thrombosis and pulmonary embolism is described by all of the following statements except:
   a. The risk factors are similar.
   b. About 90% of all pulmonary embolisms originate in the lower extremities.
   c. A history suggestive of pulmonary embolism contraindicates palpation of the lower extremities.
   d. The therapies are similar.
   e. Femoral vein thrombosis is more likely to result in pulmonary embolism than calf vein thrombosis.

5. Assessment of oxygenation is an important part of the evaluation of patients with suspected pulmonary embolism. Which of the following statements is correct?
   a. Only room air ABGs should be performed.
   b. A normal A–a gradient eliminates pulmonary embolism as a diagnosis.
   c. Acute respiratory acidosis is the most typical finding.
   d. Pulse oximeters are not generally useful in the evaluation of pulmonary embolism.
   e. An abnormal blood gas is considered a substitute for a chest radiograph.

6. Which of the following is not a reason for patients with suspected pulmonary embolism to have chest radiography?
   a. A normal radiograph rules out pulmonary embolism
   b. Other diseases mimic pulmonary embolism
   c. Westermark's sign may be noted
   d. For baseline assessment
   e. To allow interpretation of the $\dot{V}/\dot{Q}$ nuclear scan

7. Which of the following is not true about $\dot{V}/\dot{Q}$ scanning?
   a. $\dot{V}/\dot{Q}$ scans utilize radioactive isotopes to assess regional blood and air flow.
   b. Because a normal perfusion scan effectively rules out pulmonary embolism, this part is usually done first.
   c. Most $\dot{V}/\dot{Q}$ scan results are reported in ranges (i.e., low probability or high probability) based on the degree of overlap of ventilation and perfusion defects.
   d. To be definitively abnormal, a defect must have normal ventilation and no perfusion.
   e. Every patient with suspected pulmonary embolism needs a $\dot{V}/\dot{Q}$ scan.

8. The clinical significance of the $\dot{V}/\dot{Q}$ scan was specifically evaluated by PIOPED study. Which finding was not true according to this study?
   a. A negative scan effectively rules out pulmonary embolism.
   b. A low-probability scan is associated with a 16% incidence of angiographically demonstrated pulmonary embolism.

c. Interpretation of V̇/Q̇ scans is easily performed by emergency physicians.
d. The clinical implications of low and intermediate probability are similar (i.e., need to investigate further).
e. A high-probability scan is highly predictive (88% predictive) of pulmonary embolism.

9. During the clinical diagnosis of pulmonary embolism, all of the following are true except:
   a. The pretest probability heavily influences the utility of the V̇/Q̇ scan.
   b. Clear criteria for determining high from low probability patients do not exist.
   c. Most patients have normal or nonspecific ECG changes (e.g., sinus tachycardia).
   d. Tests of clot lysis, such as D-dimers, are unlikely to ever prove useful in the diagnosis of pulmonary embolism.
   e. Objective testing for deep vein thrombosis is indicated for patients with low- or intermediate-probability V̇/Q̇ scans.

10. Pulmonary angiography is considered the gold standard for the diagnosis of pulmonary embolism. Which is not true?
    a. Up to 5% of patients die during angiography.
    b. Even though it is the gold standard, disagreements over interpretation occur frequently.
    c. Pulmonary angiography is contraindicated in patients with negative V̇/Q̇ scans.
    d. Renal insufficiency is a relative contraindication because contrast is used.
    e. Most patients with high-probability V̇/Q̇ scans do not need an angiogram.

11. Which is not an acceptable therapeutic modality for patients with pulmonary embolism?
    a. Heparin 10,000 U bolus, with infusion to follow
    b. Vena cava filter
    c. Ultrasonic clot disruption
    d. Surgery
    e. Thrombolysis

12. Which piece of demographic information is incorrect about pulmonary embolism?
    a. It may account for 50,000 deaths annually in the United States.
    b. There are about 600,000 cases annually in the United States.
    c. The incidence is highest in women younger than 50 years.
    d. It is likely overdiagnosed.
    e. It is likely underdiagnosed.

13. Which can contribute to the increased A–a gradient seen in pulmonary embolism?
    a. V̇/Q̇ mismatch
    b. Intrapulmonary shunting
    c. Intracardiac shunting
    d. Hypoventilation
    e. All of the above

14. Which of the following substances is not associated with pulmonary embolism?
    a. Amniotic fluid
    b. Cartilage
    c. Air
    d. Bullets
    e. Fat

15. All of the following are typically associated with death from pulmonary embolism except:
    a. Mechanical obstruction of RV outflow
    b. Profound pulmonary vasoconstriction
    c. Hemorrhage
    d. Bronchospasm
    e. Exacerbation of underlying disease

Answers

1.d. Virchow's triad relates the risk factors for deep vein thrombosis as well as pulmonary embolism. Stasis (e.g., immobilization), intimal damage (e.g., trauma), and hypercoagulability (e.g., malignancy or protein S/C deficiency) make up the triad. The NSAIDs are not associated with pulmonary embolism. *(Emergency Medicine, Chapter 28, pp 239–251)*

2.c. Noncardiac chest pain is what is typically expected, although angina may be precipitated by the hypoxemia. Both hemoptysis and dry cough may be seen. Headache alone is not a typical complaint and should be accompanied by other, more suspicious suggestions. *(Emergency Medicine, Chapter 28, pp 239–251)*

3.d. Pulmonary embolism may be one of the most underdiagnosed disease entities. Twenty percent of patients with pleuritic chest pain may have pulmonary embolism.[1] Because there are no clinical criteria that adequately include or exclude pulmonary embolism, the diagnostic evaluation usually includes an objective test. Most patients appear asymptomatic or minimally symptomatic. Pulmonary embolism has been shown to be asymptomatic in 40% of patients with deep vein thrombosis.[2] Up to 40% of patients with the diagnosis of pulmonary embolism do not have identifiable risk factors.[3] *(Emergency Medicine, Chapter 28, pp 239–251)*

4.c. Although most pulmonary embolisms originate in the legs, they are often not noted on examination. Evaluation of the legs, however, is still useful because signs of deep vein thrombosis direct the next diagnostic test and are an indication for treatment with heparin. Clot dislodgment should not occur with gentle examination. Although clots in the calf veins alone rarely embolize, extension into the proximal venous system can occur; therefore, many clinicians choose to treat these patients with anticoagulants. *(Emergency Medicine, Chapter 28, pp 239–251)*

5.d. It is potentially dangerous to remove therapeutic oxygen to get a "baseline" room air blood gas. Calculation of the gradient can be corrected, or estimated, for patients on supplemental oxygen. Although a normal A–a gradient is comforting, it does not obviate the need for further diagnostic studies if the clinical suspicion remains high.[4] Although some patients with a pulmonary embolism will have a normal ABG, most will have hypoxia caused by $\dot{V}/\dot{Q}$ mismatching and respiratory alkalosis caused by hyperventilation. Respiratory acidosis is a late, and concerning, finding. Pulse oximeters simply record the patient's oxygen saturation and do not take into account how hard the patient is breathing to attain that saturation. Thus, both patients breathing comfortably at a rate of 14 breaths/min and those breathing deeply at 40 breaths/min may have an oxygen saturation of 96% to 100%. What differs in these patients is the work of breathing; the A–a gradient better accounts for this because the P_{CO_2} is largely proportional to ventilation. A chest radiograph is needed to assess for other causes of blood gas abnormalities.[5] *(Emergency Medicine, Chapter 28, pp 239–251)*

6.a. Most patients with pulmonary embolism have abnormal radiographic findings, at least retrospectively or if interpreted with knowledge that the patient has a pulmonary embolism. Most of these findings are nonspecific, however, although occasionally a few useful ones, such as Westermark's sign (focal oligemia), are found. Many experts argue that a "normal" or "nonspecific" radiograph may actually raise your suspicion for pulmonary embolism, because the other causes of similar symptoms (e.g., pneumonia or pneumothorax) are largely excluded. The other choices are generally considered adequate reasons for chest radiography.[5] *(Emergency Medicine, Chapter 28, pp 239–251)*

7.e. Although $\dot{V}/\dot{Q}$ scans are nuclear medicine scans using radioisotopes, patients are at little to no risk from the procedure. If the blood flow throughout the lung is normal, there cannot be an embolus, so the study is considered normal (a negative scan). Based on the PIOPED data, results are reported in nonequal ranges (i.e., not quartiles) and are meant to be combined with clinical criteria/judgment. The difficulty in the interpretation of $\dot{V}/\dot{Q}$ scans is defining overlap of defects. Ventilated areas lacking perfusion are typically called abnormal, but with time, nonperfused segments may become atelectatic, clouding the utility of this finding. Unstable patients, those with positive angiograms, and those with high clinical probability of deep vein thrombosis should not undergo $\dot{V}/\dot{Q}$ scanning.[6, 7] *(Emergency Medicine, Chapter 28, pp 239–251)*

8.c. The PIOPED study found that answers a, b, d, and e were true. Unfortunately, the ability of emergency physicians to interpret $\dot{V}/\dot{Q}$ scans is likely to be limited because even seasoned nuclear medicine radiologists could not agree on almost one third of the studies in PIOPED. Some have called for simplification of the interpretation scheme by combining low and intermediate probability scans because such patients generally require further evaluation.[4] *(Emergency Medicine, Chapter 28, pp 239–251)*

9.d. In the PIOPED study, the pretest probability significantly altered the clinical applicability of the $\dot{V}/\dot{Q}$ scan. For example, a low-probability scan in a patient with low clinical suspicion carries only a 4% chance for angiographically demonstrable pulmonary embolism, whereas a patient with a high clinical suspicion has a 40% likelihood of a positive study despite the low-probability $\dot{V}/\dot{Q}$ scan. D-dimer assay appears to be sensitive and may eventually be helpful in the evaluation of clot dissolution. The major limitation is currently technological. Patients with non–high-probability abnormal $\dot{V}/\dot{Q}$ scans should have an evaluation of the lower extremity vascular system, because this is the major source of emboli.[7, 8] *(Emergency Medicine, Chapter 28, pp 239–251)*

10.a. Although renal failure, allergy, and hemorrhage are occasionally noted, the mortality directly related to pulmonary angiography is less than 0.5%. As with most objective studies, interpretation is an art and disagreement is not uncommon (5% to 15%). Patients with high-probability scans in whom heparin is contraindicated, surgery is anticipated, or the diagnosis is in question need to have angiographic confirmation. *(Emergency Medicine, Chapter 28, pp 239–251)*

11.c. Attempting to disrupt the clot with sound waves would likely shower emboli. The other modalities are accepted. High-dose heparin is generally necessary for adequate anticoagulation. Surgery is reserved for patients in extremis. Tissue plasminogen activator is currently the thrombolytic drug of choice.[9] *(Emergency Medicine, Chapter 28, pp 239–251)*

12.c. Although men younger than 50 years are more likely to be diagnosed with pulmonary embolism than women of the same age, pulmonary embolism is seen most frequently in elderly patients, with a peak incidence in the seventh decade. However, pulmonary embolisms can occur in all age groups. It is considered overdiagnosed (by a high clinical exclusion rate) and underdiagnosed (by autopsy studies).[10–12] *(Emergency Medicine, Chapter 28, pp 239–251)*

13.e. All may contribute to the A–a gradient. $\dot{V}/\dot{Q}$ mismatching and intrapulmonary shunting probably produce most of the changes. Hypoventilation is a late finding in patients with severe pulmonary embolism. Up to 35% of the population may have a patent foramen ovale that causes intracardiac shunting and can contribute to the observed A–a gradient.[5] *(Emergency Medicine, Chapter 28, pp 239–251)*

14.b. Amniotic fluid embolus is a complication of the peripartum period. Although marrow fat may embolize after trauma, cartilage is not associated with embolization. Air embolus involves the entry of large volumes of air into the venous circulation and is often associated with underwater diving. Foreign bodies, such as bullets or bullet fragments, may enter the venous circulation, and if the vessel lumen is sufficiently wide, the object may embolize to the lungs. *(Emergency Medicine, Chapter 28, pp 239–251)*

15.c. Although the majority of deaths in patients with pulmonary embolism are caused by mechanical outflow obstruction (i.e., RV failure), pulmonary embolism is not purely a mechanical problem. Platelet-induced pulmonary vasoconstriction and bronchospasm may contribute. Hypoxemia may contribute to death, particularly in patients with underlying disease processes (e.g., coronary artery disease). Hemorrhage is generally not a factor. *(Emergency Medicine, Chapter 28, pp 239–251)*

Chronic Obstructive Pulmonary Disease

1. Which is not an indication for tracheal intubation in patients with exacerbations of COPD?
   a. The finding of a "silent chest" on physical examination
   b. The inability of the patient to speak one or two simple words
   c. An elevated P_{CO_2} with a normal pH
   d. A depressed level of consciousness
   e. Progression of symptoms despite appropriate therapy

2. Clinical evaluation of patients with acute decompensation of their COPD is likely to reveal all of the following except:
   a. Symptoms of a viral infection
   b. Noncompliance with medications
   c. Anemia
   d. Cyanosis
   e. Rhonchi or wheezes

3. Which of the following about diagnostic studies in COPD patients is true?
   a. Chest radiographs are essentially always normal.
   b. ABG assessment is necessary in all patients with COPD-related ED visits.
   c. Sputum cultures usually reveal a single infecting organism.
   d. A single FEV_1 or peak flow measurement may not accurately reflect the patient's clinical status.
   e. Elevated leukocyte counts are highly suggestive of pneumonia.

4. Which of the following statements is true regarding therapy for patients with COPD?
   a. Albuterol and epinephrine share a similar adverse effects profile.
   b. Epinephrine is contraindicated in adults.
   c. There is no role for metered-dose inhalers in the ED.
   d. BiPAP may be beneficial.
   e. The therapeutic effect of theophylline is achieved through inhibition of phosphodiesterase.

5. Which of the following should not be used in the ED management of patients with COPD?
   a. Prednisone, 40 mg PO, empirically
   b. Magnesium, 1 g IV, in patients without renal dysfunction
   c. Empiric antimicrobials if the patient is febrile
   d. Respiratory stimulants, such as doxapram, if respiratory effort is poor
   e. IV fluid, for patients without signs of dehydration

6. Which physical finding is not commonly noted in patients with COPD?
   a. Barrel chest
   b. Spider angiomata
   c. Clubbing
   d. Pulsus paradoxus
   e. Pursed-lip breathing

7. Which of the following is not a typical complication of COPD?
   a. Pneumonia
   b. Pneumothorax
   c. Heart failure
   d. Accelerated atherogenesis
   e. Hyperviscosity syndromes

8. All of the following are etiologies for COPD except:
   a. Cigarette smoking
   b. Cystic fibrosis
   c. Fibrotic lung disease
   d. Alpha$_1$-protease (antitrypsin) deficiency
   e. Asthma

9. Which of the following is not an expected occurrence during the management of patients with COPD?
   a. Hypoxemia
   b. Respiratory acidosis
   c. Barotrauma
   d. Seizures
   e. Mucus plugging

10. Which pathophysiologic mechanism best explains the acute respiratory acidosis noted after supplemental oxygen therapy in some patients with COPD?
    a. $\dot{V}/\dot{Q}$ mismatch
    b. Pneumothorax
    c. Cor pulmonale
    d. Loss of hypoxic drive
    e. Bronchospasm

Answers

1.c. Because many patients with COPD have a well-compensated chronic respiratory acidosis, an elevated P_{CO_2} noted on an ABG may not be indicative of respiratory failure. Clinical findings are generally a better indicator of the severity of the acute disease exacerbation. A silent chest suggests that the patient is unable to provide adequate air exchange to generate audible wheezes. Similarly, patients with severe airflow limitation may be unable to speak as a result of the inability to force air past the vocal cords. Altered mental status implies symptomatic hypercapnia or hypoxemia, the latter of which may present as agitation. *(Emergency Medicine, Chapter 30, pp 264–273)*

2.c. Because of chronic hypoxemia, many patients with COPD compensate by increasing their RBC mass. Thus, the finding of anemia would be unexpected. Viral infections often trigger pulmonary decompensation. As with many chronic disease states, noncompliance with medical regimens is a common cause of exacerbation. Cyanosis and adventitious pulmonary sounds are common findings in patients with chronic and decompensated COPD. *(Emergency Medicine, Chapter 30, pp 264–273)*

3.d. Pulmonary function testing, either with peak flow or FEV_1, is generally best used to follow the patient's response to therapy. These tests are useful for the initial assessment of the severity of an exacerbation only for patients in whom the baseline test values are known. Chest radiographs are abnormal in at least 15% of patients with COPD. Patients who improve rapidly with initial therapy should not undergo a painful arterial puncture because it is unlikely to provide beneficial information. Cultures are often contaminated by colonizing organisms; for this reason, Gram's stains of an adequate sputum sample may be more useful. Elevated WBC counts are often related to the use of beta-adrenergic agonists and steroids (demargination).[13] *(Emergency Medicine, Chapter 30, pp 264–273)*

4.d. BiPAP and CPAP are noninvasive respiratory assist devices to reduce the work of breathing experienced by patients with decompensated COPD. Epinephrine produces significantly more adverse effects than albuterol, particularly in older or infirm patients. Despite this, epinephrine is usually safe in children and may be useful in adults. Many EDs successfully use spacer-adapted metered-dose inhalers in place of nebulized drugs. Theophylline has demonstrated little benefit in the early management of COPD, although it may be beneficial with chronic use. It derives its therapeutic effect through the antagonism of adenosine receptors.[14] *(Emergency Medicine, Chapter 30, pp 264–273)*

5.d. Respiratory stimulants, such as doxapram or caffeine, are not beneficial and may produce significant toxicity. Steroids reduce the delayed, inflammatory component of COPD. Magnesium may function as a calcium channel inhibitor to provide bronchodilation. Antimicrobials, although not generally useful, may be indicated in patients with pneumonia or unexplained fever. Saline hydration, if done gently, may replace insensible losses and help loosen viscous sputum. *(Emergency Medicine, Chapter 30, pp 264–273)*

6.b. Spider angiomata are vascular malformations noted predominantly in patients with liver disease. The other findings are classic findings in patients with COPD. The need to accommodate increased lung volume leads to a barrel chest appearance. Clubbing of the fingertips is caused by chronic hypoxic changes in the distal extremities. Pulsus paradoxus may be seen in patients with increased intrathoracic pressure. Pursed-lip breathing increases the intrathoracic pressure to maintain smaller airway patency. *(Emergency Medicine, Chapter 30, pp 264–273)*

7.d. Pneumonia is a complication of bronchitis and altered ciliary clearance. Pneumothorax may result from altered ventilatory mechanics and air trapping. Cor pulmonale is right-sided ventricular failure caused by altered pulmonary vascular resistance. Profound elevations in RBC mass (polycythemia) caused by chronic hypoxemia may produce sludging of the blood through critical organs such as the brain (hyperviscosity syndrome). Although patients with COPD may suffer atherosclerotic disease at a rate exceeding the general population, COPD and atherosclerosis do not appear to be causally related, although they share an association with cigarette smoking. *(Emergency Medicine, Chapter 30, pp 264–273)*

8.e. There is no evidence that patients with asthma are at risk for COPD. Asthma, by definition, is reversible airway disease. All of the other choices are associated with COPD, although cigarette smoking is unquestionably the most prevalent (and preventable) cause. *(Emergency Medicine, Chapter 30, pp 264–273)*

9.d. Although most patients with $\dot{V}/\dot{Q}$ mismatches generally improve with the addition of oxygen, some patients with severe underlying COPD may decompensate in response and develop paradoxical hypoxemia. For this reason, after the addition of supplemental oxygen, repeat clinical examination or ABG analysis is mandated. "Stacking of breaths," with resultant barotrauma, may result if the patient's lungs are not allowed to fully deflate before administration of the next positive pressure (mechanically provided) breath.

Mucus plugging of the airways leads to entrance of large volumes of air, and thus pressure, into the remaining open lung segments. Hypoventilation may produce hypercapnia and respiratory acidosis. ***(Emergency Medicine, Chapter 30, pp 264–273)***

10.a. Until recently it was assumed that the acute respiratory failure occasionally seen (but always discussed) after oxygen therapy was caused by the loss of the hypoxic stimulus to breathe. These patients were believed to have a reduced sensitivity of cerebral chemoreceptors to CO_2 because of chronic hypercapnia. Thus, their stimulus to breathe was assumed not to be increasing P_{CO_2}, as in the normal patient, but rather falling P_{O_2}. It is now believed that hypoxia occurs due to $\dot{V}/\dot{Q}$ mismatching. Supplemental oxygen causes poorly perfused, diseased lung segments to become minimally oxygenated. As blood flow increases to these segments, $\dot{V}/\dot{Q}$ mismatch actually increases. The other conditions may produce respiratory failure, but they are not related to oxygen administration. ***(Emergency Medicine, Chapter 30, pp 264–273)***

REFERENCES

1. Hull RD, Raskob GE, Carter CJ, et al. Pulmonary embolism in outpatients with pleuritic chest pain. Arch Intern Med 1988; 148:838–844.
2. Moser KM, Fedullo PF, Littlejohn JK, et al. Frequent asymptomatic pulmonary embolism in patients with deep venous thrombosis. JAMA 1994; 271:223–225.
3. Giuntini C, Giorgio DR, Martini C, et al: Epidemiology. Chest 1995; 107:3S–9S.
4. PIOPED Investigators: Value of the ventilation/perfusion scan in acute pulmonary embolism: Results of the Prospective Investigation of Pulmonary Embolism Diagnosis (PIOPED). JAMA 1990; 263:2753–2759.
5. Stein PD, Terrin ML, Hales CA, et al: Clinical, laboratory, roentgenographic and electrocardiographic findings in patients with acute pulmonary embolism and no pre-existing cardiac or pulmonary disease. Chest 1991; 100:598–603.
6. Stein PD, Henry JW, Gottschalk A: Mismatched vascular defects. Chest 1993; 104:1468–1472.
7. Stein PD, Henry JW, Gottschalk A: The addition of clinical assessment to stratification according to prior cardiopulmonary disease further optimizes the interpretation of ventilation/perfusion lung scans in pulmonary embolism. Chest 1993; 104: 1472–1476.
8. Goldhaber SZ, Simons GR, Elliot G, et al: Quantitative plasma D-dimer levels among patients undergoing pulmonary angiography for suspected pulmonary embolism. JAMA 1993; 270:2819–2822).
9. Goldhaber SZ. Contemporary pulmonary embolism thrombolysis. Chest 1995; 107:45S–51S.
10. Bone RC: Ventilation/perfusion scan in pulmonary embolism: "The emperor is incompletely attired." JAMA 1990; 263:2794–2795.
11. Robin ED: Overdiagnosis and overtreatment of pulmonary embolism: The emperor may have no clothes. Ann Intern Med 1977; 87:775–781.
12. Wagenvoort CA: Pathology of pulmonary thromboembolism. Chest 1995; 107:10S–17S.
13. Emerman CL, Cydulka RK: Evaluation of high yield criteria for chronic obstructive pulmonary disease. Ann Emerg Med 1993; 22:680–684.
14. Pennock BE, Crawshaw L, Kaplan PD: Non-invasive nasal mask ventilation for acute respiratory failure: Institution of a new therapeutic technology for routine use. Chest 1994; 105:441–444.

BIBLIOGRAPHY

Olinger ML: Pulmonary embolism. *In* Howell JM, Altieri M, Jagoda AS, et al (eds): Emergency Medicine. Philadelphia, WB Saunders, 1998, pp 239–251.

Schneider SM: Chronic obstructive pulmonary disease. *In* Howell JM, Altieri M, Jagoda AS, et al (eds): Emergency Medicine. Philadelphia, WB Saunders, 1998, pp 264–273.

12 Asthma, Pneumonia, Pleurisy, Empyema, and Disorders of the Pleura and Mediastinum

LUIS RODRIGUEZ, MD

Asthma

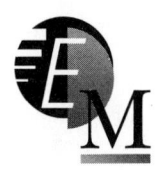

1. Warning signs of severe asthma and impending respiratory failure include all of the following except:
   a. Hypoxemia (PaO$_2$ <60)
   b. Acidosis (pH <7.25)
   c. Decreasing peak flow
   d. Altered mental status
   e. Decreasing PaCO$_2$

2. Factors that may precipitate a sudden asthma attack include all of the following except:
   a. Sinus infections
   b. Exposure to cold air
   c. Exercise
   d. Exposure to dust or pollen
   e. Overuse of inhaled steroids

3. A 23-year-old woman is brought to the ED by her husband, who reports that she has had an 8-hour history of asthma symptoms that have failed to respond to beta-agonist and steroid therapy at home. On evaluation, the patient, who is sleepy, was found to have a heart rate of 100 and RR of 16. Her O$_2$ saturation is 92% by pulse oximetry. Wheezing is noted in all lung fields, although breath sounds are diminished. She is unable to do a peak flow. An ABG is sent. Which feature of her presentation is most suggestive of impending respiratory failure?
   a. Tachypnea
   b. Hypoxia
   c. Inability to do a peak flow
   d. Sleepiness
   e. Diminished breath sounds

4. A patient with an asthma exacerbation may require ICU admission based on all of the following except:
   a. Peak expiratory flow rate below 200 L/min or 25% of baseline
   b. Heart rate greater than 100 beats/min
   c. RR greater than 30 breaths/min
   d. PaCO$_2$ greater than 40 mm Hg
   e. Pulsus paradoxus greater than 20 mm Hg

5. Asthmatic patients who require mechanical ventilation should be managed with all of the following except:
   a. Sedation
   b. Paralyzing agents
   c. Ventilator tidal volume of 8 to 10 mL/kg
   d. RRs of 20 to 25 breaths/min
   e. FIO$_2$ set to maintain oxygen saturation above 92%

6. Objective measures frequently used in the ED to assess the response of a patient with asthma to therapy include all of the following except:
   a. Pulsus paradoxus
   b. Oxygen saturation measurements
   c. Chest radiograph
   d. FEV$_1$ or peak expiratory flow rate
   e. Clinical acumen

7. Medications used in the emergency management of asthma include all of the following except:
   a. Theophylline
   b. Corticosteroids
   c. Oxygen
   d. Albuterol sulfate
   e. Anticholinergics

8. Physiologic changes that occur during an asthma attack include all of the following except:
   a. Hypercapnia
   b. Respiratory acidosis
   c. Metabolic acidosis
   d. Respiratory muscle fatigue
   e. Decreased airway pressure

9. Extrinsic asthma is characterized by:
   a. Perennial symptoms
   b. Development later in life
   c. Elevated IgE levels and eosinophilia
   d. No family history of atopy
   e. Poor response to bronchodilator therapy

10. The differential diagnosis of new-onset pediatric asthma should include all of the following except:
    a. Bronchopulmonary dysplasia
    b. Foreign body aspiration
    c. Bronchiolitis

d. CHF
e. Bacterial tracheitis

Answers

1.e. The airway obstruction caused by asthma results in V̇/Q̇ mismatching. The normal physiologic response to the resulting hypoxia is hyperventilation, which initially results in hypocapnia. Patients with severe asthma, who are at risk of impending respiratory failure, are unable to maintain adequate ventilation as a result of progressive respiratory muscle fatigue and will demonstrate a normal or increased $PaCO_2$ on arterial blood gas. (*Emergency Medicine, Chapter 29, pp 252–263*)

2.e. Sinus infections, upper respiratory infections, or exposure to cold air, dust, or pollen may contribute to or directly precipitate an attack of asthma. Although overuse of inhaled steroids and inhaled beta-agonists has been associated with increased morbidity and mortality of patients suffering an exacerbation of asthma, their overuse per se is not causally related to precipitating an attack. There is limited benefit in the isolated use of inhaled steroids immediately following an acute exposure or the isolated use of inhaled beta-agonists during prolonged attacks, during which there is likely to be significant airway inflammation. A direct relationship between the duration and severity of an attack has never been demonstrated. Patients may suddenly become apneic and suffer cardiopulmonary arrest within hours of onset of an attack or may become progressively obstructed and die after an attack that has lasted days. Because the only physician seen on a regular basis for many of these patients is the emergency physician, it is the responsibility of the emergency physician to educate them concerning the appropriate use of their medications and when to seek medical care. (*Emergency Medicine, Chapter 29, pp 252–263*)

3.d. Signs of impending respiratory failure includes hypoxemia (PaO_2 <60), acidosis (pH <7.25), decreasing pulsus paradoxus and peak flows (<25% predicted), hemodynamic instability, subjective exhaustion, and altered mental status. The elective decision to intubate and mechanically ventilate an asthmatic patient should be made based on these clinical parameters, in conjunction with ABG data, before overt respiratory arrest occurs. (*Emergency Medicine, Chapter 29, pp 252–263*)

4.b. In addition to those asthmatic patients already intubated and on mechanical ventilation, indications for admission to an ICU include signs of impending respiratory failure (as indicated by pulsus paradoxus greater than 20 mm Hg), peak flows less than 200 L/min or 25% of baseline, heart rates greater than 120 beats/min, RR greater than 30 breaths/min, or a $PaCO_2$ of 40 mm Hg or higher. (*Emergency Medicine, Chapter 29, pp 252–263*)

5.d. After intubation, the goal of mechanical ventilation is to provide adequate ventilation at safe respiratory rates and pressures, to avoid both barotrauma and air trapping. Overzealous mechanical ventilation can result in pneumothorax formation and compromised venous return. The intubated patient should be kept sedated and paralyzed to minimize the risk of accidental extubation and prevent bucking the respirator. Appropriate ventilator settings include a tidal volume between 8 and 10 mL/kg, a respiratory rate between 10 and 16 breaths/min, an inspiratory flow rate of 60 L/min, and an FIO_2 set to maintain oxygen saturations greater than 92%. At times it is not possible to fully correct a patient's hypercapnia by extrinsic ventilation without risking airway damage or shock. Under these circumstances, controlled hypoventilation, resulting in permissive hypercapnia, is appropriate. This can be achieved by decreasing the respiratory rate to allow adequate time for expiration and maintaining static lung pressures less than 30 cm H_2O and intrinsic PEEP less than 5 cm H_2O. (*Emergency Medicine, Chapter 29, pp 252–263*)

6.c. Chest radiographs are not indicated in the majority of asthmatic patients. Indications to obtain a radiograph include signs and symptoms of infection, pneumothorax or pneumomediastinum, failure to clear with treatment, and a first episode of wheezing. (*Emergency Medicine, Chapter 29, pp 252–263*)

7.a. The National Asthma Education Program currently recommends against the use of theophylline in the ED. For patients already receiving a beta-agonist, many studies have demonstrated that there is no additional benefit in using theophylline, a weak bronchodilator, which has the potential for serious side effects. (*Emergency Medicine, Chapter 29, pp 252–263*)

8.e. Although bronchial smooth muscle contraction is rapidly reversible, the inflammatory changes seen in asthma take days to weeks to resolve. Reversible changes result in increased airway resistance and work of breathing, decreased expiratory flow rates, V̇/Q̇ mismatch, and air trapping. Clinically, these physiologic changes result in respiratory muscle fatigue and subsequent metabolic acidosis; hypoventilation with resultant hypercarbia and respiratory acidosis; hypoxemia; and the complications of air trapping resulting in increased airway pressures, hypotension, and pneumothorax. (*Emergency Medicine, Chapter 29, pp 252–263*)

9.c. Approximately 10% of all asthmatic patients have extrinsic asthma, which is characterized by sensitivity to inhaled allergens, onset during childhood, seasonal occurrence, elevated IgE levels and eosinophilia, a family history of atopy, and a good response to bronchodilators. (*Emergency Medicine, Chapter 29, pp 252–263*)

10.e. Bacterial tracheitis is a medical emergency that, like epiglottitis, may suddenly result in complete airway obstruction and death. Although the initial pattern of respiratory distress seen with tracheitis closely resembles that of laryngotracheobronchitis, the degree of fever and the toxic appearance of the patient should alert the clinician to a high probability of a bacterial disease.[1] The old adage "all that wheezes is not asthma" should be remembered for all children who present with wheezing, especially the child with no previous history of asthma. Bronchiolitis, bronchopulmonary dysplasia, foreign body aspiration, and CHF all can present with tachypnea, tachycardia, wheezing, and retractions and should always be considered in the differential diagnosis. *(Emergency Medicine, Chapter 29, pp 252–263)*

Pneumonia, Pleurisy, and Empyema

1. The pathogens commonly associated with typical bacterial pneumonia include all of the following except:
   a. *Streptococcus pneumoniae*
   b. *Mycoplasma pneumoniae*
   c. *Haemophilus influenzae*
   d. *Staphylococcus aureus*
   e. *Moraxella catarrhalis*

2. Typical bacterial community-acquired pneumonia is characterized by all of the following except:
   a. Cough
   b. Fever
   c. Possible onset after a mild viral illness
   d. Insidious onset
   e. Sputum production

3. Extrapulmonary manifestations of mycoplasma infection include all of the following except:
   a. Maculopapular rash
   b. Conjunctivitis
   c. Guillain-Barré syndrome
   d. Hepatitis
   e. Thrombocytosis

4. The hallmark of *Legionella* pneumonia is:
   a. Diarrhea and vomiting with or without abdominal pain
   b. Confusion and lethargy
   c. Fever that increases daily
   d. Relative bradycardia
   e. Onset of mildly productive cough, occasionally with bloody sputum

5. All of the following are true of polyvalent pneumococcal vaccines except:
   a. Full protection is achieved in 45% to 90% of immunocompetent recipients.
   b. It is highly effective in children younger than 2 years of age.
   c. Patients can be revaccinated after 6 years.
   d. It is fully effective 3 weeks after administration.
   e. Maximum immunity occurs 3 years after administration and wanes thereafter.

6. Mortality associated with *Legionella* pneumonia increases with all of the following except:
   a. Hyponatremia
   b. Hypoxemia
   c. Sputum that is positive for *Legionella* by direct fluorescent antibody staining
   d. Respiratory failure
   e. Multilobe extension

7. All of the following organisms can cause pneumonia with cavitation except:
   a. *Mycobacterium tuberculosis*
   b. *Staphylococcus aureus*
   c. *Klebsiella pneumoniae*
   d. *Bacteroides melaninogenicus*
   e. *Coxiella burnetii*

8. The most common route of acquiring lower respiratory tract disease is:
   a. Direct inhalation of pathogenic organisms
   b. Aspiration of pathogens directly into the lung
   c. Direct penetration into the lung
   d. Dissemination from remote sites
   e. Spread from contiguous structures

9. All the following are common pathogens in pediatric pneumonia after the neonatal period except:
   a. *Haemophilus influenzae*
   b. *Streptococcus pneumoniae*
   c. *Listeria monocytogenes*
   d. Respiratory syncytial virus
   e. *Staphylococcus aureus*

10. All of the following are true regarding bronchopulmonary dysplasia except:
    a. Oxygen dependence
    b. Underlying pulmonary edema
    c. Radiographic abnormalities
    d. Airway hyperactivity
    e. Susceptibility to respiratory infections with *Pseudomonas aeruginosa*

Answers

1.b. The pathogens that are commonly associated with typical bacterial pneumonia include *Streptococcus pneumoniae, Haemophilus influenzae, Moraxella catarrhalis, Staphylococcus aureus,* enteric gram-negative bacilli (e.g., *Enterobacteriaceae* family members and *Pseudomonas* spp.), and to some extent anaerobes. *Mycoplasma pneumoniae* is among the organisms that cause atypical clinical syndromes. *(Emergency Medicine, Chapter 31, pp 274–295)*

2.d. Most patients with typical bacterial community-acquired pneumonia have cough, fever, and sputum production. The onset of the illness is generally abrupt and may follow a mild viral illness in one third to one half of patients. Pleuritic chest pain, dyspnea, and some degree of dehydration are also features of bacterial pneumonias. *(Emergency Medicine, Chapter 31, pp 274–295)*

3.e. Extrapulmonary manifestations of mycoplasma infection are common. Conjunctivitis is seen in 20% of patients and maculopapular manifestations occur in 15% to 25%. Some patients develop erythema multiforme or Stevens-Johnson syndrome (<3% of patients). Neurologic symptoms such as encephalitis, cerebral ataxia, Guillain-Barré syndrome, cranial nerve palsies, mononeuropathies, and transverse myelitis have been described. Hemolytic anemia, thrombocytopenia, hepatitis, myocarditis, and pericarditis have all been reported in less than 3% of patients. Death from *M. pneumoniae* infection is rare. *(Emergency Medicine, Chapter 31, pp 274–295)*

4.c. The hallmark of *Legionella* pneumonia is fever that increases daily. Confusion and lethargy are exhibited by 20% to 40% of patients. Diarrhea and vomiting, with or without abdominal pain, are just as common. Pulmonary symptoms occur 2 to 4 days after disease onset, manifested by a cough that is mildly productive and occasionally bloody. Relative bradycardia has been reported in as many as 40% of patients. *(Emergency Medicine, Chapter 31, pp 274–295)*

5.b. Polyvalent pneumococcal vaccine should be given to all high-risk patients. It is fully effective 3 weeks after administration, with full protection being achieved in 45% to 90% of immunocompetent recipients. Immunity is maximum for 3 years and wanes thereafter. Patients can be revaccinated after 6 years. Efficacy is reduced in children younger than 2 years of age and in patients with hypogammaglobulinemia or Hodgkin's disease and in patients who have had splenectomies or who are on chemotherapy. *(Emergency Medicine, Chapter 31, pp 274–295)*

6.a. Despite therapy, mortality from *Legionella* pneumonia remains from 10% to 20%. The likelihood of mortality increases with hypoxemia, respiratory failure, multilobe extension, degree of comorbidity, and the finding of *Legionella* on an expectorated sputum stained with direct fluorescent antibodies. Hyponatremia is seen in 30% to 50% of patients, but it is not associated with an increase in mortality. *(Emergency Medicine, Chapter 31, pp 274–295)*

7.e. Radiographic features of reactivation tuberculosis include apical lesions with cavitation, scarring, and retraction of surrounding structures. Reactivation tuberculosis often resembles primary tuberculosis on chest radiographs in patients with CD4 cell counts less than 200 mm^3. The incidence of suppurative complications is high for staphylococcal pneumonia, with both cavitation and pleural effusion, likely an empyema, commonly seen. Gram-negative bacteria have the propensity for producing necrotizing infection, cavitation, and empyema. Although the initial infection after aspiration of anaerobes is usually a simple pneumonitis or consolidation, if left untreated, empyema frequently develops. Although the typical chest radiograph seen after infection with *Coxiella burnetii* (Q fever) shows bilateral hilar infiltrates and occasionally consolidation, effusion is uncommon and cavitation is not seen. Q fever is a self-limiting illness, and it is not clear whether treatment alters its course or affects complications. *(Emergency Medicine, Chapter 31, pp 274–295)*

8.b. Aspiration of pathogens directly into the lungs is the most common route of acquiring lower respiratory tract disease. The second most common route of pneumonia acquisition is the direct inhalation of pathogenic organisms. Pneumonia also evolves from direct penetration, spread from contiguous structures, dissemination from remote sites, indwelling catheters, and colonization. *(Emergency Medicine, Chapter 31, pp 274–295)*

9.c. Pneumonia can occur at any age during childhood, from newborn to adolescence, although the peak incidence occurs between 6 months and 5 years of age. With the exception of the first 2 weeks of life, viruses are the predominant cause of pneumonia in childhood. *Streptococcus pneumoniae, Haemophilus influenzae,* and *Staphylococcus aureus* are the most common bacterial pathogens in children older than 2 weeks. *Listeria monocytogenes* is a likely pathogen in the immediate neonatal period because intrauterine infection or transmission while passing through the birth canal can occur.[2] *(Emergency Medicine, Chapter 31, pp 274–295)*

10.e. Bronchopulmonary dysphasia is a syndrome consisting of oxygen dependence, radiographic abnormalities, and chronic respiratory symptoms in infants over 28 days old. With improved survival of severely premature infants, bronchopulmonary dysplasia has become the most common form of chronic lung disease in infancy in the United States. Children with bronchopulmonary dysplasia have frequent respiratory problems because of underlying pulmonary edema, airway hyperactivity, airway inflammation, and chronic lung

Disorders of the Pleura and Mediastinum

1. The clinical presentation of a tension pneumothorax includes all of the following except:
   a. Severe dyspnea
   b. Hypotension
   c. Tachycardia
   d. Unilateral chest pain
   e. Unilateral dullness to percussion

2. Characteristics of a spontaneous pneumothorax include all of the following except:
   a. It is more common among males.
   b. Patients are usually tall, thin cigarette smokers.
   c. About 50% recur within 1 to 2 years.
   d. Initial symptoms usually occur during exercise.
   e. Tension pneumothorax is infrequently associated.

3. Absolute indications for chest tube placement include all of the following except:
   a. Tension pneumothorax
   b. Empyema
   c. Boerhaave's syndrome
   d. Traumatic pneumothorax
   e. Pneumomediastinum

4. All of the following suggest an exudative pleural effusion except:
   a. Pleural fluid protein to serum protein ratio greater than 0.5
   b. Pleural fluid lactate dehydrogenase to serum lactate dehydrogenase ratio greater than 0.6
   c. Pleural fluid glucose to serum glucose ratio greater than 0.5
   d. Pleural fluid lactate dehydrogenase level greater than 200 IU
   e. Pleural fluid WBC greater than 1000 cells/mm^3

5. Catamenial pneumothorax is associated with the following condition:
   a. Histiocytosis X
   b. Menses
   c. Marfan's syndrome
   d. Recent inhaled marijuana or cocaine
   e. Sarcoidosis

6. All of the following symptoms are usually associated with empyema except:
   a. Ill appearance with fever
   b. Tachycardia
   c. Halitosis
   d. Respiratory insufficiency
   e. Hypotension

7. Conditions associated with the development of pleural effusions include all of the following except:
   a. Mesothelioma
   b. Meigs' syndrome
   c. Hyperthyroidism
   d. Pancreatitis
   e. Sarcoidosis

8. Pleurisy is characterized by all of the following except:
   a. Fever
   b. Unilateral pleuritic chest pain
   c. Associated viral symptoms
   d. Pericardial rub
   e. History of rheumatologic disorders

9. All of the following are always present in tension pneumothorax except:
   a. Severe dyspnea
   b. Tracheal deviation
   c. Hypoxemia
   d. Hypotension
   e. Tachycardia

10. Symptomatic pneumothoraces in neonates present with all of the following except:
    a. Tachypnea
    b. Retractions
    c. Symmetric breath sounds
    d. Jugular vein distention
    e. Wheezing

Answers

1. e. Tension pneumothoraces usually present with severe dyspnea, tachycardia, hypotension, unilateral chest pain, unilaterally diminished breath sounds, and hyperresonance. Dullness to percussion is seen in hemothorax, pleural effusions, and empyema. *(Emergency Medicine, Chapter 32, pp 296–300)*

2.d. Spontaneous pneumothorax is more common among males (5:1 male to female ratio), usually in the third and fourth decades of life. Patients are typically tall and thin and smoke cigarettes. About 50% of spontaneous pneumothoraces recur within 1 to 2 years, frequently on the same side. Many patients with spontaneous pneumothorax have initial symptoms during periods of rest. Spontaneous pneumothoraces rarely progress to tension pneumothorax. *(Emergency Medicine, Chapter 32, pp 296–300)*

3.e. Adult patients with a pneumomediastinum who are stable may be observed as outpatients without specific intervention. Occasionally mediastinal air tracks into the pleural space, resulting in a pneumothorax and requiring tube thoracostomy. *(Emergency Medicine, Chapter 32, pp 296–300)*

4.c. Exudative effusions are suggested by a pleural fluid protein to serum protein ratio greater than 0.5, pleural fluid lactate dehydrogenase to serum lactate dehydrogenase ratio greater than 0.6, pleural fluid lactate dehydrogenase level greater than 200 IU, pleural fluid glucose to serum glucose ratio less than 0.5, and pleural fluid WBC greater than 1000/mm^3. *(Emergency Medicine, Chapter 32, pp 296–300)*

5.b. A catamenial pneumothorax is associated with menses and is thought to result from endometrial implants on the pleura. *(Emergency Medicine, Chapter 32, pp 296–300)*

6.c. Patients with empyema are usually ill, presenting with fever, tachycardia, respiratory insufficiency, and occasionally hypotension. Halitosis is seen in patients with anaerobic pneumonia complicated by abscess formation. These patients usually present with copious foul-smelling sputum. The characteristic odor of this infection is caused by a mixed anaerobic infection, which on chest radiography can be seen layering in the abscess cavity.[3] *(Emergency Medicine, Chapter 32, pp 296–300)*

7.c. Any patients with a pleural effusion should be asked about risk factors and symptoms for pulmonary embolus, which is associated with pleural effusions. Sarcoidosis and a history of exposure to asbestos (i.e., mesothelioma) are also risk factors for pleural effusion. Meigs' syndrome may present as a pleural effusion in the setting of ovarian cancer, occasionally even without ascites. Patients with free fluid in the peritoneum (patients with cirrhosis or on peritoneal dialysis) may also develop pleural effusion. Pancreatitis, subphrenic abscess, and hypothyroidism are also risk factors for this disorder. Hyperthyroidism is not a risk factor for pleural effusion formation. *(Emergency Medicine, Chapter 32, pp 296–300)*

8.d. Pleurisy is a pleural inflammation caused by viruses or is associated with certain rheumatologic disorders (e.g., rheumatoid arthritis). Clinical presentation includes unilateral pleuritic chest pain, fever, and a pleural rub. Chest radiograph, ECG, and pulse oximetry are generally normal. The chest radiograph may be suggestive of viral pneumonitis (e.g., interstitial pattern). Pleurisy is generally self-limiting and is usually treated on an outpatient basis with NSAIDs or by treating underlying rheumatologic disorders. *(Emergency Medicine, Chapter 32, pp 296–300)*

9.b. Rapid identification and treatment of a tension pneumothorax is critical. Patients with a tension pneumothorax will complain of unilateral chest pain and shortness of breath. On examination they may be tachycardic and hypotensive and have unilaterally diminished breath sounds. Deviation of the trachea away from the involved side and distention of jugular vein may occur, but they are not always present. *(Emergency Medicine, Chapter 32, pp 296–300)*

10.d. Neonates with symptomatic pneumothoraces will present with an acute onset of respiratory distress manifested by labored breathing, retractions, abdominal breathing, and wheezing. The most reliable clinical finding is the presence of asymmetric chest wall movement. Unilaterally diminished breath sounds, jugular vein distention, and tracheal deviation are often not appreciated. *(Emergency Medicine, Chapter 32, pp 296–300)*

REFERENCES

1. Grad R, Taussig LM: Acute infections producing upper airway obstruction. *In* Chernick V, Kendig EL, et al (eds): Disorders of the Respiratory Tract in Children. WB Saunders, 1990, pp 336–349.
2. Bortolussi R, Evans J: Listeriosis. *In* Feigin RD, Cherry JD, et al (eds): Textbook of Pediatric Infectious Diseases. WB Saunders, 1992, pp 1180–1185.
3. Finegold SM: Anaerobic Infections of Lungs and Pleura. *In* Fishman AP, et al (eds): Pulmonary Diseases and Disorders. New York, McGraw-Hill, 1988, pp 1505–1516.

BIBLIOGRAPHY

Howell JM: Disorders of the pleura and mediastinum. *In* Howell JM, Altieri M, Jagoda AS, et al (eds): Emergency Medicine. Philadelphia, WB Saunders, 1998, pp 296–300.

Pennza PT, Feller RA: Pneumonia, pleurisy, and empyema. *In* Howell JM, Altieri M, Jagoda AS, et al (eds): Emergency Medicine. Philadelphia, WB Saunders, 1998, pp 274–295.

Rodgers KG, Falcone A: Asthma. *In* Howell JM, Altieri M, Jagoda AS, et al (eds): Emergency Medicine. Philadelphia, WB Saunders, 1998, pp 252–263.

SECTION FOUR

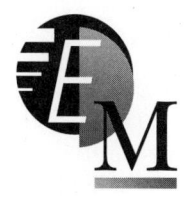

Gastrointestinal Disorders

13 Approach to the Patient with Abdominal Pain and Diarrhea

LYNNE HOLDEN, MD

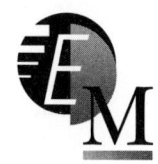

1. The abdominal condition most frequently requiring surgery in the elderly is:
   a. Appendicitis
   b. Abdominal aortic aneurysm
   c. Acute cholecystitis
   d. Large bowel obstruction
   e. Incarcerated hernia

2. All of the following are extra-abdominal conditions that may cause abdominal pain except:
   a. Streptococcal pharyngitis
   b. Diabetic ketoacidosis
   c. Herpes zoster
   d. MI
   e. Spontaneous pneumothorax

3. Which is true concerning the mechanism of abdominal pain transmission?
   a. Visceral afferent nerve endings respond to tearing or cutting.
   b. Visceral pain is sharp and well localized.
   c. Somatic pain is dull and poorly localized.
   d. Kehr's sign is an example of referred pain.
   e. Referred pain is caused by embryologically proximated neurosegments that migrate apart and change their associated innervation.

4. All of the following physical findings can be associated with appendicitis except:
   a. Blumberg's sign
   b. Rovsing's sign
   c. Murphy's sign
   d. Iliopsoas test
   e. Obturator test

5. Which of the following is associated with a higher yield of positive abdominal radiographic findings?
   a. Generalized diffuse pain
   b. History of treated ulcer disease
   c. Pain longer than a week's duration
   d. Abdominal pain with distention
   e. Gastrointestinal bleeding

6. All of the following can indicate the need for IV rehydration with isotonic fluid except:
   a. Tachycardia
   b. Hypotension
   c. Poor capillary refill
   d. Poor urine output
   e. Diarrhea

7. In cases of uncomplicated diarrhea:
   a. Stool cultures are routinely obtained.
   b. The presence of fecal leukocytes can guide therapy.
   c. A specific etiology is usually established in the ED.
   d. Preventing dehydration is the main focus.
   e. Antimicrobials are always required.

8. Which of the following is best tolerated in the patient recovering from diarrhea?
   a. Apple juice
   b. Pear juice
   c. Water
   d. Milk
   e. French fries

9. The antimicrobial agent of choice for the treatment of *Shigella* and *Salmonella* is:
   a. Ciprofloxacin
   b. Trimethoprim-sulfamethoxazole
   c. Metronidazole
   d. Penicillin
   e. Cephalexin

10. *Clostridium difficile* may be caused by all of the following antimicrobials except:
    a. Cefaclor (Ceclor)
    b. Metronidazole
    c. Ampicillin
    d. Erythromycin
    e. Clindamycin

11. Which of the following statements is true about botulism?
    a. Neurologic abnormalities occur immediately in adult botulism.
    b. Infant botulism occurs more commonly than adult botulism.
    c. Milk has been associated with cases of infant botulism.

76 GASTROINTESTINAL DISORDERS

    d. The toxin binds at the neuromuscular junction irreversibly and prevents the release of norepinephrine.
    e. Antitoxin is recommended to cure infant botulism.

12. Six hours after eating at a local seafood restaurant, a 22-year-old man complained of vomiting, diarrhea, and tremors. Two hours after arriving in the ED, he asked a nurse for ice chips. She noted that he spit them out and stated that his tongue was burning. His symptoms were most likely caused by:
    a. Scombroid poisoning
    b. Ciguatera
    c. Paralytic shellfish poisoning
    d. Neurotoxic shellfish poisoning
    e. Norwalk virus

13. A 45-year-old otherwise healthy female presents to the ED complaining of flushing, dizziness, palpitations, headache, and itching. She states that an hour ago she had tuna at an exclusive seafood restaurant. On examination, you hear wheezing. The best initial treatment is:
    a. IV epinephrine
    b. IM epinephrine
    c. IV mannitol
    d. IV diphenhydramine (Benadryl)
    e. PO diphenhydramine (Benadryl)

14. The following findings indicate dehydration in a child except:
    a. Rapid, weak pulse
    b. Hypotension
    c. Decreased urine output
    d. Sunken fontanelles
    e. Tears

15. Patients should return to the ED after discharge if they experience diarrhea along with any of the following except:
    a. Bloody stools
    b. Hematuria
    c. Severe abdominal pain
    d. Fever greater than 101.4°F
    e. Increased urine output

Answers

1.c. In patients younger than 50 years, appendicitis is the most common abdominal condition requiring surgery. However, in patients older than 50 years, cholecystitis is the most frequent cause of abdominal pain that requires surgery. Geriatric patients have more comorbid diseases complicating abdominal conditions and increasing morbidity and mortality. *(Emergency Medicine, Chapter 33, pp 301–311)*

2.e. For still unclear reasons, some well-documented extra-abdominal disease processes and metabolic derangements often cause abdominal pain. A few additional examples are pulmonary embolism, black widow spider bite, hypertensive crises, and hypothyroidism. *(Emergency Medicine, Chapter 33, pp 301–311)*

3.d. Visceral pain is caused by afferent nerve endings located in the walls of hollow organs and the capsules of solid organs that respond to rapid stretching. It is dull, diffuse, poorly localized, and perceived to be midline. On the other hand, somatic pain arises from the stimulation of afferent nerves in the parietal peritoneum and subcutaneous tissues of the anterior abdominal wall that become irritated by chemical mediators of inflammation, causing a sharp, well-localized pain. Referred pain is any pain that occurs at a distance from the primary stimulus. It is caused by embryologically proximate neurosegments that migrate apart yet keep their associated innervation. Kehr's sign is an example. Diaphragmatic irritation causes ipsilateral shoulder and neck pain. The pain stimulus that arises at the diaphragm travels via the phrenic nerve to the midcervical roots. *(Emergency Medicine, Chapter 33, pp 301–311)*

4.c. Blumberg's sign is rebound tenderness that signifies localized peritonitis. Rovsing's sign is the palpation of the left lower quadrant that results in right lower quadrant pain. Murphy's sign is inspiratory arrest with palpation over the right upper quadrant resulting from an inflamed gallbladder. An inflamed mass in contact with the particular muscle eliciting irritation with movement causes the positive iliopsoas and obturator tests, respectively. *(Emergency Medicine, Chapter 33, pp 301–311)*

5.d. Positive abdominal radiographs have been associated with the following: abdominal distention, foreign body ingestion, hematuria with flank tenderness, previous abdominal surgery, and high-pitched bowel sounds. *(Emergency Medicine, Chapter 33, pp 301–311)*

6.e. With diarrhea, the degree of dehydration is important. The patient with diarrhea and poor oral intake or simultaneous nausea and vomiting would be a candidate for IV rehydration to avert dehydration. Patients with significant degree of dehydration should be rehydrated with IV D_5 Ringer's lactate or D_5 normal saline through a large-bore IV catheter. Patients should be given an initial bolus of 10 to 20 mL/kg. *(Emergency Medicine, Chapter 38, pp 357–368)*

7.d. Stool cultures are recommended if there is a public health concern. They are not reasonable from a cost-benefit standpoint, and the patient is usually improved by the time the results are final. Studies have shown no association between fecal leukocytes and culture results. In the ED, the patient is treated based on severity and duration of illness. An etiology is rarely found. Antimicrobials are used to decrease morbidity and mortality of certain pathogens. *(Emergency Medicine, Chapter 38, pp 357–368)*

8.c. In cases of uncomplicated diarrhea, gut rest is discouraged because this results in decreased renewal of the intestinal endothelial cells, increasing dehydration, and starvation. Dairy products can cause bloating and diarrhea from lactose deficiency. Sugars such as fructose and sorbitol can promote osmotic diuresis. The breakdown products of a high-fat diet can cause an osmotic load. *(Emergency Medicine, Chapter 38, pp 357–368)*

9.a. The quinolones (ciprofloxacin, ofloxacin, and norfloxacin) have been shown to be effective and sometimes curative with a single tablet. Fluoroquinolones are contraindicated in children and pregnant women because of cartilaginous injury observed in animal models. Patients with quinolone allergies are treated with trimethoprim-sulfamethoxazole (Bactrim). Bactrim does not cover *Campylobacter* species, and resistant *Escherichia coli* and *Shigella* species have been reported. *(Emergency Medicine, Chapter 38, pp 357–368)*

10.b. Treatment is with oral metronidazole or vancomycin. *Clostridium difficile*–induced colitis results from the intestinal overgrowth of the *C. difficile* bacteria. It usually follows antimicrobial treatment. It occurs in up to 1 in 100 hospitalized patients receiving clindamycin, ampicillin, cephalosporins, lincomycin, or erythromycin. It rarely occurs during outpatient antimicrobial treatment. *C. difficile* can occur within 4 to 9 days of the antimicrobial start date or up to 10 weeks after completion. *(Emergency Medicine, Chapter 38, pp 357–368)*

11.b. Infant botulism has been associated with ingestion of honey (which is not recommended in children younger than 1 year) containing *C. botulinum* spores. Infants can present with constipation, poor feeding, weak cry, and decreased muscle tone. Antitoxin is of no benefit. *(Emergency Medicine, Chapter 38, pp 357–368)*

12.b. Ciguatera is a seafood-related illness involving the gastrointestinal, neurologic, and cardiovascular systems. A late but classic finding is reversal of hot and cold sensations. It has no specific antidote, but mannitol has been proposed to provide relief of gastrointestinal and neurologic symptoms. *(Emergency Medicine, Chapter 38, pp 357–368)*

13.d. The ingestion of dark meat fish (tuna, mackerel, bonito, and mahi-mahi) can cause scombroid, which is classically ascribed to histamine ingestion. Symptoms of diaphoresis, palpitations, flushing, dizziness, itching, and headache usually occur 5 to 10 minutes after ingestion. In addition to treatment with antihistamine, IV cimetidine can be used. *(Emergency Medicine, Chapter 38, pp 357–368)*

14.e. Infants and children with severe dehydration require IV boluses of D_5 lactated Ringer's solution or D_5 normal saline at 20 mL/kg boluses. If IV access cannot be obtained, then an IO infusion should be done. Indications for admission in children with diarrhea include inability to take oral fluids, severe dehydration, and suspected sepsis. *(Emergency Medicine, Chapter 38, pp 357–368)*

15.e. Patients should also return after ED discharge if they are unable to take oral hydration or experience a decrease in urine output, lack of resolution of symptoms after 5 days, neurologic symptoms, or rash. *(Emergency Medicine, Chapter 38, pp 357–368)*

BIBLIOGRAPHY

Lukens T: Approach to the patient with abdominal pain. *In* Howell JM, Altieri M, Jagoda AS, et al (eds): Emergency Medicine. Philadelphia, WB Saunders, 1998, pp 301–311.

Newdow M, Talan DA: Diarrhea and food-borne illness. *In* Howell JM, Altieri M, Jagoda AS, et al (eds): Emergency Medicine. Philadelphia, WB Saunders, 1998, pp 357–368.

14 Disorders of the Esophagus, Liver, Pancreas, and Gallbladder

LYNNE HOLDEN, MD

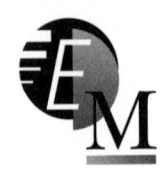

1. Esophageal reflux:
   a. May present only with cough
   b. Is relieved with lying flat
   c. Never occurs with hiatal hernias
   d. Has no association with carcinoma
   e. Is never exacerbated by bending or heavy lifting

2. Which of the following is not associated with chest pain of esophageal etiology?
   a. Pain with exertion
   b. Nocturnal pain
   c. Positional relief
   d. Onset of pain with vomiting
   e. Pain lasting for hours

3. Which of the following is not true?
   a. Button battery ingestion can be an emergency.
   b. The lower esophageal sphincter is the narrowest portion of the esophagus that a foreign object must traverse.
   c. Children are more likely to have esophageal entrapment at the cricopharyngeus muscle.
   d. Lower esophageal sphincter entrapment is easily localized.
   e. Adults are more likely to experience entrapment at the lower esophageal sphincter.

4. The following radiographic findings are consistent with esophageal perforation except:
   a. Mediastinal air
   b. Pneumothorax
   c. Pleural effusion
   d. Widened mediastinum
   e. Pleural apical capping

5. A 65-year-old female complaining of odynophagia for 1 month can be experiencing this because of all of her medications except:
   a. Hydrochlorothiazide
   b. Potassium supplementation
   c. Aspirin
   d. Iron pill
   e. Doxycycline

6. The following feature is typical of biliary colic:
   a. Lasts less than 15 minutes
   b. Can last from 1 to 5 hours
   c. Is positional
   d. Is diminished by the passage of gas
   e. Always occurs in the right upper quadrant

7. Risk factors for cholesterol gallstones include all of the following except:
   a. Female sex
   b. Nulliparity
   c. Obesity
   d. Family history
   e. Estrogen supplementation

8. Acute cholangitis can present with Reynold's pentad, which can include all of the following except:
   a. Septic shock
   b. Normal mental status
   c. Fever
   d. Jaundice
   e. Altered mental status

9. The best test to diagnose acute cholecystitis is:
   a. CT scan
   b. HIDA scan
   c. Ultrasound
   d. Plain film of the abdomen
   e. Oral cholecystography

10. In the ultrasound diagnosis of uncomplicated acute cholecystitis, all of the following may be present except:
    a. Rounded gallbladder shape
    b. Thickening in gallbladder wall
    c. Stones with sludge in gallbladder
    d. Sonographic Murphy's sign
    e. Pericholecystic fluid collection

11. All of the following statements are true about fulminant liver failure except:
    a. Viral hepatitis is a common etiology.
    b. Cerebral edema resulting in brain stem herniation is the leading cause of death.

c. Hypoglycemia is the most common metabolic abnormality.
d. Renal failure occurs in 50% of cases.
e. Liver transplantation has not been shown to be helpful.

12. In acetaminophen overdose:
    a. Encephalopathy never occurs.
    b. *N*-Acetylcysteine works by preventing glutathione deficiency.
    c. *N*-Acetylcysteine must be given within 6 hours of ingestion.
    d. Increased alkaline phosphatase indicates liver damage.
    e. Only the loading dose of *N*-acetylcysteine is required.

13. A 23-year-old sexually active male who presents to the ER with symptoms of acute hepatitis would be considered for admission for all of the following reasons except:
    a. AIDS
    b. Fever
    c. Persistent vomiting and diarrhea
    d. Encephalopathy
    e. Sepsis

14. All of the following are true concerning hepatic abscesses in adults except:
    a. It may be treated with metronidazole.
    b. It usually affects the right lobe of the liver.
    c. Diagnostic aspiration is never required.
    d. Picket-fence pattern temperature fluctuations may occur.
    e. Right-sided pleural effusion may be present on chest radiograph.

15. A 1½-day-old male delivered at home by a midwife presents to the ED icteric. All must be considered except:
    a. Physiologic jaundice
    b. Glucose-6-phosphate dehydrogenase deficiency
    c. Breast milk jaundice
    d. Rh incompatibility
    e. Sepsis

16. In acute pancreatitis, all are true except:
    a. Gallbladder disease accounts for the majority of cases.
    b. Pain often radiates to the back.
    c. Physical examination may reveal left-sided lung findings.
    d. The patient should not eat or drink.
    e. Antimicrobials are always given.

17. Serum amylase levels:
    a. Are both sensitive and specific for pancreatitis
    b. Are elevated only in pancreatitis
    c. That are normal exclude pancreatitis
    d. Have a shorter half-life than lipase
    e. That are elevated qualify as one of Ranson's criteria

18. In a patient presenting to the ED with acute pancreatitis, which of the following would not be an indicator of severe disease?
    a. Age, 65 years
    c. Serum glucose, 500 mg/dL
    c. WBC count, 30,000/mm^3
    d. Serum lactate dehydrogenase, 1000 IU/L
    e. Serum calcium, 12 mg/dL

19. Plain films may reveal all of the following in acute pancreatitis except:
    a. An ileus
    b. Abrupt termination of the gaseous transverse colon at the splenic flexure
    c. Pancreatic calcifications
    d. Left-sided effusion
    e. Left-sided atelectasis

20. Which of the following is true regarding the pancreatic pseudocyst?
    a. It usually occurs in the tail of the pancreas.
    b. It is more common in chronic pancreatitis.
    c. Surgery is always required.
    d. Ultrasound is the study of choice for detection.
    e. It most commonly develops over 6 months.

Answers

1.a. Esophageal reflux presents with burning substernal or retrosternal pain radiating to the chest associated with "acid taste," regurgitation, belching, or coughing. It is typically worse at night and after large meals. It is relieved in the upright position. Symptoms may be exacerbated by bending, heavy lifting, or wearing constrictive clothes. Reflux symptoms may be present with hiatal hernia. Long-standing reflux may be associated with Barrett's esophagus. (*Emergency Medicine, Chapter 34, pp 312–322*)

2.a. A presumption of cardiac pain must be made initially. Cardiac pain commonly presents with exertion and is associated with diaphoresis, lightheadedness, shortness of breath, nausea, and vomiting. The single most helpful historical feature is similarity to previously correctly diagnosed cardiac or esophageal pain. The symptom onset, duration, and frequency may be helpful distinguishing features. Esophageal pain can last several hours, is more typically nocturnal in onset, and may have positional relief. (*Emergency Medicine, Chapter 34, pp 312–322*)

3.d. Esophageal foreign bodies are normally trapped at one of three areas of narrowing: the cricopharyngeus muscle, which is easily localized by the patient; the area where the aorta crosses over the esophagus; and the lower esophageal sphincter. Lower esophageal foreign bodies are poorly localized by patients. (*Emergency Medicine, Chapter 34, pp 312–322*)

4.e. Esophageal perforation is associated with leakage of air and esophageal contents into the neck and mediastinum. Typically, the pleural effusion is left sided in esophageal perforation. There is intrinsic weakness in the left posterior aspect of the distal esophagus, which is the typical site of spontaneous rupture. *(Emergency Medicine, Chapter 34, pp 312–322)*

5.a. Pill-induced esophagitis can be caused by all of the above except hydrochlorothiazide. Additionally, aspirin, clindamycin, and quinidine are culprits. *(Emergency Medicine, Chapter 34, pp 312–322)*

6.b. Biliary colic occurs when a gallstone becomes impacted in the cystic duct, causing a rise in the intraluminal pressure of the gallbladder. A sudden severe pain that can be steady and constant is created in the epigastrium and right upper quadrant. It may last for several hours. It is not positional or diminished by the passage of flatus. *(Emergency Medicine, Chapter 41, pp 388–397)*

7.b. The prevalence of cholesterol stones is highest among northern European and North and South American populations and is rare among indigenous African peoples. Risk factors for gallstones include female sex, multiparity, obesity, age older than 40 years, estrogen use, and family history. Other conditions associated with increased risk of gallstone formation include Crohn's disease, diabetes mellitus, and spinal cord trauma. *(Emergency Medicine, Chapter 41, pp 388–397)*

8.b. Acute cholangitis results from complete or partial obstruction of the biliary ducts with associated gram-negative infection. It may result in liver abscess, sepsis, and death if untreated. Patients may present with the classic Charcot's triad, which includes fever (> 90% of cases), jaundice (66% of cases), and right upper quadrant pain with evidence of peritonitis (66% of cases). Reynold's pentad includes the addition of septic shock and altered mental status. *(Emergency Medicine, Chapter 41, pp 388–397)*

9.b. Because the ^{99m}Tc-labeled analogues of iminodiacetic acid are taken up by normally functioning hepatocytes and excreted in bile, an obstructed cystic duct delays gallbladder visualization. Therefore, radionuclide scanning is nearly 100% sensitive and specific in diagnosing acute cholecystitis. *(Emergency Medicine, Chapter 41, pp 388–397)*

10.e. Ancillary criteria improve the accuracy of ultrasound in making the diagnosis of acute cholecystitis, including stones or sludge in the gallbladder, gallbladder shape, wall thickening, sonographic Murphy's sign, and dilated common duct. Pericholecystic fluid collection and periportal mass may indicate complications such as gallbladder perforation and abscess. *(Emergency Medicine, Chapter 41, pp 388–397)*

11.e. Both viral hepatitis and drug toxicity are common causes of fulminant hepatic failure. Metabolic abnormalities include hypokalemia, hyponatremia, metabolic acidosis, and (most commonly) hypoglycemia. Hepatic encephalopathy is defined as hepatic failure with encephalopathy developing in less than 8 weeks without preexisting liver disease. The patient presents with jaundice, change in mental status, mild agitation, or delusions and may rapidly progress to coma and death. The encephalopathy is thought to be caused by the accumulation of ammonia and mercaptans that bypass the liver through shunts. Renal failure in liver failure is a poor prognostic sign, especially when associated with acetaminophen overdose. Early transplantation has been shown to have a significant impact on outcome. *(Emergency Medicine, Chapter 39, pp 369–380)*

12.b. After acetaminophen overdose, encephalopathy occurs within 72 hours after drug ingestion in fulminant liver failure. *N*-Acetylcysteine given as late as 36 hours after a toxic ingestion has been shown to improve survival in acetaminophen-induced liver failure in patients who present with acetaminophen detectable in the serum or any biochemical evidence of hepatic dysfunction. Serum AST and ALT may increase to more than 100 times normal. PT becomes prolonged and can determine the need for liver transplantation. The dose for *N*-acetylcysteine is 140 mg/kg oral load and then 70 mg/kg every 4 hours for the next 72 hours. *(Emergency Medicine, Chapter 39, pp 369–380)*

13.b. Admission should be considered for patients with suspected viral hepatitis if the following are present: bilirubin greater than 18 mg/dL, evidence of gastrointestinal bleeding or coagulopathy, encephalopathy, sepsis, persistent vomiting or diarrhea, pregnancy, or immunocompromised states. *(Emergency Medicine, Chapter 39, pp 369–380)*

14.c. In adults, although amebic abscesses are usually caused by *Entamoeba histolytica* cyst invasion from contaminated food or water, pyogenic liver abscesses result from bacterial (usually *Escherichia coli, Klebsiella,* and gram-negative aerobic rods) and rarely fungal infection. In children, gram-positive aerobic cocci are common causative agents. All abscesses usually affect the right lobe of the liver. Metronidazole is considered an essential component to treatment. *(Emergency Medicine, Chapter 39, pp 369–380)*

15.d. Hyperbilirubinemia is divided into two forms: unconjugated (indirect) and conjugated (direct). The goal of any therapeutic approach to unconjugated hyperbilirubinemia is to lower the serum bilirubin level and to prevent neonatal neurotoxicity. However, because it cannot cross the blood-brain barrier, conjugated bilirubin is not neurotoxic. Causes of unconjugated hyperbilirubinemia in a 2- to 3-day-old infant are as follows: physiologic, Crigler-Najjar syndrome (familial nonhemolytic icterus), congenital hemolytic disorders such as spherocytosis, G-6-phosphate dehydrogenase deficiency, breast milk jaundice, sepsis, and TORCH. (TORCH is an acronym for toxoplasmosis, rubella, cytomegalovirus, and herpes simplex virus.) In the infant 48 hours old, phototherapy is considered when bilirubin levels exceed 12 mg/dL and is recommended when levels are 15 mg/dL or greater. *(Emergency Medicine, Chapter 39, pp 369–380)*

16.e. In the Western world, pancreatitis is caused by alcohol (35%) and gallbladder disease (45%) presenting with midepigastric or left upper quadrant pain radiating to the back. Up to 20% of patients will have left-sided chest findings ranging from atelectasis to pleural effusion. However, severe disease may have findings consistent with pulmonary edema. Pancreatic rest by holding oral intake and using parenteral nutrition is the mainstay of treatment. The rate of infection in mild pancreatitis is less than 1%. Broad-spectrum antimicrobials are required in cases of necrotizing pancreatitis and infected pseudocysts. *(Emergency Medicine, Chapter 40, pp 381–387)*

17.d. Serum amylase levels are neither sensitive or specific for pancreatitis. In fact, amylase levels have a half-life of 10 hours but may not be produced at all in the "burnt out" pancreas. Amylase should be three times normal to diagnose pancreatitis. Hyperamylasemia can be caused by intra-abdominal disorders such as ectopic pregnancy or ruptured aortic aneurysm; extra-abdominal disorders causing a rise in amylase include salivary gland diseases and diabetic ketoacidosis. The pancreas, however, is the only organ to produce the isomer AMY2. Lipase is more specific and slightly less sensitive than amylase and has a longer half-life. *(Emergency Medicine, Chapter 40, pp 381–387)*

18.e. A score of three or greater in Ranson's criteria predicts moderate to severe disease and is evaluated at admission and at 48 hours. At admission, the criteria are as follows: (1) age older than 55 years; (2) leukocytosis greater than 16,000/mm^3; (3) hyperglycemia greater than 200 mg/dL; (4) serum lactate dehydrogenase greater than 400 IU/L; and (5) serum AST greater than 250 U/L. After 48 hours, the criteria are (1) hematocrit fall greater than 10%; (2) fluid deficit greater than 4 L; (3) hypocalcemia less than 8.0 mg/dL; (4) hypoxemia (Po_2 <60 mm Hg); (5) BUN rise (>5 mg/dL) after IV fluids; and base deficit greater than 4 mEq/L. *(Emergency Medicine, Chapter 40, pp 381–387)*

19.c. The hallmark of chronic pancreatitis that occurs in 33% of patients is pancreatic calcifications that require both AP and oblique views. A large pseudocyst should be suspected when there is displacement of the intestines. However, CT is the best noninvasive study to evaluate the pancreas because it detects fluid accumulation, inflammatory changes, and pseudocysts. *(Emergency Medicine, Chapter 40, pp 381–387)*

20.a. A pancreatic pseudocyst is a collection of secretions enclosed by a wall of fibrous or granulation tissue that develops over 4 to 6 weeks as a consequence of acute pancreatitis (80%), pancreatic trauma (10%), or chronic pancreatitis (10%). It usually occurs in the tail. The most common complaint is of pain, and other symptoms are related to complications such as obstruction, bleeding, or infection. A CT scan is the study of choice. A cyst that is infected, bleeding, or causing a complication should be drained percutaneously or by endoscopy. *(Emergency Medicine, Chapter 40, pp 381–387)*

BIBLIOGRAPHY

Ackrell M, Vukich D: Disorders of the pancreas. *In* Howell JM, Altieri M, Jagoda AS, et al (eds): Emergency Medicine. Philadelphia, WB Saunders, 1998, pp 381–387.

Butler K, Robinson D, Blasen A: Disorders of the liver. *In* Howell JM, Altieri M, Jagoda AS, et al (eds): Emergency Medicine. Philadelphia, WB Saunders, 1998, pp 369–380.

Cox GR: Disorders of the gallbladder. *In* Howell JM, Altieri M, Jagoda AS, et al (eds): Emergency Medicine. Philadelphia, WB Saunders, 1998, pp 388–397.

Munter DW: Disorders of the esophagus. *In* Howell JM, Altieri M, Jagoda AS, et al (eds): Emergency Medicine. Philadelphia, WB Saunders, 1998, pp 312–322.

15 Gastrointestinal Hemorrhage and Appendicitis

ANTHONY J. WEEKES, MD   MARIAN L. GAMBRELL, MD

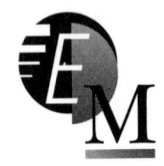

1. A 54-year-old male with a history of alcohol abuse presents with profuse hematemesis. He is lethargic with a BP of 80/60 mm Hg and a pulse of 130. Initial management should include all of the following except:
   a. Fluid resuscitation with crystalloids and blood
   b. Early surgical and gastrointestinal consultation
   c. Administration of IV somatostatin
   d. Insertion of a gastroesophageal balloon
   e. Endotracheal intubation

2. A 74-year-old male reports having black stools for a day. He has a history of hypertension and abdominal aortic aneurysmal repair 2 years ago. The stool is guaiac positive. Which of the following endoscopic findings is the strongest indicator for further radiologic studies?
   a. Nonbleeding proximal duodenal ulcer
   b. Gastric ulcer on the greater curvature
   c. Gastritis
   d. Distal duodenal ulcer
   e. Mucosal tear at the junction of the stomach and esophagus

3. Complications of transfusion with multiple units of blood include:
   a. Fluid overload
   b. Thrombocytopenia
   c. Hypothermia
   d. Dysrhythmias
   e. All of the above

4. Which of the following causes of lower gastrointestinal bleeding is more likely to occur in later childhood than in early childhood?
   a. Necrotizing enterocolitis
   b. Volvulus
   c. Polyps
   d. Anal fissures
   e. Intussusception

5. Endoscopic diagnosis of a slowly bleeding gastric ulcer in an elderly patient can be appropriately addressed with all of the following except:
   a. Biopsy and culture
   b. IV vasopressin (20 U in 200 mL of normal saline at 0.25 to 0.5 U/min)
   c. Epinephrine injection into the ulcer base
   d. Laser photocoagulation

6. A 20-year-old college student states she induced vomiting after an eating binge. She was alarmed by the blood she brought up after several retches. She now has pain when she swallows. Which of the following is true about her likely diagnosis?
   a. The lesion is primarily located at the distal esophagus.
   b. Antimicrobial therapy against *Helicobacter pylori* is indicated.
   c. It is frequently associated with excessive alcohol use.
   d. It can be identified as a transmural lesion.
   e. The majority of lesions require thoracic surgical repair.

7. Angiodysplasias are associated with which of the following?
   a. Physiologic stress such as sepsis and burns
   b. Painful bleeding
   c. Change in caliber of stool
   d. Identification with sigmoidoscopy
   e. Significant hematochezia

8. A 69-year-old retired mailman has been having maroon stools for 2 days. He has no abdominal discomfort but feels weak. Vital signs include a systolic BP of 90 mm Hg, a weak pulse of 136, and a temperature of 98°F. Following resuscitation, which of the following is a logical sequence of diagnostic evaluation?
   a. Nuclear RBC scan, colonoscopy, nasogastric aspiration
   b. Upper gastrointestinal series, upper endoscopy, colonoscopy
   c. Nasogastric aspiration, flexible sigmoidoscopy, arteriography
   d. Upper endoscopy, arteriography, nuclear scan

9. Which is the least likely source of hematochezia?
   a. Ulceration through the posterior wall of the proximal duodenum

b. Epistaxis requiring posterior nasal packing
c. Alcohol- and NSAID-induced gastritis
d. Right-sided colonic diverticulosis
e. Colonic angiodysplasias

10. All of the following statements about variceal bleeding in an adult are true except:
    a. It is characterized by painless hematemesis.
    b. The sites of major bleeding are the stomach and the esophagus.
    c. Resuscitation is usually required.
    d. It is usually provoked by sudden increases in intragastric pressure.
    e. Empiric management by balloon tamponade is directed initially at varices on the cardia of the stomach.

11. A stool guaiac test can be positive in all of the following situations except:
    a. Daily vitamin C supplementation
    b. In the absence of gastrointestinal bleeding
    c. For 10 to 12 days after a large gastrointestinal bleed
    d. Less than 90 mL of blood in the gastrointestinal tract
    e. Epistaxis

12. Risk factors for developing a major gastrointestinal bleed include all of the following except:
    a. Age greater than 60 years
    b. Alcohol intake on a frequent basis
    c. A history of gastrointestinal bleeding
    d. Psychological stress
    e. Current steroid use

13. A 14-month-old girl has been having intermittent episodes vomiting and crying as if she's having severe pain. Her father said the last time he changed the diaper there was maroon mucoid stool. The girl is now quiet but is also tired and apathetic. Appropriate diagnostic tests include all of the following except:
    a. Barium enema
    b. Plain upright abdominal radiograph
    c. Apt test
    d. Ultrasound of the abdomen
    e. CBC

14. All of the following statements about appendicitis during pregnancy are true except:
    a. During pregnancy, the appendix rotates counterclockwise.
    b. Laxity of the abdominal muscles can potentially obscure peritoneal irritation.
    c. If appendicitis is undiagnosed, mortality approaches 2% and 6%, respectively, for mother and fetus.
    d. The incidence of appendicitis is lower in pregnancy.

15. All of the following statements are typical of appendiceal perforation except:
    a. Over time, an increased localization of pain to the right lower quadrant develops.
    b. Vomiting can occur.
    c. Pain duration is typically over 36 hours.
    d. Patients can present with either constipation or diarrhea.
    e. Fever and tachycardia are not specific signs of perforation.

16. A 25-year-old woman presents to the ED after having a syncopal episode. She complains of right lower quadrant pain for 2 days, anorexia, and vomiting. In the ED she is orthostatic and has diffuse abdominal tenderness with guarding and rebound. On pelvic examination, she has isolated right adnexal tenderness. Initial management includes all except:
    a. Large-bore IV access and fluid resuscitation
    b. Stat pregnancy test
    c. PO trial with clear liquids
    d. Administration of IV antimicrobials
    e. Surgical consultation

17. A 70-year-old man with hypertension and diabetes mellitus presents with 3 days of midabdominal pain, vomiting, and fever. He is found to have abdominal distention and a right lower quadrant mass. All of the following are true except:
    a. Initial management includes ECG, cardiac telemetry, and supplemental oxygen.
    b. This patient requires surgical consultation and intensive observation.
    c. Five percent to 10% of appendicitis cases occur in the elderly.
    d. The absence of guarding, rebound, and rigidity rules out perforation in this patient.

18. All of the following statements about the MANTRELS score are false except:
    a. The maximum score is 7 points.
    b. This scoring system is more accurate in children than adults.
    c. Right lower quadrant tenderness is given 2 points.
    d. A score of 7 is definitive for appendicitis.
    e. Rebound tenderness is given 2 points.

19. Features that help differentiate pelvic inflammatory disease from appendicitis include:
    a. The majority of women with appendicitis have pain onset greater than 14 days from the last menstrual period.
    b. Cervical motion tenderness is more common in appendicitis.
    c. Pelvic inflammatory disease most often presents with unilateral adnexal tenderness.
    d. The incidence of vaginal bleeding is greater in appendicitis.
    e. WBC counts are generally higher in appendicitis than in pelvic inflammatory disease.

20. A 5-year-old boy presents with a 1-day complaint of right lower quadrant pain, dysuria, and vomiting. Initial diagnostic studies include all of the following except:
    a. Abdominal examination
    b. Rectal examination
    c. Abdominal CT

d. CBC
e. Abdominal ultrasound

21. All of the following are appropriate antimicrobial therapy for perforated appendix except:
    a. Gentamicin, clindamycin, and ampicillin in a 12-year-old boy
    b. Clindamycin and metronidazole in a 25-year-old penicillin-allergic woman
    c. Clindamycin and ceftriaxone in 45-year-old diabetic on hemodialysis
    d. Ceftriaxone and gentamicin in a 6-week gravid woman
    e. Clindamycin and metronidazole in a hypotensive patient

22. All of the following are true except:
    a. Elevated serum and urine amylase levels are specific markers for appendicitis.
    b. Acute appendicitis may present with dysuria and abnormal urine analysis.
    c. Useful radiographic signs of appendicitis include rightward scoliosis and localized ileus.
    d. Abdominal CT is 85% to 95% sensitive in identifying uncomplicated appendicitis.
    e. Ultrasound is 89% to 100% specific for diagnosing appendicitis.

23. All of the following are true except:
    a. The appendix is capable of secreting immunoglobulins.
    b. The most common organisms in appendicitis are *Bacteroides fragilis* and *Esherichia coli.*
    c. Once the appendix becomes obstructed it no longer secretes mucus.
    d. Tumors are rarely a cause of appendiceal obstruction.
    e. Appendicitis may occur in the absence of luminal obstruction.

Answers

1.d. This presentation is suggestive of a variceal bleed or hemorrhagic gastritis leading to shock. He may have lost up to 30% to 40% of his blood volume. Immediate interventions include large-bore peripheral IV infusion of crystalloids, followed by packed RBCs if 2 to 3 L of crystalloid do not improve vital signs or if bleeding continues. Airway protection with early endotracheal intubation is indicated. Pharmacotherapy with somatostatin can selectively constrict the splanchnic vascular bed. This paves the way for easier endoscopic lavage and identification of the source of bleeding. Hemostasis can often be achieved by treating varices, ulcers, or tears. The gastroesophageal balloon is indicated for variceal bleeding not controlled with pharmacotherapy and when timely endoscopy is unavailable. (*Emergency Medicine, Chapter 37, pp 347–356*)

2.d. Melena prompts a search for a source of bleeding from the gastrointestinal tract above the ligament of Treitz. The bleeding source is in this region in 95% of the cases. Nonbleeding ulcerations warrant biopsy and culture to investigate the presence of malignancy and *Helicobacter pylori* infection. Proximal duodenal ulcers and gastric erosions each account for 20% to 25% of the cases of upper gastrointestinal bleeding. Ulcerations in the third portion of the duodenum are unusual. In a patient with an aortic aneurysm repair, a connection between the vascular system and the gastrointestinal bleeding (aortoenteric fistula) must be investigated. These sentinel bleeds may be followed by massive hemorrhage within 96 hours. A CT scan of the abdomen is indicated. Unusually located duodenal ulcerations are also the sites of unusual neoplasms such as the carcinoid tumor. (*Emergency Medicine, Chapter 37, pp 347–356*)

3.e. Multiple blood transfusions for trauma and gastrointestinal hemorrhage may be needed in rapid sequence. Blood products can be stored for up to 21 days at 4°C. The rapid infusion of as little as 4 to 5 U of unwarmed blood can lead to hypothermia. This leads to venous spasm, an increased viscosity, and a lowered flow state and subsequent dysrhythmias. Although packed RBC units contain less citrate than does whole blood, the potential for hypocalcemia exists. The colloid osmotic pressure increase associated with sequential transfusions can lead to fluid overload in patients with poor renal, hepatic, or cardiac function. Reasons for the development of a transfusion coagulopathy include prolonged time in shock, tissue injury, and dilution from platelet-deficient blood. It is advised that a platelet count be obtained after 5 U of blood are transfused, and if the platelet count is less than 50,000/mm, a platelet transfusion should be started.[1] (*Emergency Medicine, Chapter 37, pp 347–356*)

4.c. Anal fissures are a common cause of rectal bleeding throughout childhood. Intussusception occurs mostly in children younger than 3 years, especially the 6- to 18-month age group. Bloody diarrhea, fever, and vomiting in a newborn are characteristic of necrotizing enterocolitis. Volvulus presents as blood-streaked stool in patients younger than 1 year old, with bilious vomiting, constant pain, and a distended abdomen. Polyps are more common as childhood progresses. (*Emergency Medicine, Chapter 37, pp 347–356*)

5.b. In a nonvariceal slowly bleeding source, hemostasis can be directly applied using any of several methods, including laser photocoagulation, electrocoagulation, heater probes, and injection with sclerosing agents and vasoconstrictors. *Helicobacter pylori* is a bacterium involved in the pathogenesis of ulcerations, gastritis, and gastric cancer. Biopsy can detect the presence of malignant cells, and culture can determine if antimicrobial therapy is also going to be included. Vasopressin is indicated in significant upper gastrointestinal bleeding, especially variceal bleeding. It is a vasoconstrictor, decreasing portal venous blood flow and pressure as well as lessening splanchnic blood flow. It also has strong peripheral vasoconstrictive effects and may lead to skin necrosis, myocardial ischemia, and bowel ischemia. Although these effects can be lessened with the administration of nitroglycerin, somatostatin can be given instead because it is more selective. If there is no hemodynamic compromise, then the risks of vasopressin administration in the elderly and those with poor physiologic reserve outweighs its benefits. *(Emergency Medicine, Chapter 37, pp 347–356)*

6.c. A history of bright red blood after repeated retching or vomiting is consistent with a Mallory-Weiss tear. Other ways of provoking increases in intragastric pressure are blunt abdominal trauma, coughing, straining, childbirth, and vigorous CPR. The lesion is usually a single mucosal tear in the proximal stomach 80% of the time and in the distal esophagus 20% of the time. Boerhaave's syndrome involves a complete tear of the wall of the esophagus. The Mallory-Weiss syndrome is frequently associated with excessive alcohol use. The bleeding is generally self-limited. Surgical repair is required in fewer than 5% of these cases. *(Emergency Medicine, Chapter 37, pp 347–356)*

7.e. Angiodysplasias are, along with diverticulosis and polyps, the most common causes of significant lower gastrointestinal bleeding. They can be found in any part of the gastrointestinal tract but are typically in the ascending colon and cecum. Angiodysplasia may present as hematochezia and melena. It is usually painless. Physiologic stress can lead to gastric or duodenal ulcers or even bowel ischemia. Decreased caliber of stool, weight loss, and changes in bowel habits suggest a left colonic malignancy. *(Emergency Medicine, Chapter 37, pp 347–356)*

8.c. Hematochezia is from the lower gastrointestinal tract 90% of the time. An active upper gastrointestinal source of the bleeding should be excluded first with nasogastric or orogastric aspiration of bilious fluid or endoscopic visualization. An upper gastrointestinal series is not prudent or helpful in a hemodynamically unstable patient. It is usually an outpatient study. When lower gastrointestinal endoscopy reveals either brisk bleeding or segments with bleeding, arteriography is indicated to localize the vessels involved. If a bleed is slow or intermittent, a nuclear-labeled RBC scan can be used to detect bleeding rates as low as 0.1 to 0.5 mL/min. The results can then direct a more selective angiography and embolization. Angiography is needed when there is a rapid bleed not controlled and before surgery to help localize the bleeding vessels so as to lessen the extent of bowel resection. Nuclear scans reveal little if done after an indicated angiogram. *(Emergency Medicine, Chapter 37, pp 347–356)*

9.b. Hematochezia represents bleeding from the colon in about 85% of cases. A source is found in the upper gastrointestinal tract 10% of the time and in the small intestine in the other 5%. Hematochezia from an upper gastrointestinal source is from a brisk bleed, often with hemodynamic instability. An ulceration perforating the posterior of the duodenum can lead to profuse bleeding from erosions into the gastroduodenal artery, as can erosions high in the gastric body eroding into the left gastric artery. Common causes of significant hematochezia include diverticulosis and acquired angiodysplasias. Severe epistaxis usually results in melena. *(Emergency Medicine, Chapter 37, pp 347–356)*

10.d. Cirrhosis of the liver leads to impeded drainage of blood from the splenic and superior mesenteric veins. Collateral vessels become engorged into varicosities. The varices found at the proximal stomach and the distal esophagus have scant supporting tissue and are prone to rupture. Bleeding is usually severe, and volume resuscitation is often required. Airway control often is indicated. Early gastrointestinal and surgical consultation should be obtained. In situations in which endoscopy is delayed or unavailable and ongoing hemorrhage surpasses volume replacement, balloon tamponade of presumed variceal bleeding is indicated. The gastric portion of the gastroesophageal balloon is inflated first and tension applied for several hours. If the bleeding does not appear to be controlled, then the esophageal balloon is also inflated to address esophageal varices. Variceal bleeding is not associated with pain. Sudden increases in intragastric pressure can cause a tear to the mucosal layer of the wall of the proximal stomach extending across the gastroesophageal junction to the distal esophagus. This is the Mallory-Weiss syndrome. *(Emergency Medicine, Chapter 37, pp 347–356)*

11.a. Stool tests for occult blood may be positive with as little as 50 to 100 mL of blood anywhere along the gastrointestinal tract. A large upper gastrointestinal bleed of 1000 to 2000 mL can yield 4 to 5 days of melena and 10 to 12 days of guaiac-positive stool. Positivity can be a result of several foods and medications such as iron preparations, bismuth subsalicylate, tomatoes, cherries, licorice, and roast beef. Vitamin C, ascorbic acid, has antioxidant properties. Tests for occult blood are premised on the pseudoperoxidase activity of heme. This activity is inhibited by low levels of reducing substances such as ascorbic acid, leading to occasional false-negative guaiac results. *(Emergency Medicine, Chapter 37, pp 347–356)*

12.d. With increased age comes an increased prevalence of colonic angiodysplasias and diverticulosis. Both are common causes of major lower gastrointestinal bleeding. Alcohol use has direct toxic effects on the intestinal mucosa and indirectly plays a role in the pathogenesis of portal hypertension and coagulopathies. Alcohol use is frequently associated with bleeding from gastritis, varices, ulcers, and mucosal tears. Steroids, like NSAIDs, inhibit the cyclooxygenase enzymes and reduce the synthesis of mucosal-protecting prostaglandins. They can lead to erosions and inflammation. Approximately 75% of patients with a prior upper gastrointestinal bleed will rebleed within 1 year if not fully compliant with prescribed medications. Psychological stress is not a risk factor for a major gastrointestinal bleed. *(Emergency Medicine, Chapter 37, pp 347–356)*

13.c. Intussusception usually presents in a previously healthy child with sudden episodes of screaming in pain and vomiting with intervals of no discomfort. The child may appear irritable, weak, lethargic, or apathetic. Ultrasonography in experienced hands can detect a "crescent in a donut" sign. The hyperechoic crescent is pathologically confirmed to be the mesentery enclosing the invaginated bowel. It has been suggested that ultrasonography can be used to screen suspected cases and may eliminate unnecessary barium enemas. The barium enema can then selectively be used for its therapeutic effects by applying hydrostatic pressure and relieving the intussusception. Newborns may have bloody stool after swallowing maternal blood during birth or from cracked nipples. Bloody stool can also have worrisome diagnostic possibilities such as necrotizing enterocolitis. The Apt test can determine if blood is of maternal origin. One part of the bloody stool or vomitus is mixed with 5 to 10 parts of water. It is centrifuged and the supernatant is mixed with 1 mL of 0.2 N to 0.25 N sodium hydroxide. The test is based on the different susceptibilities of different hemoglobins to alkaline denaturation. Within 2 to 5 minutes color changes occur; brown indicates adult hemoglobin and pink means fetal blood.[2] *(Emergency Medicine, Chapter 37, pp 347–356)*

14.d. Anatomic and physiologic changes during pregnancy include rotation of the appendix counterclockwise to a position so that as term approaches, the tip of the appendix overlies the right kidney. In the third trimester, right upper quadrant and flank pain are common symptoms. The laxity of abdominal muscles potentially obscures signs of peritoneal irritation. An increase in serum steroids diminishes the inflammatory response and may lead to a rapid development of peritonitis. These changes alter the presentation of appendicitis during pregnancy, but the incidence remains the same. *(Emergency Medicine, Chapter 36, pp 339–346)*

15.a. Patients with perforated appendix experience pain duration over 36 hours, with more diffuse pain rather than localization to the right lower quadrant. This pain is caused by peritoneal irritation from spillage of appendiceal contents. *(Emergency Medicine, Chapter 36, pp 339–346)*

16.c. This patient is in shock and requires immediate replacement of fluid deficits. Ectopic pregnancy is always the first diagnosis in a premenopausal woman with lower abdominal pain until proven otherwise. In the event of a negative serum pregnancy test, ruptured appendix or ruptured ovarian cyst is a likely diagnosis in this patient, in which case she will eventually require surgical intervention. Intravenous antimicrobials should be given in cases of suspected ruptured appendicitis. Surgical consultation should be obtained, and the patient should be kept NPO in anticipation of surgery. *(Emergency Medicine, Chapter 36, pp 339–346)*

17.d. The elderly commonly exhibit abdominal distention and a right lower quadrant mass caused by perforation and abscess formation; the more classic signs and symptoms of vomiting, fever, anorexia, and peritonitis occur less frequently. Atypical presentations and delays in seeking medical attention may account for the high perforation rates and a subsequent mortality rate of 5% to 20% in the elderly patient population. Also, all elderly patients are at risk for acute MI, ruptured aortic aneurysm, or ruptured viscus. *(Emergency Medicine, Chapter 36, pp 339–346)*

18.c. The MANTRELS score has a maximum of 10 points, with 2 points each given to right lower quandrant tenderness and leukocytosis. Each of the remaining factors of pain migration, anorexia, nausea, rebound tenderness, elevated temperature, and shift to left of WBCs receives 1 point. Although a MANTRELS score of greater than 7 is highly suspicious for appendicitis, it is not definitive. This scoring system is only a guideline. It has been found to be less accurate in children than in adults. *(Emergency Medicine, Chapter 36, pp 339–346)*

19.a. The incidence of vaginal bleeding, WBC counts, pain migration, rectal tenderness, and gastrointestinal symptoms does not differ between appendicitis and pelvic inflammatory disease. However, in women diagnosed with appendicitis, 50% to 85% develop pain more than 14 days after their last menstrual period. The majority (82%) of women with pelvic inflammatory disease have cervical motion tenderness, which is found in only 28% of women with appendicitis. *(Emergency Medicine, Chapter 36, pp 339–346)*

20.c. The most common physical finding in children with appendicitis older than 2 years is right lower quadrant tenderness. The WBC count is normal within the first 24 hours in up to 82% of children with acute appendicitis, and the neutrophil count and percentage are usually elevated. Sonography has an overall sensitivity of 85% to 95% and a specificity of 90% to 100%. Fifty percent to 80% of children with appendicitis have localized rectal tenderness, and up to 25% have a palpable rectal mass. The usefulness of CT in diagnosing uncomplicated appendicitis in children has not been proven. *(Emergency Medicine, Chapter 36, pp 339–346)*

21.d. Intravenous antimicrobials should be given to patients who are septic or have obvious perforation. The regimen must provide anaerobic coverage. However, aminoglycosides should be avoided in elderly patients, pregnant women, patients with renal disease, and hypotensive patients. *(Emergency Medicine, Chapter 36, pp 339–346)*

22.a. Elevated urine and serum amylase levels as well as other serologic markers (alpha$_1$-antitrypsin, alpha-interferon, or serotonin levels) are not specific for appendicitis. Most radiographs are nonspecific in appendicitis. Useful radiographic signs include calcified fecaliths, rightward scoliosis, soft tissue masses, free fluid, local or generalized ileus, obstruction, flank stripe and psoas obliteration, and right lower quadrant haziness. The appendix is in close proximity to the ureter, and when inflamed it can cause ureteral irritation. Abdominal CT is 87% to 96% sensitive in identifying uncomplicated appendicitis. Sensitivity of ultrasonography in the diagnosis of appendicitis ranges from 78% to 94%, and specificity ranges from 89% to 100%. *(Emergency Medicine, Chapter 36, pp 339–346)*

23.c. The appendix is a diverticulum that arises from the inferior tip of the cecum. It is lined with colonic epithelium. This epithelium contains lymphoid follicles that proliferate and are capable of secreting immunoglobulins. Luminal obstruction is the foremost cause of appendicitis. Appendicitis can also occur from mucosal ulceration and direct bacterial invasion. Subsequent to obstruction, the epithelial cells continue to secrete mucus, which results in appendiceal distention and decreased lymphatic and venous drainage. *(Emergency Medicine, Chapter 36, pp 339–346)*

REFERENCES

1. Hewson J, Neame P, Kumar N, et al: Coagulopathy related to dilution and hypotension during massive transfusion. Crit Care Med 1985; 13:387–391.
2. Del-Pozo G, Albillos J, Tejedor D: Intussusception: US findings with pathologic correlation: The crescent in donut sign. Radiology 1996; 199:688–692.

BIBLIOGRAPHY

McGuirk T, Munter DW: Gastrointestinal hemorrhage. *In* Howell JM, Altieri M, Jagoda AS, et al (eds): Emergency Medicine. Philadelphia, WB Saunders, 1998, pp 347–356.

Rothrock S: Appendicitis: *In* Howell JM, Altieri M, Jagoda AS, et al (eds): Emergency Medicine. Philadelphia, WB Saunders, 1998, pp 339–346.

16 Gastrointestinal Obstruction and Anorectal Disorders

ERNST PAUL, Jr, MD   MARY RYAN, MD

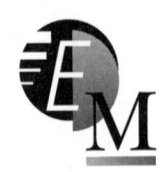

1. In patients with small bowel obstruction, delayed and feculent vomiting signifies:
    a. Gastric outlet obstruction
    b. Volvulus
    c. Hernia
    d. Ileal obstruction
    e. Fecal impaction

2. An 18-year-old patient presents with sudden, severe epigastric pain and distention, retching, and an inability to vomit. Multiple attempts at passing a nasogastric tube are unsuccessful. The most likely diagnosis is:
    a. Strangulated hernia
    b. Ogilvie's disease
    c. Gastric volvulus
    d. Large bowel obstruction
    e. Gastritis

3. The management is paired correctly with the disease entity in each of the following statements except:
    a. Immediate surgery for gastric volvulus
    b. Conservative therapy in patients with small bowel obstruction and no abdominal scars or hernia
    c. Increased dietary fiber and liquids in functional constipation
    d. Attempted at reduction of incarcerated, nonstrangulated hernias by gentle manual manipulation
    e. Endoscopy for gastric outlet obstruction

4. Plain radiography confirms what percentage of small bowel obstruction?
    a. 20%
    b. Nondiagnostic
    c. 90%
    d. 60%
    e. None of the above

5. Which of the following statements is correct?
    a. Indirect hernias are more frequently seen in adulthood.
    b. Sigmoid volvulus is not a common cause of bowel obstruction.
    c. The most common cause of large bowel obstruction is inflammatory intestinal disease.
    d. Adult hypertrophic pyloric stenosis causes most gastric outlet obstruction.
    e. Biliary and gastric surgery are the most common causes of small bowel obstruction.

6. Common presenting symptoms/findings of intussusception include all of the following except:
    a. Vomiting
    b. Sausage-shaped abdominal mass
    c. Lethargy
    d. Abdominal tenderness
    e. "Currant jelly" stools

7. A pathognomonic finding in pyloric stenosis is:
    a. Hypochloremic metabolic alkalosis
    b. Jaundice
    c. Olive-shaped mass in abdomen
    d. Visible gastric peristalsis
    e. Vomiting

8. Which of the following statements about Hirschsprung's disease is correct?
    a. It is caused by abnormally innervated bowel that becomes hypertonic and stenotic.
    b. The entire colon may be involved.
    c. A family history of 3% to 7% can occur.
    d. It can present as foul-smelling diarrhea.
    e. All the above are correct.

9. The most common source of constipation in children is:
    a. Anatomic
    b. Neurologic
    c. Endocrine
    d. Functional
    e. Metabolic

10. Ultrasonography is most diagnostic in which disease entity?
    a. Constipation
    b. Midgut volvulus
    c. Hirschsprung's disease
    d. Pyloric stenosis
    e. Hernia

11. A 48-year-old woman presents to the ED complaining of constipation. Today she noticed a mass protruding from her rectum when straining at stool. She also noticed some painless bleeding per rectum. Both the mass and bleeding disappeared when she stood up. Anoscopy in the ED revealed internal hemorrhoids only. This woman's hemorrhoids are classified as:
    a. First degree
    b. Second degree
    c. Third degree
    d. Fourth degree

12. A 35-year-old man complains of rectal pain and tenesmus for 5 days. He now has bloody discharge per rectum and a low-grade fever. A foreign body is suspected, although the patient denies the possibility. Management of this patient includes all of the following except:
    a. IV fluids, blood cultures, antimicrobials
    b. Digital rectal examination to confirm the presence of a foreign body and determine if it is low-lying or high-lying
    c. Abdominal and pelvic radiographs
    d. Surgical consult
    e. Anoscopy before and after removal of the foreign body

13. Regarding anorectal abscess, all of the following are true statements except:
    a. Most begin in the intersphincteric space.
    b. Most result from cryptoglandular infection.
    c. Urinary retention may occur from centrally mediated inhibition.
    d. Pain and bleeding are generally present.
    e. Approximately 10% result from an underlying disease process (e.g., inflammatory bowel disease)

14. The classic triad for chronic anal fissure includes which of the following?
    a. Sentinel pile, postanal dimple, and proximal papilla
    b. Postanal dimple, proximal papilla, and fissure
    c. Fissure, severe pain, and sentinel pile
    d. Severe pain, fissure, and postanal dimple
    e. Fissure, sentinel pile, and proximal papilla

15. Match the following disease entity with the best treatment option.
    a. Rectal prolapse
    b. Pilonidal cyst
    c. Fourth-degree internal hemorrhoids
    d. Simple perianal abscess
    e. Acute external thrombosed hemorrhoids

    i. Marsupialization
    ii. Emergent surgical consult
    iii. Excision
    iv. Reduction and outpatient surgical referral
    v. Incision and drainage

16. A patient with a history of chronic constipation, mucus per rectum, and soiling now complains of painless mass per rectum. Physical examination shows a large pink mass per rectum with circumferential folds. The mass is nontender and reduces with manual pressure. All of the following are true of this condition except:
    a. It is more common at extremes of age.
    b. It is associated with cystic fibrosis in some cases.
    c. It is likely to recur despite successful manual reduction.
    d. A stat surgical consult is needed.
    e. The fold pattern helps differentiate this condition from mucosal prolapse.

Answers

1.d. A common complaint in patients with small bowel obstruction is nausea and vomiting. Vomiting usually follows episodic, crampy, and poorly localized abdominal pain. Proximal small bowel obstruction presents with vomiting that is early, voluminous, and bilious. Ileal or distal small bowel obstruction is associated with vomiting that is delayed and feculent. The vomiting caused by gastric outlet obstruction is voluminous in undigested food and relieves the abdominal pain associated with this condition. Volvulus, hernias, and fecal impaction are uncommonly associated with vomiting as a presenting feature. *(Emergency Medicine, Chapter 35, pp 323–337)*

2.c. Borchardt's triad consists of severe epigastric pain and distention, vomiting followed by violent retching with an inability to vomit, and difficulty or inability to pass a nasogastric tube. This symptom complex is classic for gastric volvulus. Hernias most commonly present as nonpainful masses of bowel that are reducible through a peritoneal defect. Incarcerated hernias are irreducible and can gradually progress to an ischemic or infarcted loop of bowel or strangulation. Strangulated bowel is associated with nonepigastric pain, vomiting, peritonitis, and the development of a toxic appearance. Large bowel obstruction presents as constipation, obstipation, abdominal distention, and less severe, vague abdominal pain. This is also the presentation of Ogilvie's disease or colonic pseudo-obstruction. Gastritis is associated with copious vomiting, dyspepsia, hematemesis, and a nondistended abdomen. *(Emergency Medicine, Chapter 35, pp 323–337)*

3.b. Patients with clinical and radiographic signs of small bowel obstruction but with no surgical scars or obvious hernias should be suspected of having an internal hernia or closed-loop volvulus. These patients should not be managed conservatively because they require immediate celiotomy to prevent bowel ischemia and necrosis. Gastric volvulus is a surgical emergency to prevent gastric necrosis. Correction of functional constipation requires increased fiber and fluids in the diet with development of regular bowel habits by adhering to defecation reflexes. Attempted reduction of incarcerated hernias should occur, preferably with the patient given analgesia and being well sedated. In gastric outlet obstruction, although a barium swallow is diagnostic in the majority of cases, endoscopy allows for diagnosis as well as for biopsy of the gastric tissue to determine the cause. *(Emergency Medicine, Chapter 35, pp 323–337)*

4.d. Plain radiographs can confirm 60% of small bowel obstructions. Typically, gas is not visualized in the small bowel, compared with the stomach or large bowel. Plain films show air-fluid levels at varying heights in a stepladder pattern or the "string of pearls sign" (chain of radiolucent bubbles) in the small bowel. The diagnosis of small bowel obstruction is further supported by minimal or absent gas in the large bowel, suggesting either partial or complete obstruction, respectively. Plain films have a false-negative rate of 20%. **(Emergency Medicine, Chapter 35, pp 323–337)**

5.b. Sigmoid volvulus is not a common cause of bowel obstruction. It accounts for approximately 0.8% to 3.4% of all episodes. Large bowel obstruction is most commonly caused by carcinoma of the colon and rectum. Less common causes include inflammatory bowel disease, benign colonic stricture, and ischemic colitis. Small bowel obstruction is most frequently caused by surgery of the bowel or gynecologic procedures. Biliary or gastric operations are a rare cause. Indirect hernias occur most commonly in infancy, not adulthood, and adult hypertrophic pyloric stenosis is a rare cause of gastric outlet obstruction. **(Emergency Medicine, Chapter 35, pp 323–337)**

6.e. Intussusception most commonly occurs in infants younger than 2 years of age, with a male predominance and a summer prevalence. Only 10% of children do not present with a history of intermittent drawing up of the legs with screaming or pain for several minutes, then returning to baseline. The presentation may also include vomiting (85%), a right upper quadrant sausage-shaped mass (62%), lethargy (50%), and abdominal tenderness (61%). "Currant jelly" stools are rare, and only 43% to 53% of patients have guaiac-positive stools. **(Emergency Medicine, Chapter 35, pp 323–337)**

7.c. Pyloric stenosis occurs in 1 of 300 births and typically presents at 5.1 weeks in term infants. Common presenting symptoms include increasingly frequent vomiting, becoming projectile. This may lead to a hypochloremic metabolic alkalosis and dehydration. Jaundice may also occur (8%), caused by deficiency of hepatic glucuronyl transferases and caloric insufficiency. Visible gastric peristalsis can be seen in the relaxed, fed infant. But the most significant (pathognomonic) finding is the palpation of an olive-shaped mass anywhere between the right upper abdomen and the umbilicus, indicating the hypertrophic pylorus. **(Emergency Medicine, Chapter 35, pp 323–337)**

8.e. Hirschsprung's disease or aganglionic megacolon is caused by the absence of ganglionic cells at submucosal and myenteric plexus of the colon. The aganglionic bowel becomes stenotic, with dilation of the proximal, normally innervated segment. The extent of colon involvement may be variable, with most cases involving the anus to the sigmoid colon. Rarely, the entire colon is affected. Common presentations include failure of meconium passage in the neonate, persistent or recurrent constipation, bowel obstruction, abdominal distention, and enterocolitis. Enterocolitis presents in a child with a history of constipation who develops fever, foul-smelling diarrhea, and abdominal distention. This presentation is ominous. Hirschsprung's disease has a family incidence of 3% to 7%. **(Emergency Medicine, Chapter 35, pp 323–337)**

9.d. Constipation is defined as fewer than three stools per week with straining and passage of hard, small stools. Constipation can be caused by organic (anatomic, neurologic, endocrine, metabolic) or functional causes. Functional constipation is the most common cause of constipation in children and is not associated with physical abnormalities or medications. Causes include poor toilet habits, voluntary withholding, low-fiber diet, and depression. Functional causes dominate in early childhood as a result of the psychosocial events surrounding early schooling. **(Emergency Medicine, Chapter 35, pp 323–337)**

10.d. Ultrasonography is 97% sensitive and 100% specific for the diagnosis of pyloric stenosis. This accuracy is due to direct visualization of the hypertrophied pylorus muscle with this procedure. The diagnosis of constipation is mainly based on history, and plain radiographs can be used to confirm diffuse stool throughout the bowel. A suspicion of midgut volvulus should be confirmed with an upper gastrointestinal series (100% sensitive). Other supportive studies include plain films showing the "double bubble" sign or a paucity of gas in the small and large bowels. A number of studies can be used to diagnose Hirschsprung's disease, including a barium enema, ultrasonography, anorectal manometry, or rectal biopsy. The diagnosis of hernias is based on history and clinical exam, with plain film studies if bowel obstruction is suspected. **(Emergency Medicine, Chapter 35, pp 323–337)**

11.b. Hemorrhoids are classified as either internal or external. External hemorrhoids are located below the dentate line and are covered by skin. Internal hemorrhoids arise above the dentate line and have a mucous membrane covering. Internal hemorrhoids are classified as follows:
First degree—the hemorrhoids are seen above the dentate line in the submucosal vascular tissue and appear as a bulge into the lumen.
Second degree—the hemorrhoids are visible protruding through the anus on straining but reduce spontaneously.
Third degree—the hemorrhoids prolapse through the anal margin and require manual reduction
Fourth degree—the hemorrhoids are prolapsed through the anus but cannot be reduced. They are now at risk of thrombosis and strangulation. **(Emergency Medicine, Chapter 42, pp 398–409)**

12.b. It is important to include foreign body in the differential diagnosis when managing such patients. As in this case, patients often deny the possibility of a foreign body. When dealing with rectal foreign bodies, it is important to establish the type and location of the foreign body and the time of insertion. Also assess for the possibility of complications (e.g., perforation or sepsis). When the presence of a sharp object cannot be excluded, digital rectal examination is contraindicated. Anoscopy can be helpful to identify the type and location of the foreign body and determine the presence and extent of tissue injury. Radiographs can be helpful to define the type, size, and location of a suspected foreign body and also assess the possibility of perforation. If a complication is suspected (perforation/sepsis), as in this case, IV fluids, blood culture, and antimicrobials are recommended. Soft, low-lying anorectal foreign bodies may be removed in the ED. All others should have surgical or gastrointestinal consult for evaluation and foreign body removal. Anoscopy is important after removal to look for additional foreign bodies and identify tissue damage caused by the foreign body itself or by its removal. *(Emergency Medicine, Chapter 42, pp 398–409)*

13.d. Bleeding is not typical of anorectal abscess. Its presence suggests an accompanying fissure. Pain is the most common presenting symptom. There are cases where pain is minimal or absent, for example, neuropathy, immune compromise, or draining abscess. Constipation caused by pain is common. Centrally mediated urinary retention can occur.

Most anorectal abscesses result from cryptoglandular infection in the intersphincteric space. From there, infection may spread and involve other spaces (e.g., ischiorectal abscess from horizontal spread, supralevator abscess from upward spread, perianal abscess from downward spread). In the remainder of cases (10%), an underlying disease process can be identified, such as inflammatory bowel disease or malignancy.

Physical findings largely depend on the space involved. Rectal examination is important to delineate the site and extent of infection. Pain is a limiting feature, and examination under anesthesia may be needed. As with abscesses elsewhere, treatment consists of incision and drainage. Antimicrobials are generally not indicated, except in patients with immune compromise, valvular heart disease, and prosthetic devices.

Aggressive treatment is needed when the patient has immune compromise or when necrotizing infection is suspected. In these cases, spread can be rapid and outcome fatal.

In neutropenic patients, rectal manipulation should be avoided. Early antimicrobial therapy is essential, and surgical intervention is reserved for cases in which medical management has failed. *(Emergency Medicine, Chapter 42, pp 398–409)*

14.e. In chronic anal fissure, there is typically a single midline fissure with well-defined edges. White diagonal fibers of the anal sphincter may be visible in the base. The second feature, the sentinel pile, represents an edematous skinfold and is found at the distal end of the fissure. In chronic fissures the papilla, which is proximal, becomes hypertrophic and prominent; it typically measures about 1 to 3 cm. Chronic fissures result from inadequate treatment of acute fissures. Unlike acute fissures, pain is not a major feature. The symptoms of bleeding, mucous discharge, and pruritus are common and are often intermittent.

Management consists of measures to relieve constipation and promote healing—stool softeners and sitz baths. For definitive management, referral to a surgeon is recommended.

Postanal dimples are typically associated with developmental cysts and not fissures. *(Emergency Medicine, Chapter 42, pp 398–409)*

15.a. iv; b. i; c. ii; d. v; e. iii

Rectal prolapse: Manual reduction is often successful but generally only temporary. These patients can be discharged home from the ED with outpatient surgical referral. Surgical consult in the ED is needed if the prolapse cannot be reduced or if there is evidence of ischemia.

Pilonidal cyst: Although incision and drainage are helpful to manage abscess formation of a pilonidal cyst, the abscess will tend to recur as long as the cyst exists. Definitive management of the pilonidal cyst itself is marsupialization of the cyst.

Fourth-degree internal hemorrhoids: This implies that the prolapsed hemorrhoids cannot be reduced and as such are at risk of thrombosis or infarction. Once this diagnosis is made, emergent surgical consult is needed.

Simple perianal abscess: This is treated like abscess anywhere else—incision and drainage. Antimicrobials are generally not indicated.

Acute external thrombosed hemorrhoids: External hemorrhoids occur below the dentate line and are covered by skin. When thrombosis occurs, pain can be severe. If symptoms are present for less than 48 hours, local excision of the thrombus is recommended. If symptoms are present for more than 48 hours, medical management and symptomatic relief are generally sufficient. *(Emergency Medicine, Chapter 42, pp 398–409)*

16.d. The history of constipation, mucus, and soiling with painless mass per rectum suggests rectal prolapse or internal hemorrhoids. The physical finding of a large painless mass with circumferential folds is consistent with complete rectal prolapse. It occurs at the extremes of age. In the elderly it occurs because of weakening of the supporting structures from aging and in association with chronic constipation and straining. In children, rectal prolapse occurs primarily in patients younger than 5 years. Constipation or acute diarrhea is often seen. Risk factors include cystic fibrosis, polyps, and Hirschsprung's disease. In about 15% of cases, no cause can be found.

In adults, prolapse tends to recur after manual reduction, necessitating outpatient surgical referral. If the prolapse is not reducible or evidence of ischemia exists, surgical consult should be requested immediately. In children, rectal prolapse usually resolves with resolution of the underlying problem, such as acute diarrhea. About 10% will fail medical therapy and need surgical management.

Rectal prolapse can be classified as complete prolapse, internal prolapse, or mucosal prolapse. In a complete prolapse, all layers of the rectum are involved, and circumferential folds of tissue are seen protruding through the anus. Internal prolapse represents intussusception of the rectum without prolapse through the anal sphincter. Mucosal prolapse is not a true rectal prolapse because it involves the mucosal layer of the rectum only. This is seen as a radial fold configuration on examination. *(Emergency Medicine, Chapter 42, pp 398–409)*

BIBLIOGRAPHY

Clark M: Gastrointestinal obstruction. *In* Howell JM, Altieri M, Jagoda AS, et al (eds): Emergency Medicine. Philadelphia, WB Saunders, 1998, pp 323–337.

Groleau G, Perpall A: Anorectal disorders. *In* Howell JM, Altieri M, Jagoda AS, et al (eds): Emergency Medicine. Philadelphia, WB Saunders, 1998, pp 398–409.

SECTION FIVE

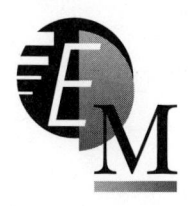

Serious Infections

17 Febrile Child

ROBBY MAHADEO, MD

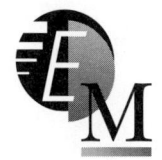

1. A 3-week-old, full-term infant presents to the ED with a rectal temperature of 96.0°F. Which management decision would be the most appropriate?
   a. Partial sepsis diagnostic evaluation without IV antibiotic
   b. Partial sepsis diagnostic evaluation with IV antibiotics
   c. Complete sepsis diagnostic evaluation without IV antibiotics
   d. Complete sepsis diagnostic evaluation with IV antibiotics
   e. Overhead warmer and discharge after temperature normalizes

2. At what temperature is a fever considered to be "harmful"?
   a. 103°F
   b. 104°F
   c. 105°F
   d. 106°F
   e. 107°F

3. Which body site is most appropriate in determining the presence of a fever in a young child?
   a. Axilla
   b. Mouth
   c. Rectum
   d. Tympanic membrane
   e. Any of the above

4. Noninfectious causes of fever include:
   a. Thyrotoxicosis
   b. Cerebral palsy
   c. Serum sickness
   d. Leukemia
   e. All of the above

5. A 2-week-old infant born at 36 weeks presents for a routine clinic visit bundled in blankets and has a temperature of 101°F. No antipyretics were given. The child appears well, and a repeat rectal temperature was 98.7°F. Which of the following would be the most appropriate management decision?
   a. Partial sepsis diagnostic evaluation without IV antibiotics
   b. Partial sepsis diagnostic evaluation with IV antibiotics
   c. Complete sepsis diagnostic evaluation without IV antibiotics
   d. Complete sepsis diagnostic evaluation with IV antibiotics
   e. Good discharge instructions with follow-up visit in 24 hours

6. Which of the following organisms can commonly cause infections in infants?
   a. *Streptococcus pneumoniae*
   b. Group B streptococcus
   c. *Escherichia coli*
   d. *Listeria monocytogenes*
   e. All of the above

7. Factors associated with sepsis in the newborn include all of the following except:
   a. Low birth weight
   b. Prolonged rupture of membranes
   c. A heart rate of 160
   d. Maternal fever
   e. Meconium-stained amniotic fluid

8. Which of the following statements about infants is false?
   a. A single episode of fever may be the only sign of meningitis.
   b. Late-onset group B streptococcus has a peak occurrence at about 4 weeks of age.
   c. *Streptococcus pneumoniae* infection occurs commonly.
   d. *Listeria monocytogenes* infection occurs infrequently.
   e. Irritability and fussiness are common complaints in this age group.

9. Which of the following is not an independent variable that describes an infant's appearance according to the Yale Infant Observation Scale?
   a. Color

b. Hydration state
c. Reaction to parental stimulation
d. Quality of infant's cry
e. Fever

10. Which of the following regarding children in the 3-month to 3-year age range is false?
    a. Half of this group seeking medical attention for fever will be diagnosed with upper respiratory infections or otitis media.
    b. They will experience a febrile illness 3 to 6 times during this time period.
    c. Sixty-five percent of all febrile children seek medical care.
    d. Febrile children represent 25% of all pediatric ED visits.
    e. Most children with fever without a source appear well.

11. Which of the following is the most accurate description of "paradoxical irritability"?
    a. Failure of the baby to be comforted by the nurse
    b. Failure of the baby to be comforted by the doctor
    c. Failure of the baby to be comforted by the mother
    d. Irritability during phlebotomy
    e. Crying during feeding

12. A 1-year-old male presents to the ED with rhinorrhea and a temperature of 103°F. He received a measles-mumps-rubella vaccination 12 days earlier. On examination, he appears well with no obvious source of fever. Which of the following would be the most appropriate medical management decision?
    a. Partial sepsis evaluation and discharge without antibiotics
    b. Decongestants for rhinorrhea
    c. Partial sepsis evaluation with IM antibiotics
    d. Discharge with antipyretics
    e. Full sepsis evaluation with IV antibiotics

13. The mother of a 2-year-old boy reports that her son has been spiking fevers for 1 week. Which of the following statements is false?
    a. Multiple courses of antimicrobials may be a source of the fever.
    b. The majority of viral illnesses produce fever of only a few days' duration.
    c. The parents may be reporting afebrile temperature.
    d. Malignancies are not usually included in the differential diagnosis.
    e. Two separate viral illnesses can account for the fever.

14. Which organisms are most likely to infect children 3 months to 3 years of age?
    a. *Haemophilus influenzae* and *Neisseria meningitidis*
    b. *Haemophilus influenzae* and *Escherichia coli*
    c. Group B streptococcus and *Neisseria meningitidis*
    d. Group B streptococcus and *Escherichia coli*
    e. *Streptococcus pneumoniae* and group A streptococcus

15. Which of the following statements about meningitis is false?
    a. A normal child may have a full fontanelle while supine.
    b. Soft pulsations of the fontanelle may occur without obvious pathology.
    c. A stiff neck is a reliable sign in children older than 1 year.
    d. A stiff neck is present in only 3% to 27% of infants less than 6 months of age with meningitis.
    e. It is possible to elicit meningismus in babies.

16. Children with the following foreign bodies are prone to serious consequences as a result of a febrile illness except:
    a. Ventriculoperitoneal shunt
    b. Central venous catheters
    c. Cystostomy tubes
    d. Arterial catheters
    e. Mitral valve prosthesis

17. A 7-week-old full-term baby presents to the ED with a temperature of 104°F. Physical examination is unremarkable. Cultures for blood and urine are obtained. No abnormalities are noted on urinalysis. A CBC reveals a WBC count of 12,000. Appropriate management decisions include all of the following except:
    a. Discharge without antimicrobials but appropriate follow-up care
    b. Discharge after receiving 50 mg/kg ceftriaxone IM
    c. Discharge only after normal results from a lumbar puncture are obtained
    d. Full sepsis evaluation with IV antibiotics until cultures are negative
    e. Chest radiography and admission if an infiltrate is present

18. Which of the following statements regarding urinary tract infections is false?
    a. A normal urinalysis excludes pyelonephritis.
    b. Males with urinary tract infections are seen most often in the first 6 months of life.
    c. Females have a higher frequency of urinary tract infections than males.
    d. White females are more at risk for urinary tract infections than black females.
    e. Tumor necrosis factor predicts bacteremia and sepsis.

19. In studies of children with clear-cut cases of meningitis on presentation, how long has it taken to administer antibiotics after arrival to the ED?
    a. ½ hr
    b. 1 hr
    c. 1½ hr
    d. 2 hr
    e. 2½ hr

20. Which of the following is least likely to cause a fever in an infant less than 2 months of age?
    a. Urinary tract infection
    b. Congenital syphilis
    c. *Listeria* sepsis
    d. Viral sepsis
    e. Mononucleosis

Answers

1.d. Hypothermia (a temperature of <96.5°F or 36.5°C) has the same significance as fever (≥100.4°F or 38°C) in infants. Blood, urine, and spinal fluid must be cultured, and a CBC, urinalysis, and cerebrospinal fluid cell count and chemistry obtained. The patient should be admitted after starting IV antimicrobials pending culture results. (*Emergency Medicine, Chapter 43, pp 411–420*)

2.e. A harmful fever is a temperature of 107°F, which is the temperature at which brain damage begins to occur as a result of disruption of enzyme function. (*Emergency Medicine, Chapter 43, pp 411–420*)

3.c. The four sites routinely used to measure a patient's temperature are the axilla, mouth, rectum, and tympanic membrane. Although oral temperatures can accurately reflect the core body temperature, results are influenced by both mouth breathing and the temperature of any recently ingested food or drink. Although the temperature of the vascular tympanic membrane should also reflect the core body temperature, tympanic thermography requires that the probe be oriented toward the tympanic membrane and not at the ear canal or any cerumen within it. This is often difficult in the small child because of both lack of cooperation and the shape of the ear canal. The axillary temperature is a surface temperature with a low sensitivity for detecting fever, because the temperature of skin is subject to the effect of both physiologic vasoconstriction and environmental warming and cooling. The rectal temperature is the only site that reliably reflects a child's core body temperature and therefore has become the gold standard for measurement of temperature in children. (*Emergency Medicine, Chapter 43, pp 411–420*)

4.e. Noninfectious causes of fever include malignancies and autoimmune disorders such as serum sickness and drug fever. Endocrine causes, particularly thyrotoxicosis, are rare but important causes of fever because they have substantial morbidity and even mortality if they remain unrecognized and untreated. A neurologically impaired child may have a dysfunctioning hypothalamus that causes recurrent fevers, as is seen in various congenital anomalies and cerebral palsy and after radiation therapy. (*Emergency Medicine, Chapter 43, pp 411–420*)

5.e. An infant who is overdressed and blanketed may experience fevers up to 101.5°F without ill effects and without an infectious cause. If the temperature returns to normal within 15 to 30 minutes after unbundling and without antipyretics and if the infant appears well, nothing further need be done. (*Emergency Medicine, Chapter 43, pp 411–420*)

6.e. Infections from group B streptococcus and *Escherichia coli* are perinatally acquired and may present in the first week of life. Late-onset group B streptococcus or *E. coli* infections have a peak occurrence at about 4 weeks of life and have a high potential for severe morbidity and mortality. *Listeria monocytogenes*, *Salmonella* species, and *Streptococcus pneumoniae* infections occur less frequently. (*Emergency Medicine, Chapter 43, pp 411–420*)

7.c. The presence of maternal fever is an important clue to sepsis in the baby, as are a history of prematurity, low birth weight, prolonged or premature rupture of membranes, and meconium staining of the amniotic fluid. The normal heart rate of an infant varies from 120 to 180. (*Emergency Medicine, Chapter 43, pp 411–420*)

8.c. Children between 1 and 8 weeks of age with fevers are less likely to be septic than are febrile neonates, but they may have only a single episode of fever as the only sign of a serious bacterial infection or meningitis. Late-onset group B streptococcus or *E. coli* infections have a peak occurrence at about 4 weeks of life and have a high potential for severe morbidity and mortality. *Listeria monocytogenes*, *Salmonella* species and *Streptococcus pneumoniae* infections occur less frequently. Irritability, fussiness, and poor sleeping are common complaints in infancy; however, if the mother, especially one who is experienced, reports these complaints to be more marked with fever or significantly different from normal behavior, they cannot be dismissed as mere colic. (*Emergency Medicine, Chapter 43, pp 411–420*)

9.e. The McCarthy or Yale Observation Scale is useful in describing an infant's appearance because there is no universally accepted definition of toxic-appearing infants. This scale is made up of six independent variables that measure (1) the quality of an infant's cry; (2) reaction to parental stimulation; (3) the state of arousal from aware to unarousable; (4) color; (5) hydration status; and (6) response to social overtures. Although not absolutely predictive in an individual case, lower scores have been correlated with increased risk of serious infection. (*Emergency Medicine, Chapter 43, pp 411–420*)

10.d. Children will experience fever an average of 3 to 6 times between the age of 3 months and 3 years. During this period, approximately 65% of them will be brought to medical attention for a febrile illness. At least half of this group of children will receive a diagnosis of upper respiratory infection or otitis media. In the ED, febrile children in this age group represent 10% of all pediatric visits. Those who appear ill or have an obvious focus of infection do not present a diagnostic problem; however, most children will appear well and without a source for this fever. (*Emergency Medicine, Chapter 43, pp 411–420*)

11.c. Paradoxical irritability is the failure of a baby to be comforted by his or her mother or father. (*Emergency Medicine, Chapter 43, pp 411–420*)

12. d. A history of vaccination within the past 48 hours (diphtheria-pertussis-tetanus or *Haemophilus influenzae* type B) or 10 to 14 days (measles-mumps-rubella) is an adequate explanation of a fever up to 104°F (lower for measles-mumps-rubella) and does not require further evaluation provided the infant appears well. The risk of bacteremia is not increased in such infants. *(Emergency Medicine, Chapter 43, pp 411–420)*

13. d. The duration of fever is important. The majority of viral illnesses and occult bacteremia produce fever of only a few days' duration. If the fever has persisted for more than a week, it is important to find out how the parents are taking the temperature and what they are reporting as fever. Parents may report afebrile temperatures (99°F to 100.4°F) as fever, thereby giving the impression that two separate mild illnesses may be a single, more worrisome illness. Prolonged fever generally occurs with more serious conditions such as osteomyelitis, endocarditis, malignancies, and autoimmune disorders. Children with repeated febrile illnesses such as otitis media and sinusitis who have been on multiple courses of antibiotics may develop drug fever that stops only after cessation of treatment. *(Emergency Medicine, Chapter 43, pp 411–420)*

14. a. The bacterial organisms most likely to infect children 3 months to 3 years of age are *Streptococcus pneumoniae, Neisseria meningitidis,* and *Haemophilus influenzae. (Emergency Medicine, Chapter 43, pp 411–420)*

15. c. A bulging fontanelle may indicate the presence of increased intracranial pressure. However, a normal child may have a full fontanelle while supine that disappears when sitting. Soft pulsations of the fontanelle may occur without obvious pathology. A stiff neck is a reliable sign in children older than 18 months, but it is present in only 3% to 27% of infants younger than 6 months with meningitis. It is possible to elicit meningismus in babies by supporting the trunk and watching for pain or failure to support the head. *(Emergency Medicine, Chapter 43, pp 411–420)*

16. c. Children with chronic, underlying medical conditions, most commonly immunodeficiency or implanted catheters (ventriculoperitoneal shunts or central venous catheters), are more likely to have serious consequences from infections of typically less virulent organisms. Vegetations may form at the ends of catheters and produce septic emboli. A child with a mitral valve prosthesis is at increased risk for endocarditis. Common organisms include *Staphylococcus aureus, Staphylococcus epidermidis,* and streptococcal species. Gastrostomy and cystostomy do not place the child at risk for these infections because they are not in direct contact with the blood stream. *(Emergency Medicine, Chapter 43, pp 411–420)*

17. e. There are a number of options available for the management of febrile infants in the 4- to 12-week age group. Ill-appearing infants require a full sepsis evaluation and treatment, but well-appearing infants may require no more than a CBC, urinalysis, and cultures of blood and urine. If those studies are normal (WBC between 5000 and 15,000 and the urinalysis has less than 10 WBC per high-power field), the risk of a serious bacterial infection approaches zero. Some physicians consider it safe to discharge these infants with good follow-up on no antimicrobials or after parenteral ceftriaxone. Others recommend that discharge be allowed only after a normal lumbar puncture is obtained. Still other physicians would recommend a full sepsis evaluation and admission on IV antimicrobials pending negative culture results. A chest radiograph is not part of the evaluation unless there are specific signs or symptoms suggesting lower respiratory tract infections. *(Emergency Medicine, Chapter 43, pp 411–420)*

18. a. A normal urinalysis does not exclude the presence of a urinary tract infection or even pyelonephritis. Pyuria is present in just over 50% of children with urinary tract infection. Positive cultures from a bagged urine specimen should be confirmed by a catheterized or suprapubic aspiration specimen. Males with urinary tract infections present most often in the first 6 months of life. These infections are usually associated with congenital anomalies of the urinary tract. Females have a higher frequency of urinary tract infections than males, and white females have a higher risk than black females. Early indicators of inflammation such as interleukin-6 or tumor necrosis factor have been shown to predict bacteremia and sepsis, but these tests are not readily available. *(Emergency Medicine, Chapter 43, pp 411–420)*

19. d. The mean time to administer antimicrobials in cases of clear-cut meningitis has been measured at 2 hours after ED arrival, compared with a more desirable 30-minute interval. The time it takes to perform a lumbar puncture is the most common cause of this delay. Thus, the current recommendations are to administer antimicrobials before head CT and lumbar puncture, if meningitis is suspected. *(Emergency Medicine, Chapter 43, pp 411–420)*

20. e. Mononucleosis is included in the differential diagnosis of fever in children older than 2 years. Urinary tract infection, congenital syphilis, *Listeria* species, and viral sepsis should be included in the differential diagnosis of fever of infants younger than 2 months. *(Emergency Medicine, Chapter 43, pp 411–420)*

BIBLIOGRAPHY

Orenstein JB: Approach to the febrile child. *In* Howell JM, Altieri M, Jagoda AS, et al (eds): Emergency Medicine. Philadelphia, WB Saunders, 1998, pp 411–420.

18 Approach to the Patient with HIV Infection and AIDS

RICHARD J. WONG, MD

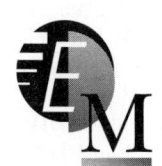

1. All of the following statements concerning *Cryptococcus neoformans* are true except:
   a. *Cryptococcus neoformans* is one of the most common causes of meningitis in AIDS patients.
   b. In patients with suspected cryptococcal meningitis the opening pressure will rarely be elevated.
   c. The drug of choice for cryptococcal meningitis is amphotericin B.
   d. Fungal cerebrospinal fluid cultures are positive in essentially 100% of patients with cryptococcal meningitis.
   e. India ink preparation of the cerebrospinal fluid is less sensitive than cryptococcal antigen.

2. All are true regarding cytomegalovirus retinitis except:
   a. More than 25% of AIDS patients develop cytomegalovirus retinitis.
   b. Fundoscopy may reveal perivascular white granular infiltrates and hemorrhages.
   c. Emergency ophthalmologic referral is mandatory in any AIDS patient with new visual symptoms.
   d. The drug of choice for cytomegalovirus retinitis is acyclovir, 10 mg/kg IV every 8 hours.

3. All of the following clinical features are characteristic of *Pneumocystis carinii* pneumonia except:
   a. *Pneumocystis carinii* is the most common cause of pulmonary disease in the late stage of HIV infection.
   b. *Pneumocystis carinii* is the most common cause of bilateral diffuse infiltrates on chest radiographs.
   c. Up to 10% of patients with *Pneumocystis carinii* can develop a pneumothorax.
   d. The patient commonly complains of a dry, nonproductive cough, malaise, fever, and night sweats.
   e. The patient's CD4+ is greater than 400 cells/mm^3.

4. All of the following are reasonable guidelines regarding evaluating a patient with suspected *Pneumocystis carinii* pneumonia except:
   a. Copious purulent sputum argues strongly against *Pneumocystis carinii* pneumonia.
   b. The suspicion of *Pneumocystis carinii* pneumonia should be entertained in HIV patients with complaints of dyspnea on exertion.
   c. An elevated serum lactate dehydrogenase and an elevated A–a gradient with a Pao$_2$ less than 80 mm Hg are nonspecific findings that should increase suspicion for *Pneumocystis carinii* pneumonia.
   d. *Pneumocystis carinii* pneumonia may be associated with cavitary lesions on chest radiography.
   e. Corticosteroids are contraindicated in patients with moderate to severe *Pneumocystis carinii* pneumonia (Pao$_2$ <70 mm Hg).

5. All of the following are adult AIDS-related pneumonias except:
   a. Lymphoid interstitial pneumonitis
   b. *Pneumocystis carinii*
   c. *Mycobacterium tuberculosis*
   d. *Staphylococcus aureus*
   e. *Cryptococcus neoformans*

6. All of the following are true regarding AIDS except:
   a. Ninety percent of AIDS-defining illnesses occur in patients with a CD4+ T-lymphocyte count greater than 300 cells/mm^3.
   b. Cytomegalovirus and *Mycobacterium avium-intracellulare* infections rarely occur in AIDS patients with a CD4+ greater than 50 cells/mm^3.
   c. In the United States, Kaposi's sarcoma is much more common in homosexual and bisexual men than in IV drug users.
   d. Among women, Kaposi's sarcoma is rare except among female sexual partners of bisexual men.
   e. Tuberculosis is more common in IV drug users than in homosexual and bisexual men.

7. The most common cause of AIDS retinitis is:
   a. *Toxoplasma gondii*
   b. *Candida albicans*
   c. *Treponema pallidum*
   d. Herpes zoster virus
   e. Cytomegalovirus

8. The most common cause of meningitis in AIDS is:
   a. *Cryptococcus neoformans*
   b. *Histoplasma capsulatum*

c. *Listeria monocytogenes*
d. *Mycobacterium tuberculosis*
e. *Haemophilus influenzae*

9. A 22-year-old male is brought to the ED by ambulance. He is awake, alert, and oriented. Vital signs reveal a temperature of 101.4°F. The patient complains that bright lights bother him and that he has mild neck stiffness. He also indicates that he is HIV positive, but he does not know his CD4+ lymphocyte count. An emergent CT scan with contrast is negative for mass lesions or evidence of increased intracranial pressure. The opening pressure on lumbar puncture is greater than 300 mm Hg. The cerebrospinal fluid cryptococcal antigen is positive. The best initial management of the increased intracranial pressure is:
   a. Serial lumbar puncture to remove approximately 20 mL of cerebrospinal fluid
   b. Ventriculoperitoneal shunt placement
   c. Treatment with high-dose dexamethasone
   d. Treatment with IV amphotericin B (1 mg/kg per day)
   e. Treatment with acetazolamide

10. Which is least likely to cause intracranial mass effect in an AIDS patient?
    a. *Toxoplasma gondii*
    b. Non-Hodgkin's lymphoma
    c. Kaposi's sarcoma
    d. Progressive multifocal leukoencephalopathy
    e. *Cryptococcus neoformans*

11. All of the following are true regarding AIDS-related mass lesions except:
    a. Prophylactic anticonvulsant therapy is recommended.
    b. CNS lymphoma carries a poor prognosis despite radiation therapy.
    c. Patients with toxoplasmosis and lymphoma may require steroids to control cerebral edema and increased intracranial pressure.
    d. These patients usually have altered mental status, focal neurologic deficits, and seizures.
    e. Toxoplasmosis characteristically appears as multiple ring-enhancing lesions on head CT. If these are seen, patients should be presumptively started on pyrimethamine, sulfadiazine, and folinic acid.

12. A 35-year-old HIV-positive male presents with a history of watery, bloody diarrhea for 6 days. He also complains of mild, crampy abdominal pain and has had a subjective fever at home. He has not traveled outside New York City in more than 5 years. On physical exam, he is a thin, well-developed, well-dressed male in no acute distress. His oral temperature is 100.9°F, his heart rate is 112, and he is mildly orthostatic. His physical exam is remarkable only for a rectal exam that reveals guaiac-positive mucus. All of the following are important diagnostic tests or treatment options except:
    a. IV rehydration with normal saline
    b. Blood cultures
    c. Antimotility agents to control his gastrointestinal symptoms.
    d. Stool culture
    e. Stool for ova and parasites

13. Regarding HIV and health care workers, all of the following are true except:
    a. The transmission of HIV from patients to health care workers is rare.
    b. Percutaneous injuries from needles or other sharp instruments contaminated with HIV-infected blood carry a risk of infection of approximately 0.5%.
    c. The risk of HIV transmission is greatest if infected blood is in direct contact with mucous membranes or nonintact skin.
    d. Workers in inner-city EDs have a higher risk of HIV infection compared with workers in suburban EDs.
    e. Universal Precaution protocols are based on the premise that the blood and body fluid from all patients is potentially hazardous.

14. Match the following AIDS-associated pulmonary condition with the likely radiographic pattern (a choice may be used more than once or not at all):
    a. Diffuse interstitial reticulonodular infiltrate
    b. Focal infiltrate
    c. Nodular infiltrate
    d. Pneumothorax
    e. Cavitary lesions

    i. *Streptococcus pneumoniae*
    ii. *Pneumocystis carinii*
    iii. *Mycobacterium tuberculosis*
    iv. *Staphylococcus aureus*
    v. *Mycobacterium avium* complex

Answers

1.b. *Cryptococcus neoformans*, a yeast-like fungus, is the most common cause of meningitis in patients with AIDS. The opening pressure, measured during lumbar puncture, is elevated (>200 mm H₂O) in approximately 70% of patients. Although the traditional method of identifying *Cryptococcus* is an India ink preparation, it is less sensitive than cryptococcal antigen. Fungal cerebrospinal fluid cultures are positive in nearly 100% of cases. The initial treatment of suspected cryptococcal meningitis is usually amphotericin B. *(Emergency Medicine, Chapter 44, pp 421–444)*

2.d. Cytomegalovirus, a member of the herpes family, infects the retina in more than 25% of AIDS patients. Symptoms depend on the area of the retina involved; although central lesions cause scotomas or visual field defects, the impression of floaters may be the only complaint. The classic lesions seen on fundoscopy are perivascular white granular infiltrates and hemorrhage. To minimize the potential for further vision loss, emergency referral to an ophthalmologist is mandatory in any AIDS patients with visual symptoms. Hospitalization for IV ganciclovir or foscarnet may be required to limit disease progression. *(Emergency Medicine, Chapter 44, pp 421–444)*

3.e. *Pneumocystis carinii* is the most common cause of pulmonary disease in late HIV infection, usually appearing as diffuse bilateral infiltrates on chest radiography. Pneumothoraces occur in up to 10% of patients with *Pneumocystis carinii* pneumonia. Although *Pneumocystis* may cause fulminant pulmonary disease, the more common presentation is an indolent onset of a dry cough, malaise, fever, and night sweats. AIDS patients with CD4+ counts above 200 to 300 cells/mm^3 are unlikely to have *Pneumocystis carinii* pneumonia. *(Emergency Medicine, Chapter 44, pp 421–444)*

4.e. *Pneumocystis carinii* is an organism with both fungal and protozoan features. The cough of patients with *Pneumocystis carinii* pneumonia is usually nonproductive. Cavitary lesions are seen with fulminant disease. Nonspecific findings, such as an elevated serum lactate dehydrogenase or an elevated A–a gradient, should increase the suspicion for *Pneumocystis carinii* pneumonia. Corticosteroids reduce both mortality and the risk of progression to respiratory failure in patients with *Pneumocystis carinii* pneumonia. Steroids are therefore indicated in a patient with moderate to severe infection, suggested by a Pao$_2$ on room air less than 70 mm. *(Emergency Medicine, Chapter 44, pp 421–444)*

5.a. Lymphoid interstitial pneumonitis is common only in children. A disease of unknown cause, lymphoid interstitial pneumonitis occurs in up to 40% of children with HIV infection. *(Emergency Medicine, Chapter 44, pp 421–444)*

6.a. Ninety percent of AIDS-defining illnesses occur in patients with a CD4+ T-lymphocyte count less than 200 cells/mm^3. *(Emergency Medicine, Chapter 44, pp 421–444)*

7.e. The most common cause of AIDS retinitis is cytomegalovirus. More than 25% of AIDS patients develop cytomegalovirus retinitis. Other causes of retinitis in AIDS patients include *Toxoplasma gondii, Candida albicans, Treponema pallidum,* herpes zoster virus, and *Pneumocystis carinii.* *(Emergency Medicine, Chapter 44, pp 421–444)*

8.a. *Cryptococcus neoformans*, a yeast-like fungus, is the most common cause of meningitis in the AIDS patient, affecting approximately 10% of all AIDS patients. *Histoplasma capsulatum* is a fungus that causes meningitis in a limited geographic area. *Listeria monocytogenes, Mycobacterium tuberculosis,* and *Haemophilus influenzae* are relatively uncommon causes of meningitis in AIDS patients. *(Emergency Medicine, Chapter 44, pp 421–444)*

9.a. Therapy for cryptococcal meningitis is usually begun with amphotericin B 0.7 mg/kg/day, but this is unlikely to reduce an elevated cerebrospinal fluid pressure. The increased intracranial pressure (opening pressure >200 mm Hg) caused by cryptococcal infection can be treated with serial lumbar punctures to remove large volumes (20 mL) of cerebrospinal fluid. When serial lumbar punctures do not control the increased intracranial pressure, a ventriculoperitoneal shunt should be considered. Glucocorticoids, osmotic agents, and acetazolamide are not generally recommended in the management of cryptococcal-induced increased intracranial pressure. *(Emergency Medicine, Chapter 44, pp 421–444)*

10.c. *Toxoplasma gondii,* non-Hodgkin's lymphoma, and progressive multifocal leukoencephalopathy account for 80% of all CNS mass lesions in late-stage HIV infection. *Cryptococcus neoformans* can cause cryptococcoma-type lesions. Kaposi's sarcoma is a very rare cause of HIV-related CNS mass lesions. *(Emergency Medicine, Chapter 44, pp 421–444)*

11.a. *Toxoplasma*, a protozoan, causes a characteristic ring-enhancing lesion on CT scan and MRI of the head. Toxoplasmosis and lymphoma may require a short course of steroids to control cerebral edema and increased intracranial pressure. If seizures occur, they can be treated with anticonvulsants; however, the prophylactic use of anticonvulsants is not recommended. Despite treatment, CNS lymphoma carries a poor prognosis. *(Emergency Medicine, Chapter 44, pp 421–444)*

12.c. The incidence of infectious diarrhea, both bacterial and parasitic, is higher in the HIV-positive population. The incidence of infection with *Entamoeba histolytica, Giardia lamblia,* and *Blastocystis hominis* is considerably higher in homosexual men. The management of acute diarrheal illness in an HIV-positive patient is similar to that of other patients. In all patients with febrile diarrheal illnesses, antimotility agents should be avoided and blood cultures should be considered as part of the diagnostic evaluation. *(Emergency Medicine, Chapter 44, pp 421–444)*

13.c. The transmission of HIV from infected patients to health care workers is rare. Although the risk of infection after percutaneous exposure is low (<0.5%), the risk of infection after mucous membrane or nonintact skin exposure is even lower (0.05%). The seroprevalence rate of HIV varies from 0.2% among suburban ED patients to 8.9% among inner-city ED patients. *(Emergency Medicine, Chapter 44, pp 421–444)*

14.a. ii, iii, v; b. i, iv; c. iii; d. ii; e. ii, iii, iv *(Emergency Medicine, Chapter 44, pp 421–444)*

BIBLIOGRAPHY

Miller KD, Polis MA: Approach to the patients with HIV infection and AIDS. *In* Howell JM, Altieri M, Jagoda AS, et al (eds): Emergency Medicine. Philadelphia, WB Saunders, 1998, pp 421–444.

19 Sepsis

DONALD BARTON, MD

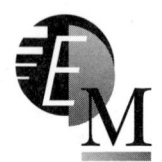

1. Agents useful in the management of hypotension caused by septic shock include all but:
    a. Dopamine
    b. Norepinephrine
    c. Phenylephrine
    d. Dobutamine
    e. IV fluids

2. The physiologic response to sepsis generally occurs in the following order:
    a. Hypotension, tachycardia, tachypnea
    b. Hypotension, tachypnea, tachycardia
    c. Tachycardia, tachypnea, hypotension
    d. Tachypnea, hypotension, tachycardia
    e. Tachypnea, tachycardia, hypotension

3. Which of the following is true of sepsis?
    a. The incidence of sepsis seen in the ED is increasing.
    b. The mortality rate of sepsis is as high as 60%.
    c. The onset of multiple organ dysfunction syndrome is a bad prognostic sign.
    d. Early recognition and treatment of sepsis may reduce both morbidity and mortality.
    e. All the above are true.

4. Which therapy for the indicated clinical condition is less than optimal?
    a. Ceftriaxone plus gentamicin for urinary tract infection
    b. Cefoxitin for a presumed abdominal source
    c. Nafcillin for abscess
    d. Vancomycin for endocarditis
    e. Ceftazidime and an aminoglycoside for neutropenia

5. An agitated 62-year-old presents to the ED with a history of cough and fever. Vital signs are temperature 101°F, heart rate 110, RR 20, and BP 80/60. On physical examination, the patient is found to have labored breathing, right-sided rales, and cold, clammy skin. Despite administration of oxygen by face mask, the patient remains dyspneic, with an oxygen saturation of 89% noted. The best choice of management at this point would be to:
    a. Intubate immediately without rapid-sequence intubation
    b. Establish IV access and intubate immediately using ketamine
    c. Bolus with normal saline and plan intubation using etomidate
    d. Bolus with Ringer's lactate and plan intubation using ketamine
    e. Bolus with Ringer's lactate and plan intubation using thiopental

6. Factors that contribute to the hypotension seen in septic shock include all of the following except:
    a. Systemic vasodilation
    b. Intravascular pooling
    c. Third spacing
    d. Evaporative losses from fever
    e. All of the above

7. A 70-year-old nursing home patient is brought to the ED with a history of fever and change in mental status. On presentation, vital signs are temperature 38.6°C, heart rate 100, RR 22, and BP 100/60. On examination, the patient is found to be confused with evidence of dehydration, but no source of infection is found. The following labs are obtained: CBC: H/H 11.1/33; WBC 13,500 with 15% bands; ABG pH 7.30; Pao$_2$ 80; Paco$_2$ 30; urinalysis 2+ leukocytes and nitrates with bacteria on microscopic examination. Which of the following abnormalities found in this patient are not included in the definition of sepsis?
    a. Hyperthermia
    b. Tachycardia
    c. Hypotension
    d. Hypocapnia
    e. Leukocytosis

8. Which of the following suggests a poor prognosis in a patient with sepsis?
    a. Preexisting dementia
    b. Elevated fibrin split products
    c. Guaiac-positive stools
    d. BUN to creatinine ratio greater than 10
    e. All of the above

9. True statements concerning volume deficits seen in sepsis include all of the following except:
   a. Subtle findings include cold or clammy extremities and delayed capillary refill.
   b. As much as 6 to 8 L of IV fluids may be required to obtain a euvolemic state.
   c. Sources of fluid loss include third spacing and insensible fluid loss.
   d. Blood transfusions should be given to hypotensive septic patients to maintain a hemoglobin between 12 and 14.
   e. Volume deficits may complicate the management of respiratory distress.

Answers

1.d. The initial management of any hypotensive septic patient should include fluids, either crystalloid or blood. Dopamine (5 to 10 µg/kg per minute) is the best first-line agent for treating hypotension caused by septic shock in the euvolemic or near-euvolemic patient. Having both inotropic and vasopressor properties, it should be titrated to maintain a mean arterial pressure of approximately 80 mm Hg. High-dose dopamine (up to 20 µg/kg per minute) may be attempted if hypotension remains refractory to lower doses. Norepinephrine (0.5 to 5.0 µg/kg per minute), which has predominately vasopressor properties, may be more reliable than high-dose dopamine at raising arterial pressure in the refractory patient. With significant tachycardia, phenylephrine may be useful because it exerts its effect predominately through alpha-receptors, increasing BP and inotropy without increasing heart rate. Epinephrine, which has both alpha and beta effects, can also be attempted in the refractory patient. Although dobutamine increases cardiac output, it is inherently vasodilatory and may in fact decrease BP. For this reason, dobutamine should probably not be given to the hypotensive septic patient. (*Emergency Medicine, Chapter 45, pp 445–450*)

2.e. The physiologic progression from sepsis to septic shock may occur rapidly, depending on multiple host factors. The earliest vital sign abnormality seen is usually tachypnea, because of the central effects of inflammatory mediators and as a response to acidosis. Because falling BP usually triggers an increase in heart rate, tachycardia usually precedes the onset of measurable hypotension, which appears only after normal compensatory mechanisms fail. Moreover, hypotension also results from the direct vasodilatory effect of inflammatory mediators (e.g., cytokines). (*Emergency Medicine, Chapter 45, pp 445–450*)

3.e. The combination of an aging population and advances in the outpatient management of a number of disease states (e.g., HIV, malignancy) has resulted in an increased number of patients presenting to the ED with sepsis. The death rate of septic patients has been estimated to be from 40% to 60% and may be as high as 90% among those who develop multiple organ dysfunction. Although extensive research has been done on identifying and characterizing the mediators of the inflammatory response to sepsis, the complexity of the interplay of these mediators has, to date, prevented the introduction of effective therapy directed at altering the inflammatory response. Short of this, the early detection and stabilization of the septic patient as well as use of appropriate broad-spectrum antimicrobials may go a long way in reducing both morbidity and mortality. (*Emergency Medicine, Chapter 45, pp 445–450*)

4.c. The early use of appropriate antimicrobial therapy in septic patients, preferably within 30 minutes of arrival to the ED, may reduce morbidity and mortality. Preexisting medical conditions, clinical history, and physical or laboratory findings may point to a source of infection. Although nafcillin is usually effective coverage for the bacterial pathogens present in most abscesses (*Staphylococcus aureus* and other streptococcal species), the treatment of choice of any abscess is drainage. (*Emergency Medicine, Chapter 45, pp 445–450*)

5.c. Although this patient with impending septic shock clearly requires intubation, it is advisable to administer an IV fluid bolus before intubation to prevent catastrophic hypotension. Both pharmacologic induction, which decreases venous tone, and positive pressure ventilation, which decreases venous return, adversely affect BP. Normal saline is preferred over Ringer's lactate because patients with severe systemic hypoperfusion may be unable to metabolize the lactate contained in Ringer's solution. Induction for rapid-sequence intubation should be with the smallest reasonable dose of an induction agent. Etomidate has been shown to have the least cardiovascular side effects of all the sedative agents used in rapid-sequence intubation. The dose of etomidate (0.3 mg/kg) should be reduced in the elderly. (*Emergency Medicine, Chapter 45, pp 445–450*)

6.e. Patients with septic shock can have significant volume deficits and may require as much as 6 to 8 L of IV fluid to be brought to a euvolemic state. A number of factors contribute to this volume deficit. The inflammatory mediators released in sepsis cause both systemic vasodilation, resulting in intravascular pooling, and increased capillary leakage, resulting in third space losses. Increased insensible losses occur because of fever and tachypnea. Septic patients often have had a period of decreased fluid intake because of anorexia and decreased mobility, preexisting medical conditions, and sepsis itself. In addition, the frequently associated vomiting and diarrhea directly contribute to fluid loss. (*Emergency Medicine, Chapter 45, pp 445–450*)

7.c. Sepsis is defined by the presence of two or more of the following: body temperature above 38°C or below 36°C; heart rate greater than 90; RR greater than 20; $PaCO_2$ less than 32; or total WBC count of more than 12,000 or less than 4000 cells/mm^3 or more than 10% band forms on the manual differential count. Hypotension can result from septic shock but is not part of the definition of sepsis. Although not all patients who meet this definition of sepsis are found to be septic, this definition is purposely broad to be certain that this diagnosis is not missed. *(Emergency Medicine, Chapter 45, pp 445–450)*

8.e. The onset of multiple organ dysfunction syndrome in the septic patient is associated with significantly increased mortality. Decreased tissue perfusion results in hypoxia, acidosis, and ultimately end-organ dysfunction and damage. Findings include pulmonary insufficiency and ARDS, myocardia dysfunction and decreased ejection fraction, hepatic and renal insufficiency, disseminated intravascular coagulation, adynamic ileus, and stress ulcers of the gut. An altered mental status is a poor prognostic factor in the septic patient. Changes that immediately precede the onset of sepsis suggest CNS infection, whereas changes that are rapid in onset or severe suggest overwhelming infection. Interestingly, preexisting alterations of mental status also portend a poor prognosis. *(Emergency Medicine, Chapter 45, pp 445–450)*

9.d. Volume deficits in sepsis can be significant and may require huge amounts of intravenous crystalloid solution to correct. If fluid requirements become large, a blood transfusion may be required to maintain a hemoglobin between 10 and 12, offsetting hemodilution and maintaining tissue oxygen delivery. Transfusing patients to higher hemoglobin levels has been proven to confer no additional benefit. Skin findings of impending or existing shock include cold or clammy extremities, diaphoresis, delayed capillary refill, and cyanosis. Alterations of mental status suggest decreased cerebral perfusion. Decreased tissue perfusion causes acidosis. Respiratory distress can result from direct lung injury (pneumonia), from lung injury caused by hypoperfusion (ARDS), or from centrally mediated attempts to correct acidosis. Management of respiratory distress, e.g., intubation and ventilation, is complicated by the fact that the induction agents used for rapid-sequence intubation are vasodilators and that positive pressure ventilation decreases venous return, both of which can exacerbate hypotension. *(Emergency Medicine, Chapter 45, pp 445–450)*

BIBLIOGRAPHY

Rothenhuis TC: Sepsis. *In* Howell JM, Altieri M, Jagoda AS, et al (eds): Emergency Medicine. Philadelphia, WB Saunders, 1998, pp 445–450.

20 CNS Infections (Meningitis and Encephalitis)

FRANK LoVECCHIO, DO

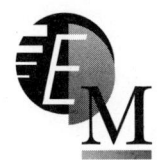

1. All of the following are true except:
   a. Fever may be absent in up to 44% of cases of adult meningitis.
   b. Petechial skin lesions may be noted in cases of meningitis.
   c. A Gram's stain may be positive in 80% of patients with untreated bacterial meningitis.
   d. Dexamethasone, if given early in the course in children with meningitis, may decrease the incidence of neurosensory hearing loss.
   e. *Listeria* meningitis classically presents with a lymphocytic predominance in the cerebrospinal fluid.

2. All are consistent with meningitis except:
   a. A flat anterior fontanelle
   b. Awake and a normal mental status
   c. Left arm paralysis
   d. Poor feeding
   e. Frontal headache

3. A lumbar puncture is contraindicated in all of the following except:
   a. A neonate with cardiorespiratory compromise
   b. A patient with papilledema
   c. Cellulitis involving the lumbosacral area
   d. Gastrointestinal hemorrhage caused by alcoholic hepatitis
   e. Scoliosis or severe degenerative joint disease

4. Which of the following cerebrospinal fluid values would be considered abnormal in a 1-week-old infant?
   a. 20 WBC/mm^3
   b. Sixty percent polymorphonuclear leukocytes
   c. Protein equal to 90 mg/dL
   d. 300 RBC/mm^3
   e. A cerebrospinal fluid glucose greater than two thirds of the serum glucose

5. Likely pathogens in the 1- to 3-week-old infant include all of the following except:
   a. *Escherichia coli*
   b. Group B streptococcus
   c. *Haemophilus influenzae*
   d. *Listeria monocytogenes*
   e. *Enterococcus* species

6. Which of the following organisms is most likely to cause infection of a shunt implanted for the treatment of hydrocephalus?
   a. *Pseudomonas aeruginosa*
   b. *Candida albicans*
   c. *Staphylococcus epidermidis*
   d. *Haemophilus influenzae*
   e. *Staphylococcus aureus*

7. The best indication for chemoprophylaxis against meningitis is in which of the following situations?
   a. Day care personnel after a brief contact with a child who eventually develops meningococcal meningitis
   b. Household members of a 3-year-old child with *H. influenzae* meningitis
   c. Medical personnel who briefly examined a patient with meningococcal meningitis but had no contact with oral secretions
   d. An HIV-infected employee after brief contact with a patient with meningococcal meningitis
   e. A sibling of a patient with meningitis who develops headache and fever

Answers

1.e. Fever may be absent in 44% of adults and 50% of infants with meningitis. Petechial rash may be a clue to infection with *Neisseria meningitidis*. A Gram's stain is positive in 80% of cases of bacterial meningitis. A decreased incidence of neurosensory hearing loss has been noted when dexamethasone therapy is instituted at the time of the initial dose of antimicrobials. *Listeria monocytogenes* is characterized by a monocytic, not lymphocytic, predominance in the cerebrospinal fluid WBCs. (*Emergency Medicine*, Chapter 46, pp 451–458)

2.c. The presentation of meningitis varies significantly with age. The clinician should have a high index of suspicion in order to make a prompt diagnosis, particularly in the extremes of age. An infant may present with a flat fontanelle caused by underlying dehydration. A bulging fontanelle is classically described; however, this is neither sensitive nor specific for meningitis. Patients are often awake and alert during their initial presentation of meningitis. Poor feeding may be the only presenting sign in children younger than 3 months and the elderly. A global headache is more common, although any location of cephalgia can be seen in meningitis. Focality of symptoms or findings is usually inconsistent with the diagnosis of meningitis and should raise the suspicion of an intracranial lesion. *(Emergency Medicine, Chapter 46, pp 451–458)*

3.e. There are four scenarios in which a lumbar puncture is contraindicated. First, any patient, particularly the neonate, with clinically significant cardiorespiratory compromise can be made worse by positioning for a lumbar puncture. Second, any patient with signs of increased intracranial pressure on physical examination (i.e., papilledema) should undergo cranial CT before lumbar puncture to exclude an intracranial lesion. Third, infection in the tissue to be traversed by the spinal needle should be avoided because the study may introduce organisms into the cerebrospinal fluid. Fourth, any patient with a history or clinical signs of a bleeding disorder should have the coagulopathy corrected before lumbar puncture. Spinal scoliosis and degenerative joint disease may make lumbar puncture more technically challenging but are not a contraindication. *(Emergency Medicine, Chapter 46, pp 451–458)*

4.d. During the first week of life, the cerebrospinal fluid WBC count can be as high as 32 cells/mm^3 with 60% polymorphonuclear leukocytes, although the typical range of a term neonate is 0 to 22 WBCs/mm^3. The cerebrospinal fluid protein of a newborn is significantly higher than that of an adult or older child, averaging 90 mg/dL, whereas cerebrospinal fluid glucose is similar to the adult value, averaging 70% to 80% of a serum glucose drawn in the same time frame. An elevated RBC count in the cerebrospinal fluid should raise the clinician's suspicion of child abuse or a CNS bleed. A traumatic lumbar puncture can be excluded by noting lack of clearing of RBCs in the terminal cerebrospinal fluid sample. *(Emergency Medicine, Chapter 46, pp 451–458)*

5.c. Making the diagnosis of meningitis in neonates is especially difficult because of the lack of specific diagnostic signs and symptoms in this age group. It is likely that pathogens are transferred to the infant transvaginally during delivery. Ampicillin is adequate coverage for group B streptococcus and has some activity against *Listeria monocytogenes* and *Enterococcus* species. An aminoglycoside or cefotaxime is necessary for coverage of *Escherichia coli* and other coliforms. *Haemophilus influenzae* is a more common pathogen in older children and adults and is not usually seen in neonates. *(Emergency Medicine, Chapter 46, pp 451–458)*

6.c. *Staphylococcus epidermidis* is the most frequent cause of infections involving CNS shunts. It frequently colonizes the skin and is thought to have an ability to stick to foreign surfaces. Although infections with the other organisms mentioned may occur, they are not the most likely. *(Emergency Medicine, Chapter 46, pp 451–458)*

7.b. Chemoprophylaxis is recommended for day care center personnel if exposure includes children younger than 2 years of age and contact is greater than 25 hours a week. When a meningococcus is the offending agent, prophylaxis is recommended for all household members, day care personnel, or medical personnel with a history of contact with the patient's oral secretions. No current recommendations exist for immunosuppressed individuals in contact with patients with meningitis; however, close observation is prudent. A sibling who exhibits symptoms consistent with meningitis should undergo prompt evaluation and treatment if necessary. Simply prescribing rifampin for patients with symptoms consistent with meningitis is not adequate. Chemoprophylaxis is recommended for all household members if the child with *H. influenzae* is younger than 4 years old. *(Emergency Medicine, Chapter 46, pp 451–458)*

BIBLIOGRAPHY

Ten Eyck R: Meningitis and encephalitis. *In* Howell JM, Altieri M, Jagoda AS, et al (eds): Emergency Medicine. Philadelphia, WB Saunders, 1998, pp 451–458.

21 Mycobacterial and Tick-Borne Infections

FRANK LoVECCHIO, DO

Mycobacterial Disease

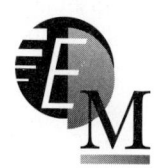

1. Administration of isoniazid for the treatment of tuberculosis is associated with all of the following except:
   a. Peripheral neuropathy
   b. Dizziness and ataxia
   c. Muscle fasciculations
   d. Hepatitis
   e. Photodermatitis

2. All of the following are considered high-risk groups for active tuberculosis except:
   a. Persons with diabetes mellitus
   b. Homeless inner-city residents
   c. Southeast Asian immigrants
   d. Alcohol and drug abusers
   e. Nursing home residents

3. All of the following statements concerning drugs used to treat tuberculosis are true except:
   a. Rifampin may accelerate the metabolism of other drugs.
   b. The most common adverse effect of pyrazinamide is renal insufficiency.
   c. Ethambutol can cause retrobulbar neuritis.
   d. Streptomycin should be given only parenterally.
   e. Isoniazid can cause seizures in overdose.

4. All of the following are true concerning pediatric tuberculosis except:
   a. Adults transmit the disease more easily than children.
   b. Reactivated tuberculosis is rare in children.
   c. Tuberculosis meningitis is the leading cause of death.
   d. Children younger than age 4 years have the highest rates of disease.
   e. Extrapulmonary tuberculosis is rare in children.

5. All of the following should be considered in the ED during stabilization of the hypotensive tuberculosis patient except:
   a. Crystalloids followed by vasopressors as needed
   b. Pericardiocentesis for acute pericardial tamponade
   c. Hydrocortisone
   d. Isoniazid, rifampin, and pyrazinamide therapy
   e. Oxygen for hypoxia

Answers

1.e. The most severe side effect of isoniazid therapy is hepatitis. The risk of hepatitis increases with age, daily ethanol use, and history of previous liver injury. Isoniazid-induced hepatitis is rare in patients younger than 20 years of age. Hepatitis is reported in 1.2% of 20- to 34-year-olds and in 2.3% of the population over age 50 receiving isoniazid. Peripheral neuropathy may occur, but vitamin B_6 can ameliorate this effect. Drug-induced lupus is reported in 20% of patients receiving isoniazid therapy having a positive antinuclear antibody. Isoniazid rarely produces a number of nonspecific neurologic sequelae, including convulsions, optic neuritis, muscle twitching, dizziness, and ataxia. Photodermatitis does not occur. *(Emergency Medicine, Chapter 47, pp 459–468)*

2.a. A high index of suspicion is necessary for the early diagnosis of tuberculosis. Tuberculosis is spread via inhalation; it is therefore not surprising to note an increased incidence in crowded habitats. Patients who are at high risk for tuberculosis and who have suspicious symptoms should be admitted for evaluation. Patients with HIV infection are at considerably higher risk for tuberculosis. Diabetes mellitus is not a risk factor for acquiring tuberculosis. *(Emergency Medicine, Chapter 47, pp 459–468)*

3.b. Rifampin is a potent inducer of the cytochrome P450 system. Before starting rifampin, all of a patient's current medications should be reviewed for potential interactions and whether they are metabolized in the liver. Because the most common and serious adverse effect of ethambutol therapy is retrobulbar neuritis, patients receiving ethambutol should be routinely questioned about visual symptoms. Streptomycin is available only in injectable form. Overdoses of isoniazid can present as status epilepticus. In the setting of isoniazid-induced seizures, pyridoxine should be given parenterally, 1 g for each gram of isoniazid ingested or 5 g if the amount ingested is unknown. Liver abnormalities are the most common adverse effect of pyrazinamide therapy. Renal disease is rarely reported with pyrazinamide chemotherapy. *(Emergency Medicine, Chapter 47, pp 459–468)*

4.e. Adults have a more forceful cough than children, making them more infectious. Most cases of pediatric tuberculosis arise from contact with adults. Tuberculosis meningitis is the leading cause of tuberculosis-related death in children. Young children suffer the greatest morbidity from tuberculosis infection. Extrapulmonary disease is present in 25% of children, compared with 15% of adults. *(Emergency Medicine, Chapter 47, pp 459–468)*

5.d. The initial approach to all patients in the ED with hypotension should include a fluid trial followed by vasopressors based on response. The underlying disease and cardiac status often dictate the quantity of IV fluids and timing of vasopressors. Patients with tuberculosis may develop pericardial tamponade that may present with hypotension, distant heart sounds, jugular venous distention, and/or pulsus paradoxus. Oxygen is indicated for all hypoxic patients. Hydrocortisone is indicated for adrenal insufficiency. The institution of antituberculous chemotherapy will have no impact on mortality, and although therapy should be instituted early, it should not take priority in initial stabilization of the hypotensive patient. *(Emergency Medicine, Chapter 47, pp 459–468)*

Tick-Borne Disease: Rocky Mountain Spotted Fever and Ehrlichiosis

1. Which of the following are useful in differentiating Rocky Mountain spotted fever from ehrlichiosis?
   a. A petechial rash is present in Rocky Mountain spotted fever and not ehrlichiosis.
   b. Rocky Mountain spotted fever causes fever, and ehrlichiosis does not.
   c. Hepatitis occurs only in ehrlichiosis.
   d. The rash of Rocky Mountain spotted fever involves the palms and soles, in contrast to the rash of ehrlichiosis, which does not.
   e. Ehrlichiosis may cause headache, whereas Rocky Mountain spotted fever rarely does.

2. The typical rash of Rocky Mountain spotted fever can best be described as:
   a. Erythema migrans
   b. A rash that begins on the abdomen and spreads peripherally
   c. Macules that progress to petechiae
   d. Painful erythematous pustules
   e. Necrotic lesions that begin at the site of the tick bite

3. The causative organism of Rocky Mountain spotted fever is:
   a. *Rickettsia rickettsii*
   b. *Francisella tularensis*
   c. *Borrelia burgdorferi*
   d. *Dermacentor andersoni*
   e. *Dermacentor variabilis*

4. Which of the following is not a component of the classic triad of Rocky Mountain spotted fever?
   a. Hyperpyrexia
   b. Arthralgias
   c. Headache
   d. Rash

5. A 7-year-old with Rocky Mountain spotted fever should be treated with:
   a. Ceftriaxone
   b. Erythromycin
   c. Streptomycin
   d. Chloramphenicol
   e. Amoxicillin

6. All of the following should be considered in the differential diagnosis of Rocky Mountain spotted fever except:
   a. Meningococcemia
   b. Sepsis
   c. Measles
   d. Tick paralysis
   e. Viral illness

7. All of the following statements concerning Rocky Mountain spotted fever and ehrlichiosis are true except:
   a. Early antimicrobial therapy has no proven effect on mortality.
   b. Patients with asymptomatic tick bites do not require prophylactic antibiotics.
   c. It is more common in the Atlantic states than the Rocky Mountain states.
   d. *Ehrlichia chafeensis* is the etiologic agent in ehrlichiosis.
   e. Repeat infection with ehrlichiosis is rare.

Answers

1.d. The most helpful clue in differentiating Rocky Mountain spotted fever from ehrlichiosis is that the rash of ehrlichiosis involves the palms and soles in less than 5% of cases. The remainder of the history and physical examination is essentially identical. Although hepatitis is reported more commonly with ehrlichiosis, with elevation of transaminases in 75% of cases, it also occurs with Rocky Mountain spotted fever. *(Emergency Medicine, Chapter 50, pp 484–488)*

2.c. The classic rash of Rocky Mountain spotted fever is present in 90% of patients and is described as pink macules 2 to 5 mm in diameter that progress to petechiae, ecchymosis, and palpable purpura. The rash begins on the wrist and ankles and spreads centripetally to the arms, legs, and trunk. Erythema migrans, also known as erythema chronica migrans, is pathognomonic for Lyme disease. Painful pustules are associated with herpes infection. The rash of Rocky Mountain spotted fever is painless and may go unnoticed. *Loxosceles* species envenomation by the brown recluse spider causes a central area of necrosis, typically 3 to 6 days after a "bite." *(Emergency Medicine, Chapter 50, pp 484–488)*

3.a. The causative organism of Rocky Mountain spotted fever is *Rickettsia rickettsii*. It is transmitted by arthropod vectors, most notably the mountain wood tick, *Dermacentor andersoni*, in the Rocky Mountain states. *Amblyomma americanum* is the main vector in the south central United States. *Francisella tularensis* causes tularemia; it is associated with rabbits and vermin; it can also be transmitted by the same tick species as Rocky Mountain spotted fever. *(Emergency Medicine, Chapter 50, pp 484–488)*

4.b. The classic triad of Rocky Mountain spotted fever is fever, frontal headache, and rash. The triad is present in only 60% of patients. Although these symptoms are described as classic for Rocky Mountain spotted fever, they are not specific, and other diseases should be considered in the differential diagnosis, including meningitis, sepsis, and endemic typhus. Although arthralgias as well as malaise are also common in Rocky Mountain spotted fever, they are nonspecific and are not part of the classic triad. *(Emergency Medicine, Chapter 50, pp 484–488)*

5.d. Doxycycline is the drug of choice for Rocky Mountain spotted fever but is not recommended for lactating or pregnant females and children younger than 9 years. The use of doxycycline in children is controversial at best and should be avoided. The drug of choice for treatment of Rocky Mountain spotted fever in children younger than 9 years is chloramphenicol. The side effects of chloramphenicol include aplastic anemia, reversible bone marrow suppression, and an increased risk of gray baby syndrome. Ceftriaxone is the drug of choice for disseminated Lyme disease and meningitis of unknown etiology. Streptomycin is used for tularemia. Amoxicillin is an alternative drug for the treatment of the acute phase of Lyme disease, but it is not an alternative choice for Rocky Mountain spotted fever. *(Emergency Medicine, Chapter 50, pp 484–488)*

6.d. Tick paralysis is a rare toxin-mediated illness seen with prolonged attachment of the female tick. The toxin affects both central and peripheral nerves. Initially patients may complain of paresthesias that evolve into an ascending, symmetric, flaccid paralysis over 48 hours. All patients with suspected Guillain-Barré syndrome should undergo thorough evaluation for the presence of a tick because of the similarity in symptoms and difficulty in differentiating these diseases. Complete recovery of tick-induced paralysis is rapid following the removal of the tick. Meningococcemia and sepsis should be considered in any patient with a fever and rash. Benign viral infections, which present with fever and a petechial rash, are a common source of confusion. The rash of measles usually begins on the face and spreads down the trunk. The rash of Rocky Mountain spotted fever spares the face and begins on the arms and spreads centrally. *(Emergency Medicine, Chapter 50, pp 484–488)*

7.a. Early recognition and treatment of Rocky Mountain spotted fever is crucial. The mortality of untreated infection approaches 25%. Antibiotics have been shown to decrease morbidity, including neuropathies and ischemic changes of distally perfused skin. Rocky Mountain spotted fever was first reported in Montana and Idaho; however, it is more prevalent in Oklahoma, the Carolinas, Tennessee, and middle and southern Atlantic states. The causative agent of ehrlichiosis is *Ehrlichiosis chafeensis*, and it is transmitted by the brown dog tick. Prior infection with ehrlichiosis appears to offer lifelong immunity. *(Emergency Medicine, Chapter 50, pp 484–488)*

Lyme Disease

1. Lyme disease is caused by what organism?
   a. *Ixodes* tick species
   b. *Borrelia burgdorferi*
   c. *Rickettsia rickettsii*
   d. *Treponema pallidum*
   e. *Hantavirus* species

2. The pathognomonic skin rash of Lyme disease is:
   a. *Borrelia* lymphocytoma
   b. Acrodermatitis chronica atrophicans
   c. Erythema marginatum
   d. Erythema migrans
   e. Erythema nodosum

3. All of the following statements concerning the cardiac manifestations of Lyme disease are true except:
   a. Steroids may be of benefit for severe cardiac involvement.
   b. The most common presentation is pericarditis.
   c. Antimicrobials shorten the course of cardiac inflammation.
   d. An important clue to cardiac involvement is alternating bradycardia and tachycardia.
   e. Carditis occurs in up to 10% of patients with Lyme disease.

4. All of the following are indications for antimicrobial treatment of Lyme disease except:
   a. Cranial nerve involvement
   b. A gravid female with erythema migrans
   c. An asymptomatic patient with positive serology for Lyme disease
   d. Children younger than 9 years old
   e. Knee pain without erythema or effusion

5. Diagnostic studies of patients with Lyme disease may reveal all of the following except:
   a. Elevated liver function studies
   b. Elevated ESR
   c. Ultrasound-confirmed lymphadenopathy around the parotid gland
   d. Cerebrospinal fluid characterized by a neutrophilic pleocytosis
   e. A positive ELISA

6. All of the following patients should be admitted for treatment of Lyme disease except:
   a. A patient with unresolving symptoms after 2 months of oral therapy
   b. A patient with arthritic involvement
   c. A pregnant patient with Bell's palsy
   d. A patient with a PR interval longer than 3 seconds occurring 2 months after an initial untreated tick bite
   e. A patient with disseminated disease with photophobia and nuchal rigidity

Answers

1.b. The spirochete *Borrelia burgdorferi* is the causative organism of Lyme disease. It is transmitted via a tick vector, particularly the ixodid species. An *Ixodes* tick by itself does not cause disease. Rocky Mountain spotted fever is caused by *Rickettsia rickettsii*; its major vector is the wood tick, *Dermacentor andersoni*. *Treponema pallidum,* also a spirochete, is the cause of syphilis. *Hantavirus* is spread via the inhalation of contaminated rodent droppings. Although *Hantavirus* species is being reported sporadically throughout the country, the majority of cases are seen in the southwestern United States. (*Emergency Medicine, Chapter 49, pp 475–483*)

2.d. Although *Borrelia* lymphocytoma and acrodermatitis chronica atrophicans are late manifestations of Lyme disease, they are rare. *Borrelia* lymphocytoma are bluish red subcutaneous nodules occurring on the breasts or earlobes. Acrodermatitis chronica atrophicans is a bluish red skin discoloration with edema present on the extensor surface of extremities. Erythema migrans, also known as erythema chronicum migrans, is the pathognomonic skin lesion that occurs in 60% to 80% of cases of Lyme disease. Erythema marginatum and erythema nodosum should be considered in the differential diagnosis of skin lesions resembling erythema migrans. Erythema marginatum, a rash with raised margins and a clear center, may erupt in patients with acute rheumatic fever, glomerulonephritis, and drug reactions, whereas the margins of erythema migrans are not raised and expand peripherally over 3 weeks. Erythema nodosum often presents as bilateral, tender nodules, unlike erythema migrans, which is painless. (*Emergency Medicine, Chapter 49, pp 475–483*)

3.b. Cardiac involvement is essentially the only manifestation of Lyme disease that requires emergent intervention. The most common presentation is AV block that may rapidly progress to clinical deterioration. Unexplained fluctuations in cardiac rate are reported in Lyme-induced cardiac disease. An ECG is recommended for all patients with suspected Lyme disease in the ED. All patients with cardiac involvement should be admitted to an electrocardiographically monitored setting. Steroids and antimicrobials may improve the clinical course of carditis. Steroids have no proven benefit for Lyme-induced Bell's palsy. (*Emergency Medicine, Chapter 49, pp 475–483*)

4.c. Positive serology in an asymptomatic patient is not an indication for treatment. Any patient with suspected or documented Lyme disease and evidence of neurologic involvement requires treatment with antimicrobials. All pregnant patients should also be treated: those with early localized disease only, i.e., erythema migrans, can be treated with amoxicillin; those with any other manifestation should be admitted for IV antimicrobial therapy. Doxycycline should be avoided in children less than 9 years old and in pregnancy for fear of permanent binding to calcium and inducing discoloration of teeth and growth inhibition if deposited in bone. Lyme-induced arthritis causes pain out of proportion to swelling. The knee is the most commonly affected joint in Lyme disease. Knee pain should heighten the clinician's suspicion for Lyme arthritis, because prompt antimicrobial therapy can minimize adverse sequelae. The affected joints are characteristically lacking objective signs, with pain often the only symptom of arthritic involvement. (*Emergency Medicine, Chapter 49, pp 475–483*)

5.d. Lyme disease affects multiple organ systems when it progresses from its first to its third stage. An elevated ESR is the most common laboratory abnormality noted; unfortunately it is nonspecific. With CNS involvement, cerebrospinal fluid is characterized by lymphocytic predominance. An ultrasound may be helpful in cases of Bell's palsy by revealing unilateral nonpalpable lymphadenopathy in the caudal area of the parotid gland.

An ELISA may provide false-positive results because of cross-reactivity with other spirochetes and other disease states. A false-negative ELISA result is rare. *(Emergency Medicine, Chapter 49, pp 475–483)*

6.b. All patients with early disseminated disease or late disease require intravenous antimicrobial therapy. Patients with early localized disease, focal cranioneuropathies, and arthritis can be treated with oral antimicrobials. All pregnant patients with anything other than early localized rash should be admitted. Cardiac involvement in Lyme disease requires hospitalization and monitoring for the potential complications of carditis and heart block. A prolonged PR interval may be the earliest ECG sign of cardiac involvement. Disseminated disease with signs of meningeal irritation is an indication for hospitalization for IV antimicrobial therapy. *(Emergency Medicine, Chapter 49, pp 475–483)*

BIBLIOGRAPHY

Hemphill R, Polis MA: Mycobacterial disease. *In* Howell JM, Altieri M, Jagoda AS, et al (eds): Emergency Medicine. Philadelphia, WB Saunders, 1998, pp 459–468.

Jolin SW: Lyme disease. *In* Howell JM, Altieri M, Jagoda AS, et al (eds): Emergency Medicine. Philadelphia, WB Saunders, 1998, pp 475–483.

Jolin SW: Rocky Mountain spotted fever and ehrlichiosis. *In* Howell JM, Altieri M, Jagoda AS, et al (eds): Emergency Medicine. Philadelphia, WB Saunders, 1998, pp 484–488.

22 Parasitic and Exotic Illnesses (Malaria, Dengue Fever, and Trypanosomiasis) and Syphilis and Leptospirosis

CHARLES DiMAGGIO, PA-C, MPH   FRANK LoVECCHIO, DO

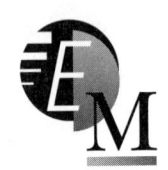

Parasitic Diseases (Malaria, Dengue Fever, and Trypanosomiasis)

CHARLES DiMAGGIO, PA-C, MPH

1. In evaluating a febrile patient for malaria, dengue fever, or trypanosomiasis, the most important piece of information is a history of:
   a. Recurrent chills and sweats
   b. Dark urine
   c. Travel to an endemic area
   d. Severe arthralgias
   e. Periorbital swelling

2. The most effective method of diagnosing Chagas' disease is:
   a. Xenodiagnosis
   b. Serologic testing
   c. Thin and thick peripheral smears
   d. Polymerase chain reaction
   e. Chest radiograph

3. The mortality rate of dengue shock syndrome is:
   a. 90%
   b. 50%
   c. 20%
   d. 10%
   e. Minimal to no mortality

4. Which of the following is usually diagnosed with a peripheral blood smear?
   a. Dengue fever
   b. Malaria
   c. Trypanosomiasis
   d. Schistosomiasis
   e. All of the above

5. A history of recent travel to which of the following areas would most raise your index of suspicion for dengue fever?
   a. Papua New Guinea
   b. Vietnam
   c. China
   d. Puerto Rico
   e. Brazil

6. Prospective travelers to areas endemic for chloroquine-resistant *Plasmodium falciparum* should receive:
   a. Vaccination
   b. Prophylaxis with chloroquine phosphate starting 1 week before departure
   c. Prophylaxis with mefloquine starting 1 week before departure
   d. Prophylaxis with Fansidar starting 2 weeks before departure
   e. Prophylaxis with doxycycline starting 4 weeks before departure.

Answers

1.c. Only a history of travel to an endemic area can be elicited in all these diseases. A travel history should be obtained from any febrile patient. Each of the other choices can be attributed to a particular disease. Recurrent chills and sweats are characteristic of malaria. The dark urine of blackwater fever is caused by massive hemolysis and is associated with *P. falciparum*. The severe arthralgias associated with dengue fever account for the name "breakbone fever." The conjunctiva is frequently the portal of entry for *Trypanosoma cruzi*, the parasite responsible for Chagas' disease. The trypanosome is transmitted by the bite of the reduviid or "kissing" bug, which often drops from the thatched roof of rural dwellings. The insect usually attacks at night and bites at the mucocutaneous junction of the outer canthus of the eye, resulting in painless, *unilateral* periorbital swelling (Romaña's sign). **(Emergency Medicine, Chapter 52, pp 493–498)**

2.d. Polymerase chain reaction provides nearly 100% accuracy in diagnosing Chagas' disease. Although it is possible to demonstrate parasites in the peripheral blood, thin and thick smears are more commonly associated with the diagnosis of malaria. Serologic testing is useful but not as accurate as polymerase chain reaction. Xenodiagnosis is a method used in endemic areas and involves demonstrating parasites in the intestines of reduviid bugs that have fed upon a patient with suspected infection. There are no characteristic chest radiographic findings associated with acute cases of Chagas's disease. *(Emergency Medicine, Chapter 52, pp 493–498)*

3.b. Classic dengue or breakbone fever tends to occur in nonindigenous, nonimmune individuals. Typical symptoms include a severe, splitting, retro-orbital headache as well as lower back, leg, and joint pain. Dengue shock syndrome is the most severe form of dengue hemorrhagic fever and is associated with a 50% mortality. Prior exposure and immunity to dengue is a common feature of this syndrome, which affects children more frequently than adults. *(Emergency Medicine, Chapter 52, pp 493–498)*

4.b. Although serologic or polymerase chain reaction methods are required for the definitive diagnosis of dengue and trypanosomiasis, a blood smear treated with Wright's or Giemsa's stain will often allow the identification of the plasmodium species responsible for malaria because of the characteristic appearance of each species in peripheral erythrocytes. For example, the gametocytes (merozoites) of *Plasmodium falciparum* are relatively large and banana shaped, and because the parasite tends to migrate to areas of low oxygen concentration, they can usually be diagnosed with blood obtained from a fingerstick. Although *P. vivax* and *P. ovale* can persist in extra-erythrocytic forms (hepatic) for months to years after the initial infection, these species re-invade the blood stream, allowing identification. *(Emergency Medicine, Chapter 52, pp 493–498)*

5.d. Dengue's distribution in tropical and warm temperate zones, which include Puerto Rico and the southern United States, corresponds to the distribution of its main vector, the *Aedes aegypti* mosquito. Malaria has a wide distribution throughout Africa, Central and South America, Asia, and Oceania and is usually transmitted by a female anopheline mosquito during a blood meal. The vector for Chagas' disease is the reduviid bug, which is found in South and Central America, from Chile and Argentina northward to Mexico. *(Emergency Medicine, Chapter 52, pp 493–498)*

6.c. The drug of choice for chemoprophylaxis against chloroquine-resistant *P. falciparum* is mefloquine started 1 week before departure. Although Fansidar is also effective, the possibility of Stevens-Johnson syndrome associated with its use makes it a poor choice. The regimens suggested in the other choices are ineffective. In addition to pharmacologic prophylaxis, the importance of personal protective measures should not be overlooked. Patients should be advised to remain in well-screened areas between dusk and dawn, use mosquito netting while sleeping, cover most of the body with clothes, and use insect repellent containing moderate concentrations of diethyltoluamide (DEET) on exposed skin. *(Emergency Medicine, Chapter 52, pp 493–498)*

Syphilis and Leptospirosis

FRANK LoVECCHIO, DO

1. Syphilis is caused by:
   a. *Haemophilus ducreyi*
   b. *Treponema pallidum*
   c. *Chlamydia trachomatis*
   d. Human papilloma virus
   e. *Trichomonas vaginalis*

2. Leptospirosis is transmitted to human beings by:
   a. Sexual intercourse
   b. Inhalational exposure
   c. Dermal contact
   d. Retained tampons in menstruating females
   e. Tick bite

3. Which of the following lesions are compatible with primary syphilis?
   a. Macular rash involving the palms
   b. Painless papules
   c. Multiple painful vesicles
   d. Chancroid
   e. Condylomata lata

4. All of the following are compatible with tertiary syphilis except:
   a. Gummas
   b. Cardiovascular involvement
   c. Ataxia
   d. Condylomata lata
   e. Poorly reactive pupils

5. All of the following statements are true concerning leptospirosis except:
   a. Elevated amylase is common.
   b. Fever, myalgias, and headache are common.

c. Serious infection may involve the liver and kidneys.
d. Pericarditis may be present.
e. A high mortality is associated with untreated disease.

6. The gold standard for diagnosing syphilis is:
   a. VDRL
   b. Rapid plasma reagin
   c. FTA-ABS
   d. Western blot test
   e. Blood culture

7. All are true concerning treatment of syphilis except:
   a. Primary syphilis should be treated with one dose of 2.4 million units of benzathine penicillin G.
   b. Alternative treatment for the penicillin-allergic patient includes doxycycline or erythromycin.
   c. All patients with suspected meningeal involvement should be hospitalized.
   d. Neurosyphilis requires treatment with penicillin for 14 days.
   e. All sexual partners should be referred for evaluation.

Answers

1.b. The causative organism of syphilis is *Treponema pallidum,* a spirochete also responsible for yaws and pinta. *Haemophilus ducreyi* is a gram-negative bacillus that causes lymphadenopathy and genital ulcers. *Chlamydia trachomatis* causes urethritis, epididymitis, and proctitis in men and urethritis, cervicitis, and pelvic inflammatory disease in women. Specific serotypes of *C. trachomatis* that are more prevalent in Caribbean countries can cause lymphogranuloma venereum. Genital warts are caused by direct transmission of the human papilloma virus. *Trichomonas vaginalis* is a flagellated protozoan that causes urogenital infection in women and men. *(Emergency Medicine, Chapter 48, pp 469–474)*

2.c. Leptospirosis is not transmitted by sexual contact or the tick vector. Leptospirosis is transmitted to humans through breaks in the skin barrier. It then gains access to the blood stream and reproduces in the liver. Outbreaks of leptospirosis are often linked to exposure to natural waterways contaminated by infected animals. Animal reservoirs for leptospirosis include cattle, dogs, and rodents. Toxic shock syndrome has been associated with the colonization of *Staphylococcus aureus* and tampon use. Some common tick-borne diseases include Lyme disease, Rocky Mountain spotted fever, tularemia, and ehrlichiosis. *(Emergency Medicine, Chapter 48, pp 469–474)*

3.b. A painless chancre is characteristic of primary syphilis. It occurs on the penis, vulva, or area of sexual contact. Painless papules develop into a chancre. Condylomata lata and a rash involving the palms and soles are characteristic of secondary syphilis. Multiple painful vesicles should alarm the clinician of the possibility of herpes simplex. Chancroid is caused by infection with *H. ducreyi* and is associated with painful lymphadenopathy. *(Emergency Medicine, Chapter 48, pp 469–474)*

4.d. Tertiary syphilis is rare; however, patients with HIV infection are at increased risk. Gummas are granulomas on the head, neck, extremities, and mucous membranes. Neurologic and cardiovascular involvement is characteristic of latent or tertiary syphilis. An Argyll Robertson pupil is described as a pupil with normal accommodation but poor response to light. It is noted in tertiary syphilis. Condylomata lata are flat mucous patches coated with a gray exudate. They can be seen in 70% of patients with secondary syphilis. *(Emergency Medicine, Chapter 48, pp 469–474)*

5.e. Most patients with leptospirosis do not develop life-threatening illness. It is usually self-limiting, but antimicrobials may shorten the course of illness. An important finding is icterus, present in 10% of patients, which is associated with a 10% mortality. Constitutional symptoms are common. Hyperamylasemia, pericarditis, and pericardial friction rubs have all been reported in leptospirosis. *(Emergency Medicine, Chapter 48, pp 469–474)*

6.c. The VDRL and rapid plasma reagin should be used only as screening tests because false-positive results occur. The Western blot test is used in the detection of HIV. Blood cultures are of no value in diagnosing syphilis. FTA-ABS detects specific antibodies to *T. pallidum* and is the most specific test available. *(Emergency Medicine, Chapter 48, pp 469–474)*

7.b. Most authors recommend one dose of 2.4 million units of benzathine penicillin G for primary and secondary syphilis. Some patients may require similar doses at weekly intervals for 3 weeks. Any patient with suspected CNS involvement should be admitted. The treatment for neurosyphilis is daily IM or IV penicillin therapy for 2 weeks. As with any sexually transmitted disease, referral of partners for medical evaluation should be standard practice. Alternative therapy includes doxycycline, ceftriaxone, and in-hospital desensitization to penicillin. Erythromycin has a high failure rate in the treatment of syphilis and is not recommended. *(Emergency Medicine, Chapter 48, pp 469–474)*

BIBLIOGRAPHY

Howell JM: Malaria, dengue fever, and trypanosomiasis. *In* Howell JM, Altieri M, Jagoda AS, et al (eds): Emergency Medicine. Philadelphia, WB Saunders, 1998, pp 493–498.

Monico E: Syphilis and leptospirosis. *In* Howell JM, Altieri M, Jagoda AS, et al (eds): Emergency Medicine. Philadelphia, WB Saunders, 1998, pp 469–474.

SECTION SIX

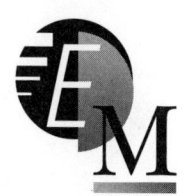

Immune Disorders

23 Autoimmune Disorders

PING WONG, MD   DONALD BARTON, MD

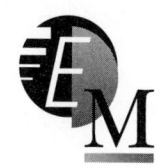

1. All of the following are consistent with Reiter's syndrome except:
   a. Arthritis
   b. Carditis
   c. Conjunctivitis
   d. Dactylitis
   e. Urethritis

2. All of the following may be complications of sarcoidosis except:
   a. Cardiac arrhythmias
   b. Cranial nerve palsies
   c. Hypocalcemia
   d. Lupus pernio
   e. Pulmonary fibrosis

3. A 61-year-old female with a history of rheumatoid arthritis is involved in a minor head-on auto collision. She is complaining of mild neck pain. What spinal cord level would be most likely suspected to be injured?
   a. C1–C2
   b. C2–C3
   c. C3–C4
   d. C4–C5
   e. C5–C6

4. Which of the following combinations is incorrect?
   a. Dermatomyositis—heliotrope rash
   b. Felty's syndrome—hepatomegaly
   c. Sarcoidosis—noncaseating granuloma
   d. Scleroderma—Raynaud's phenomenon
   e. Systemic lupus erythematosus—erythema nodosum

5. A 29-year-old female presents to the ED with fever, malaise, and arthralgias. On physical examination her temperature is 102°F and she appears lethargic with a bilateral cheek rash. Urinalysis reveals proteinuria and hematuria. All of the following may be complications of her disease except:
   a. Fetal loss
   b. Pericarditis
   c. Psychosis
   d. Sepsis
   e. Thrombocytosis

6. When treating the patient described in the previous question, which of following therapies is least helpful in the management of her disease and its complications?
   a. Antimicrobials
   b. Antimalarials
   c. Glucocorticoids
   d. NSAIDs
   e. Phototherapy

7. All of the following are characteristic of rheumatoid arthritis except:
   a. Baker's cyst
   b. Boutonnière deformity
   c. Heberden nodes
   d. Subcutaneous nodules
   e. Swan-neck deformity

8. Which of the following is classified as a vasculitic syndrome?
   a. Polymyositis
   b. Sarcoidosis
   c. Scleroderma
   d. Sjögren's syndrome
   e. Wegener's granulomatosis

9. All of the following are likely to present with ophthalmologic manifestations except:
   a. Giant cell arteritis
   b. Polymyalgia rheumatica
   c. Rheumatoid arthritis
   d. Sarcoidosis
   e. Sjögren's syndrome

10. A 55-year-old woman presents with weakness lasting for several months that she describes as difficulty in arising from a seated position and in climbing and descending stairs. She also describes difficulty in swallowing and a rash over her knuckles. She denies any visual changes or facial muscle weakness. Serum creatine phosphokinase and ESR are elevated. Considering her most likely diagnosis, all of the following are true except:

a. Deep tendon reflexes are intact.
b. Edrophonium improves weakness.
c. Glucocorticoids are first-line therapy.
d. Malignant tumors may be associated.
e. Muscle biopsy confirms the diagnosis.

11. A 25-year-old Japanese male presents to the ED with painful genital ulcers of several days' duration. Upon further questioning, the patient reports periodic mouth sores and eye pain. On examination, shallow ulcers are seen on the gums, buccal mucosa, and scrotum. Tzanck smears are negative. The most likely diagnosis is:
    a. Behçet's disease
    b. Erythema multiforme
    c. Dormant herpes simplex
    d. Inflammatory bowel disease
    e. Reiter's syndrome

12. Significant renal complications are found in each of the following pediatric rheumatologic conditions except:
    a. Systemic lupus erythematosus
    b. Scleroderma
    c. Polyarteritis nodosa
    d. Henoch-Schönlein purpura
    e. Juvenile rheumatoid arthritis

13. Which of the following pediatric rheumatologic diseases does not have fever as one of its presenting symptoms?
    a. Juvenile rheumatoid arthritis
    b. Systemic lupus erythematosus
    c. Juvenile dermatomyositis
    d. Scleroderma
    e. Polyarteritis nodosa

14. All of the following statements are true of juvenile rheumatoid arthritis except:
    a. Pauciarticular disease is the most common type.
    b. The onset of pauciarticular disease is usually in early childhood.
    c. Uveitis usually occurs in polyarticular type.
    d. Juvenile rheumatoid arthritis is predominantly seen in females.
    e. Rheumatoid factor is usually negative in juvenile rheumatoid arthritis.

15. Which combination of childhood rheumatologic disorder and rash is incorrect?
    a. Polymyositis—heliotrope rash
    b. Systemic lupus erythematosus—malar rash
    c. Henoch-Schönlein purpura—palpable purpura
    d. Systemic juvenile rheumatoid arthritis—Gottron's papules
    e. Polyarteritis nodosa—nodular rash

16. Raynaud's phenomenon is a feature of each of the following except:
    a. Systemic lupus erythematosus
    b. Polymyositis
    c. Polyarteritis nodosa
    d. Scleroderma
    e. Juvenile rheumatoid arthritis

17. Which of the following pediatric rheumatologic diseases might be confused with child abuse?
    a. Systemic lupus erythematosus
    b. Juvenile rheumatoid arthritis
    c. Polymyositis
    d. Henoch-Schönlein purpura
    e. Systemic sclerosis

18. A 6-year-old with juvenile rheumatoid arthritis presents with a 2-day history of right knee pain and swelling associated with a low-grade fever. The evaluation least likely to help in determining the cause of the problem is:
    a. Physical examination of the knee
    b. Radiograph of the affected knee
    c. WBC count and differential
    d. Detailed history of previous flares of disease
    e. Arthrocentesis of the affected knee

19. All of the following are emergent situations for patients with pediatric rheumatologic conditions except:
    a. A patient with juvenile rheumatoid arthritis complaining of new-onset paresthesias of the hand
    b. A patient with scleroderma complaining of loss of sensation in the fingertips
    c. Hoarseness and inspiratory stridor in a patient with juvenile rheumatoid arthritis
    d. Abdominal pain in a patient with systemic lupus erythematosus
    e. Drooling in a patient with juvenile dermatomyositis

20. Concerning pericarditis in patients with juvenile rheumatoid arthritis, all the following stratments are true except:
    a. Pericarditis may precede the onset of arthritis.
    b. Episodes typically last from 1 to 8 weeks.
    c. Pericardial effusions are common.
    d. Tamponade is rare.
    e. Tachycardia out of proportion to fever is characteristic.

21. Which complaint or finding is incorrectly associated with a pediatric rheumatologic disease?
    a. Henoch-Schönlein purpura—intussusception
    b. Juvenile dermatomyositis—paresthesia of fingers
    c. Polyarteritis nodosa—renal infarction
    d. Scleroderma—honeycombed appearance on chest radiograph
    e. Systemic lupus erythematosus—pseudotumor cerebri

Answers

1.b. Although the classic presentation of Reiter's syndrome consists of the triad of polyarthritis, urethritis (or cervicitis), and conjunctivitis, less than one third of patients with this disorder present with all elements of the triad. Dactylitis, or "sausage digit," results from inflammatory swelling of the digits and is a distinctive feature of both Reiter's syndrome and psoriatic arthritis. Carditis is not known to be a feature of Reiter's syndrome. *(Emergency Medicine, Chapter 54, pp 505–515)*

2.c. Sarcoidosis is a chronic granulomatous disease with multisystemic involvement. Because the main target organ is the lung, most patients first present with respiratory symptoms such as dry cough and dyspnea. Pulmonary manifestations are the result of granulomas, small airway obstructive disease, fibrosis, and a mass effect of mediastinal lymphadenopathy impinging on the large airways. Myocardial nodules can cause various degrees of heart block, arrhythmias, pericarditis, and eventually CHF. Multiple cranial nerve neuropathies are the most frequent manifestation of neural involvement. Although the most commonly found dermatologic lesion is erythema nodosum, other lesions seen include lupus pernio, plaques, and maculopapular eruptions. Hypercalcemia, believed to be associated with enhanced intestinal calcium absorption caused by an abnormally high level of 1,25-dihydroxyvitamin D produced by macrophages in the granulomas, will result in hypercalciuria and nephrolithiasis if left untreated. (*Emergency Medicine, Chapter 54, pp 505–515*)

3.a. Cervical spine instability is common because of inflammation and laxity of the transverse ligament of the atlantoaxial joint. Subluxation may occur after trivial trauma or even atraumatically. Any patients with rheumatoid arthritis presenting with new neurologic symptoms or in whom cervical spinal trauma is suspected should be considered at risk of cord compression and should be appropriately stabilized and evaluated. Care must be taken during manipulation of the neck, especially when applying a cervical collar or during intubation. (*Emergency Medicine, Chapter 54, pp 505–515*)

4.b. Felty's syndrome consists of the triad of chronic rheumatoid arthritis, neutropenia, and splenomegaly. Patients with this disease are especially prone to infection and sepsis. Dermatomyositis is a polymyositis with a characteristic rash consisting of heliotrope (bluish-purplish) lesions over the eyelids and dorsum of the hands. The painful, taut fingers of Raynaud's phenomenon are a common presentation of scleroderma but can also occur as the result of other autoimmune disorders or idiopathically. Erythema nodosum is a common hypersensitivity reaction found in various systemic disorders and infections including systemic lupus erythematosus, sarcoidosis, Behcet's disease, inflammatory bowel disease, streptococcal infection, and tuberculosis. (*Emergency Medicine, Chapter 54, pp 505–515*)

5.e. This patient's presentation is most consistent with a flare of systemic lupus erythematosus. Because lupus is a multisystemic autoimmune disorder, patients often present with nonspecific complaints and are at risk for a myriad of complications, including acute psychosis and seizure from cerebritis, chest pain from pleuritis or pericarditis, fever from opportunistic infections, and hypertension from renal involvement. Pregnant patients are at increased risk for spontaneous abortions and preeclampsia. Hematologic findings include anemia, leukopenia, and thrombocytopenia. The gastrointestinal, dermatologic, vascular, and musculoskeletal systems are also frequently involved. (*Emergency Medicine, Chapter 54, pp 505–515*)

6.e. All of the therapies may be appropriate except for phototherapy. In fact, patients with systemic lupus erythematosus often manifest photosensitivity, resulting in exacerbation of rash (e.g., the malar rash of lupus). Sunscreens and especially the avoidance of ultraviolet light are recommended. Hydroxychloroquine (400 mg PO every day) is often prescribed for discoid lupus. The presence of fever in a patient with lupus should prompt a sepsis evaluation, after which broad-spectrum antimicrobials should be initiated. Systemic high-dose glucocorticoids and plasmapheresis are reserved for life-threatening and severely disabling cases. NSAIDs (i.e., indomethacin) usually suffice for mild cases of pleurisy, arthritis, and myalgias. (*Emergency Medicine, Chapter 54, pp 505–515*)

7.c. Heberden nodes are seen in osteoarthritis, not rheumatoid arthritis. Posterior knee pain and swelling may result from a ruptured Baker's cyst, leaking synovium into an inflamed popliteal space. Boutonnière deformity is a deformity of the finger with flexion of the proximal interphalangeal joint and extension of the distal one. The swan-neck deformity of the digit is the opposite of the boutonnière deformity. Other musculoskeletal manifestations of rheumatoid arthritis include symmetric arthritis and rheumatoid nodules. (*Emergency Medicine, Chapter 54, pp 505–515*)

8.e. Wegener's granulomatosis is characterized by granulomatous vasculitis of the upper and lower respiratory tracts and evidence of glomerulonephritis. Patients present with paranasal sinus pain, purulent or bloody nasal drainage, cough, dyspnea, and hemoptysis. The proximal limb muscle weakness found in patients with polymyositis is the result of inflammatory lymphocytic infiltration. In patients with sarcoidosis, aggregates of mononuclear inflammatory cells and noncaseating granulomas are found in affected organs. Scleroderma, a disorder of abnormal collagen production, results in diffuse pathologic fibrosis of the skin and visceral organs. Its more common features can be remembered by the acronym CREST (calcinosis, Raynaud's phenomenon, esophageal dysmotility, sclerodactyly, and telangiectasia). In Sjögren's syndrome, the exocrine glands (salivary and lacrimal) are the main targets of tissue destruction from immune-complex deposition and lymphocytic infiltration. (*Emergency Medicine, Chapter 54, pp 505–515*)

9.b. Suspected giant cell arteritis (or temporal arteritis) should be treated with prednisone (40 to 60 mg/day) even before the diagnosis is confirmed by temporal artery biopsy. Without prompt therapy, patients with temporal arteritis can develop ischemic optic neuritis and eventual irreversible blindness. Features of polymyalgia rheumatica are pain and morning stiffness of the proximal muscle groups (i.e., neck, shoulders, pelvic girdle), age older than 50 years, ESR greater than 35, anemia, and depression. Although polymyalgia rheumatica is frequently associated with temporal arteritis, ocular involvement is not characteristic of this disorder. Any patient suspected of having polymyalgia rheumatica should be evaluated for temporal arteritis. Ocular lesions in patients with sarcoid are common and include conjunctivitis, uveitis, and cataracts. Patients with Sjögren's syndrome commonly present with keratoconjunctivitis sicca and xerostomia. The rheumatoid process can affect the eye, leading to episcleritis and scleritis, and up to 20% of patients with rheumatoid arthritis develop Sjögren's syndrome. ***(Emergency Medicine, Chapter 54, pp 505–515)***

10.b. This patient's clinical picture of proximal muscle weakness and skin rash and the laboratory findings suggest dermatomyositis. Definitive diagnosis is confirmed by a muscle biopsy in an area of abnormal electromyographic activity. Because the pathology is destruction of skeletal muscle fibers by inflammatory cell infiltration, edrophonium (an anticholinesterase inhibitor) has no role in the evaluation. High-dose prednisone (1 to 2 mg/kg per day) is the recommended treatment. Patients with severe disease or who fail to respond to glucocorticoids may warrant a course of cytotoxic drugs (i.e., azathioprine). Other manifestations of dermatomyositis and polymyositis include esophageal dysmotility, cardiac arrhythmias, heart failure, pneumonitis, and ARDS as well an association with malignant neoplasms. ***(Emergency Medicine, Chapter 54, pp 505–515)***

11.a. Major diagnostic criteria for Behçet's disease include recurrent oral (aphthous) ulcers, uveitis, genital ulcers, and skin lesions (i.e., folliculitis, erythema nodosum). Its etiology is thought to be autoimmune and vasculitic in nature. The prevalence of Behçet's disease is highest in Japan and Mediterranean countries. Although usually self-limited, serious complications such as glaucoma, blindness, CNS involvement, and venous thrombosis may occur. Treatment is palliative and includes topical and systemic corticosteroids. In addition to the classic triad of polyarthritis, urethritis, and conjunctivitis, Reiter's syndrome may manifest with mouth ulcers and circinate balanitis, painless shallow ulcerations of the glans penis. Aphthous ulcers are found in both Crohn's disease and ulcerative colitis. ***(Emergency Medicine, Chapter 54, pp 505–515)***

12.e. Renal disease, presenting as either nephrotic syndrome or renal failure, is the second most common cause of morbidity and mortality among patients with systemic lupus erythematosus. Findings include proteinuria, urinary casts (RBC, granular and mixed), and an elevated serum creatinine. Initial management is with corticosteroids, but severe or progressive disease may require admission and more aggressive intervention. Although the renal disease of scleroderma is usually manifested by mild to moderate systemic hypertension, a small number of patients can present with malignant hypertension, with systolic BPs ranging from 150 to 200 mm Hg. Despite their mild presenting symptoms, often just a mild headache, these children are at significant risk for rapid deterioration of renal function and death within weeks of onset and require admission and intensive treatment, including ACE inhibitors, minoxidil, beta-blockers, and, in refractory cases, bilateral nephrectomy. Most patients with polyarteritis nodosa (90% of patients with generalized polyarteritis nodosa and 50% of patients with the cutaneous form) are hypertensive. Although their hypertension can usually be controlled with diuretics, hydralazine, and beta-blockers, some patients develop severe hypertension that results in encephalopathy and CHF. The vasculitis seen in polyarteritis nodosa can cause infarction of the renal vessels (resulting in renal ischemia, hematuria, hypertension, and uremia) or aneurysmal dilation and rupture of the renal artery (presenting with the sudden onset of flank pain, gross hematuria, hypotension, and an expanding abdominal mass). The most common renal manifestations of Henoch-Schönlein purpura are hematuria, with or without casts, and proteinuria, which usually occurs during the first weeks of illness. Although most children with nephritis have complete resolution, a small number go on to develop chronic renal disease within a few years of their initial presentation. Despite the multiorgan involvement of juvenile rheumatoid arthritis, the kidneys are not usually affected. ***(Emergency Medicine, Chapter 56, pp 529–547)***

13.d. Fever is not typically seen in patients with scleroderma. In juvenile rheumatoid arthritis, fever can result from a recurrence of disease or an intercurrent infection. A noninfectious etiology is suggested by the presence of characteristic rash, typical joint involvement, and a fever pattern resembling earlier bouts of the disease, in the absence of other localizing signs, symptoms, or findings. Patients with systemic lupus erythematosus are immunosuppressed as result of the immune abnormalities associated with the disease itself (including leukopenia, functional asplenia, hypocomplementemia, lymphocytotoxic serum factors, decreased leukocyte chemotaxis, and defective phagocytosis) and the drugs used to treat it (corticosteroids and cytotoxic agents) and are therefore at increased risk for infection by both opportunistic organisms and common bacterial pathogens. Fever can result from intercurrent infections, the disease process itself, or both. In general, children with temperatures over 38.5°C should be admitted for IV antimicrobials and close observation pending culture results. Children on steroids should be given stress doses during acute infections. Juvenile dermatomyositis usually presents with malaise, easy fatigability, muscle weakness, rash, and fever. High fever and chills are seen in patients with juvenile dermatomyositis during formation of inflamed, tender subcutaneous calcium nodules (calcinosis). These patients also develop pneumonia as a result of palatal muscle weakness, pooling of oral secretions, and aspiration. Polyarteritis nodosa often first presents as a fever of unknown origin associated with unexplained joint, pulmonary, cardiac, or renal findings.

As with the other childhood rheumatologic diseases, treatment with steroids and cytotoxic agents place the child at increased risk for infection, further complicating the evaluation of fever. *(Emergency Medicine, Chapter 56, pp 529–547)*

14.c. Childhood juvenile rheumatoid arthritis presents in three typical patterns: polyarticular, pauciarticular, and systemic. The most common form, representing 50% of cases, is the pauciarticular type. This form, which involves four or fewer joints, occurs predominantly in females (5:1 female to male ratio) in early childhood (peak, 1 to 2 years old) and has an excellent prognosis except for chronic uveitis, which occurs in 20% of the cases. There is no systemic involvement with this form. The polyarticular form, involving five or more joints, also occurs predominantly in females (3:1 ratio) but presents throughout childhood, although the peak incidence is also in early childhood (1 to 3 years old). Its prognosis is more guarded because systemic involvement is more common. The least common form, systemic juvenile rheumatoid arthritis, which presents throughout childhood, has no peak age of incidence and no sex predominance. It involves a variable number of joints and has a moderate to poor prognosis. Rheumatoid factor is positive in 10% of patients with the polyarticular form but is otherwise uncommon. The antinuclear antibody test is frequently positive in both polyarticular and pauciarticular disease. *(Emergency Medicine, Chapter 56, pp 529–547)*

15.d. Skin manifestations of polymyositis include a typical violaceous heliotrope rash in the periorbital region; atrophic lesions over the extensor surfaces of the knees, elbows, and knuckles (Gottron's papules); and periungual erythema. Although the rashes of systemic lupus erythematosus are extremely variable in character and distribution, typical lesions include the characteristic butterfly rash that appears on both malar eminences and the bridge of the nose and a maculopapular rash that typically occurs on sun-exposed areas of the body. The finding of palpable purpura is essential to making the diagnosis of Henoch-Schönlein purpura. These lesions occur on dependent and pressure-bearing areas of the body, typically the lower extremities and buttocks, appearing in crops as a mixture of petechial and purpuric lesions. The typical rash of scleroderma is called morphea, a firm white fibrotic patch of skin with an erythematous rim, which can occur either as a single lesion or more generally distributed. Diffuse skin involvement can occur with or without visceral involvement, although visceral involvement is more common in children with diffuse skin disease. Polyarteritis nodosa occurs in both cutaneous and generalized forms, with livedo reticularis and nodular rashes more common in the cutaneous form and urticarial, petechial, and ischemic rashes more common in the systemic form. As noted, Gottron's papules are seen in polymyositis and not juvenile rheumatoid arthritis. *(Emergency Medicine, Chapter 56, pp 529–547)*

16.e. Raynaud's phenomenon is characterized by a triphasic color change of the distal extremities, usually upon exposure to cold, the result of chronic vascular injury and impaired circulation. Severe episodes can result in excruciating pain, digital ulceration, and autoamputation. Wound healing of paronychia is impaired by poor circulation, and digital cellulitis is frequently seen. Calcium channel blockers may decrease the frequency and severity of attacks, whereas sympathetic blockade may be necessary to treat impending gangrene. Raynaud's phenomenon is seen in patients with systemic lupus erythematosus, polymyositis, polyarteritis nodosa, and scleroderma, but not in juvenile rheumatoid arthritis. *(Emergency Medicine, Chapter 56, pp 529–547)*

17.d. The only disease that could be confused with child abuse among the choices offered is Henoch-Schönlein purpura. Henoch-Schönlein purpura is the most common vasculitis of childhood, with a peak incidence in the 5- to 15-year-old age group and occurring more commonly in boys than girls. It has been associated with preceding upper respiratory tract infections and occurs most frequently in the winter. On presentation, patients have ecchymotic lesions over dependent and pressure-bearing areas of the body, especially the lower extremities and buttocks, and usually complain of pain in the large joints of the lower extremity, such as the knees and ankles. Because the ecchymotic lesions superficially resemble bruises and usually occur over the buttocks or a tender swollen joint, child abuse may be suspected. However, examination of the rash will reveal a mixture of petechial and purpuric lesions that have appeared in crops and are in different stages of evolution. None of the other rashes are likely to be confused with child abuse. *(Emergency Medicine, Chapter 56, pp 529–547)*

18.c. The diagnosis of acute arthritis can be made only if, on examination, there are findings of either swelling or effusion of the joint with limited range of motion, warmth, tenderness, or pain on motion. A radiograph of the knee will help rule out a traumatic injury or osteomyelitis. Because patients with juvenile rheumatoid arthritis often have recurrent inflammation of the same joints, history will help determine whether the current episode is similar to those in the past. As it is impossible to rule out a septic arthritis on purely clinical grounds, if septic arthritis is suspected clinically, aspiration of joint fluid for cell count and culture is necessary. Because patients with juvenile rheumatoid arthritis frequently have leukocytosis during flares of their disease, a WBC count is unlikely to help exclude an infectious etiology. *(Emergency Medicine, Chapter 56, pp 529–547)*

19.b. Cervical spine involvement is a common complication of systemic and polyarticular type juvenile rheumatoid arthritis. Apophyseal joint disease, accompanied by bony fusion, occurs most commonly at the C2–C3 level and can result in atlantoaxial subluxation and cord compression. Although one of the earliest symptoms of cord compression is paresthesia of the fingers, weakness of the extremities or inability to control the bladder can also occur. Appropriate stabilization of the neck and radiographic evaluation are indicated. Children with juvenile rheumatoid arthritis are also at risk for cricoarytenoid arthritis. Although rare, it should be considered in a child with juvenile rheumatoid arthritis who presents with the acute onset of stridor and hoarseness, usually associated with dysphonia or dysphasia. Because acute airway obstruction can occur, it should be evaluated by direct laryngoscopy and treated aggressively with large doses of corticosteroids in an effort to avoid intubation or tracheostomy. Although minor gastrointestinal complaints (anorexia and nausea) are common in systemic lupus erythematosus, the onset of abdominal pain requires careful evaluation, because the usual signs and symptoms of peritonitis (fever, vomiting, diarrhea, abdominal distention, diffuse tenderness, and decreased bowel sounds) can be masked by corticosteroids. These patients are at increased risk for bowel vasculitis, ischemia, infarction, and perforation, because of both their intrinsic disease and the treatment they receive. They should therefore be carefully examined, started on IV hydration, and closely monitored for signs of shock. Patients with dermatomyositis have progressive muscle involvement characterized by pain, tenderness, and weakness. In patients with advanced disease, involvement of the muscles of the palate and pharynx causes difficulty with swallowing, resulting in pooling of oral secretions, frequent aspiration, and, compounded by a weak cough, pneumonia. Because of the risk of aspiration, patients with marked palatal muscle weakness should have a nasogastric tube placed and steroids started. The loss of sensation to the fingertips in a patient with scleroderma is a manifestation of Raynaud's phenomenon. Treatment with nifedipine is urgent, not emergent. Long-standing vascular compromise can result in gangrene, which can usually be prevented by using systemic or topical vasodilators, but if gangrene progresses and is not infected, it should be left to autoamputate, because the morbidity after spontaneous separation is significantly less than after surgical amputation. *(Emergency Medicine, Chapter 56, pp 529–547)*

20.e. Pericarditis, often complicated by pericardial effusion, is most commonly seen in children with systemic-onset juvenile rheumatoid arthritis. It may precede the onset of arthritis or occur anytime during the course of the disease, usually during exacerbations of systemic disease. Episodes typically last from 1 to 8 weeks. Despite the presence of effusion, tamponade is rare. Although myocarditis can also occur in juvenile rheumatoid arthritis, it is far less common than pericarditis. Tachycardia out of proportion to fever is characteristic of myocarditis, not pericarditis. Evaluation should include an electrocardiogram, a chest radiograph, and echocardiography. Myocarditis is treated with steroids. The initial management of pericarditis is with bed rest and NSAIDs. Corticosteroids are indicated if pericardial effusion is present, when cardiac output is compromised, or in cases refractory to treatment. *(Emergency Medicine, Chapter 56, pp 529–547)*

21.b. In patients with Henoch-Schönlein purpura, segmental edema and hemorrhage into the bowel wall can act as lead points for intestinal intussusception. Diagnosing this potentially life-threatening complication is made more difficult by the fact that both colicky abdominal pain and guaiac-positive stools are common even in the absence of intussusception. Vasculitis of the renal vessels in patients with polyarteritis nodosa may lead to renal infarction and ischemia manifested by hematuria, hypertension, and uremia. Diffuse interstitial pulmonary fibrosis in patients with scleroderma initially results in diffusion abnormalities and restrictive lung disease that progresses to irreversible pulmonary fibrosis, right-sided heart failure, and respiratory failure. A "honeycombed" appearance on chest radiograph is typical of advanced disease. Patients with systemic lupus erythematosus may develop blurring or loss of vision associated with headaches and vomiting. These patients are at risk for meningitis, severe hypertension, pseudotumor cerebri, and ophthalmic disorders (uveitis, retinal vasculitis, and vascular occlusion) and should be evaluated both by an ophthalmologist and by lumbar puncture after CT scan. Patients with juvenile dermatomyositis have both acute and chronic non-suppurative inflammation of striated muscle and skin, with muscular involvement characterized by symmetric pain and weakness of proximal muscles. Paresthesias of the fingers seen in juvenile rheumatoid arthritis are the result of early cord compression caused by apophyseal joint disease, most commonly at the C2–C3 level. *(Emergency Medicine, Chapter 56, pp 529–547)*

BIBLIOGRAPHY

Jain AM: Autoimmune emergencies. *In* Howell JM, Altieri M, Jagoda AS, et al (eds): Emergency Medicine. Philadelphia, WB Saunders, 1998, pp 505–515.

Lipnick R: Pediatric rheumatologic emergencies. *In* Howell JM, Altieri M, Jagoda AS, et al (eds): Emergency Medicine. Philadelphia, WB Saunders, 1998, pp 529–547.

24 Hypersensitivity and Related Disorders

FRED F. TILDEN, MD

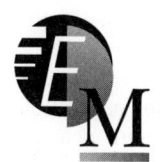

1. In the prehospital setting, for a patient who has presumed anaphylaxis to an insect sting, all of the following statements are true except:
   a. Intubate a patient with stridor.
   b. Intubate a patient who is drooling.
   c. Intubate a patient who has decreased mentation.
   d. Intubate a patient with voice changes.
   e. Patients with mild pruritus can rapidly deteriorate to airway obstruction.

2. In the prehospital setting, appropriate treatment for severe anaphylaxis (hypotension, stridor) caused by an insect bite in a 70-year-old male with known coronary artery disease includes all of the following except:
   a. A 1- to 2-L fluid challenge
   b. Epinephrine, SQ or IV
   c. Removal of the insect's stinger with tweezers
   d. Establishing an airway
   e. Diphenhydramine, 50 mg IV

3. Concerning ED treatment of acute anaphylaxis, which of the following is true?
   a. In patients with severe laryngeal edema and an established IV, a bolus of a crystalloid should be given.
   b. In patients with moderate hypotension, epinephrine 0.3 mL 1/10,000 SQ is generally sufficient to prevent immediate deterioration.
   c. H_2-blockers are beneficial.
   d. IV cimetidine is likely to potentiate the effect of epinephrine.
   e. IV steroids are thought to potentiate the effect of epinephrine.

4. Concerning the presentation of acute anaphylaxis, which of the following is false?
   a. Acute hypotension is the key life-threatening sign.
   b. Voice changes are an ominous sign.
   c. Facial flushing may precede hypotension.
   d. The rapidity of onset is not related to the severity of symptoms.
   e. The inciting allergen is often not identified.

5. Concerning allergic reactions to antimicrobials, which of the following statements is false?

   a. Trimethoprim-sulfamethoxazole tends to not cause severe anaphylaxis.
   b. Trimethoprim-sulfamethoxazole can cause Stevens-Johnson syndrome.
   c. Ceftazidime tends to cause fewer allergic cross-reactions than cefazolin in patients with allergy to penicillins.
   d. Activated charcoal can help decrease the allergic reaction in an acute ingestion.
   e. It is wise to refer a patient with an upper respiratory infection and a history of an allergic reaction to cefazolin to an allergist for skin testing.

6. Concerning anaphylactic reactions to radiocontrast media, which of the following is false?
   a. Prednisone is part of the pretreatment regimen in those patients known to be at high risk.
   b. These reactions are not IgE mediated.
   c. IV cimetidine and diphenhydramine are used in emergent pretreatment regimens in patients known to be at high risk for an anaphylactic reaction.
   d. High cost limits the use of low osmolar contrast.
   e. Pretreatment in those with a history of anaphylaxis to radiocontrast media significantly reduces the risk of reaction.

7. Concerning hypersensitivity to thrombolytics, which of the following is false?
   a. Recombinant tissue plasminogen activator (rt-PA) should be used instead of streptokinase in the setting of AMI if the patient has received streptokinase within the past month.
   b. Most patients with hypersensitivity-mediated hypotension respond to rapid volume repletion.
   c. One should discontinue streptokinase therapy if a rash occurs.
   d. In those receiving streptokinase for an AMI, a severe anaphylactic reaction should be treated with epinephrine.
   e. Pretreatment with IV steroids decreases the incidence of allergic reactions to streptokinase.

8. Concerning allergic reactions to insect bites, which of the following statements is false?

124 IMMUNE DISORDERS

   a. Always check closely for stingers imbedded in the skin.
   b. Anaphylaxis occurs in up to 80% of patients who have been previously stung.
   c. All patients with an allergic reaction to insect stings should be referred to an allergist.
   d. Swelling of the forearm 2 to 3 days after a bee sting should not be treated with prednisone.
   e. Lowering an extremity that has been stung and using ice help attenuate anaphylaxis.

9. In a 3-year-old boy with a severe early anaphylactic reaction, which of the following is false?
   a. This patient is probably not a good candidate for 4 to 6 hour ED observation and discharge, even if he responds promptly to treatment.
   b. The patient should eventually be seen by an allergist.
   c. The dose of IV epinephrine is 0.1 mL/kg of a 1:10,000 solution.
   d. IO injection of epinephrine requires higher dosage of medications.
   e. Nonmedical personnel should begin treatment of children with acute anaphylaxis.

10. Concerning pathophysiology of allergic reactions, which of the following is false?
    a. Histamine causes vasodilation.
    b. Histamine causes bronchospasm.
    c. The complement cascade may be activated.
    d. The reaction caused by radiocontrast media is IgE mediated.
    e. ACE inhibitors cause angioedema.

Answers

1.d. In the prehospital setting, severe anaphylaxis manifested by airway obstruction and profound hypotension needs aggressive resuscitation. Establishing an airway is of paramount importance. Although patients with mild allergic symptoms (pruritus, urticaria, intraoral edema) need to be monitored closely for rapid deterioration, voice changes per se do not mandate intubation. *(Emergency Medicine, Chapter 55, pp 516–528)*

2.c. Although epinephrine is relatively contraindicated in those with coronary artery disease, it should not be withheld in a patient who is dying. Imbedded insect stingers should not be squeezed; instead, flick them out with a credit card. *(Emergency Medicine, Chapter 55, pp 516–528)*

3.b. Most patients with moderate anaphylaxis respond quickly to SQ epinephrine. In severe anaphylaxis, many clinicians will give SQ epinephrine while an IV is being established, but absorption may be erratic in the hypotensive patient. H$_2$-blockers and steroids have no effect in the acute setting. *(Emergency Medicine, Chapter 55, pp 516–528)*

4.d. Hypotension suggests a profound systemic process requiring aggressive resuscitation, and it can be present without urticaria. Possible harbingers of complete airway obstruction include voice changes and perioral edema. The rapidity of onset is directly related to the severity of symptoms. *(Emergency Medicine, Chapter 55, pp 516–528)*

5.e. Reactions to sulfonamides are not IgE mediated and therefore do not tend to cause acute hypersensitivity reactions. Stevens-Johnson syndrome (erythema multiforme with fever and mucocutaneous lesions) is a lymphocyte-mediated lesion that occurs 1 to 2 weeks after sulfa drug therapy has begun. Later-generation cephalosporins are not as cross-reactive with penicillins as earlier ones. Activated charcoal helps eliminate persistent allergen. If there are several treatment options, skin testing is not necessary and should be considered a poor utilization of resources. *(Emergency Medicine, Chapter 55, pp 516–528)*

6.a. Between 17% and 35% of patients with a history of previous reaction to radiocontrast media will have subsequent reactions. Radiocontrast media should therefore be avoided, and other modalities should be used whenever possible in these patients. IV medications are used in emergent pretreatment regimens, which includes H$_1$- and H$_2$-blockers and corticosteroids. In high-risk patients, the reaction rate is reduced from about 9% to less than 1%. Oral corticosteroids such as prednisone have a slow onset of action. *(Emergency Medicine, Chapter 55, pp 516–528)*

7.c. Streptokinase should not be used again in patients who have recently been treated. Tissue plasminogen activator and acute angioplasty are good alternatives. Mild reactions to streptokinase do not require discontinuation; rather, give antihistamines and steroids. Hypotension usually responds to discontinuation of streptokinase and IV fluids. Pretreatment has not been shown to be helpful. *(Emergency Medicine, Chapter 55, pp 516–528)*

8.c. Patients who call the ED for advice after a bee sting should be told to use ice, place the affected extremity in a dependent position, take diphenhydramine, and use self-injectable epinephrine if available. Reactions that are obviously mild need no further medical attention unless the clinical picture worsens. Mild reactions to single bites need not be referred for allergy testing, but severe and multiple stings should. Delayed swelling is not a hypersensitivity reaction and does not require systemic therapy. *(Emergency Medicine, Chapter 55, pp 516–528)*

9.d. Most patients with anaphylaxis can be treated, observed, and discharged from the ED. However, those with severe reactions of very rapid onset are at higher risk for late reaction and should probably be monitored for a day or so as an inpatient and electively seen by an allergist. IO dosages are the same as IV dosages.

Quick outpatient treatment by laypersons en route to the hospital improves outcomes significantly. *(Emergency Medicine, Chapter 55, pp 516–528)*

10.d. Radiocontrast media causes endothelial injury, which stimulates factor XII and the coagulation cascade. It is not IgE mediated. Classic hypersensitivity reactions are IgE mediated, causing mast cell degranulation and release of histamine, prostaglandins, leukotrienes, and other substances. Histamines cause vasodilation, increased endothelial cell permeability, and increased smooth muscle tone in the lungs. *(Emergency Medicine, Chapter 55, pp 516–528)*

BIBLIOGRAPHY

Gin-Shaw SL: Hypersensitivity and related disorders. *In* Howell JM, Altieri M, Jagoda AS, et al (eds): Emergency Medicine. Philadelphia, WB Saunders, 1998, pp 516–528.

SECTION SEVEN

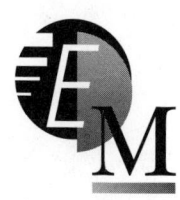

Endocrine and Fluid and Electrolyte Disorders

25 Fluid and Electrolyte Management

DAVID H. DORFMAN, MD   JOHN C. BRANCATO, MD

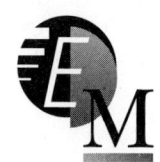

1. A 10-month-old child presents to the ED with a history of multiple episodes of vomiting and diarrhea over the past day. The child appears tired, with dry mucous membranes and slight tachycardia. Blood pressure and capillary refill are normal. Of the following, the best rehydration solution is:

Route	Na (mEq/L)	Glucose (g/L)
a. Oral	40	2
b. IV	34	5
c. Oral	75	2
d. IV	154	10
e. Oral	40	10

2. Which of the following is most likely to cause hypernatremic dehydration in an infant?
   a. Acute glomerulonephritis
   b. Incorrect formula preparation
   c. Pituitary tumor
   d. Congenital adrenal hyperplasia
   e. Excessive salt intake in foods

3. A child being treated for hypernatremic dehydration develops seizures. The most likely explanation is:
   a. Rapid change in blood pH
   b. Hyperglycemia
   c. Rapid change in serum sodium concentration
   d. Rapid drop in calcium concentration
   e. Intracranial hemorrhage

4. A 7-year-old boy who presents with vomiting and marked dehydration has a serum sodium of 125 mEq/L and a serum osmolality of 325 mOsm/kg H_2O. The low serum sodium is from an abnormal amount of another solute in the serum. Your diagnosis is based on an abnormality of which of the following:
   a. Glucose
   b. Creatinine
   c. Chloride
   d. Potassium
   e. Bicarbonate

5. A 12-month-old girl presents to the ED with fever and lethargy. She has poor capillary refill, weak pulses, a heart rate of 190, and BP of 60/20. An IO needle is placed. Which of the following initial therapies is most appropriate?
   a. Transfuse with whole blood.
   b. Administer epinephrine, 0.01 to 0.02 mg/kg.
   c. Normal saline, 20 mL/kg rapidly. Reassess and repeat if BP and capillary refill have not normalized.
   d. Administer dopamine, 5 µg/kg per minute, and titrate up until BP normalizes.
   e. Administer Ringer's lactate solution, 20 mL/kg over 45 minutes, and reassess. Repeat if necessary.

6. An 8-month-old infant has had diarrhea for 3 days. He has received only water and diluted apple juice during this time. The child is listless with dry mucous membranes and delayed capillary refill. The most likely electrolyte abnormality of this child is:
   a. Hyperglycemia
   b. Hyperkalemia
   c. Hypoglycemia
   d. Hyponatremia
   e. Hypocalcemia

7. A 15-month-old child with severe dehydration caused by diarrhea and vomiting presents with tachycardia, hypotension, lethargy, and delayed capillary refill. Of the following, the most appropriate IV fluid for resuscitation is:
   a. D_5 0.2% saline
   b. 0.45% saline
   c. D_5 0.45% saline
   d. Whole blood
   e. 0.9% saline

8. Mild dehydration is characterized by all of the following except:
   a. Alert sensorium
   b. A sunken fontanelle
   c. Capillary refill less than 2 seconds
   d. Decreased urine output
   e. Moist mucous membranes

9. All of the following are found with hyponatremia except:

a. Irritability
b. Lethargy
c. Doughy skin texture
d. Nausea
e. Muscle cramps

10. Hypocalcemia may cause all of the following signs and symptoms except:
    a. Muscle weakness
    b. Tetany
    c. Laryngospasm
    d. Trousseau's sign
    e. Shortened QTc interval on ECG

11. Children with significant dehydration from diarrhea may start on a regular diet:
    a. After 48 hours of no diarrhea
    b. After tolerating a BRAT diet for 24 hours
    c. After tolerating a challenge with 10% sucrose solution
    d. As soon as it is tolerated
    e. When stool cultures prove to be negative

12. An 12-year-old child weighing 50 kg presents with a 3-day history of gastroenteritis and vomiting. He is tachycardic, orthostatic, and lethargic. He has tenting of his skin. His labs reveal a sodium of 170, with a potassium of 3.6. What is his total body water (TBW) deficit, and over what amount of time would you replace his fluids?
    a. 10.3 L, over 4 hours
    b. 10.3 L, over 6 hours
    c. 10.3 L, over 24 hours
    d. 5.3 L, over 24 hours
    e. 5.3 L, over 1 to 2 hours

13. A renal failure patient arrives weak and confused. He has a widened QRS complex and peaked T waves on his ECG. The most appropriate initial therapy would be:
    a. IV insulin and glucose
    b. IV bicarbonate
    c. Calcium gluconate, 1 g IV
    d. Kayexalate, 30 g PO
    e. Magnesium sulfate, 1 g IV

14. Hypokalemia may caused by all of the following except:
    a. Diuretic administration
    b. Beta-agonist therapy
    c. Diabetic ketoacidosis
    d. Laxative use
    e. Metabolic acidosis

15. A patient receiving vincristine for acute leukemia is brought by her family to the ED because of lethargy and mild agitation. Her vital signs are normal but her serum sodium level is found to be 118 mEq/L. Initial therapy should include which of the following?
    a. D_5 one quarter–normal saline
    b. D_5 half-normal saline
    c. D_5 normal saline
    d. Normal saline
    e. 3% normal saline

16. Central pontine myelinolysis may result from the aggressive treatment of which of the following?
    a. Hypernatremia
    b. Hyponatremia
    c. Hyperkalemia
    d. Hypokalemia
    e. None of the above

17. A 28-year-old man is rescued after being lost for several days in the desert. He is mildly agitated and anorexic and his peripheral pulses are thready. He is found to have a serum sodium of 160 mEq/L. The most appropriate type of therapy is:
    a. Isotonic saline followed by hypotonic saline
    b. Hypotonic saline
    c. Water
    d. Parenteral vasopressin and hypotonic saline

Answers

1.c. Children with mild to moderate dehydration may be treated with oral rehydration therapy. Oral rehydration therapy has been advocated by the American Academy of Pediatrics and may be used in children with vomiting as well as in those with dehydration caused by diarrhea. Glucose absorption is enhanced by sodium; likewise, sodium absorption is augmented by glucose and related sugars. Maximum transport occurs when the molar concentration of carbohydrate to sodium is less than 2 to 1. Therefore, solutions containing about 2% glucose in half-isotonic (77 mEq/L) sodium chloride allow maximal transport across the small bowel. Oral solutions containing more glucose may lead to osmotic diarrhea caused by incomplete absorption of glucose. Intravenous therapy is not indicated in this mildly dehydrated patient. If the child is unable to tolerate oral fluids, none of the IV solutions listed would be appropriate: the solution of normal saline containing 10% dextrose would lead to osmotic diuresis. The other IV solution is too hypotonic to treat dehydration effectively. *(Emergency Medicine, Chapter 57, pp 549–571)*

2.c. Central diabetes insipidus causes hypernatremia because of disruption in the production, storage, or release of vasopressin (antidiuretic hormone). Any illness or injury that affects the hypothalamic-hypophyseal axis, such as tumors, trauma, or congenital defects, may lead to decreased vasopressin and loss of free water with resulting hypernatremia. Pituitary tumors are the most common neoplastic cause of diabetes insipidus.

Acute glomerulonephritis causing renal failure leads to water retention and hyponatremia. Excessive salt intake leads to increased serum sodium, but not dehydration. Improperly dilute formula will lead to hyponatremia. Congenital adrenal hyperplasia causes hypoaldosteronism with hyponatremia and hyperkalemia. *(Emergency Medicine, Chapter 57, pp 549–571)*

3.c. The development of hypernatremic dehydration generally occurs over the course of hours to days. During this time, the brain produces intracellular osmolytes that help maintain the water balance between extracellular and intracellular compartments. If hypernatremia and osmolality of the extracellular space are lowered rapidly, there may be a rapid shift of fluid to the intracellular space. This can cause cerebral edema and seizures. Hypernatremic dehydration is therefore treated with fluids distributed equally over the course of 48 to 72 hours. Hypocalcemia and hyperglycemia may accompany hypernatremia. The mechanism of hypocalcemia is unclear, but serum calcium should be monitored and supplemented as needed. Mild hyperglycemia during rehydration would not cause neurologic deterioration. (*Emergency Medicine, Chapter 57, pp 549–571*)

4.a. This child has diabetes mellitus with marked hyperglycemia. He has a measured hyponatremia and a serum osmolality of 325 mOsm/kg H_2O. Serum osmolality may be calculated by the formula 2(Na) + BUN/2.8 + glucose/18. Factitious hyponatremia occurs when a nonpermeating solute such as glucose is increased in the extracellular space. Water moves into the extracellular compartment and decreases the measured sodium and chloride concentrations. The equation used to correct for this effect is as follows: for every 100 mg/dL of glucose above 200 mg/dL, add 1.6 mEq/L to the measured serum sodium. Thus, if this child's serum glucose were 800 mg/dL, his adjusted serum sodium would be $(800-200)/100 \times 1.6 + 125 = (6 \times 1.6) + 125 = 135$. (*Emergency Medicine, Chapter 57, pp 549–571*)

5.c. This child is in shock and needs rapid fluid resuscitation. A rapid bolus of normal saline or Ringer's lactate at 20 mL/kg, followed by reassessment and another bolus if needed, is most appropriate. This child likely has distributive shock from sepsis. If the child remains in shock after receiving fluids, pharmacologic support is necessary. The American Heart Association recommends epinephrine if the child remains hypotensive after appropriate fluid administration. Dopamine may also be used. (*Emergency Medicine, Chapter 57, pp 549–571*)

6.d. Hyponatremia is the most likely electrolyte disturbance. The child has received fluids insufficient to replace his ongoing sodium losses from diarrhea. Hyponatremia may lead to lethargy in this dehydrated child. (*Emergency Medicine, Chapter 57, pp 549–571*)

7.e. The child has hypovolemic shock and requires rapid administration of parenteral fluids to restore losses from her intravascular space. It is important to realize that hypotension is not synonymous with shock and that hypotension is a late finding in shock that occurs when compensatory mechanisms have been overcome. Vasoconstriction of the vascular beds of the kidneys, intestines, skin, and muscle help maintain blood flow to the brain and heart. If shock is not reversed quickly it may progress to "irreversible shock." With dehydration, shock may occur when the child has lost fluid equal to 10% to 15% of initial body weight. Of the fluids mentioned, normal saline is most appropriate. Crystalloids, such as normal saline or lactated Ringer's, are given in a dose of 20 mL/kg as a rapid bolus. Crystalloids, lacking colloids, are distributed to the intravascular space and the extravascular interstitial space. The volume of the extravascular space is approximately three times that of the intravascular space. Thus, one fourth of the volume of crystalloids given is distributed to the intravascular space, and three fourths is eventually distributed to the extravascular space. After the initial bolus of saline or Ringer's lactate, the child must be reevaluated and given another bolus if she has not improved significantly. Once she is no longer in shock, fluids should be continued at a slower rate to correct her deficit and supply maintenance needs.

The other crystalloid fluids listed as answers are too hypotonic and would rapidly dissipate from the intravascular space. Whole blood is not indicated unless hypotension is the result of blood loss. With hypovolemic shock from hemorrhage, whole blood should be used if the patient does not stabilize after 40 mL/kg of isotonic crystalloid or if there is significant ongoing bleeding. (*Emergency Medicine, Chapter 57, pp 549–571*)

8.b. A sunken fontanelle is associated with moderate to severe dehydration. The other findings listed are found in mild dehydration. Children with mild dehydration are alert. They may become irritable as they become more significantly dehydrated, and lethargic with extreme dehydration. Capillary refill reflects peripheral perfusion and is usually normal in mild dehydration. Capillary refill is, however, dependent on many variables (including ambient room temperature). Urine output decreases with mild dehydration, although significant decreases may be a sign of more pronounced dehydration. (*Emergency Medicine, Chapter 57, pp 549–571*)

9.c. A decline in serum sodium concentration produces a reduction in plasma osmolality and leads to an osmotic gradient across the blood-brain barrier. Movement of water along this gradient may lead to cerebral edema and the neurologic symptoms associated with hyponatremia. These symptoms include apathy, headache, nausea, vomiting, altered consciousness, coma, and seizures. Most patients with hyponatremia have normal muscle tone and function. Occasionally, however, muscle cramps may occur but respond quickly to correction of the serum sodium. Soft, doughy skin texture is a classic finding of marked hypernatremic dehydration (greater than 10%). It is not found with hyponatremic dehydration.

The most common cause of hyponatremic dehydration in children is viral gastroenteritis causing diarrhea and vomiting. Other causes in the pediatric population include adrenal insufficiency, diuretic use, administration of hypotonic fluids, and renal disorders. Causes of hyponatremia in the adult population include adrenal insufficiency, hypothyroidism, thiazide diuretic use, certain drugs, and pulmonary disease. There are a variety of instances in which the measured sodium may be low but does not reflect true hyponatremia (pseudohyponatremia). Illnesses that cause excessive plasma proteins or lipids (e.g., nephrotic syndrome) in the blood decrease the percentage of plasma that is water. Laboratories that report the serum sodium concentration as milliequivalents per liter of plasma will report artificially low values in these disease states. *(Emergency Medicine, Chapter 57, pp 549–571)*

10.e. Hypocalcemia is relatively common in critically ill children, especially neonates. Other causes include disorders of vitamin D metabolism, parathyroid function, renal failure, and hypernatremic dehydration. Calcium in the plasma is distributed among three compartments: free calcium ions (ionized calcium), complexed calcium, and protein-bound calcium. Only the ionized fraction is a physiologically active component of blood calcium. The clinical effects of hypocalcemia largely result from the effects on the neuromuscular system. Hypocalcemia may cause muscle weakness, tetany, laryngospasm, Trousseau's sign, and Chvostek's sign. Seizures may occur. In addition, severely diminished cardiac function may result from decreased ionized calcium levels. Prolonged QTc is seen with hypocalcemia. *(Emergency Medicine, Chapter 57, pp 549–571)*

11.d. Children being treated for dehydration may begin a regular diet as soon as they are able to tolerate it. There is little or no advantage to keeping children on "clears" or slowly advancing them to solid foods through the use of special diets such as the BRAT (bananas, rice, apples, toast) diet. Delaying feeding to provide bowel rest after a diarrheal illness may have deleterious effects on the nutritional status of the children. Although stool output is increased in infants placed on early feedings, the duration of the diarrhea is not affected. Infants may be started on formula or breast milk after they are rehydrated. Lactose intolerance develops in only a small minority of patients with gastroenteritis. *(Emergency Medicine, Chapter 57, pp 549–571)*

12.d. This patient is moderately to severely dehydrated. He is hypernatremic from free water loss. His free water deficit (FWD) (in liters) can be calculated by using the following formula:

$$FWD = normal\ TBW - current\ TBW$$
$$Normal\ TBW = .6\ (wt\ in\ kg)$$
$$Current\ TBW = normal\ Na \times normal\ TBW/measured\ Na$$
$$Normal\ Na = 140$$
$$FWD = .6(wt) - (140 \times .6(wt)/measured\ Na)$$
$$= .6(wt) \times (1 - 140/measured\ Na)$$
$$= .6(50) \times (1 - 140/170)$$
$$= 30 \times .18$$
$$= 5.4\ L$$

Once the patient is hemodynamically stable, half of the deficit should be replaced over the first 24 hours. Once fluids are replaced, maintenance fluids can be calculated as 100 mL/kg per day for the first 10 kg of body weight, 50 mL/kg per day for the second 10 kg of body weight, and 20 mL/kg per day for every additional kilogram of body weight. If the serum sodium is decreased too rapidly, CNS edema may occur (see answer to question 3). *(Emergency Medicine, Chapter 57, pp 549–571)*

13.c. This patient has severe hyperkalemia (potassium greater than 8 mEq/dL) from either medication noncompliance or missed dialysis. The elevated extracellular concentration of the ion decreases the transcellular membrane potential, causing delayed depolarization, faster repolarization, and a slower conduction velocity. Hyperkalemia can lead to ECG findings of peaked T waves, widened QRS complexes, and life-threatening arrhythmias or asystole. In the patient with widened QRS, ventricular arrhythmia, or asystole, rapid infusion of calcium gluconate (or calcium chloride) can be lifesaving. Calcium increases the threshold potential and allows excitable cells to repolarize, thereby stabilizing neuromuscular membranes and preventing cardiac arrhythmias. The dose of calcium gluconate for hyperkalemia is 5 to 30 mL of a 10% solution (0.5 to 3 g) IV over 1 to 5 minutes. Although calcium chloride may also be used, it is more irritating to the veins. Calcium works immediately and has a duration of action of 20 to 40 minutes. Bicarbonate works within 5 to 10 minutes by shifting potassium into cells by changing the serum pH. The duration of action is approximately 2 hours. Insulin and glucose decrease serum potassium by promoting movement of potassium into the cells and out of the extracellular space. Onset of action is 30 minutes and duration is 4 to 6 hours. Kayexalate (sodium polystyrene sulfonate resin) decreases total body potassium by exchanging potassium for sodium in the small intestine, thus increasing excretion. Its relatively slow time of onset—approximately 1 hour—makes it inappropriate in an emergent situation Finally, hemodialysis or peritoneal dialysis may be used to increase potassium excretion. *(Emergency Medicine, Chapter 57, pp 549–571)*

14.e. Most clinically important causes of hypokalemia result from a net loss of potassium from the body. Diuretics increase urine flow rates and delivery of sodium to the distal nephron. Laxatives cause intestinal potassium loss. Illnesses causing significant vomiting may also lead to hypokalemia. In diabetic ketoacidosis, excess potassium is lost via the urine. The increased aldosterone released in response to the accompanying dehydration exacerbates renal loss of potassium. However, since potassium is particularly responsive to pH changes, metabolic acidosis causes potassium ions to shift into the extracellular space and may result in hyperkalemia, despite total body decrease of potassium. Thus, serum potassium may be high, low, or normal in diabetic ketoacidosis. *(Emergency Medicine, Chapter 57, pp 549–571)*

15.e. This patient's hyponatremia is most likely the result of the syndrome of inappropriate antidiuretic hormone induced by her vincristine. Many other pharmacologic agents may produce a similar effect, such as oral hypoglycemics (tolbutamide and chlorpropamide), psychoactive drugs (carbamazepine, amitriptyline, and haloperidol), and other antineoplastic/immunosuppressives (vinblastine and cyclophosphamide). Patients with hyponatremia of any origin most commonly become symptomatic when their serum sodium falls below 120 to 125 mEq/L. With normal vital signs and no other history to suggest hypovolemia, the most appropriate initial therapy for this patient would be 3% normal saline. Enough should be administered to raise the sodium to approximately 125 mEq/L, after which the remaining correction may be completed more slowly with normal saline or even 0.5% normal saline. The volume (in milliliters) of 3% normal saline is determined by (125 − measured sodium) × wt (kg) × 1.2. *(Emergency Medicine, Chapter 57, pp 549–571)*

16.b. Cerebral demyelination (formerly known as central pontine myelinolysis) is an irreversible complication of treatment of hyponatremia. Although uncommon, it is thought that both the rate and the magnitude of the initial sodium correction influence its development. Patients present with cranial nerve findings, quadriplegia, and coma. Most reports are associated with rapid correction of chronic hyponatremia, such as in alcoholic and malnourished patients. Limiting the initial sodium correction to a minimum level likely to relieve symptoms (approximately 125 mEq/L) may reduce the risk of demyelination. *(Emergency Medicine, Chapter 57, pp 549–571)*

17.a. It is essential to remember the basics when treating hypernatremia. This patient has intravascular volume depletion and should be treated with isotonic saline until his vital signs are stable. This should be followed by hypotonic saline over 48 hours until both intracellular and extracellular compartments are repleted (see answer to question 12). *(Emergency Medicine, Chapter 57, pp 549–571)*

BIBLIOGRAPHY

Berry PL, Belsha CW: Hyponaetremia. Pediatr Clin North Am 1990; 37:351–363.

Conley SB: Hypernaetremia. Pediatr Clin North Am 1990; 37:365–372.

Tayal VS, Conners GP: Fluid and electrolyte disorders. *In* Howell JM, Altieri M, Jagoda AS, et al (eds): Emergency Medicine. Philadelphia, WB Saunders, 1998, pp 549–571.

26 Endocrine Disorders

RON MEDZON, MD   TODD C. ROTHENHAUS, MD

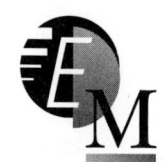

1. All of the following abnormalities are associated with diabetic ketoacidosis except:
   a. Total body potassium depletion
   b. Hyperkalemia
   c. Hyperphosphatemia
   d. Metabolic acidosis
   e. Measured hyponatremia

2. The most important initial goal of therapy for diabetic ketoacidosis is:
   a. Restoration of intravascular volume
   b. Bicarbonate administration to correct metabolic acidosis
   c. Rapid normalization of blood glucose
   d. Determination of the underlying cause
   e. Assessment of renal function to guide potassium replacement.

3. Symptoms of acute pituitary necrosis (apoplexy) include all of the following except:
   a. Headache
   b. Visual field defects
   c. Ocular palsy
   d. Paresthesias
   e. Vomiting and photophobia

4. The most common cause of primary adrenal insufficiency in the United States and developed nations is:
   a. Abrupt discontinuation of exogenous corticosteroids
   b. Autoimmune adrenalitis
   c. Malignancy
   d. Sepsis
   e. Tuberculosis

5. Patients with adrenal insufficiency may present with all of the following signs and symptoms except:
   a. Weakness
   b. Hypertension
   c. Back or flank pain
   d. Fever
   e. Nausea and vomiting

6. The classic triad of pheochromocytoma includes all of the following signs and symptoms except:
   a. Sweating
   b. Headache
   c. Fever
   d. Palpitations

7. Acceptable treatments for hypertension associated with pheochromocytoma include all of the following except:
   a. Beta-blockers
   b. Calcium channel blockers
   c. Sodium nitroprusside
   d. Prazosin
   e. Phentolamine

8. Treatment of patients with adrenal crisis (insufficiency) should include all of the following except:
   a. Restoration of intravascular volume
   b. Maintenance of normal blood glucose
   c. Supplemental corticosteroids
   d. Intravenous potassium
   e. Vasopressors—for hypotension that remains after restoration of intravascular volume

9. The drug of choice for empiric therapy in patients with unconfirmed or suspected adrenal insufficiency is:
   a. ACTH
   b. Hydrocortisone
   c. Dexamethasone
   d. Prednisone
   e. None of the above

10. All of the following statements about the treatment of myxedema coma are true except:
    a. Administration of L-thyroxine should generally be accompanied by supplemental glucocorticoid.
    b. Empiric therapy is exceedingly safe and should be considered in all patients who present to the ED with coma and hypotension.
    c. Hyponatremia should be treated initially with isotonic or hypertonic fluids.
    d. Aggressive rewarming may be hazardous.
    e. Patients should be closely monitored in the ICU for hypoventilation and the need for intubation.

11. Signs and symptoms associated with thyroid storm include all of the following except:

a. Fever
b. Tachycardia
c. Rales
d. Loss of reflexes
e. Anxiety

12. Laboratory abnormalities associated with adrenal insufficiency include:
    a. Hypernatremia
    b. Hypokalemia
    c. Hypoglycemia
    d. Hypermagnesemia
    e. Hypercalcemia

13. All of the following statements about thyrotoxicosis are true except:
    a. Diarrhea and hyperdefecation may foreshadow impending thyroid storm.
    b. Atrial fibrillation is the most common electrocardiographic abnormality.
    c. Temperature is often greater than 100°F in the absence of infection.
    d. CNS dysfunction such as anxiety and tremors is present in nearly every patient.
    e. Pulse pressure is widened.

14. Treatment of thyroid storm includes all of the following except:
    a. Propylthiouracil, PO initially, to inhibit thyroid hormone synthesis
    b. Lugol's solution (iodide), PO, to inhibit thyroid hormone release
    c. Supportive care including oxygen, cardiac monitoring, and electrolyte analysis
    d. Propranolol IV up to 10 mg total to block the hormone's peripheral conversion of T4 to T3
    e. Lithium to block the release of thyroid hormone

15. All of the following statements about patients with adrenal insufficiency are true except:
    a. Adrenal crisis can be precipitated by trauma.
    b. Critically ill patients with a history of adrenal insufficiency should receive IV dexamethasone.
    c. Patients may present with hypertension, headache, and sweating.
    d. Adrenal crisis can be precipitated by cessation of inhaled steroids.
    e. Patients may present with hyperpigmentation of extensor surfaces, palms, and soles.

16. Which of the following statements about pheochromocytoma is false?
    a. Patients classically present with hypertension, headache, sweating, and palpitations.
    b. Psychological stress is rarely a trigger for an attack.
    c. It is associated with multiple endocrine neoplasia type II.
    d. Diagnosis is made by a spot urinalysis for the catecholamine metabolite vanillylmandelic acid.
    e. It may often be confused with other illnesses.

17. Signs or symptoms of myxedema include all of the following except:
    a. Tachycardia
    b. Cold intolerance
    c. Delayed relaxation phase of deep tendon reflexes
    d. Weakness and fatigue
    e. Dry, waxy, nonpitting swelling of the skin

18. Which of the following is not consistent with secondary adrenal insufficiency?
    a. Tachycardia
    b. Abdominal pain and vomiting
    c. Hypotension
    d. Hyperpigmentation
    e. Orthostatic hypotension

19. You are called to see a patient with changes in mental status. A fingerstick glucose reads greater than 400 mg/dL. Urinalysis reveals very high glucose, but no ketones. The patient has a past medical history of cardiac disease only. Before further labs are available, the most appropriate initial management should include:
    a. Immediate fluid resuscitation with IV normal saline and potassium chloride at 10 mEq/hour
    b. Administration of 10 units of regular insulin IV, fluid resuscitation with normal saline, and IV potassium chloride at 10 mEq/hour
    c. Administration of 10 units of regular insulin IV and fluid resuscitation with half-normal saline
    d. Immediate fluid resuscitation with normal saline, decreasing the rate of infusion once urine output is established
    e. Immediate fluid resuscitation with normal saline

20. In hyperosmolar nonketotic coma, which statement is true?
    a. Serum sodium correlates with the volume of fluid replacement required.
    b. Urine output is an accurate initial assessment of hydration status.
    c. Severity of mental status change correlates with the degree of hyperosmolarity.
    d. Plasma osmolarity correlates with the volume of fluid replacement required.
    e. Cerebral edema is common, and caution should be used in replacing volume.

21. Which statement about pheochromocytoma is false?
    a. It may be part of the multiple endocrine neoplasia syndrome.
    b. 10% of hypertensives harbor a pheochromocytoma.
    c. 10% of pheochromocytomas are malignant.
    d. 10% of pheochromocytomas are bilateral.
    e. 10% of pheochromocytomas are extra-adrenal.

22. A 37-year-old woman presents with complaints of weight gain and fatigue. On physical exam she is noted to be obese and to have a round or moon-shaped face, excess facial hair, and fat deposits between her shoulders ("buffalo hump"). The most common etiology for this constellation of symptoms would be:
    a. Pheochromocytoma
    b. Pituitary adenoma
    c. Prolonged use of prednisone

d. ACTH-secreting carcinoma
e. Adrenal tumor

23. A 5-year-old girl with type 1 diabetes mellitus presents with Kussmaul's respirations, altered mental status, glucosuria, and ketonuria. Which of the following statements is false?
    a. Venous blood gas will reveal an anion gap metabolic acidosis.
    b. Ketone levels are useful in guiding treatment over time.
    c. Potassium replacement will be required.
    d. Normal saline is the fluid of choice for initial resuscitation.
    e. An insulin drip will be required.

24. A 62-year-old woman presents with weakness, depression, and numbness and tingling around her mouth and in her fingertips. Her past medical history is significant for a recent thyroidectomy for thyroid cancer. Physical examination is remarkable for hyperactive deep tendon reflexes. Laboratory results are as follows: Na$^+$, 132; K$^+$, 3.6; Cl$^-$, 109; CO$_2$, 23; BUN, 12; creatinine, 0.7; total calcium, 6.8 mg/dL; Mg^{++}, 2.3; albumin, 3.0. Which statement is correct?
    a. She is probably suffering from hyperventilation syndrome.
    b. Her symptoms are probably a result of her thyroidectomy.
    c. She is not hypocalcemic because her corrected calcium is normal.
    d. Treatment includes calcitonin initially IV, then subcutaneously.
    e. She is probably hypothyroid.

25. A 26-year-old woman presents in diabetic ketoacidosis. Laboratory values are as follows: Na$^+$, 129; K$^+$, 3.2; Cl$^-$, 116; HCO$_3^-$, 16; glucose, 806. The corrected value of the sodium is:
    a. 118
    b. 130
    c. 140
    d. 151
    e. 135

26. A 56-year-old woman presents to the ED complaining of headache. She admits to having taken 10 tablets of her diabetes pill, which is confirmed by her husband to be chlorpropamide, 5-mg tablets. Vital signs are BP, 170/85; heart rate, 98; temperature, 98.5°F; RR, 18. Blood glucose is 145 mg/dL. She denies any other ingestion. She is treated with 50 g of activated charcoal and sorbitol. The psychiatry service consulting believes she is not suicidal or a threat to others and believes she can be discharged and followed as an outpatient. The most appropriate disposition is:
    a. Discharge home with close medical and psychiatric follow-up
    b. Admit to psychiatry for suicide attempt
    c. Give the patient something to eat and recheck the blood glucose in 1 hour
    d. Observe with hourly blood glucose checks and discharge after 6 hours if asymptomatic
    e. Admit overnight for frequent glucose checks

27. A 52-year-old woman presents with diaphoresis, tachycardia, confusion, and headache. A fingerstick glucose is 45 mg/dL. All of the following are possible causes for her low blood glucose level except:
    a. Starvation
    b. Exercise
    c. Type 2 diabetes mellitus
    d. Thyroid storm
    e. Insulin overdose

28. A 78-year-old man who lives alone is found on the floor of his apartment. He has been too weak to eat for at least 24 hours. Once he has used up his plasma glucose, what is his next source of endogenous glucose in his state of starvation?
    a. Gluconeogenesis in the liver from amino acid breakdown
    b. Triglyceride breakdown products (i.e., free fatty acids)
    c. Glycogenolysis in the liver
    d. Gluconeogenesis by the kidney
    e. Lactate transformation into glucose

29. A 47-year-old male presents with abdominal pain, nausea, and vomiting for 3 days, which has been worsening over the past 10 to 12 hours. He admits to occasional alcohol use, but none for 3 days. He has not been eating for the past 3 days. Vital signs are BP, 120/70; heart rate, 120; temperature, 99°F; RR, 22; Na$^+$, 138; K$^+$, 3.1; Cl$^-$, 91; HCO$_3^-$, 16. Urine shows 3+ ketones, and the ethanol level is 0. The patient's chart arrives and the patient has a documented history of alcohol abuse. What is the best course of initial therapy?
    a. Administer normal saline IV
    b. Administer D$_5$ normal saline IV
    c. Administer normal saline IV and 10 units of regular insulin IV
    d. Administer 100 mg of thiamine IV and D$_5$ normal saline IV
    e. Administer Valium

30. A 46-year-old woman presents with progressive weakness and constipation over several weeks. Laboratory analysis reveals a calcium of 12.2 mg/dL with a normal albumin. All of the following may account for the hypercalcemia except:
    a. Hyperparathyroidism
    b. Rickets
    c. Paget's disease
    d. Sarcoidosis
    e. Metastatic breast cancer

31. A 71-year-old woman with Paget's disease presents with a complaint of confusion and weakness. Physical exam is unremarkable except that the patient is somewhat disoriented. Laboratory results are as follows: Na$^+$, 134; K$^+$, 4.2; Cl$^-$, 107; CO$_2$, 23; BUN, 15; creatinine, 0.6;

Ca^{++}, 13.1; albumin, 3.9. The most appropriate ED actions include all of the following except:
a. Admission to a monitored bed
b. Aggressive hydration with IV normal saline
c. Diuresis with IV Lasix
d. Mithramycin by slow IV infusion

32. Which of the following is therapy for hypercalcemia?
a. Aggressive administration of normal saline with Lasix as needed
b. Calcitonin initially IV, then subcutaneously
c. Etidronate disodium by slow IV infusion
d. Mithramycin by slow IV infusion
e. All of the above

Answers

1.c. In patients with diabetic ketoacidosis, hyperglycemia results in a profound osmotic diuresis, leading to volume depletion as well as loss of potassium, chloride, calcium, magnesium, and phosphate through the kidneys. Cellular buffering of accumulated acids within the blood stream results in the transfer of hydrogen ions into cells and transfer of potassium into the extracellular fluid, leading to a paradoxical hyperkalemia in the presence of total body potassium depletion. Distributive hyponatremia occurs because of the additional solute load from glucose, which dilutes the measured serum sodium. *(Emergency Medicine, Chapter 58, pp 573–584)*

2.a. Volume depletion in patients with diabetic ketoacidosis may be severe and can lead to lactic acidosis, shock, and cardiovascular collapse. Fluid deficits may be assumed to be between 10% and 20% total body water. Initial replacement should be made with normal saline until vital signs are stabilized. Eventually, hypotonic fluids (i.e., half-normal saline) may be employed to address free water losses. Normalization of blood glucose should proceed slowly to avoid cerebral edema. Bicarbonate therapy should rarely be used in the management of patients with diabetic ketoacidosis, except in cases in which the pH is dangerously low (i.e., below 6.9). Although determination of the etiology of diabetic ketoacidosis is important, this should not supersede stabilization of the patient. *(Emergency Medicine, Chapter 58, pp 573–584)*

3.d. Necrosis of the pituitary within the sella turcica results in a constellation of symptoms, including headache from irritation of the meninges and pressure on the optic chiasm resulting in visual field defects. Cranial nerve palsies, most commonly of the third nerve but also affecting the fourth, fifth, and sixth, are also common. Paresthesias are not associated with pituitary apoplexy. *(Emergency Medicine, Chapter 59, pp 585–592)*

4.b. Primary adrenal insufficiency occurs when secretion of hormones by the adrenal gland is insufficient to meet the needs of the body. The most common cause worldwide is tuberculosis. However, autoimmune adrenalitis accounts for up to 60% of adult cases of primary adrenal insufficiency in the United States and the industrialized world. Administration of exogenous corticosteroids suppresses ACTH production by the pituitary gland; hence, abrupt discontinuation results in secondary adrenal insufficiency. *(Emergency Medicine, Chapter 59, pp 585–592)*

5.b. Low levels of circulating adrenal hormones (cortisol and aldosterone) result in inadequate gluconeogenesis by the liver, hypoglycemia, and generalized weakness. Aldosterone deficiency results in renal sodium loss and volume depletion, and cortisol deficiency results in decreased cardiac contractility. Hypotension may be severe. Back pain is a frequent complaint in patients with adrenal insufficiency and is thought to occur as a direct result of inflammation of the adrenal glands. Nausea, vomiting, and anorexia may be seen. Fever is rare. *(Emergency Medicine, Chapter 59, pp 585–592)*

6.c. Headache, sweating, and palpitations are the most common symptoms of pheochromocytoma and occur in 80%, 70%, and 60% of patients, respectively. Presence of all three symptoms has a sensitivity of 89% and specificity of 67% for the diagnosis. Fever is rarely associated with pheochromocytoma. *(Emergency Medicine, Chapter 59, pp 585–592)*

7.a. Calcium channel blockers, peripheral alpha-blockers, and nitrates are all acceptable alternatives in the management of hypertension associated with pheochromocytoma. Their use should be dictated by the severity of hypertension, the patient's mental status, and the urgency of the situation. Alpha-blockers (prazosin and phentolamine) may cause postural hypotension and should be used in small doses. Beta-blockers, including labetalol, should never be used alone in the management of pheochromocytoma, because blockade of beta-receptor–mediated vasodilation may result in paradoxical worsening of hypertension. *(Emergency Medicine, Chapter 59, pp 585–592)*

8.d. Inadequate circulating cortisol results in inadequate gluconeogenesis by the liver and in hypoglycemia. Patients with adrenal crisis are often between 15% and 20% volume depleted. Prompt administration of supplemental corticosteroids may be lifesaving. Patients with adrenal insufficiency are frequently hyperkalemic; therefore, supplemental potassium is rarely warranted. *(Emergency Medicine, Chapter 59, pp 585–592)*

9.c. Supplemental corticosteroids are the mainstay in the management of adrenal insufficiency. Both dexamethasone and hydrocortisone are suitable for the treatment of adrenal crisis. Hydrocortisone has the advantage of having both mineralocorticoid and glucocorticoid activity. However, hydrocortisone cross-reacts with the assay for cortisol and interferes with subsequent endocrinologic testing. Therefore, dexamethasone (Decadron) is the preferred agent when the diagnosis of adrenal insufficiency is unconfirmed. *(Emergency Medicine, Chapter 59, pp 585–592)*

10.b. Patients with myxedema coma present with weakness, lethargy, and impaired thermal regulation. Hypothermia is common, and although occasionally severe, it is best managed with passive rewarming measures alone. Volume depletion, hypotension, and hyponatremia are also seen and should be managed with isotonic or, if exceedingly severe, hypertonic fluids. Administration of replacement thyroid hormone is the mainstay of management of the patient with myxedema coma. L-Thyroxine is the recommended agent. Because large doses of thyroid hormone may precipitate cardiac ischemia, treatment should be reserved for patients in whom one strongly suspects hypothyroidism. Adrenal insufficiency commonly accompanies myxedema coma; therefore, adrenal testing and empiric treatment with glucocorticoids are essential. *(Emergency Medicine, Chapter 60, pp 593–596)*

11.d. Symptoms and signs of thyrotoxicosis or thyroid storm are numerous. Fever is quite common and may be greater than 105°F. Cardiovascular manifestations include tachycardia, frequently out of proportion to coexistent fever; a widened pulse pressure; atrial fibrillation; and CHF. Neurologic manifestations include tremor, anxiety, and hyperreflexia. *(Emergency Medicine, Chapter 60, pp 593–596)*

12.c. Hyponatremia is the most common laboratory abnormality associated with adrenal insufficiency and results from both impaired cortisol and aldosterone secretion. Hyperkalemia results from aldosterone deficiency and is associated with primary adrenal insufficiency. Hypoglycemia from cortisol deficiency is the most common laboratory abnormality in secondary adrenal insufficiency. Anemia, eosinophilia, and prerenal azotemia are also common. *(Emergency Medicine, Chapter 59, pp 585–592)*

13.b. Thyrotoxicosis can affect multiple systems. Sinus tachycardia is the most common cardiac abnormality. Atrial fibrillation, premature ventricular contractions, and complete heart block are possible. Fever is commonly present, with temperatures ranging from 100°F to 106°F. CNS findings are found in 90% of patients and range from anxiety and restlessness to obtundation and coma. Neuromuscular findings, including tremor and generalized weakness, can also be present. The average pulse pressure in thyrotoxicosis is widened to 80 mm, and there is increase in stroke volume, cardiac output, and myocardial oxygen consumption. Congestive heart failure may be a presenting sign of thyrotoxicosis. *(Emergency Medicine, Chapter 60, pp 593–596)*

14.d. There are four facets to the treatment of thyroid storm. Supportive care should include IV access, oxygen for increased metabolic requirements, and correction of electrolyte abnormalities. Inhibition of thyroid hormone synthesis is accomplished by administering propylthiouracil or methimazole. Iodide preparations prevent the release of thyroid hormone. The oral form of iodine is Lugol's solution. Sodium iodide is given IV. Lithium carbonate also blocks release of thyroid hormone. Beta-adrenergic blockade is used to dampen the adrenergic excess of thyrotoxicosis. It has no direct effect on the conversion of T4 to T3. *(Emergency Medicine, Chapter 60, pp 593–596)*

15.c. Adrenal crisis can be precipitated by trauma as well as by cessation of exogenous corticosteroids, including inhaled steroids. Hypertension, headache, and sweating are signs of catecholamine excess that are classically associated with pheochromocytoma and not hypoadrenalism. *(Emergency Medicine, Chapter 59, pp 585–592)*

16.d. Clinical manifestations of pheochromocytoma include headache, sweating, palpitations, and a sense of anxiety or impending doom. Psychological stress is not a trigger for an attack. The diagnosis of pheochromocytoma is made using a 24-hour urine collection for free catecholamines or vanillylmandelic acid, a catecholamine metabolite. Definitive diagnosis of pheochromocytoma in the ED is impossible, and treatment should be initiated when suggested by history and physical exam. *(Emergency Medicine, Chapter 59, pp 585–592)*

17.a. Myxedema is a manifestation of hypothyroidism. Patients either have primary hypothyroidism, as in Hashimoto's disease, or have been treated for hyperthyroidism by surgery or radioactive iodine (ablation) and are, hence, functionally hypothyroid. Symptoms of hypothyroidism include cold intolerance, weight gain, fatigue, and weakness. Signs include scant body hair, thin eyebrows, and a thick tongue. Deep tendon reflexes have a slowed relaxation phase. The heart may be enlarged, and a pericardial effusion may be present. An ECG may show low voltage. The patient may experience ileus, which can occasionally progress to megacolon. Temperatures tend to run low. Electrolyte abnormalities include hyponatremia, hypoglycemia, hypochloremia, and hypercholesterolemia. *(Emergency Medicine, Chapter 60, pp 593–596)*

18.d. Primary adrenal insufficiency is a rare disease. Symptoms do not appear until 90% of the gland is destroyed. Most commonly, the cause is idiopathic autoimmune adrenalitis. Other causes range from bacterial and granulomatous diseases to infiltrative diseases such as sarcoid and amyloid. Without the feedback inhibition from the hormones produced by the adrenal gland, the pituitary gland produces an excess of ACTH as well as excess melanocyte-stimulating hormone; thus, patients with primary adrenal disease show evidence of hyperpigmentation. Secondary adrenal insufficiency is most commonly caused by suppression of the adrenal-pituitary-hypothalamic axis by glucocorticoid therapy. Any process that damages the pituitary can result in decreased production of ACTH and, hence, decreased adrenal function. Etiologies include tumors, infarction (pituitary apoplexy), and hemorrhage (Sheehan's syndrome) of the pituitary gland. Hyperpigmentation does not occur in secondary adrenal insufficiency because there is no excess of ACTH and melanocyte-stimulating hormone. *(Emergency Medicine, Chapter 59, pp 585–592)*

19.e. Hyperosmolar nonketotic coma is a state of dehydration that results from a prolonged osmotic diuresis. Two thirds of patients have no prior history of diabetes mellitus. It can occur in the presence of pneumonia, gram-negative sepsis, chronic renal insufficiency, and MI. It has a mortality rate of 20% to 60%, and quick action is required once the diagnosis is suspected. Although ketosis is not universally absent, in this case the patient is extremely hyperglycemic without ketosis in the setting of altered mental status. Laboratory analysis reveals an elevated blood glucose, elevated BUN/creatinine ratio, low potassium (total body potassium is depleted), a high-anion-gap acidosis, and high, normal, or low sodium. Initial management includes vigorous volume resuscitation and rehydration with normal saline. Not all cases of hyperosmolar nonketotic coma require the use of insulin. The glucose level will drop considerably by dilution alone during rehydration. Most patients are depleted of total body potassium and will require potassium repletion. However, renal function must be assessed before starting infusion of potassium to ensure that the patient is not in renal failure. Urine output is not a good measure of volume status in management of hyperosmolar nonketotic coma, because continued osmotic diuresis may give a false impression of adequate hydration. *(Emergency Medicine, Chapter 58, pp 573–584)*

20.c. Neither serum sodium nor plasma osmolarity accurately predicts the volume of fluid replacement required for resuscitation in hyperosmolar nonketotic coma. Urine output should not be used in initial assessment of hydration status because as long as the patient remains hyperglycemic, ongoing osmotic diuresis will occur. The severity of mental status changes happens to correlate well with the degree of hyperosmolarity. Cerebral edema is rare and probably results from inappropriate administration of hypotonic fluids and severe disease. *(Emergency Medicine, Chapter 58, pp 573–584)*

21.b. Epinephrine and norepinephrine are released into the blood stream by the chromaffin cells of the adrenal medulla. Tumors of theses cells are called pheochromocytomas. The "10%" rule of pheochromocytomas is that 10% are malignant, 10% are extra-adrenal, and 10% are bilateral. More than 90% of patients with pheochromocytoma present with hypertension, headache, and other signs of excess epinephrine and norepinephrine. Sipple syndrome, or multiple endocrine neoplasia type II, consists of pheochromocytoma, medullary carcinoma of the thyroid, and parathyroid adenoma. *(Emergency Medicine, Chapter 59, pp 585–592)*

22.c. Cushing's syndrome, or hypercortisolism, is a result of symptomatic glucocorticoid excess. Patients most commonly present with fat deposits in the face (moon facies), shoulders and back (buffalo hump), hirsutism, menstrual disorders, hypertension, muscular weakness, purple striae, and acne. Prolonged excess exogenous steroid use is the most common cause of hypercortisolism. Other causes include pituitary adenomas, ACTH-secreting carcinomas (e.g., small cell bronchogenic cancer and pancreatic cancer), and adrenal neoplasms. Pheochromocytomas cause excess secretion of epinephrine and norepinephrine. *(Emergency Medicine, Chapter 59, pp 585–592)*

23.b. Once hyperglycemia greater than 250 mg/dL has been verified by dextrose stick, this patient will require insulin to treat diabetic ketoacidosis. Initial fluid of choice is normal saline to replace intravascular volume as well as restore sodium balance. Patients in diabetic ketoacidosis are depleted of total body potassium and require careful monitoring of potassium. Initial acidemia will cause a shift of potassium from the intracellular to the extracellular-intravascular compartment, and care must be taken not to mistake a normal to high initial potassium level for high or normal potassium stores. Cardiac monitoring and ECG are prudent until the patent's potassium is restored. Ketoacidosis is a result of increased production of beta-hydroxybutyrate and acetoacetate in the liver. Beta-hydroxybutyrate has a concentration three times that of acetoacetate. However, the laboratory test used to measure ketones in serum measures acetoacetate only. Therefore, it is not helpful to follow ketone levels to guide treatment over time. Venous blood gases are easier to draw than arterial blood gases in children. Serial venous pH measurements are adequate to assess the acidosis. *(Emergency Medicine, Chapter 58, pp 573–584)*

24.b. Parathyroid hormone increases serum calcium by increasing bone resorption of calcium, enhancing intestinal absorption of calcium via vitamin D, and enhancing calcium resorption by the kidney. There is a risk in thyroidectomy surgery that all four parathyroid tissues are removed, thus creating a patient who is clinically hypoparathyroid and who ultimately becomes hypocalcemic. One of the parathyroid glands is usually implanted into the patient's forearm to prevent hypocalcemia. Total plasma calcium is present in the form of free (ionized) calcium and calcium bound to proteins (albumin and globulins). Only the ionized form is physiologically active. For every decrease in serum albumin of 1 g/dL, the total serum calcium decreases by 0.8 mg/dL without changing the ionized calcium. Therefore, this patient's corrected calcium is 7.6 mg/dL. It is unlikely that this patient is hypothyroid, given the hyperactive tendon reflexes. Calcitonin increases calcium absorption by bone and hence lowers the serum calcium. *(Emergency Medicine, Chapter 60, pp 593–596)*

25.c. The presence of glucose in the serum causes a dilutional effect when measuring serum sodium. For every

100 mg/dL of glucose greater than 100 mg/dL, the actual serum sodium is 1.6 mEq higher. The patient's glucose is 706 mg/dL higher than a baseline of 100 mg/dL. There is 7 × 1.6 mg/dL more sodium than the lab has measured (1.6 × 7 = 11.2). The corrected sodium is 129 + 11.2 = 140.2 mg/dL. **(Emergency Medicine, Chapter 57, pp 558)**

26.e. Chlorpropamide has a half-life of 36 hours, the longest of the sulfonylurea oral hypoglycemic medicines. Profound hypoglycemia can occur at any time during the elimination half-life of the drug, especially in an overdose situation. Although this patient has been cleared by psychiatry and has no signs or symptoms of hypoglycemia, she must be admitted overnight to observe for hypoglycemia. **(Emergency Medicine, Chapter 58, pp 573–584)**

27.d. Exercise and starvation can cause states of low blood glucose. Excess insulin will also cause hypoglycemia, whether from endogenous sources like an islet cell tumor of the pancreas or exogenously by administration of too much insulin. Early diabetes, especially of the type 2 kind, is characterized by a state of relative insulin resistance. Patients with type 2 diabetes early in their illness may have a delayed release of excess insulin after eating, causing a transient 20-minute episode of hypoglycemia. Hyperglycemia is a common finding in thyroid storm, not hypoglycemia. **(Emergency Medicine, Chapter 58, pp 573–584)**

28.c. In the starvation state, as plasma glucose and insulin levels fall, a number of rescue mechanisms occur. First is the breakdown of glycogen to glucose by the liver. Once the insulin level is low, proteolysis and lipolysis are no longer inhibited. The amino acids from proteolysis are reconstructed into glucose in the liver, i.e., gluconeogenesis. This process is aided by the presence of glucagon. Triglycerides are broken down into free fatty acids and glycerol; however, the brain and the formed elements of the blood cannot use free fatty acids as an energy source. The released glycerol can be converted to glucose by the liver. Lactate can also be converted to glucose but is a minor source of glucose in the starvation state. **(Emergency Medicine, Chapter 58, pp 573–584)**

29.d. Alcoholic ketoacidosis usually occurs after a heavy binge of alcohol drinking accompanied by little food intake for several days. It is postulated that during increased lipolysis, the liver produces a substantial amount of the ketone bodies acetoacetate and beta-hydroxybutyrate. Furthermore, acetate from the breakdown of alcohol is degraded to ketones. To compound matters, chronic malnutrition contributes to the ketoacidosis. The typical patient experiences abdominal pain 24 to 72 hours prior to presenting to the ED. In the ED, the patient presents with dehydration, tachycardia, and diffuse abdominal pain. Urine will be positive for ketones and frequently the ethanol level is 0 because the binge ended days before. Treatment with IV normal saline alone is adequate; however, patients recover faster if dextrose is added to the fluids. In order to avoid Wernicke's encephalopathy, 100 mg of thiamine should be administered prior to starting any dextrose-containing solution. Insulin is rarely required in alcoholic ketoacidosis. Glucose levels are frequently normal or low, and insulin may in fact be dangerous. **(Emergency Medicine, Chapter 58, pp 573–584)**

30.b. Hypercalcemia can be caused by malignancy, Paget's disease, granulomatous diseases, hyperparathyroidism, and a number of rare causes, including vitamin D intoxication in food faddists. Rickets results from a lack of vitamin D and causes hypocalcemia. **(Emergency Medicine, Chapter 60, pp 593–596)**

31.d. Aggressive hydration is the first line of therapy in hypercalcemia. Diuretics help reduce the calcium load and avoid fluid overloading. Since large amounts of fluids can cause electrolyte shifts of sodium, potassium, and magnesium, close observation is crucial. If aggressive hydration and loop diuretics fail to lower the calcium sufficiently, then calcitonin is a treatment option before resorting to mithramycin. Mithramycin is the most potent agent for management of hypercalcemia. Its use should be restricted to emergency treatment of severe hypercalcemia because of its toxicity to the liver and kidneys, and its potential to lower the platelet count. **(Emergency Medicine, Chapter 60, pp 593–596)**

32.e. Normal saline increases urinary calcium excretion and the loop diuretic further inhibits calcium and sodium transport downstream from the proximal tubule. Calcitonin increases calcium deposition in the bone, increases calcium excretion and phosphate reabsorption by the kidneys, and increases phosphate absorption from the gut. It should be used if hydration and diuresis fail. Mithramycin is the most potent antihypercalcemia medication. It lowers serum calcium by inhibiting bone reabsorption. Etidronate is a diphosphonate that inhibits bone resorption by osteoclasts and is especially effective for lowering hypercalcemia in patients with malignancy. **(Emergency Medicine, Chapter 60, pp 593–596)**

BIBLIOGRAPHY

Ferraro CM: Thyroid and parathyroid glands. *In* Howell JM, Altieri M, Jagoda AS, et al (eds): Emergency Medicine. Philadelphia, WB Saunders, 1998, pp 593–596.

Raney LH: Disorders of glucose metabolism. *In* Howell JM, Altieri M, Jagoda AS, et al (eds): Emergency Medicine. Philadelphia, WB Saunders, 1998, pp 573–584.

Rothenhaus TC: Disorders of the adrenal and pituitary systems. *In* Howell JM, Altieri M, Jagoda AS, et al (eds): Emergency Medicine. Philadelphia, WB Saunders, 1998, pp 585–592.

Tayal VS, Conners GP: Fluid and electrolyte disorders. *In* Howell JM, Altieri M, Jagoda AS, et al (eds): Emergency Medicine. Philadelphia, WB Saunders, 1998, pp 549–572.

SECTION EIGHT

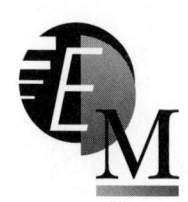

Head and Neck Disorders

27 Traumatic and Nontraumatic Eye Disorders

SYNDEE J. GIVRE, MD

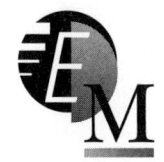

1. A patient presents to the ED after a chemical splash to the right eye. The first course of action is to:
   a. Determine the nature of the chemical and then begin irrigation
   b. Determine the nature of the chemical and then begin irrigation with a neutralizing solution
   c. Check the patient's visual acuity
   d. Irrigate the eye
   e. Check the pH of the inferior conjunctival fornix

2. A 32-year-old man is brought to the ED by ambulance. He is complaining of left eye pain and cannot give a clear history (a strong odor of alcohol is noted). A glance at the patient reveals lacerations of the left upper and lower eyelids and a scleral laceration with uveal prolapse in that eye. Which of the following statements is false?
   a. A primary survey for life-threatening conditions should proceed before the open globe is attended to.
   b. Because the mechanism of globe injury cannot be ascertained by history, a CT of the orbits should be obtained to exclude an intraocular foreign body; MRI, if available, is preferable for better resolution of orbital and ocular contents.
   c. Appropriate medications to be administered are tetanus prophylaxis, IV antimicrobials, and, if needed, antiemetics.
   d. Once the open globe has been diagnosed, an eye shield (Fox shield) should be placed and ophthalmologic consultation requested.
   e. The lid lacerations should probably be repaired in the operating room.

3. A 52-year-old woman presents to the ED after the wind caused a tree branch to hit her in the left eye. She is complaining of severe eye pain. Complete ocular examination is normal except for a left corneal abrasion. Which of the following statements is true?
   a. The patient may be treated with topical antimicrobial drops to prevent infection and, if needed, topical anesthetic drops for pain control.
   b. The patient may be treated by instillation of an antimicrobial ointment and then placement of a pressure patch.
   c. Both oral and topical antimicrobials are indicated for a large corneal abrasion in the visual axis (in front of the pupil).
   d. The patient may be treated with a topical steroid–antimicrobial combination drop to prevent traumatic iritis and infection.
   e. The patient may be treated with topical antimicrobial drops to prevent infection and, if needed, cycloplegic drops for photophobia.

4. Match each of the following visual symptoms with its most likely etiology. (Each etiology may be used more than once or not at all.)
   a. Uniocular flashing lights and shower of floaters (black spots)
   b. Persistent uniocular curtain or veil across the field of view
   c. Uniocular single black spot floating through field of view, present 2 years
   d. Uniocular, transient graying of vision lasting 10 minutes
   e. Uniocular blurred vision associated with pain and tearing

   i. Retinal detachment
   ii. Corneal abrasion
   iii. Posterior vitreous detachment
   iv. Transient ischemic attack—anterior circulation
   v. Transient ischemic attack—posterior circulation

5. A 40-year-old woman falls two stories, suffering severe blunt trauma. Which of the following statements is false?
   a. Once the diagnosis of retrobulbar hemorrhage has been made, lateral canthotomy/cantholysis is required.
   b. Examination reveals proptosis of the globe, decreased visual acuity, and an afferent pupillary defect in the right eye; the most likely diagnosis is retrobulbar hemorrhage.
   c. Examination reveals periorbital swelling, restriction of elevation, and hypoesthesia below the lower right eyelid; the most likely diagnosis is orbital floor fracture.

d. Retinal hemorrhages may be present without blunt trauma directly to the globe.
e. The presence of vitreous hemorrhage should prompt careful examination for an open globe injury.

6. Which of the following statements concerning hyphema is false?
   a. Complications of hyphema include increased intraocular pressure and corneal staining.
   b. Rebleeding most commonly occurs within the first few days after the hyphema.
   c. Therapy most commonly consists of bed rest and cycloplegic drops.
   d. Hyphemas involving 80% or more of the anterior chamber should be washed out to avoid prolonged raised intraocular pressure and blood staining of the cornea in the visual axis.
   e. In cases of total (eight-ball) hyphema, it is important to promptly examine the posterior segment (e.g., lens, retina, and optic nerve) of the globe for damage.

7. Adverse effects of topical corticosteroids include all of the following except:
   a. Elevation of intraocular pressure
   b. Episcleritis
   c. Cataracts
   d. Exacerbation of bacterial keratitis
   e. Exacerbation of viral and fungal keratitis

8. A 19-year-old woman is brought to the ED after engaging in a knife fight with a fellow inmate. She has multiple lacerations to the left eyelids and a conjunctival laceration. Which of the following is true?
   a. The lower eyelid margin laceration lateral to the lacrimal punctum should not require repair by an ophthalmologist.
   b. The linear laceration down to the level of the orbicularis oculi may result in permanent ptosis if not repaired correctly.
   c. The 1.0-mm laceration to the conjunctiva requires repair with one or two absorbable sutures.
   d. The through-and-through upper lid laceration requires a multilayered closure and no further evaluation.
   e. The lower eyelid margin laceration medial to the lacrimal punctum should be repaired by an ophthalmologist.

9. A 23-year-old metal worker presents to the ED complaining of pain in her right eye. Which of the following statements is false?
   a. A corneal foreign body is detected; it can be removed with a cotton-tipped applicator stick or a fine needle.
   b. Multiple vertical corneal abrasions are detected; eversion of the eyelid should be performed.
   c. A corneal foreign body and cataract are detected; the foreign body should be removed and the patient referred for routine evaluation by an ophthalmologist regarding cataract extraction.
   d. A corneal foreign body is detected and removed; however, the rust ring cannot be removed successfully. Follow-up the next day for removal of the remainder of the rust ring by an ophthalmologist is acceptable.
   e. Examination of both eyes reveals multiple punctate areas of uptake after administration of fluorescein; the patient should be questioned about the possibility of recent arc-welding.

10. Vitreous hemorrhage can be seen commonly in all of the following situations except:
    a. Diabetic retinopathy
    b. Blunt trauma to the globe
    c. Ocular perforation
    d. Posterior vitreous detachment
    e. Retinal tear

11. Each of the following constitutes an ophthalmic emergency requiring rapid intervention in the ED except:
    a. Central retinal artery occlusion
    b. Temporal arteritis
    c. Acute optic neuritis
    d. Orbital cellulitis
    e. Increased retrobulbar pressure

12. Match the eye emergency with the signs and symptoms with which it usually presents. (Each diagnosis may be paired with more than one presentation.)
    a. Central retinal artery occlusion
    b. Temporal arteritis
    c. Acute narrow-angle glaucoma
    d. Increased retrobulbar pressure
    e. Orbital cellulitis

    i. Eyelid edema and injection, conjunctival chemosis and injection, decreased adduction, and afferent pupillary defect in an 18-month-old boy
    ii. Decreased vision, orbital pain, afferent pupillary defect, myalgias, weight loss, and jaw claudication in a 79-year-old woman
    iii. Red, painful eye with a hazy cornea, dense cataract, and poor vision in a 65-year-old woman
    iv. Painless decrease in vision to hand motion in a hypertensive 62-year-old man
    v. Gradual loss of vision and afferent pupillary defect in a 57-year-old man with prostate cancer

13. Match the type of conjunctivitis with its commonly encountered features.
    a. Viral
    b. Gonococcal
    c. Allergic
    d. Staphylococcal
    e. Chlamydial

    i. Small, white ulcerations at the limbus associated with erythematous eyelid margin
    ii. Itchy eye; injected, chemotic conjunctiva with splinter hemorrhages and preauricular adenopathy
    iii. Itchy eyes, injected and chemotic conjunctivae, recurring every spring
    iv. Red eye with profuse purulent discharge accompanied by corneal infiltration and thinning
    v. Mild conjunctivitis with lid edema, conjunctival chemosis, and mucous discharge persisting despite 3 weeks of broad-spectrum topical antimicrobial coverage

14. A 72-year-old woman with hypertension and type 2 diabetes mellitus presents to the ED with acute, painless loss of vision in the right eye for the past 1.5 hours. Examination reveals visual acuity of light perception, normal anterior segment, intraocular pressure of 25, and an opaque, white retina with cherry-red spot in the macula. Which of the following statements is false?
    a. It is too late for reperfusion of the retina to result in improved vision.
    b. Emergent, noninvasive treatment includes digital massage of the globe and having the patient breathe into a paper bag, though likelihood of visual improvement is small.
    c. The history and examination are most consistent with a central retinal artery occlusion.
    d. Steroids may be given emergently.
    e. The mildly elevated intraocular pressure is likely unrelated to the acute visual loss.

15. Which of the following statements concerning lid pathology is true?
    a. Initial treatment for an external hordeolum consists of incision and drainage.
    b. Hemifacial spasm is a benign disorder that can be treated with injections of botulinum toxin.
    c. Chronic blepharitis can be staphylococcal or seborrheic.
    d. Ptosis can be associated with conjunctivitis, aging, cranial nerve VII palsy, and Horner's syndrome.
    e. Ectropion frequently leads to chronic irritation from eyelashes rubbing against the cornea.

16. A 27-year-old woman presents to the ED with a complaint of a red left eye. Which of the following statements is true?
    a. A subconjunctival hemorrhage is noted in the left eye. With no history of trauma, a CBC and PT/PTT are the only labs indicated initially.
    b. Examination reveals mildly dilated ocular surface blood vessels that blanch after application of a drop of 10% phenylephrine. The patient is likely to have an associated, identifiable rheumatologic disorder.
    c. Examination reveals flare and cells in the anterior chamber of the left eye. Pain on shining a light into the right eye is probably due to early iritis in this eye as well.
    d. Blurred vision in a patient with iritis implies a coexisting posterior uveitis and retinitis.
    e. Examination reveals a tender, bluish purple quadrant of inflamed ocular vessels that do not blanch on administration of topical phenylephrine. Emergent/urgent consultation with an ophthalmologist is required for scleritis.

17. A 32-year-old man presents to the ED with vesicles on the right upper eyelid. The conjunctiva is mildly injected and the cornea exhibits multiple areas of staining after instillation of fluorescein. Which statement about this patient is false?
    a. The patient's condition may be a result of herpes simplex virus or herpes zoster virus.
    b. There is an increased incidence of herpes virus infection and reactivation in patients with AIDS.
    c. Topical antivirals are indicated for keratitis caused by herpes zoster keratitis.
    d. Oral acyclovir may be indicated.
    e. Steroids may severely exacerbate herpes simplex keratitis.

18. An 11-month-old boy is brought to the ED by his mother, who complains that he tears constantly from the right eye and wakes up each morning with the lashes matted together. Which of the following statements is false?
    a. Dacryocystitis may progress to orbital cellulitis.
    b. The patient's symptoms are consistent with dacryoadenitis.
    c. A trial of massage and topical antimicrobials is indicated in this case.
    d. Reflux of mucus from the punctum with massage over the nasolacrimal sac is virtually diagnostic of nasolacrimal duct obstruction.
    e. A similar set of symptoms can be seen in adults with dacryoliths.

19. A 71-year-old man presents to the ED complaining of pain in his right eye, nausea, and vomiting. Which of the following statement regarding this patient is true?
    a. The intraocular pressure in the right eye is 50. The eye is injected and the anterior chamber appears narrow on slit-lamp examination; the patient should have immediate laser iridectomy.
    b. The intraocular pressure in the right eye is 50. The eye is injected and the hazy cornea precludes determination of anterior chamber depth; the patient should have immediate iridectomy for presumed acute narrow-angle glaucoma.
    c. The intraocular pressure in the right eye is 50. The pupil is mid-dilated and the cornea is slightly hazy; the patient should be treated with ocular hypotensive medications including topical beta-blockers, low-concentration pilocarpine (1 or 2 percent), and systemic medication such as acetazolamide and osmotic agents as needed to lower the pressure.
    d. The intraocular pressure in the right eye is 50. The eye is injected and the cornea is hazy. The intraocular pressure in the left eye is 32. High pressure in the left eye points to a diagnosis of primary open-angle glaucoma rather than narrow-angle glaucoma.
    e. Osmotic agents decrease aqueous humor production.

20. A 2-year-old girl is brought to the ED with a history of a recent upper respiratory infection and 2 days of right eyelid swelling and erythema. Which of the following statements regarding the management of this patient is true?
    a. A distinction between preseptal and orbital cellulitis cannot be made clinically in preverbal children.
    b. Periorbital cellulitis is more common in adults than in children.
    c. In a reliable, compliant patient, orbital cellulitis may be treated with oral antimicrobials and daily follow-up.

d. On examination, the patient exhibits markedly decreased adduction of the right eye and mildly decreased abduction; the diagnosis of orbital cellulitis is made, the patient is admitted for IV antimicrobial treatment, and CT scan is not necessary.
e. Therapy for periorbital cellulitis should cover *Haemophilus influenzae, Streptococcus pneumoniae, Staphylococcus aureus,* and beta-hemolytic streptococcus.

Answers

1.d. In all cases of chemical injury to the eye, the first action should be irrigation with the nearest IV solution. The faster irrigation is begun, the more quickly the agent will be removed from contact with the ocular surface, thus minimizing damage. Irrigation should continue at least until pH paper placed in the inferior conjunctival fornix reads neutral (around 7.0). History can be obtained during irrigation, and the remainder of the examination can proceed after irrigation is completed. *(Emergency Medicine, Chapter 63, pp 626–638)*

2.b. Life-threatening injuries take precedence over sight-threatening injuries. Once an open globe has been diagnosed, an eye shield should be placed over the eye against the bony orbit margins (**not touching the globe itself; any pressure on the globe could lead to further extrusion of intraocular contents**). Tetanus prophylaxis, IV antimicrobials, and, if needed, antiemetics should be given and an ophthalmology consultation requested. Lid lacerations should be attended to after the globe is closed in the operating room (again, to prevent any pressure on the globe and further extrusion of intraocular contents). In cases of possible foreign body, a CT scan should be obtained. MRI is contraindicated because of the possibility of a metallic foreign body. *(Emergency Medicine, Chapter 63, pp 626–638)*

3.e. Corneal abrasions should be treated with topical antimicrobials. Oral antimicrobials are not indicated. Topical cycloplegic agents may help to decrease photophobia. When the abrading agent (in this example a tree branch) is potentially "dirty," a pressure patch should not be placed because this could accelerate infection. **Topical anesthetic drops are never indicated as therapy—the resulting corneal anesthesia could cause severe trauma and infection.** *(Emergency Medicine, Chapter 63, pp 626–638)*

4.a. i, iii; b. i; c. iii; d. iv; e. ii. Complaints of floaters coupled with flashes of light or a curtain/veil in the visual field are strongly suggestive of retinal detachment. Patients with such complaints should have a detailed retinal examination. Patients who see floaters without flashes or a curtain are less likely to have a retinal detachment; however, such patients should also have a detailed retinal examination (perhaps less urgently). Anterior circulation transient ischemic attacks produce monocular visual loss. Posterior circulation transient ischemic attacks produce bilateral visual loss. Other causes of transient visual loss include papilledema, migraine, giant cell arteritis, impending central retinal vein occlusion, and ischemic optic neuropathy. Ocular surface pathology (i.e., corneal and conjunctival) is often accompanied by symptoms of pain, tearing, and photophobia. *(Emergency Medicine, Chapter 63, pp 626–638)*

5.a. Retrobulbar hemorrhage can increase intraocular pressure. Mild elevations in pressure may be well tolerated by the patient without any therapy. More severe elevations in pressure may require treatment. The first attempts at lowering intraocular pressure should be pharmacologic (e.g., topical beta-blocker, oral or IV acetazolamide, and hyperosmotic agents such as mannitol). If these are unsuccessful, lateral canthotomy/cantholysis will be necessary. If lateral canthotomy/cantholysis is unsuccessful, orbital decompression surgery may be necessary. *(Emergency Medicine, Chapter 63, pp 626–638)*

6.d. The most acute danger of a hyphema of any size is elevated intraocular pressure. (Also, the higher the intraocular pressure, the higher the risk of corneal blood staining.) Treatment depends on the level of intraocular pressure, not on the amount of hyphema. When a total hyphema is present, the posterior segment of the globe must be examined indirectly (e.g., with ultrasound B scan). *(Emergency Medicine, Chapter 63, pp 626–638)*

7.b. Topical corticosteroids should not be given without the advice of an ophthalmologist. Adverse effects can be sight-threatening. *(Emergency Medicine, Chapter 63, pp 626–638)*

8.e. Any eyelid margin laceration requires precise repair to prevent notching and merits consultation by an ophthalmologist. Eyelid margin lacerations medial to the punctae may involve the lacrimal canaliculi. Canalicular laceration requires surgical repair by an ophthalmologist to prevent chronic tearing. The orbicularis oculi is the superficial muscular layer in the eyelid. The orbicularis is a large muscle responsible for closing the eyelid. A laceration down to the level of orbicularis should not dramatically affect eyelid function. The levator palpebrae muscle, responsible for opening the eyelid, is deep to the orbicularis. Damage to the levator commonly results in ptosis and requires repair by an ophthalmologist. Through-and-through eyelid lacerations should alert the examiner to possible open globe injuries. A thorough ocular examination is needed in the case of full-thickness lacerations. Small conjunctival lacerations (up to 1.5 cm) do not require closure. *(Emergency Medicine, Chapter 63, pp 626–638)*

9.c. Superficial corneal foreign bodies are removed with an applicator stick or a fine needle (26 or 30 gauge).

If the foreign body is sitting on the corneal surface it can be irrigated off. It may not be possible to completely remove deeply embedded foreign bodies or rust rings at the first visit. They can be removed the next day, because they migrate more superficially. Any history suggestive of possible ocular perforation such as working with machinery, metal striking metal, or explosion warrants complete ocular examination to exclude a foreign body (symptoms can be minimal). The finding of a cataract in this patient is extremely suggestive of ocular perforation. A complete examination and imaging study are necessary, in addition to ophthalmology consultation. Fine, vertical, linear scratches with fluorescein uptake suggest a foreign body under the eyelid. Multiple areas of punctate staining in both eyes suggests a burn from a welding lamp. This is often extremely painful. Treatment is with topical antimicrobials and cycloplegics. *(Emergency Medicine, Chapter 63, pp 626–638)*

10. d. Vitreous hemorrhage is rarely seen in posterior vitreous detachment. If vitreous hemorrhage is present, an extensive search for a retinal tear or detachment must be made by an ophthalmologist. *(Emergency Medicine, Chapter 63, pp 626–638)*

11. c. Treatment of central retinal artery occlusion is aimed at moving the embolus further downstream, so that more retina is perfused. Digital massage and anterior chamber paracentesis cause fluctuations in intraocular pressure that may dislodge the embolus. Increased carbon dioxide levels from breathing into a paper bag leads to dilation of the retinal vessels, which may dislodge the embolus. Irreversible damage to the retina occurs after approximately 90 to 120 minutes of nonperfusion. Temporal arteritis is an inflammatory condition resulting in arterial obstruction. Prompt treatment with steroids can prevent further visual loss in the involved eye and prevent visual loss in the uninvolved eye. Orbital cellulitis requires prompt delivery of antimicrobials to the infected orbital regions, which may include the cranial nerves (including the optic nerve). Treatment is also aimed at preventing the spread of infection to the CNS. Increased retrobulbar pressure may compress the optic nerve, permanently damaging it, or may increase IOP, permanently damaging intraocular structures. Prompt lowering of retrobulbar pressure is indicated in these situations. Optic neuritis can cause acute visual loss, for example, in multiple sclerosis. Studies have demonstrated that prompt treatment with IV steroids does not affect the final visual recovery of affected patients (although speed of recovery may be increased with IV steroid treatment). *(Emergency Medicine, Chapter 62, pp 609–625)*

12. a. ii, iv—Central retinal artery occlusion may be the result of temporal arteritis.
    b. ii, iv—Any patient over the age of 50 with a central retinal artery occlusion should have an ESR done and should be questioned about symptoms of temporal arteritis.
    c. iii—Large, cataractous lenses may shallow the anterior chamber, contributing to a congenitally narrow angle; alternatively, anterior segment ischemia from repeated narrow-angle attacks may contribute to cataract formation.
    d. v—Retrobulbar masses, such as metastases, may increase retrobulbar pressure, leading to compression of the optic nerve and gradual visual loss.
    e. i—If infection is posterior to the orbital septum, visual acuity, ocular motility, and pupillary responses can be affected. *(Emergency Medicine, Chapter 62, pp 609–625)*

13. a. ii—Viral conjunctivitis is often bilateral and may be hemorrhagic; a history of recent upper respiratory infection or contact with someone with a red eye may be obtained.
    b. iv—*Gonococcus* is one of the few bacteria that can penetrate the cornea.
    c. iii—Allergic conjunctivitis presents with bilateral chemosis, itching, and watery discharge.
    d. i—Staphylococcal blepharitis is commonly associated with conjunctivitis and peripheral corneal infiltrates. Treatment is eyelid hygiene (lid scrubs with baby shampoo) and topical steroid–antimicrobial combination (steroids should be given only in consultation with an ophthalmologist).
    e. v—Chlamydial conjunctivitis should be suspected when conjunctivitis does not resolve in 3 to 4 weeks. Sexual history should be obtained and partners treated. *(Emergency Medicine, Chapter 62, pp 609–625)*

14. a. The patient has a central retinal artery occlusion. This could be secondary to temporal arteritis (in which case steroids are indicated). The patient gives a history of 1.5 hours of visual loss. This is within the time frame of possible beneficial results of reperfusion of the retina. At a minimum, noninvasive treatment should be instituted. Anterior chamber paracentesis (invasive) should be discussed with an ophthalmologist. *(Emergency Medicine, Chapter 62, pp 609–625)*

15. c. The initial treatment for external hordeolum is warm soaks and topical antimicrobials. Hemifacial spasm is characterized by unilateral spasm of the entire side of the face, including during sleep. It is most commonly caused by damage to cranial nerve VII in the brain stem. Neuroimaging is indicated to exclude a tumor. This is in contrast to benign essential blepharospasm, which involves the eyelid only and can be bilateral. Benign essential blepharospasm disappears during sleep. Ptosis occurs with cranial nerve III palsy. Ectropion refers to eversion of the eyelid. Entropion refers to inversion of the eyelid margin, including the eyelashes. Inversion of the eyelashes can cause chronic corneal irritation. *(Emergency Medicine, Chapter 62, pp 609–625)*

16. e. Subconjunctival hemorrhage does not require evaluation unless it is recurrent. Answer b describes a patient with episcleritis. In the majority of patients with episcleritis, an underlying disorder cannot be found. In

iritis or anterior uveitis, pain occurs on shining a light into the uninvolved eye because this induces a consensual pupillary response in the involved eye. Patients with anterior uveitis or iritis without posterior involvement may have blurred vision caused by inflammatory material in the anterior chamber or from malfunctioning of the ciliary muscle, which controls accommodation of the lens. Answer e describes a patient with nodular scleritis. In some cases, scleritis can lead to scleral thinning and perforation or optic nerve involvement. The inflammation must be reduced in a timely manner to avoid these complications. Emergent/urgent consultation with an ophthalmologist is needed to treat the scleritis and to evaluate the patient for an underlying etiology (e.g., connective tissue diseases such as rheumatoid arthritis, Wegener's granulomatosis, and lupus; sarcoidosis; syphilis; and tuberculosis). *(Emergency Medicine, Chapter 62, pp 609–625)*

17. c. Topical antiviral medication is the treatment for herpes simplex conjunctivitis or keratoconjunctivitis. Antiviral drops are not indicated for herpes zoster ophthalmicus; however, if given early in the course, high-dose oral acyclovir may shorten the course of the disease, and, in nonimmunocompromised patients, oral corticosteroids may minimize postherpetic neuralgia. Corticosteroids (topical or oral) should not be used in herpes simplex keratoconjunctivitis, as they may worsen the infection. *(Emergency Medicine, Chapter 62, pp 609–625)*

18. b. The patient's complaints are consistent with a diagnosis of nasolacrimal duct obstruction. This occurs congenitally in children (more than 90% of ducts open spontaneously within the first 6 months of life) or in older adults whose passages may be obstructed by stones. In children, the initial attempt to open the duct consists of gentle massage over the nasolacrimal duct (just medial to the medial canthus) and topical antimicrobials. If this is not successful, nasolacrimal duct probing is usually curative. Rarely, an infected nasolacrimal apparatus can progress to orbital cellulitis. Dacryoadenitis refers to inflammation of the lacrimal gland, located in the superior, lateral orbit. It is most commonly caused by viral infections and usually does not cause excessive tearing. *(Emergency Medicine, Chapter 62, pp 609–625)*

19. c. The patients in answers a through d have acute narrow-angle glaucoma. The patient will present with some or all of the following signs and symptoms: pain, decreased vision, injection, corneal haze (corneal edema due to high intraocular pressure), mid-dilated and sluggish pupil, and elevated intraocular pressure. The first line of treatment is to abort the attack by opening up the angle and restoring the flow of aqueous out of the eye. Pilocarpine constricts the pupil and will move the peripheral iris out of the angle so that aqueous can flow out of the eye. However, when the pressure is high, as in acute angle closure, the ischemic iris constrictor muscle is much less responsive to medication. For this reason, pilocarpine must be given simultaneously with medications that lower intraocular pressure. Beta-blockers and acetazolamide lower intraocular pressure by decreasing the production of aqueous. Osmotic agents lower intraocular pressure by shrinking the vitreous. Once the acute attack is broken and the inflammation ameliorated, the patient can have laser iridectomy. Laser iridectomy is not indicated during an acute attack of angle closure because it would severely exacerbate the inflammation already present from the attack itself. (Also, the procedure requires a clear view of the iris through the cornea, which is usually not present.) Primary narrow-angle glaucoma is a bilateral disease. It is common for patients with narrow angles to have recurrent subclinical attacks with elevated pressure. This leads to chronic changes in and malfunctioning of the angles, which cause further chronic pressure elevation. Thus, it would not be surprising if a patient with primary narrow-angle glaucoma had a high pressure in the eye not involved in the acute attack. *(Emergency Medicine, Chapter 62, pp 609–625)*

20. e. Preseptal cellulitis involves the periorbital structures anterior to the orbital septum. It is more common in children than adults and more commonly progresses to orbital cellulitis in children than adults. When infection is present posterior to the orbital septum, vital structures such as muscles and nerves may be affected. This is indicated by findings of decreased vision, afferent pupillary defect, and restriction of ocular motility. Spread to the CNS is possible. An afferent pupillary defect and restriction of ocular motility are easily demonstrated in preverbal children. Orbital cellulitis is always treated with IV antimicrobials, and CT of the orbits and sinuses is indicated to exclude an abscess, which would need to be drained surgically. *(Emergency Medicine, Chapter 62, pp 609–625)*

BIBLIOGRAPHY

Bessman ES: Nontraumatic eye disorders. *In* Howell JM, Altieri M, Jagoda AS, et al (eds): Emergency Medicine. Philadelphia, WB Saunders, 1998, pp 609–625.

Love JN, Bertram-Love N: Traumatic eye disorders. *In* Howell JM, Altieri M, Jagoda AS, et al (eds): Emergency Medicine. Philadelphia, WB Saunders, 1998, pp 626–638.

28 Disorders of the Ears, Nose, and Sinuses

PAUL A. ANDRULONIS, MD   ELIZABETH M. DATNER, MD

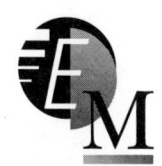

1. Thirty minutes after placement of an anterior nasal pack, a 52-year-old man continues to have epistaxis with blood flow down the posterior pharynx. What is the next step?
   a. Removal of the anterior pack and placement of a posterior pack
   b. Topical 2% tetracaine and 1% phenylephrine
   c. Silver nitrate
   d. Gelfoam and 1% phenylephrine
   e. Surgicel

2. A 6-year-old girl is brought to the ED after her parents noted recurrent foul-smelling nasal discharge. A small bead is found in her right nasal cavity. While the physician is attempting to remove the bead with a Fogarty catheter, the child begins to cough and wheeze. What is the most likely cause?
   a. Irritation of the vocal cords
   b. Irritation of the vagus nerve
   c. Aspiration of the bead
   d. Precipitation of an asthma flare
   e. All of the above

3. After 6 days of treatment with phenylephrine for viral rhinitis, a 20-year-old college student notices worsening congestion after an initial improvement. He is afebrile and has congested turbinates. The most likely cause of his condition is:
   a. Exposure to allergen
   b. Rhinitis medicamentosa
   c. Bacterial superinfection
   d. Noncompliance
   e. Cocaine insufflation (causing the refractory rhinorrhea)

4. A 43-year-old female with poorly controlled diabetes mellitus presents to the ED with complaint of fever and black nasal discharge. A necrotic nasal turbinate is visualized on examination. Appropriate treatment should include:
   a. Gentamicin
   b. Vancomycin
   c. Levofloxacin
   d. Amphotericin B
   e. Beclomethasone

5. All of the following are common bacterial agents responsible for sinusitis except:
   a. *Mycoplasma*
   b. *Staphylococcus aureus*
   c. *Moraxella catarrhalis*
   d. *Streptococcus pneumoniae*
   e. *Haemophilus influenzae*

6. All of the following are causes of anterior epistaxis except:
   a. Trauma
   b. Neoplasm
   c. Foreign body
   d. Dry mucosa
   e. Cystic fibrosis

7. Match the sinus with the approximate age of significant aeration.
   a. Frontal sinus   i.   6 months
   b. Sphenoid sinus   ii. 3 years
   c. Maxillary sinus   iii. 7 years
                               iv. 10 years
                               v.   15 years

8. A 60-year-old veteran presents with progressive hearing loss. A vibrating tuning fork is held on her maxillary incisor and she reports that the sound is predominantly in her right ear. Which of the following is compatible with this finding?
   a. Left sensorineural hearing loss
   b. Right sensorineural hearing loss
   c. Left conductive hearing loss
   d. Right conductive hearing loss
   e. Both a and d

9. A 10-year-old returns to the ED after a 10-day course of amoxicillin for otitis media with worsening earache. He is febrile and his tympanic membrane is bulging and immobile with pneumatic otoscopy. The most likely cause of treatment failure is:
   a. *Streptococcus pneumoniae* infection
   b. Viral otitis media

c. Amoxicillin-resistant bacteria
d. Development of a cholesteatoma
e. Both c and d

10. A 20-year-old college wrestler presents to the ED complaining of acute swelling of his ear. A large otohematoma is noted on examination. There are no lacerations and his hearing is intact. After drainage by needle aspirate, the next therapeutic step is:
    a. Moist heat
    b. Application of a pressure dressing
    c. Prophylatic antibiotics
    d. Both b and c
    e. All of the above

11. An alkaline button battery requires urgent removal from the external auditory canal because of its ability to cause:
    a. Otitis media
    b. Tympanic membrane perforation
    c. Granulation reaction
    d. Liquefaction necrosis
    e. Otitis externa

12. The cartilage of the pinna is highly vascularized and is the source of otohematomas.
    True or False

13. A patient presents with a 2-year history of intermittent vertigo, progressive hearing loss, and ringing in his right ear. The most likely diagnosis is:
    a. Acoustic neuroma
    b. Meniere's disease
    c. Benign positional vertigo
    d. Suppurative labyrinthitis

14. A 5-year-old girl is brought to the ED by her father after she stuck a pencil into her external auditory canal. On examination she has both hearing loss and nystagmus. The most likely cause of these findings is:
    a. Otitis externa
    b. Perforated tympanic membrane
    c. Ear canal foreign body
    d. Hematoma occluding the ear canal
    e. Ossicle injury

15. All of the following are signs or symptoms of otitis media in infants except:
    a. Nausea and vomiting
    b. Diarrhea
    c. Irritability
    d. Diplopia
    e. Poor feeding

16. Malignant otitis externa, a potentially fatal infection in diabetics, is caused by which pathogen?
    a. *Pseudomonas aeruginosa*
    b. Herpes simplex virus
    c. *Mycoplasma* spp.
    d. *Mucor* spp.
    e. *Aspergillus* spp.

17. Detergents useful for cerumen removal include which of the following?
    a. Acetic acid
    b. Mineral oil
    c. Hydrogen peroxide
    d. Carbamide peroxide
    e. All of the above

18. Possible complications of a cholesteatoma include all of the following except:
    a. Malignant transformation
    b. Recurrent otitis media
    c. Erosion of the ossicles
    d. Intracranial extension
    e. Facial nerve paralysis

19. Which of the following is a potential complication of otitis media?
    a. Meningitis
    b. Mastoiditis
    c. Tympanic membrane perforation
    d. Both b and c
    e. All of the above

20. A 52-year-old male with HIV presents complaining of dizziness. He is febrile and has a vesicular eruption on the left auricle, nystagmus, and a left facial droop. There are no other significant findings on examination. Appropriate treatment should include all of the following except:
    a. Prednisone
    b. Augmentin
    c. Acyclovir
    d. NSAIDs
    e. Both a and c

21. Which drug listed below does not have the potential to cause hearing loss?
    a. Rifampin
    b. Tobramycin
    c. Furosemide
    d. Ibuprofen
    e. Erythromycin

22. An inconsolable 8-year-old girl is brought to the ED by her parents. A live cockroach is found in her right ear. Prior to removal of the insect, which of the following should be instilled in the external auditory canal?
    a. 2% lidocaine
    b. Sterile saline
    c. Aqueous bupivacaine
    d. Mineral oil
    e. Either a or d

Answers

1.a. Continued bleeding (visualized in the posterior pharynx) despite placement of an anterior pack is evidence of a posterior bleed. Posterior bleeds originate from branches of the internal and external carotid artery and may cause significant hemorrhage and hypotension. Therapy consists of obtaining IV access, giving fluids if indicated, and placing both posterior and anterior packing. Packing remains in place for 3 to 5 days. Several methods of posterior packing have been developed. These include placement of rolled gauze attached to long heavy sutures, a Nasostat balloon, or a modified Foley catheter with the end removed. Patients with posterior packs are prone to sinus infection and hypoxia. Otolaryngology should be consulted, and the patient should be admitted. The patient should be given prophylactic antimicrobials and supplemental oxygen. Approximately 5% of all episodes of posterior epistaxis continue bleeding despite packing and require embolization or surgery. *(Emergency Medicine, Chapter 66, pp 659–663)*

2.c. Children and the mentally retarded are particularly prone to having foreign bodies lodged in their nasal cavity. A topical vasoconstrictor and an anesthetic should precede any attempt at removal. Extraction may be accomplished in a cooperative patient by having the patient occlude the patent nasal airway and then instructing the patient to blow out the nose. Parents can do this for a small child by blowing forcefully in the child's mouth. More invasive measures consist of alligator forceps, a Foley catheter, suction, and hooked instruments. Occasionally, removal may be complicated by aspiration of the foreign body, resulting in wheezing and coughing and then necessitating bronchoscopy for removal. *(Emergency Medicine, Chapter 66, pp 659–663)*

3.b. Sympathomimetics are a mainstay of treatment for rhinitis. However, prolonged use for more than 3 days may cause rebound vasodilation and subsequent engorgement of the nasal turbinates known as rhinitis medicamentosa. Discontinuation of the sympathomimetic for 2 to 3 weeks is curative. *(Emergency Medicine, Chapter 66, pp 659–663)*

4.d. Mucormycosis is a potentially lethal invasive fungal infection caused by 1 of 10 different fungi. Microscopically, the hyphae are characteristically broad and nonseptate, with 90-degree branches. Patients with poorly controlled diabetes and patients with impaired neutrophil function are most susceptible to this infection. Rhinocerebral mucormycosis typically presents with black nasal discharge, necrotic nasal turbinates, cranial nerve palsies, or bony involvement on sinus films. High-dose IV amphotericin B and aggressive surgical débridement by an experienced otolaryngologist is the treatment of choice. Amoxicillin and clarithromycin are antimicrobials useful for bacterial sinusitis. Beclomethasone and sympathomimetics are adjuncts that maintain the patency of the ostia, thereby allowing drainage of the sinuses. *(Emergency Medicine, Chapter 66, pp 659–663)*

5.a. Bacterial sinusitis arises from blockage of the sinus ostia, impaired ciliary functioning, or highly viscous secretions. These abnormalities lead to fluid accumulation in the sinuses and eventual colonization and infection by nasal bacteria. *Haemophilus influenzae* and *Streptococcus pneumoniae* are the predominant organisms, accounting for up to 75% of all adult acute sinus infections and up to 60% of pediatric cases. *Moraxella catarrhalis* is much less prevalent in the adult population (approximately 5%) compared to the pediatric age group (approximately 20%). *Staphylococcus aureus* is found predominantly after adolescence in 2% to 8% of cases. Anaerobic organisms may be present in cases of chronic sinusitis. Fungal sinusitis, although rare, may be seen in immunocompromised patients and requires surgical débridement. *(Emergency Medicine, Chapter 66, pp 659–663)*

6.e. Anterior epistaxis is the result of bleeding from the vessels of Kiesselbach's plexus located on the anterior nasal septum. Numerous etiologies have been identified. One of the most common causes is trauma resulting from direct blows, digital manipulation, orbital fractures, and basilar skull fractures. A deviated septum results in turbulent air flow, drying the mucosa and leaving the superficial vessels exposed. Subsequent insignificant trauma will disrupt the vessels with resultant epistaxis. Foreign bodies are especially common in children and the mentally retarded. These patients present with unilateral foul-smelling nasal discharge and frequent bleeding after extraction of the foreign body. Coagulopathies and growths, such as angiofibromas and paranasal tumors, are other potential etiologic factors. Debate still exists regarding the association between hypertension and epistaxis. *(Emergency Medicine, Chapter 66, pp 659–663)*

7.a. iii; b. iv; c. i. The paranasal sinuses originate from out-pouching of the nasal chamber. Development begins during the third month of gestation and continues through adolescence. The ethmoid sinus is the only significantly aerated sinus at birth. The largest sinus, the maxillary, measures only several cubic millimeters at birth and quickly expands during the early months of life. The frontal sinus develops from an anteriorly located ethmoid cell at approximately 7 years but is not fully aerated until after puberty. Finally, the sphenoid becomes aerated at around 10 years of age and is of clinical importance because of its proximity to the ophthalmic nerve. *(Emergency Medicine, Chapter 66, pp 659–663)*

8.e. The Weber and Rinne tests are used in conjunction to help determine the site of conductive versus sensorineural hearing loss. The Weber test is performed by placing a vibrating 512-Hz tuning fork on the patient's maxillary incisors or glabella. The sound will localize either to the side of conductive loss or to the side opposite of a sensorineural loss. The Rinne test consists of holding the tuning fork on the mastoid process adjacent to that ear until the sound is no longer audible, and then placing the tuning fork outside the patient's ear. Normally, air conduction is greater than bone conduction—if a conductive loss is present the sound of the tuning fork through bone conduction will be greater, whereas if a sensorineural loss is present, hearing is reduced by both routes. *(Emergency Medicine, Chapter 64, pp 639–651; Chapter 65, pp 652–657)*

9.c. Common pathogens responsible for otitis media include *Streptococcus pneumoniae* (30% to 35%), *Haemophilus influenzae* (20% to 22%), *Moraxella catarrhalis* (10% to 15%), *Streptococcus pyogenes* (5%), and *Staphylococcus aureus* (5%); however, recent studies reflecting a probable decreasing incidence of *H. influenzae* are not yet available. First-line therapy consists of a 10-day course of amoxicillin, trimethoprim-sulfamethoxazole, or erythromycin-sulfisoxazole. Resistance to amoxicillin and other first-line antibiotics has become an important cause of failed therapy. Thirty percent of *H. influenzae* and 80% of *M. catarrhalis* organisms produce beta-lactamase and are resistant to amoxicillin. *S. pneumoniae* is increasingly becoming multidrug resistant. Second-line therapy for resistant organisms and after treatment failure with first-line drugs includes amoxicillin plus clavulanate, second- or third-generation cephalosporins, and macrolides. Another alternative is to use trimethoprim-sulfamethoxazole if amoxicillin fails, and vice versa. Azithromycin is the only second-line antimicrobial prescribed for 5 days and may be useful in suspected cases of noncompliance. Decongestants have no proven role in the treatment of otitis media. *(Emergency Medicine, Chapter 64, pp 639–651)*

10.b. An otohematoma is a collection of blood between the perichondrium and the cartilage of the auricle. This type of injury is common after blunt or penetrating trauma to the area. Spontaneous otohematomas may also occur in hypertensive patients. Appropriate treatment includes either needle aspiration or surgical incision and drainage followed by a pressure dressing to prevent reaccumulation of the hematoma. Recheck in 24 hours to assess for reaccumulation is essential because repeat drainage may be necessary. In general, prophylactic antibiotics are not recommended; however, this remains controversial. Poorly treated or recurrent hematomas often result in the "cauliflower ear" deformity. *(Emergency Medicine, Chapter 65, pp 652–657)*

11.d. Alkaline button batteries contain potassium hydroxide, which is capable of producing liquefaction necrosis. The necrosis may extend into adjacent bony structures and the middle ear. Low-voltage burns and pressure necrosis are other potential mechanisms of damage. Treatment requires prompt removal and débridement of any necrotic tissue. Steroid drops may improve healing but only after the battery is removed. Consult otolaryngology if removal is unsuccessful or if the battery contents have spilled into the external ear canal. *(Emergency Medicine, Chapter 64, pp 639–651)*

12. False. The pinna consists of three important layers: the skin, the perichondrium, and the avascular cartilage. The deep cartilage is dependent on the vascular perichondrium for its supply of nutrients. Therefore, any laceration involving the cartilage must be carefully repaired, ensuring that the perichondrium covers all of the cartilage. Failure to do so may result in avascular necrosis of the cartilage. *(Emergency Medicine, Chapter 65, pp 652–657)*

13.b. Meniere's disease has a peak incidence between the ages of 40 and 60 years and is defined by the triad of peripheral vertigo, tinnitus, and sensorineural hearing loss. Pathologically, there is inadequate absorption of endolymph, resulting in hydrops. Attacks may last from minutes to hours and recur for 5 to 6 years with progressive loss in hearing. Management consists of a low-salt diet with or without hydrochlorothiazide, which reduces endolymph volume and relieves vertigo associated with Meniere's disease. Symptomatic treatment is with antivertigo medications such as diphenhydramine, meclizine, droperidol, and prochlorperazine. Patients should follow up with otolaryngology for long-term care and possible surgery for those failing medical therapy. Acoustic neuromas are tumors of the vestibulocochlear nerve that present with progressive hearing loss followed by vertigo lasting several days. Benign positional vertigo is characterized by sudden brief episodes (5–15 seconds) of vertigo associated with change in head position. The Hallpike maneuver is performed by quickly moving the patient from a sitting to a supine position with the head turned to the side. This is then repeated with the head turned to the opposite side. The occurrence of delayed rotary nystagmus while in the supine position is indicative of benign positional vertigo. Suppurative labyrinthitis presents with unremitting vertigo, nausea, vomiting, purulent otitis media, and hearing loss. *(Emergency Medicine, Chapter 64, pp 639–651)*

14.e. Tympanic membrane perforations are a relatively common complication of otitis media, middle ear squeeze, and foreign bodies. Perforations usually heal spontaneously and do not cause vertigo or a decrease in hearing. In evaluating perforations, especially those caused by trauma, the physician must determine if associated damage occurred to the inner and middle ear structures. Ossicle injury will cause both hearing loss and vertigo. External auditory canal foreign bodies and otitis externa are pathologic processes involving only the ear canal. Neither is a cause of vertigo. *(Emergency Medicine, Chapter 65, pp 652–657)*

15.d. Otitis media is an inflammation of the middle ear secondary to either a bacterial or viral infection. The pathogenesis is influenced mainly by eustachian tube dysfunction. A number of other factors also play a role, including upper respiratory infection and immunocompromised states. Infants and young children can present with localized complaints such as ear tugging (due to otalgia) or nonspecific signs such as nausea, vomiting, diarrhea, irritability, fever, and poor feeding. Any child presenting with these nonspecific complaints mandates proper otologic examination. On examination, the tympanic membrane is bulging and red or yellow and has decreased movement with a pneumatic otoscope. If the tympanic membrane ruptures, otitis media can present as otorrhea. Loss of the light reflex is not predictive of otitis media. Older children and adults present with more localized complaints of ear pain, vertigo, tinnitus, and diminished hearing. *(Emergency Medicine, Chapter 64, pp 639–651)*

16.a. Malignant otitis externa is an invasive *Pseudomonas aeruginosa* infection originating in the fissures of Santorini at the junction of the bony and cartilaginous sections of the external auditory canal. The infection may progress along the base of the skull, resulting in meningitis, cranial nerve palsies (most often the facial nerve), osteomyelitis, and cavernous sinus thrombosis. Findings on evaluation include an elevated erythrocyte sedimentation rate, variable WBC count, and bony extension on CT or MRI. Antimicrobial treatment requires a 6- to 8-week course of an oral quinolone, third-generation cephalosporin, or IV aminoglycoside combined with an antipseudomonal penicillin. Surgical débridement is also important. Diabetics over the age of 65 years are most commonly afflicted. Immunocompromised patients with HIV and leukemia are also susceptible to this life-threatening infection. *(Emergency Medicine, Chapter 64, pp 639–651)*

17.e. Cerumen impaction is one of the most common otologic problems. Cerumen is a combination of secretions from sebaceous and ceruminous glands with hair and sloughed epithelial cells from the tympanic membrane. Lysosomes and immunoglobulins in the cerumen act as a protectant against infection. Lipids are the main constituent of cerumen. Their hydrophobic properties prevent water from stagnating and causing maceration of the epithelial cell layer. Excessive cerumen in the external ear canal can be removed directly with a curet, by lukewarm water irrigation, or by softening detergents. Solutions used include acetic acid, mineral oil, hydrogen peroxide, carbamide peroxide (Debrox), and triethanolamine polypeptide oleate-condensate (Cerumenex). A careful history in an attempt to exclude tympanic membrane perforation should be taken prior to irrigation or introduction of detergents. *(Emergency Medicine, Chapter 64, pp 639–651)*

18.a. A cholesteatoma is a nonmalignant growth of keratinizing epithelial cells in the middle ear or mastoid. The cholesteatoma may be congenital or occur because of injury of the tympanic membrane. The tumor can be aggressive, destroying the nearby ossicles and the mastoid bone, and can extend to the facial nerve canal or intracranially. Its location may impede middle ear drainage through the eustachian tube, predisposing to recurrent otitis media. Progressive hearing loss is also common. Surgical resection is the only treatment. *(Emergency Medicine, Chapter 65, pp 652–657)*

19.e. Complications of otitis media are rare when proper antimicrobial therapy is instituted. However, noncompliance and undertreatment can allow extension of the infection into the mastoid and intracranial structures, producing meningitis, brain abscesses, and subdural empyemas. Labyrinthitis and tympanic membrane perforation with resulting cholesteatoma are other potential complications of otitis media. However, perforations usually heal without complications or intervention. *(Emergency Medicine, Chapter 64, pp 639–651)*

20.b. Ramsay Hunt syndrome is a varicella zoster virus infection of the geniculate ganglion and facial nerve. A painful erythematous rash on the outer ear is an early manifestation. The later stages present with a vesicular eruption on the pinna, the external ear canal, and the tympanic membrane. Central vertigo, hearing loss, and tinnitus may also be present. Involvement of the facial nerve producing a facial nerve paralysis carries a poor prognosis for complete recovery. The goal of treatment is to prevent permanent facial nerve paralysis and hearing loss. Oral prednisone for at least 1 week is the mainstay of therapy. NSAIDs for pain control and acyclovir for its antiviral properties have also been used with some success. Acyclovir has been shown to improve facial nerve function. Augmentin is used for advanced cases of bacterial otitis externa and is not indicated for Ramsay Hunt syndrome. *(Emergency Medicine, Chapter 64, pp 639–651)*

21.a. Many medications have been implicated as etiologic agents of sensorineural hearing loss. Some of the more common ototoxic drugs include loop diuretics, aminoglycosides, vancomycin, erythromycin, antimalarials, NSAIDs, salicylates, and cisplatin. Patients at high risk for hearing loss include those with impaired renal function, over the age of 65 years, taking combinations of ototoxic agents, and with elevated serum levels of the medication. Rifampin is an antituberculous drug and is not associated with hearing loss. *(Emergency Medicine, Chapter 64, pp 639–651)*

22.e. Insects are among the most challenging foreign bodies to remove from the external auditory canal. Insects crawl into the ear canal while the patient is sleeping and are then unable to maneuver their way out. Patients may quickly become terrorized by the insect's constant scratching at the tympanic membrane. In these situations it is important to quickly subdue the insect by killing it with either mineral oil or 2% lidocaine. The death of the insect will stop the irritating noise and pain and will simplify extraction. Sterile saline irrigation will assist in removing the insect's carcass and other foreign bodies but will not kill the insect. Aqueous bupivacaine, which has a prolonged half-life and a low viscosity, has not been recommended as an aid in insect removal. *(Emergency Medicine, Chapter 65, pp 652–657)*

BIBLIOGRAPHY

Bailey BJ: Head and Neck Surgery—Otolaryngology. Philadelphia, JB Lippincott, 1993.

Brook I: Otitis media: Microbiology and management. J Otolaryngol 1994; 23(4):269–275.

Drake-Lee A: Clinical Otorhinolaryngology. New York, Churchill Livingstone, 1996.

Fritz S, Kelen G, Sivertson K: Foreign bodies of the external auditory canal. Emerg Med Clin North Am 1987; 5(2):183–192.

Hughes GB, Pensak ML: Clinical Otology, 2nd ed. New York, Thieme, 1997.

Johnson JT, Yu VL: Infectious Diseases and Antimicrobic Therapy of the Ear, Nose, and Throat. Philadelphia, WB Saunders, 1997.

Perretta L, Denslow B, Brown C: Emergency evaluation and management of epistaxis. Emerg Med Clin North Am 1987; 5(2):265–278.

Reich J: Ear infections. Emerg Med Clin North Am 1987; 5(2):227–242.

Reich JJ: Otitis and nontraumatic ear disorders. *In* Howell JM, Altieri M, Jagoda AS, et al (eds): Emergency Medicine. Philadelphia, WB Saunders, 1998, pp 639–651.

Stair TO: Medical disorders of the nose and sinuses. *In* Howell JM, Altieri M, Jagoda AS, et al (eds): Emergency Medicine. Philadelphia, WB Saunders, 1998, pp 659–663.

Turbiak T: Ear trauma. *In* Howell JM, Altieri M, Jagoda AS, et al (eds): Emergency Medicine. Philadelphia, WB Saunders, 1998, pp 652–657.

29 Disorders of the Oropharynx and Throat

STEVEN C. LARSON, MD

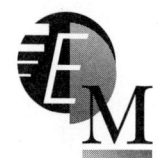

1. A 20-year-old student presents with a 2-week history of a low-grade fever, sore throat, swollen lymph nodes, and fatigue. Your examination reveals enlarged erythematous tonsils, generalized adenopathy, and splenomegaly. The most likely diagnosis is:
   a. Coxsackievirus
   b. Diphtheria
   c. Mononucleosis
   d. Group A beta-hemolytic streptococcus
   e. Oral candidiasis

2. A 16-year-old migrant worker presents with a sore throat, nausea, vomiting, chills, and a headache. He is ill-appearing, and on examination of his oropharynx you discover a blue-white exudate that forms an adherent pseudomembrane on the palatine tonsils and extends down the pharynx. The diagnosis is confirmed by:
   a. Rapid strep test
   b. Rapid plasma reagin
   c. Monospot test
   d. Bedside cold agglutinins
   e. Laboratory immunofluorescence

3. A 13-year-old patient presents with a fever, sore throat, headache, and abdominal pain. He has a fine scarlatiniform rash distributed uniformly about his body. He has beefy-red pharyngeal and tonsillar mucosae covered with a white exudate and tender cervical adenopathy. To minimize secondary complications from this illness, therapy must be delayed no later than how many days from symptom onset?
   a. None; the disease is self-limiting
   b. 1 day
   c. 3 days
   d. 6 days
   e. 9 days

4. A 33-year-old male presents complaining of jaw and neck pain. He is febrile and appears toxic. Your examination reveals poor dentition, trismus, and medial bulging of the lateral pharyngeal wall. He has soft tissue swelling and tenderness around the angle of his mandible. A CT scan confirms the presence of a lateral pharyngeal abscess. This patient is at risk for developing all of the following except:
   a. Cavernous sinus thrombosis
   b. Retropharyngeal space infection
   c. Suppurative jugular thrombosis
   d. Laryngeal edema
   e. Carotid artery erosion and rupture

5. A child with an inhaled foreign body most frequently presents with:
   a. Dyspnea
   b. Stridor
   c. Wheezing
   d. Coughing
   e. All of the above

6. The "cafe coronary," or sudden upper airway obstruction, is associated with which of the following?
   a. Caffeine
   b. Tobacco
   c. Cocaine
   d. Ethanol
   e. None of the above

7. A 39-year-old man presents with tooth pain and difficulty swallowing. He is febrile, toxic, sitting upright, and leaning forward. He has brawny, submandibular swelling. His oropharyngeal examination reveals trismus and elevation of his tongue to the roof of his mouth. The clinical diagnosis is:
   a. Diphtheria
   b. Tonsillitis
   c. Vincent's angina
   d. Ludwig's angina
   e. Retropharyngeal abscess

8. Radiographically, bronchial obstruction by a radiolucent foreign body may be inferred by which of the following?
   a. Hyperexpansion of one lung during inspiration
   b. Ipsilateral flattening of the diaphragm
   c. Contralateral mediastinal shift
   d. Atelectasis
   e. All of the above

9. A 34-year-old man presents complaining of a stiff neck, sore throat, and fever. Forty-eight hours earlier he noted a foreign body sensation in his throat while eating fish. Examination now reveals an irritable, febrile male with minimal pharyngeal erythema and mild unilateral swelling of the posterior wall of the pharynx. He has tender anterior cervical lymph nodes with asymmetric anterolateral neck swelling on the affected side. The most likely diagnosis is:
   a. Supraglottitis
   b. Laryngitis
   c. Retropharyngeal abscess
   d. Ludwig's angina
   e. Diphtheria

10. A 26-year-old woman presents with a sore throat, fever, and hoarse voice for 48 hours. She has not slept for the past 24 hours due to difficulty breathing when lying flat. On examination she is febrile and ill-appearing. She is sitting upright and uses her accessory muscles to breathe. Her pharyngeal examination is unrevealing. Appropriate management includes all of the following except:
   a. Intravenous antimicrobials
   b. Lateral neck films
   c. Admission to a critical care unit
   d. Immediate pharyngeal evaluation with laryngoscopy
   e. Emergent otolaryngology consult

11. A 4-year-old child has had several days of a low-grade fever, diminished oral intake, and malaise. On examination of her soft palate, several shallow vesicular ulcers appear visible. The most likely diagnosis is:
    a. Vincent's angina
    b. Coxsackievirus
    c. Thrush
    d. Infectious mononucleosis
    e. Adenovirus

12. A 3-year-old presents with a cold of 48 hours' duration. The patient now has a worsening seal-like barking cough, diffuse wheezes, and inspiratory stridor. Despite her ominous pulmonary findings, she remains active and playful and is eating and drinking normally. The most likely diagnosis is:
    a. Viral pharyngitis
    b. Supraglottitis
    c. Croup
    d. Retropharyngeal abscess
    e. Community-acquired pneumonia

13. An 18-year-old female presents with a fever, sore throat, and dysphagia. She speaks with a "hot potato" voice and on examination has an enlarged right palatine tonsil that displaces her uvula to the left. The most likely diagnosis is:
    a. Uvulitis
    b. Infectious mononucleosis
    c. Peritonsillar abscess
    d. Ludwig's angina
    e. Sialoadenitis

14. A homeless man presents complaining of painful, bleeding gums. He is febrile and appears toxic. On examination of his oropharynx you discover diffuse ulceration of the gingiva with a thick fibrinous exudate. A potential complication from this disorder includes:
    a. Brain abscess
    b. Gangrene of the face and oral tissue
    c. Pneumonia
    d. Bacteremia
    e. All of the above

15. A 25-year-old male presents complaining of a sore mouth for several weeks. On examination you note a thick, white, loosely adherent plaque on the tongue and soft palate with an underlying erythematous base. This disease is commonly seen in all of the following except:
    a. Infants
    b. Immunosuppressed patients
    c. Patients with poor oral hygiene
    d. Patients taking inhaled steroids
    e. Hemodialysis patients

16. A 26-year-old male complains of a painful, swollen lump under his chin. He appears nontoxic and on examination his dental hygiene appears well-maintained. He has a tender area of fluctuance on palpation of the floor of his mouth but his tongue is nondisplaced. He is in no respiratory distress. This most likely represents:
    a. Ludwig's angina
    b. Retropharyngeal abscess
    c. Sialolithiasis
    d. Actinomycosis
    e. None of the above

17. A 17-year-old female complains of difficulty breathing. She is febrile and her oropharyngeal examination is notable for a swollen, erythematous uvula. The most likely diagnosis is:
    a. Angioneurotic edema
    b. Allergic reaction
    c. Trauma
    d. Infection
    e. None of the above

18. Children often attempt to ingest small objects. All of the following are true about the ingestion of foreign bodies except:
    a. Coins in the stomach and intestine may be allowed to pass on their own.
    b. The child with a button battery in the esophagus should be monitored with daily radiographs: Most will pass, as they are small.
    c. The position of a coin (esophagus vs. trachea) can often be distinguished by a plain radiograph of the chest.
    d. Removal of a coin impacted in the esophagus can be attempted with a Foley catheter.
    e. Complications of esophageal coin impaction include airway obstruction, esophageal perforation, and fistula formation.

19. A 33-year-old patient presents complaining of persistent retrosternal pain that began during a meal that included

a large sirloin steak. She is now unable to swallow her secretions and appears markedly uncomfortable. Appropriate therapeutic intervention would include administering either sublingual nitroglycerin or IV glucagon.
True or False

20. A 4-year-old girl has just had a witnessed generalized tonic clonic seizure. In the immediate postictal phase she appears to be having difficulty with her breathing. The most likely cause for upper airway obstruction in this child is secondary to the relaxation of her tongue and the posterior pharyngeal muscles.
True or False

21. Compared to the adult airway, the child's tongue and posterior pharyngeal muscles are proportionally smaller.
True or False

Answers

1. c. Mononucleosis can cause marked tonsillar edema with exudate, palatal petechiae, fever, generalized adenopathy, and splenomegaly. The two most common symptoms are exudative pharyngitis and fever. The diagnosis is made with a monospot or heterophile antibody test. The positive heterophile antibody can be delayed up to 4 weeks from onset of symptoms. The Monospot test is positive in the first month of the illness but reverts to negative after 3 to 4 months of the illness. Treatment is supportive. Coxsackievirus is commonly seen in children less than age 4 and is manifested by fever, malaise, flulike symptoms, and a sore throat with 1- to 2-mm vesicles with a surrounding red areola on the posterior pharynx. It has a self-limited course of approximately 1 week. Diphtheria presents clinically as a pharyngitis with severe dysphagia, nausea, vomiting, chills, and headache and is most often found in unimmunized or underimmunized individuals. Untreated, it is associated with peripheral neuropathy or myocarditis. The classic "strep" throat associated with group A beta-hemolytic streptococcus presents with swollen, beefy-red pharyngeal and tonsillar mucosae with exudate in the tonsillar crypts, palatine petechiae, fever, and anterior cervical adenopathy. Oral candidiasis manifests as mucosal white patches covering shallow, friable ulcerations. It is more common in the immunosuppressed and in individuals taking broad-spectrum antimicrobials or inhaled steroids. (*Emergency Medicine, Chapter 67, pp 665–680*)

2. e. Diphtheria is usually seen in unimmunized or underimmunized individuals such as migrant workers, recent immigrants, and the homeless. It presents with severe dysphagia, nausea, vomiting, chills, and headache. Clinically one finds a blue-white, thick exudate that forms an adherent pseudomembrane and obscures the borders of the palatine tonsil. In addition to the potential airway complications presented by diphtheria pharyngitis, the organism also produces a potent exotoxin that affects both the cardiac smooth muscle and peripheral nervous system. Cranial neuropathy and myocarditis typically develop 12 weeks following the onset of initial infection. The diagnosis is made by immunofluorescence testing performed in the laboratory on a sample of the pseudomembrane. Treatment is based on empiric diagnosis and should not await culture results. Diphtheria antitoxin is the mainstay of therapy and should be administered immediately. Some advocate additional use of either penicillin or erythromycin. The rapid streptococcal antigen agglutination test detects group A beta-hemolytic streptococcus with 72% to 96% sensitivity and 90% to 100% specificity. The rapid plasma reagin test detects syphilis. The Monospot test detects infectious mononucleosis. Bedside cold agglutinins test for mycoplasma. (*Emergency Medicine, Chapter 67, pp 665–680*)

3. e. The presence of fever, sore throat with beefy-red pharyngeal and tonsillar mucosae covered with a white exudate, and anterior cervical adenopathy describes the classic strep throat. Less than 10% of cases of streptococcal pharyngitis present with all of the classic findings. However, the scarlatiniform rash (scarlet fever) that appears on the trunk and spreads centrifugally is a specific clinical feature of group A streptococcal infection. Although group A beta-hemolytic streptococcus comprises less than 30% of all cases of acute pharyngitis, it remains clinically concerning because of the risk for development of acute rheumatic fever. Treatment of group A beta-hemolytic streptococcus pharyngitis must be initiated within 9 days of symptom onset to prevent rheumatic fever.

4. a. The patient described has a lateral pharyngeal abscess. This presents clinically with trismus, induration, swelling at the angle of the mandible, medial bulging of the pharyngeal wall, and systemic toxicity. Lateral pharyngeal abscesses commonly arise from a dental abscess. Presentation is often delayed until there are complications such as suppurative jugular thrombosis, carotid artery erosion and rupture, laryngeal edema, and retropharyngeal space infection. Suppurative jugular venous thrombosis is the most common vascular complication. It manifests as the abrupt onset of fever, chills, and prostration with tenderness at the angle of the mandible or along the sternocleidomastoid muscle. Head and neck CT is useful for finding any abscess cavity but may miss an isolated jugular venous thrombosis. Patients with lateral pharyngeal abscesses require IV antimicrobials, surgical drainage, and hospitalization. Cavernous sinus thrombosis is associated with orbital cellulitis and otitis media. It is typified by spiking fever, obtundation, and increased intracranial pressure. (*Emergency Medicine, Chapter 67, pp 665–680*)

5. e. In children, the inhalation of a foreign body causes coughing, stridor, dyspnea, and wheezing. The clinician needs to be aware of the cardinal signs of upper airway obstruction, because 7% of inhalations are unwitnessed, resulting in a delay in diagnosis. Unless moderate to severe, initial management includes

avoiding stimulation of the airway and agitation of the patient, which theoretically can precipitate complete obstruction. *(Emergency Medicine, Chapter 67, pp 665–680)*

6.d. The "cafe coronary" describes sudden upper airway obstruction in adults that commonly occurs after the victim drinks ethanol, which blunts swallowing reflexes and results in food aspiration, obstructing the airway. In contrast to the sudden collapse of a patient in true cardiac arrest, the patient with a foreign body obstruction usually has a history of choking before collapse. It also occurs if the patient fails to chew food enough or cuts off a chunk of food that is larger than the esophagus can accommodate. Caffeine may exacerbate reflux esophagitis but is not implicated in airway obstruction. Tobacco smoke has been associated with an increased incidence of respiratory infection and increased airway obstruction in asthmatics but is not associated with cafe coronary. Cocaine is associated with sudden cardiac arrest from MI and myocardial ischemia. *(Emergency Medicine, Chapter 67, pp 665–680)*

7.d. Ludwig's angina is a nonfluctuant, rapidly spreading cellulitis of the tissue planes below the tongue. It most commonly arises from an abscessed lower molar. There is firm, nonfluctuant swelling of the floor of the mouth, and the patient appears toxic. Progressive soft tissue swelling forces the tongue upward and forward and eventually occludes the posterior hypopharynx, resulting in airway obstruction. Multiple organisms are associated with Ludwig's angina, and often a variety of mixed pathogens are isolated. The diagnosis of Ludwig's angina is clinical, and management should quickly focus on airway control and the potential for rapid occlusion. Intravenous broad-spectrum antimicrobials and consultation with an otolaryngologist as well as admission to a critical care bed are indicated. Diphtheria presents with severe dysphagia and a toxic appearance; however, the hallmark of this infection is the presence of a blue-white adherent pseudomembrane that extends down the pharynx. Tonsillitis presents most commonly with odynophagia, tender anterior cervical adenopathy, and erythema of the palatine tonsils. It is usually self-limiting and lasts about 1 week. Vincent's angina presents as severe gnawing gingival pain associated with fever and malaise. Examination reveals ulceration of the gingiva with a thick fibrinous exudate. A retropharyngeal abscess is associated with a fever, sore throat, dysphagia, and drooling. There is often asymmetric anterolateral neck swelling on the affected side. *(Emergency Medicine, Chapter 67, pp 665–680)*

8.e. An aspirated foreign body can be a clinically challenging diagnosis. Near-complete bronchial obstruction may cause localized stridor or wheezing. Complete obstruction of one bronchus may cause an absence of breath sounds on that side. If the foreign body is acting as a ball-valve, decreased lung sounds and hyperexpansion may result. A plain film of the chest may reveal a radiodense foreign body; however, up to 75% of objects inhaled by children will not be visualized on plain radiograph. Indirect evidence of aspiration can be inferred radiographically by hyperexpansion of the affected lung, most pronounced during expiration, ipsilateral flattening of the diaphragm, and contralateral mediastinal shift. If the obstruction is complete and prolonged, the lung may become atelectatic. *(Emergency Medicine, Chapter 67, pp 665–680)*

9.c. Retropharyngeal abscesses in children are frequently associated with an antecedent pharyngitis; in adults they frequently result from direct trauma or a retained foreign body. Clinically, patients are febrile, dyspneic, and irritable. In children, the neck is held rigid, and it is difficult to see or palpate the retropharyngeal mass. Swelling may be to one side, and the child tilts the head away from the infected side. In adults, however, there is usually variable unilateral swelling of the posterior wall of the pharynx with associated asymmetric neck swelling. Diagnosis is made by soft tissue lateral neck films, which show prevertebral soft tissue widening, air or air-fluid levels, loss of cervical lordosis, or foreign body. In adults and children, the upper limit of normal retropharyngeal tissue at C2 is 7 mm; at C6, it is 22 mm for adults and 14 to 16 mm for children. Supraglottitis occurs at all ages, and in adults it manifests as a sore throat, dysphagia, and fever. The patient is often hoarse and unable to lie supine. Clinical examination of the pharynx is frequently normal. Severe supraglottitis may cause respiratory distress manifested clinically by use of accessory muscle, stridor, drooling, and trismus. Laryngitis is described as a hoarseness, sometimes associated with dysphagia, odynophagia, and occasionally stridor. The clinical examination is often unremarkable, although occasionally stridorous breathing may be auscultated. The patient with Ludwig's angina is febrile and toxic. Firm, nonfluctuant swelling of the floor of the mouth with elevation of the tongue is present. Diphtheria presents with fever, severe dysphagia, nausea, and vomiting. A blue-white adherent pseudomembrane is found extending down the pharynx. *(Emergency Medicine, Chapter 67, pp 665–680)*

10.d. The clinical scenario described is consistent with severe supraglottitis. In children and adults with moderate to severe supraglottitis, pharyngeal examination should be deferred until the airway is protected. The patient should be placed in the critical care area of the ED and closely monitored for clinical deterioration. A lateral soft tissue film of the neck may reveal thickening of the epiglottis and aryepiglottic folds. Intravenous antimicrobials should be started with coverage for *Haemophilus influenzae* in children and gram-positive cocci in adults. An otolaryngologist should be consulted early in the course of patient management; laryngoscopy and intubation should be undertaken in the operating room using general anesthesia. *(Emergency Medicine, Chapter 67, pp 665–680)*

11.b. The clinical scenario described is classic for coxsackievirus. It occurs most commonly from June through

October. Also known as herpangina, coxsackievirus manifests as fever, malaise, flulike symptoms, and a sore throat associated with vesicles 1 to 2 mm in size with a surrounding red areola on the posterior pharynx. After 1 to 2 days the vesicles rupture, leaving shallow ulcers. The course is self-limited, lasting approximately 1 week. Vincent's angina, also known as trench mouth, is caused by multiple organisms and presents as acute gum pain worsened with spicy foods and accompanied by bleeding, fetid odor, and taste alteration. The patient appears toxic with fever and malaise. Thrush, or oral candidiasis, causes white cheesy patches throughout the oral cavity. When scraped, the oral mucosa demonstrates shallow bleeding ulcers. It is common in immunosuppressed or immunocompromised individuals. Infectious mononucleosis usually occurs between the ages of 10 to 35 years and is associated with an exudative pharyngitis and fever. Younger children are usually asymptomatic. Adenovirus infections cause symptoms of pharyngitis, conjunctivitis, and fever. Rarely, they can cause pneumonia, bronchiolitis, croup, a pertussis-like syndrome, and hemorrhagic cystitis. *(Emergency Medicine, Chapter 67, pp 665–680)*

12.c. Croup (laryngotracheobronchitis) is the most common upper airway infection in children. It primarily affects younger children—6 months to 6 years—with a peak incidence at 2 years. Most commonly, the disease occurs during late fall and early winter. Parainfluenza virus is the most likely causative organism, although respiratory syncytial virus and influenza virus may be causative as well. Inflammation of bronchial and smaller airways causes bronchial constriction, edema, and atelectasis. Wheezing, tachypnea, and a prolonged expiratory phase may be prominent components. Cold symptoms usually precede the onset of the classic croupy cough (described as a worsening seal-like barking sound) by 1 to 3 days. Despite these symptoms, most patients are active, playful, and drinking and eating normally. The vast majority of patients have mild symptoms and can be discharged safely to home. More severe cases improve with either nebulized racemic epinephrine or regular levo-epinephrine. Systemic steroids also decrease symptoms in croup, although the action is delayed several hours. Viral pharyngitis is associated with sore throat, fever, lymphadenopathy, and sometimes tonsillar exudate. It is generally self-limiting and untreatable. Supraglottitis has become relatively rare since the advent of *H. influenzae* B immunization. Supraglottitis is the preferred term for epiglottitis because most of the supraglottic structures are inflamed and edematous as well. Preschool children are the most susceptible, but nearly any age can be affected. Retropharyngeal abscesses are complications of pharyngitis and other local infections that spread to the retropharyngeal lymph nodes. Symptoms are frequently confused with those of supraglottitis. Community-acquired pneumonias, manifested by fever, chills, and productive cough, are frequently preceded by a virus-like prodrome. *(Emergency Medicine, Chapter 67, pp 665–680)*

13.c. Peritonsillar abscess forms when organisms from a preexisting tonsillitis rupture through the tonsillar capsule into the surrounding areolar tissue. It is largely a disease of young adults, and 70% of cases occur during winter months. Patients complain of increasing fever, sore throat, and dysphagia. Key symptoms include ipsilateral ear fullness, otalgia, trismus, drooling, and speaking in a muffled, "hot potato" voice. On examination, pharyngeal erythema, exudate, and tonsillar enlargement with deviation of the uvula to the opposite side are hallmarks of the diagnosis. Because the tonsils can extend inferiorly to the hypopharynx and cause obstruction, the inferior poles should be visualized. If not visualized, a lateral neck radiograph may be helpful to determine the degree of soft tissue swelling. Infectious uvulitis is caused by *H. influenzae* and *Streptococcus*. Patients appear febrile and their uvula appears red and swollen. Infectious mononucleosis presents with exudative pharyngitis, fever, diffuse adenopathy, and hepatosplenomegaly. Ludwig's angina presents with nonfluctuant cellulitis of the tissue planes below the tongue. On examination, there is firm, nonfluctuant swelling of the floor of the mouth with elevation of the tongue. Sialoadenitis produces palpable, fluctuant swelling of the floor of the mouth. Most cases are caused by obstruction of the salivary gland. Patients are nontoxic. *(Emergency Medicine, Chapter 67, pp 665–680)*

14.e. Vincent's angina, or trench mouth, is an acute necrotizing gingivostomatitis that clinically presents as the acute onset of gum pain accompanied by bleeding, fetid odor, and taste alteration. The patient appears toxic, with fever and malaise. It is caused by multiple organisms, including streptococci and oral treponemes such as *Borrelia vincentii*, *Bacteroides melaninogenicus*, and *Fusobacterium* species. It causes ulcers of the gingiva and a thick fibrinous exudate. Complications include tooth loss, gangrene of the face and oral tissues, pneumonia, bacteremia, and brain abscess. *(Emergency Medicine, Chapter 67, pp 665–680)*

15.e. Moniliasis, or overgrowth of the oral cavity by *Candida* organisms, occurs most often in immunosuppressed patients, patients with poor oral hygiene or poor nutrition, patients using inhaled steroids, and infants. Patients complain of a burning sensation in the mouth. White, cheesy patches that are loosely adherent and have an underlying base of erythema are found throughout the oral cavity. When scraped, a shallow bleeding ulceration forms. The diagnosis is confirmed by scraping the oral lesions and making a smear with potassium hydroxide to identify yeast or hyphae. Hemodialysis patients are not generally immunocompromised. *(Emergency Medicine, Chapter 67, pp 665–680)*

16.c. Sialolithiasis, or salivary calculi, presents with unilateral swelling and pain of the affected gland. The submandibular gland is affected in 75% of cases, followed by the parotid gland in 20%. Clinically, there is outward swelling that appears as a lump under the chin and palpable swelling of the floor of the mouth with a fluctuant or cystic quality. The patient appears nontoxic and has good oral hygiene. Treatment includes antimicrobials if there is concurrent infection, analgesics, and sialogogues such as lemon drops. Ludwig's angina presents with brawny painful edema of the submandibular region and elevation of the tongue. Patients appear toxic and can rapidly develop complete airway compromise. Retropharyngeal abscesses present with fever, odynophagia, neck swelling, and cervical adenopathy. Actinomycosis is an indolent suppurative infection caused by anaerobic actinomycetes. Oropharyngeal lesions result from poor dental hygiene and abscesses. Clinically, patients present with red, indurated subcutaneous masses typically in the submandibular region. Fistula tracts are common, and there is diminished pain with palpation. The diagnosis is made on tissue demonstration of tightly knit clusters, called grains. *(Emergency Medicine, Chapter 67, pp 665–680)*

17.d. Uvular edema may be caused by infection, angioneurotic edema, allergies, and chemical or physical trauma. Symptoms of uvular edema vary from a feeling of fullness to complete upper airway obstruction. The patient with infectious uvulitis is febrile and the uvula appears red and swollen. This is in contrast to the pale, boggy uvula seen with allergic reactions and angioneurotic edema. Infections of the uvula should be treated with antimicrobials active against *H. influenzae* and *Streptococcus*. *(Emergency Medicine, Chapter 67, pp 665–680)*

18.b. Preverbal children often ingest foreign bodies. Signs and symptoms of ingestion include stridor and asymmetric wheezing. Among the most commonly ingested are coins (pennies) and button batteries. Foreign body location (trachea vs. esophagus) can often be determined by a plain radiograph of the chest. Tracheal coins will be oriented in the sagittal plane, because of the orientation of the tracheal rings (the tracheal rings are not complete posteriorly, so the coin will orient in the AP direction). Esophageal foreign bodies will often be oriented in the coronal plain. Children who are asymptomatic with esophageal coins can be followed expectantly; however, this is rarely acceptable to the parents. Methods of removal include a Foley catheter inserted beyond the foreign body, then partially inflated and removed, and endoscopic removal. Foley catheter removal is controversial and carries with it the risk of tracheal aspiration as the foreign body is removed. Button batteries contain corrosive materials that may leak over time and therefore should be removed from the esophagus by endoscopy. Batteries in the stomach and intestine may be allowed to pass spontaneously but should be followed with weekly radiographs. Batteries should be removed either endoscopically or surgically if not passing beyond the stomach. Signs of bowel perforation are an indication for removal. Complications of foreign body ingestion include airway obstruction, esophageal perforation, and fistula formation. *(Emergency Medicine, Chapter 67, pp 665–680)*

19. True. Esophageal food impaction presents with the sudden onset of sharp, retrosternal pain associated with dysphagia. The patient with minimal symptoms who can swallow secretions has a partial impaction and can be managed expectantly for up to 12 hours, at which time food removal should be attempted endoscopically. The patient who cannot swallow secretions has a complete impaction and requires emergent treatment. Use of a smooth muscle relaxant such as sublingual nitroglycerin or IV glucagon (1 mg) may be effective in relaxing the lower esophageal sphincter and allowing impacted esophageal foreign bodies to pass. If there is no improvement after such treatment, endoscopic removal should be attempted. All patients should be assessed for esophageal perforation, which manifests as worsening chest pain that radiates to the neck. *(Emergency Medicine, Chapter 67, pp 665–680)*

20. True. The most common cause of upper airway obstruction is relaxation of the tongue and posterior pharyngeal muscles. Patients with depressed mental status (e.g., postictal, head trauma, overdose) may have partial obstruction of the airway. The jaw thrust should be performed to open the airway; a head tilt may be added if there is no evidence of cervical spine injury. Nasal airways are well tolerated in the semiconscious patient. Oral airways are reserved for those without a gag reflex. *(Emergency Medicine, Chapter 67, pp 665–680)*

21. False. Compared with the adult airway, the child's airway is smaller. The tongue and posterior pharyngeal soft tissue are proportionally larger and tend to occlude the airway. The epiglottis is relatively short, narrow, and floppy and the larynx is relatively high. The narrowest diameter of the airway is at the cricoid cartilage in the subglottic area. *(Emergency Medicine, Chapter 67, pp 665–680)*

BIBLIOGRAPHY

Herr RD, Ochsenschlager DW: Disorders of the oropharynx and throat. *In* Howell JM, Altieri M, Jagoda AS, et al (eds): Emergency Medicine. Philadelphia, WB Saunders, 1998, pp 665–680.

30 Dental Emergencies

WILLIAM O'CALLAHAN, MD

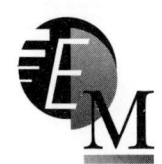

1. The prehospital care of the patient with significant maxillofacial and dental trauma includes all of the following except:
   a. Cervical spine immobilization
   b. Maintenance of adequate airway patency
   c. Control of bleeding
   d. Removal of loosened teeth for transport in appropriate preservation solution
   e. Recovery of any fractured tooth fragments, avulsed teeth, or dental prostheses

2. Traumatic injuries to the mouth and/or face may result in all of the following except:
   a. Tooth concussion
   b. Tooth avulsion
   c. Dental caries
   d. Alveolar fracture
   e. Root fracture

3. An avulsed permanent tooth that has been dry for 3 hours should be:
   a. Replanted immediately
   b. Soaked in Hank's solution for 30 minutes, then replanted
   c. Soaked in Hank's solution for 60 minutes followed by 5% doxycycline solution for 5 minutes, then replanted
   d. Soaked in Hank's solution for 30 minutes followed by a rinse in 5% doxycycline solution, then replanted
   e. Treated by a dentist and not replanted in the ED setting

4. The most appropriate antimicrobial for prophylactic coverage in extensive oral lacerations is:
   a. Ciprofloxacin
   b. Erythromycin
   c. Trimethoprim-sulfamethoxazole
   d. Penicillin
   e. Metronidazole

5. The most appropriate treatment of a superficial laceration to the intraoral mucosal surface includes:
   a. Débridement and delayed primary closure
   b. Irrigation and primary repair with absorbable suture material
   c. No repair; the patient should be instructed to irrigate the wound with swish-and-spit saline solution after meals
   d. Immediate referral to a dentist or oral surgeon for primary repair
   e. Urgent referral to a dentist or oral surgeon (within 48 hours) for delayed primary repair

6. When an avulsed tooth is successfully replanted in the ED setting, the discharge instructions should include all of the following except:
   a. Soft solid or liquid diet
   b. Appropriate analgesics, including narcotics if necessary
   c. Rinse with 5% doxycycline solution after each meal
   d. Oral penicillin or erythromycin for 10 to 14 days
   e. Urgent dental follow-up within 24 hours

7. Pericoronitis is:
   a. Inflammation of the gingiva seen in association with primary herpes simplex type 1 infection
   b. Inflammation of the mucosal surface of the hard palate
   c. Infection of the pulp of the tooth that extends to the periapical area
   d. Inflammation of the oral mucosal covering of an erupting molar
   e. Infection extending from a molar to the lateral pharyngeal space

8. A patient with extensive dental caries presents to the ED with rapidly progressing toothache. The tooth is somewhat loosened with exquisite percussion tenderness, but there is no gum swelling or fluctuance. The most likely diagnosis is:
   a. Periapical abscess
   b. Alveolar osteomyelitis
   c. Pericoronitis
   d. Gingivitis
   e. Masticator space infection

9. The appropriate ED management of an 8-year-old patient presenting with an avulsion of a permanent tooth, with an extraoral time of 1 hour, would include all of the following except:
   a. Handling the tooth by the crown only
   b. Inspection of the socket for fracture fragments and gentle irrigation of clot and debris
   c. Gently rinsing the tooth with saline followed by immediate replantation
   d. Soaking the tooth in Hank's solution for 30 minutes followed by 5% doxycycline for 5 minutes, then replanting
   e. Obtaining emergent dental consultation after appropriate replantation

10. Burns of the palate that occur as a result of hot food should be treated with all of the following except:
    a. Warm saline or dilute hydrogen peroxide rinses
    b. Débridement of burned tissue
    c. Topical anesthetics such as benzocaine-containing dental emollients
    d. Appropriate prophylactic antimicrobials
    e. Liquid or soft solid diet

11. A patient presents to the ED at night, 7 hours after a dental extraction procedure, complaining of intraoral hemorrhage. Initial evaluation and treatment may include all of the following except:
    a. Suction of clots and rinsing with saline solution
    b. Application of pressure to the bleeding site
    c. Injection of local anesthesia containing epinephrine
    d. Electrocautery of the bleeding site
    e. Placement of absorbable coagulant such as Gelfoam to the socket with an absorbable suture to hold it in position

12. All of the following statements regarding tooth eruptions in children are true except:
    a. They begin at approximately 6 months of age.
    b. They result in fever.
    c. They begin with the central incisors.
    d. They are easily treated with analgesia and hydration.
    e. They may be treated with the judicious use of topical anesthetic agents.

13. A patient presents to the ED 3 days after the removal of a tooth. He states he initially had little discomfort but now has rapidly worsening pain and a foul taste in his mouth. The most likely diagnosis is:
    a. Dental caries
    b. Alveolar osteitis (dry socket)
    c. Periapical abscess
    d. Gingivitis
    e. Peritonsillar abscess

14. A patient presents to the ED after being struck in the mouth with a baseball. There is no obvious soft tissue or dental injury, but there is percussion sensitivity of the maxillary central incisors. Appropriate management would include:
    a. Soft diet and dental follow-up
    b. Radiographic evaluation of the maxilla
    c. Antimicrobial coverage
    d. Emergent dental intervention for tooth stabilization
    e. Narcotic analgesic agents

15. Ellis class I tooth fractures:
    a. Extend into the dentin
    b. Are associated with exquisite thermal sensitivity
    c. Are typically not painful
    d. Extend into the pulp
    e. Have a poor prognosis for long-term cosmesis and function

16. All of the following are useful in the ED management of a periapical abscess except:
    a. Infiltration with a long-acting local anesthetic
    b. NSAIDs
    c. Manual extraction of loosened tooth for abscess drainage
    d. Oral penicillin or erythromycin
    e. Urgent dental referral

17. A patient presents to the ED with fever, difficulty moving the tongue, and swelling of the floor of the mouth and submandibular region. Appropriate management would include:
    a. IV penicillin in the ED followed by a 10-day course of oral penicillin
    b. Oral penicillin with urgent (within 2 days) dental follow-up
    c. Incision and drainage at point of maximal fluctuance followed by oral penicillin
    d. IV penicillin and inpatient admission
    e. Oral clindamycin and urgent dental follow-up

18. A patient reports a 2-week history of toothache and thermal sensitivity involving the mandibular third molar followed by a 2-day history of fevers, chills, and increasing difficulty opening the mouth (trismus). The most likely diagnosis is:
    a. Masticator space infection
    b. Periapical abscess
    c. Alveolar osteomyelitis (dry socket)
    d. Ludwig's angina
    e. Peritonsillar abscess

19. A 25-year-old alcoholic man presents to the ED with a complaint of fatigue, mouth pain, and bleeding with brushing. Inspection of the oral cavity reveals erythema of the gingiva as well as ulcerations of the interdental papilla with a gray membrane formation. The most likely diagnosis is:
    a. Stomatitis
    b. Mucocutaneous herpes simplex
    c. Wegener's granulomatosis
    d. Vincent's infection (trench mouth)
    e. Aphthous ulcers

20. A 23-year-old woman presents to the ED unable to close her mouth. She states she was yawning immediately before the onset of this problem and appears quite distressed. The most appropriate ED management involves:
    a. Manual reduction of the dislocated mandible

b. Emergent dental or oral surgical intervention
   c. Elliptical radiographic evaluation of the mandible
   d. Admission for operative reduction of the dislocated mandible under general anesthesia
   e. Immediate control of the airway with orotracheal intubation

21. Stensen's duct:
    a. Arises from the parotid gland and opens to the buccal mucosa at the floor of the mouth
    b. Arises from the submandibular and sublingual glands and opens to the buccal mucosa opposite the maxillary molars
    c. Arises from the parotid gland and opens to the buccal mucosa opposite the maxillary molars
    d. Arises from the submandibular and sublingual glands and opens to the buccal mucosa on the anterior floor of the mouth
    e. Arises from the parotid, sublingual, and submandibular glands and opens to the buccal mucosa both opposite the maxillary molars and the anterior floor of the mouth

22. Wharton's duct:
    a. Arises from the parotid gland and opens to the buccal mucosa at the floor of the mouth
    b. Arises from the submandibular and sublingual glands and opens to the buccal mucosa opposite the maxillary molars
    c. Arises from the parotid gland and opens to the buccal mucosa opposite the maxillary molars
    d. Arises from the submandibular and sublingual glands and opens to the buccal mucosa on the anterior floor of the mouth
    e. Arises from the parotid, sublingual, and submandibular glands and opens to the anterior floor of the mouth, and the buccal mucosa opposite the maxillary molars

23. Management of dental trauma resulting in a tooth with minimal loosening (<2 mm) includes:
    a. Wire fixation
    b. Elliptical radiograph to assess the alveolar bone
    c. No treatment
    d. Soft diet and dental follow-up
    e. Prophylactic penicillin

24. Appropriate transport media for avulsed teeth include all of the following except:
    a. Milk
    b. Tap water on ice
    c. pH balanced solution (Hank's solution)
    d. Saline-moistened gauze
    e. Saliva under the tongue of an alert patient

25. A mother presents with her 2-year-old daughter who has sustained an avulsion of her right primary maxillary central incisor. She has transported the tooth in milk and states the accident occurred 45 minutes before arrival. You should:
    a. Immediately replant the tooth with correct orientation
    b. Soak the tooth in Hank's solution for 30 minutes followed by 5% doxycycline for 5 minutes, then replant
    c. Soak the tooth in 5% doxycycline for 30 minutes followed by Hank's solution for 5 minutes, then replant
    d. Not replant the tooth
    e. Obtain emergent dental consultation for replantation and wire fixation

26. Discharge instructions after the successful reduction of a mandible dislocation should include all of the following except:
    a. Avoidance of gum chewing
    b. Soft solid or liquid diet
    c. Pain control with NSAIDs
    d. Application of ice packs to the temporomandibular joints for 48 hours
    e. Urgent dental or oral surgical referral (within 48 hours)

27. A patient presents to the ED with toothache of a left maxillary bicuspid and erythema and swelling of the face below the left eye. The most likely diagnosis is:
    a. Pericoronitis
    b. Periapical abscess
    c. Canine space infection
    d. Ludwig's angina
    e. Masticator space infection

28. Using the standard numerical classification system, the 11th tooth is the:
    a. Right maxillary canine
    b. Right mandibular canine
    c. Left maxillary central incisor
    d. Left maxillary canine
    e. Left mandibular canine

29. Using the standard numerical classification system, the right mandibular first molar is tooth number:
    a. 28
    b. 17
    c. 29
    d. 18
    e. 30

30. A 40-year-old patient involved in an motor vehicle accident during which he struck his mouth on the steering wheel is found to have a tooth that is 75% impacted into the alveolar bone of the maxilla. The tooth is not fractured. Appropriate management would include all of the following except:
    a. Analgesia and prophylactic antimicrobials
    b. Radiographic evaluation
    c. Urgent dental referral
    d. Extraction of the tooth and immediate replantation in anatomic position
    e. Instructions for soft diet and warm saline rinses

31. A college student calls the ED for advice after sustaining an avulsion of one of her teeth. She states it occurred approximately 5 minutes ago and she has the tooth.

166 HEAD AND NECK DISORDERS

Appropriate advice would include all of the following except:
a. Rinse the tooth gently in tap water
b. Use a toothbrush to cleanse the root of any adherent tissue
c. Replant the tooth immediately and bite down on gauze while coming to a dentist or ED for more definitive treatment
d. Handle the tooth by the crown only
e. Rinse the socket with swish-and-spit warm salt water before replantation to remove debris and clot

32. A 55-year-old man known to the ED staff for frequent bouts of alcohol abuse is brought in by ambulance after a fall during which he struck his head and face, resulting in avulsion of multiple teeth. The patient is intermittently combative and lethargic. The teeth were not transported with the patient. Appropriate ED management would include all of the following except:
a. Immobilization of the cervical spine
b. Assessment of the airway
c. Continuing neurologic assessment and head CT scan if appropriate
d. Attempt to find avulsed teeth and replant
e. Obtain radiographic studies to evaluate the cervical spine and to search for possibly ingested or aspirated teeth or teeth fragments

33. A 22-year-old college student is involved in a debate with a patron of a local bar, who strikes the student in the mouth with a pool cue. The student has fractures of the maxillary lateral incisor and canine that extend through the enamel and dentin, revealing exposed pulp. The injury is best described as:
a. Ellis class I tooth fracture
b. Ellis class II tooth fracture
c. Ellis class III tooth fracture
d. Root fracture
e. Alveolar bone fracture

34. The appropriate management of the student's injuries in question 33 include all of the following except:
a. Coverage of the exposed surface with calcium hydroxide paste, dental foil, or wax
b. Urgent referral to a dentist (within 48 hours) for a shallow pulpotomy
c. Instruction to avoid hot and cold liquids
d. Prescription of adequate analgesia
e. Prescription of prophylactic antimicrobials

35. A patient is referred to the ED from the dentist's office after an extracted tooth was lost during the procedure. Appropriate management would include all of the following except:
a. Discharge to home with instructions to check stools daily for 1 week
b. Chest radiograph to localize potentially aspirated tooth
c. Kidney-ureter-bladder views to localize potentially swallowed tooth
d. Pulmonary consultation for the bronchoscopic removal of tooth if aspiration is confirmed by chest radiograph
e. Discharge to home to check stools if ingestion of tooth is confirmed by kidney-ureter-bladder

Answers

1.d. As with any trauma, protection of the airway and control of hemorrhage are primary concerns in the prehospital setting. Maxillofacial trauma places the patient at risk for both head injury and cervical spine injury. Cervical immobilization should be undertaken. Fractured or avulsed teeth and dental prostheses should always be recovered by the prehospital personnel for replantation or to serve as a template for definitive care. Partially avulsed teeth should be replanted immediately with gentle pressure, and the patient should bite on gauze during transport to maintain the position of the replanted teeth if neurologic status and airway control allow. *(Emergency Medicine, Chapter 68, pp 681–691)*

2.c. Dental caries are not a traumatic condition. They are caused by acid-forming bacteria present in plaque that erode the enamel and dentin. Tooth concussion, tooth avulsion, root fracture, and alveolar bone fracture are all possible manifestations of traumatic dental injury. *(Emergency Medicine, Chapter 68, pp 681–691)*

3.e. An avulsed permanent tooth that has remained dry for more than 2 hours will almost certainly have necrosis of the periodontal ligament, and this necrotic tissue will require débridement before reimplantation. This débridement process involves chemical preparation of the tooth. This should be performed as an emergent procedure by a consulting dentist or oral surgeon. *(Emergency Medicine, Chapter 68, pp 681–691)*

4.d. Penicillin is generally considered first-line therapy for prophylaxis of oral wounds and lacerations. In the penicillin-allergic patient, erythromycin may be used. Other appropriate choices may include clindamycin, Augmentin, or metronidazole. *(Emergency Medicine, Chapter 68, pp 681–691)*

5.c. Superficial lacerations of the intraoral mucosal surface that are not associated with facial nerve, ductal, or glandular injuries and that do not extend as "through and through" injuries do not require specific repair. They will heal without complication or cosmetic deformity. Patients can be instructed to cleanse the wound with warm saline or dilute hydrogen peroxide rinsing solution after meals. Wounds in children can be cleansed with the same solutions applied to a cotton-tipped applicator if they cannot rinse. Antimicrobial prophylaxis is controversial in this setting. *(Emergency Medicine, Chapter 68, pp 681–691)*

6.c. The discharge plan after successful replantation would include a soft solid or liquid diet; pain control, including narcotic analgesia if necessary; prophylactic antimicrobial therapy with penicillin or erythromycin in the penicillin-allergic patient; and most importantly, emergent (<24 hr) dental referral for definitive care. There is no role for topical antimicrobial therapy. *(Emergency Medicine, Chapter 68, pp 681–691)*

7.d. Pericoronitis is inflammation and infection of the mucosal tissue overlying the erupting mandibular third molar in a teenager or a young adult. The tissue (pericoronal flap) is damaged by contact with the occlusal surface of the opposing molar and becomes infected by accumulation of food debris. Treatment may involve analgesics or local anesthetics, oral antimicrobials, and dental or oral surgical referral for removal of the flap and possibly the involved tooth. *(Emergency Medicine, Chapter 68, pp 681–691)*

8.a. This patient has a periapical or alveolar abscess. The necrotic pulp of carious teeth becomes contaminated with oral flora, resulting in infection spreading to the root (apex), causing pain and instability to percussion. Periapical abscesses may be associated with some gum swelling but usually not with fluctuance of the gum. *(Emergency Medicine, Chapter 68, pp 681–691)*

9.c. The root apex of permanent teeth in young children (ages 6 to 10) is immature, retaining a large pulpal blood supply that may reestablish vascularity and complete root formation after replantation. If the tooth is avulsed, with an extraoral time of less than 15 minutes, it should be soaked in 5% doxycycline solution to decrease the risk of apical abscess formation and then be replanted immediately. If the extraoral time is 15 minutes to 2 hours, the tooth should be soaked in physiologically balanced medium (Hank's solution) for 30 minutes in order to replenish depleted nutrients in the periodontal ligament cells and then in 5% doxycycline solution for 5 minutes and replanted. *(Emergency Medicine, Chapter 68, pp 681–691)*

10.b. Burns to the palate caused by hot food (pizza palate) typically require only supportive care with warm saline or diluted hydrogen peroxide rinses and analgesia with topical anesthetics and oral agents. Prophylactic antimicrobials may be useful. Débridement is not required in this setting. *(Emergency Medicine, Chapter 68, pp 681–691)*

11.d. When faced with intraoral hemorrhage after oral surgical procedures, one must first cleanse the bleeding site with saline and soft suction to properly visualize. Small areas of bleeding may be controlled with pressure alone or in combination with epinephrine-containing local anesthetics. In extensive hemorrhage from a socket, an absorbable anticoagulant can be sutured in position with an absorbable suture material. Cautery is rarely needed and should be performed by an appropriate dental or oral surgical consultant. *(Emergency Medicine, Chapter 68, pp 681–691)*

12.b. Tooth eruptions in children begin with the central incisors at approximately 6 months of age. Children may become irritable and have decreased oral intake. Low-grade fever may be associated with teething, but normally there is no fever without visible local gingival inflammation. Significant fever in the infant should never be attributed to teething alone and should always initiate a search for a source of infection. The discomfort of teething is easily relieved with oral analgesics, hydration with cooled solutions, and, if necessary, the judicious use of topical anesthetic agents. *(Emergency Medicine, Chapter 68, pp 681–691)*

13.b. The most likely diagnosis is alveolar osteitis, or "dry socket," which presents with pain increasing 2 to 3 days after a tooth extraction procedure, usually accompanied by a foul taste or odor from the mouth. It occurs as a result of lysis of the socket blood clot, leading to osteomyelitis of the underlying alveolar bone. This is a dental emergency and should be treated with pain control, oral antimicrobials, and urgent (<24 hr) dental follow-up. *(Emergency Medicine, Chapter 68, pp 681–691)*

14.a. A tooth concussion is adequately treated with a soft diet. Most concussions will heal without complication. Occult injury may, however, lead to pulpal necrosis, so timely dental follow-up should be part of the discharge plan. *(Emergency Medicine, Chapter 68, pp 681–691)*

15.c. Ellis type I fractures involve only the enamel, sparing the dentin and pulp. As such, they are typically not painful, exhibiting only minimal thermal sensitivity. Any jagged edges should be smoothed with a file or emery board. Dental referral should be made. These injuries have an excellent prognosis for cosmesis and function when treated appropriately. *(Emergency Medicine, Chapter 68, pp 681–691)*

16.c. The management of a periapical abscess involves pain control and antimicrobial therapy followed by dental referral. Although definitive dental care may require tooth extraction, these are more typically treated with root canal. There is no indication for manual extraction of a tooth in the ED setting. *(Emergency Medicine, Chapter 68, pp 681–691)*

17.d. Ludwig's angina is cellulitis of the floor of the mouth arising from mandibular infections. There is induration of the sublingual, submental, and submandibular spaces. If diagnosed early, it can be treated with large doses of IV antimicrobials in the inpatient setting. Careful observation is required because extension of infection posteriorly or inferiorly can rapidly threaten the airway, requiring emergent surgical intervention. There is no role for outpatient management in this setting. *(Emergency Medicine, Chapter 68, pp 681–691)*

18.a. Infections of the mandibular molars may extend into the masticator space between the internal pterygoid and masseter muscles. Localized pain and swelling results in spasm of these muscles, producing trismus.

168 HEAD AND NECK DISORDERS

Treatment requires surgical drainage and IV antimicrobials. *(Emergency Medicine, Chapter 68, pp 681–691)*

19.d. This represents Vincent's infection (trench mouth), or acute necrotizing ulcerative gingivitis. It is seen in young adults in association with smoking, alcohol abuse, and poor oral hygiene. Treatment is generally aimed at symptomatic relief and includes saline rinses, topical anesthetics, and oral antimicrobials. Dental follow-up is necessary to débride the lesions and avoid further tissue destruction. *(Emergency Medicine, Chapter 68, pp 681–691)*

20.a. Dislocation of one or both of the mandibular condyles can result from trauma, laughing, or yawning, and although quite distressing to the patient, it does not threaten the airway. These injuries are usually reduced with gentle forward and downward pressure applied to the molar region. In difficult cases, IV sedation with benzodiazepines or narcotics may be helpful. Radiographic evaluation is unnecessary in the absence of trauma when the diagnosis is certain. *(Emergency Medicine, Chapter 68, pp 681–691)*

21.c. See answer to question 22. *(Emergency Medicine, Chapter 68, pp 681–691)*

22.d. When assessing trauma to the dentition, mouth, and face, especially after laceration, the patency of Stensen's duct, which arises from the parotid gland and opens to the buccal mucosa opposite the maxillary molars, and Wharton's duct, which arises from the submandibular and sublingual salivary glands and opens to the anterior floor of the mouth, must be confirmed by expressing saliva. Suspicion of glandular or ductal injuries should trigger consultation with an oral or maxillofacial surgeon for repair. *(Emergency Medicine, Chapter 68, pp 681–691)*

23.d. A concussive injury that leaves the tooth minimally mobile (<2 mm) but otherwise normal with regard to alignment and dental occlusion requires nothing more than a soft diet. The patient should be instructed that occult injury can result in pulpal necrosis and discoloration of the tooth. Dental follow-up should be part of the discharge plan. *(Emergency Medicine, Chapter 68, pp 681–691)*

24.b. The success of replantation depends on the extraoral time and the tooth storage environment. Appropriate transport media include milk, commercially available pH balanced solution (Hank's solution), saline-moistened gauze, or the saliva under the tongue of an alert patient. For obvious reasons, the last of these should not be attempted in very young or intoxicated patients or in those with an altered level of consciousness. *(Emergency Medicine, Chapter 68, pp 681–691)*

25.d. It is unnecessary, and perhaps even detrimental, to replant primary teeth in children aged 6 months to 6 years, because success is rare and complications include ankylosis to the alveolar bone and/or damage to the underlying tooth follicle. Cosmetic concerns can be addressed by a pediatric dentist in follow-up. *(Emergency Medicine, Chapter 68, pp 681–691)*

26.e. This patient should avoid excessive jaw movement and should take only liquids and soft solids by mouth. Pain control is adequately achieved with local ice packs and NSAIDs. Urgent dental follow-up is unnecessary if the reduction is successful. In the rare case of frequent recurrent temporomandibular joint dislocation, oral surgical consultation and follow-up may be considered. *(Emergency Medicine, Chapter 68, pp 681–691)*

27.c. Canine space infection is seen in conjunction with infections of the anterior maxillary teeth and may be complicated by periorbital and orbital infections, cavernous sinus thrombosis, airway obstruction, or mediastinal infections if not adequately treated with drainage and antimicrobials. *(Emergency Medicine, Chapter 68, pp 681–691)*

28.d. See answer to question 29. *(Emergency Medicine, Chapter 68, p 683, Table 68–3)*

29.e. The standard numerical tooth identification system begins with the right maxillary (upper) third molar as tooth number 1 and progresses to the left maxillary third molar as tooth number 16, beginning again at the left mandibular (lower) third molar as tooth number 17 and progressing to the right mandibular third molar as tooth number 32. It is also appropriate to describe teeth anatomically when discussing care with a consultant (e.g., right or left, maxillary or mandibular, molar, canine). *(Emergency Medicine, Chapter 68, p 683, Table 68–3)*

30.d. Replantation is the appropriate ED management of avulsed teeth in most settings, but attempts to replant impacted teeth (both primary and secondary) should not be undertaken. Analgesia, antimicrobials, and urgent dental follow-up for repositioning and stabilization is the treatment of choice. Radiographic studies may assist in determining the extent of tooth penetration and underlying alveolar bone injury. *(Emergency Medicine, Chapter 68, pp 681–691)*

31.b. A tooth that is replanted within 30 minutes has an excellent (>90%) chance for retention without root resorption. The tooth should be handled only by the crown and never by the root; it should be rinsed with tap water; the periodontal ligament strands should be left in place; the socket should be cleansed of any blood clot; and the tooth should be replanted with correct orientation. The patient should then be instructed to bite on gauze to splint the tooth in position while obtaining emergent definitive care for stabilization. *(Emergency Medicine, Chapter 68, pp 681–691)*

32.d. Although success with replantation is time dependent, it should always be remembered that life-threatening emergencies take precedence over cosmesis. In this case, maintenance of the airway, control and evaluation of the cervical spine, assessment of potential head injury, and the potential for aspiration of avulsed teeth and tooth fragments should be addressed before concerns about replantation. *(Emergency Medicine, Chapter 68, pp 681–691)*

33.c. Ellis type I fractures involve only the enamel. Ellis type II fractures extend to the dentin. Ellis type III fractures extend into the pulp. Root fractures and alveolar bone fractures cannot be seen on visual inspection and require radiographic evaluation for diagnosis. *(Emergency Medicine, Chapter 68, pp 681–691)*

34.b. The management of Ellis types II and III tooth fractures are similar and include coverage of the exposed surface with calcium hydroxide paste, dental foil, or wax. Patients should be instructed to avoid hot and cold beverages. Class III fractures require more urgent follow-up care with root canal to prevent the formation of periapical abscess. In primary teeth, shallow pulpotomy is the treatment of choice for a class III fracture, but it has no role in this patient. *(Emergency Medicine, Chapter 68, pp 681–691)*

35.a. Although a lost tooth is not a life-threatening emergency, the location of the extracted tooth must be further evaluated by radiographic study. An aspirated tooth must be emergently removed by bronchoscopy, but a swallowed tooth can generally be allowed to pass without invasive attempts at retrieval. The position of the lost tooth must not be assumed without radiographic confirmation. *(Emergency Medicine, Chapter 68, pp 681–691)*

BIBLIOGRAPHY

Andreasen JO: Traumatic Injuries of the Teeth, 2nd ed. Philadelphia, WB Saunders, 1981.

Braham RL, Morris ME: Textbook of Pediatric Dentistry, 2nd ed. Baltimore, Williams & Wilkens, 1985.

Berry HM: Emergency Physicians Guide to Dental Care. Philadelphia, University of Pennsylvania Press, 1983.

Bringhurst C, Herr R, Aldous A: Oral trauma in the emergency department. Am J Emerg Med 1993; 11:486–490.

Cvek M, Cleaton-Jones P, Austin J, et al: Effect of topical application of doxycycline on pulp revascularization and periodontal healing in reimplanted monkey incisors. Endod Dent Traumatol 1990; 6:170–176.

Derbay JP: Dental disorders. *In* Howell JM, Altieri M, Jagoda AS, et al (eds): Emergency Medicine. Philadelphia, WB Saunders, 1998, pp 681–691.

Falace DA: Emergency Dental Care. Philadelphia, Williams & Wilkins, 1995.

Graham CJ: Stroke following oral trauma in children. Ann Emerg Med 1991; 20:1029–1030.

Goorhuis H, Rothrock S: Cervicofacial and thoracic barotrauma following a minor dental procedure. Pediatr Emerg Care 1993; 9:29–32.

Hammarstron L, Pierce A, Blomlof L, et al: Tooth avulsion and replantation—A review. Endod Dent Traumatol 1986; 2:1–8.

Krasner P: Modern treatment of avulsed teeth by emergency physicians. Am J Emerg Med 1994; 12(2):241–245.

Mackie IC, Warren VN: Dental trauma: general aspects of management, and trauma to the primary dentition. Dent Update 1988; 5:151.

Matsson L, Andreasen J, Cvek M, et al: Ankylosis of experimentally reimplanted teeth related to extra-alveolar period and storage environment. Pediatr Dent 1982; 4:327–329.

Medford HM: Temporary stabilization of avulsed or luxated teeth. Ann Emerg Med 1982; 68(11):490–492.

Roberts J, Hedges J: Clinical Procedures in Emergency Medicine, 2nd ed. Philadelphia, WB Saunders, 1991.

Shackelford D, Casani J: Diffuse subcutaneous emphysema, pneumomediastinum, and pneumothorax after dental extraction. Ann Emerg Med 1993; 22:248–250.

Simon RR: Emergency Procedures and Techniques, 2nd ed. Baltimore, Williams & Wilkins, 1987.

Thaller SR: Guide to Dental Problems for Physicians and Surgeons. Baltimore, Williams & Wilkins, 1988.

SECTION NINE

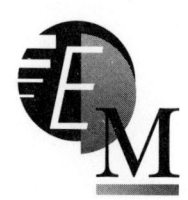

Oncology and Blood Disorders

31 Oncologic Emergencies, Red Blood Cell Disorders, and White Blood Cell Disorders

MARK J. SAGARIN, MD   ROBERT J. VISSERS, MD

Oncologic Emergencies

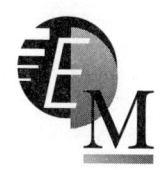

1. A 67-year-old man with small cell lung cancer presents with a gradual onset of dyspnea and swelling of his right arm and face. His jugular veins are distended and breath sounds are equal bilaterally. The most useful initial therapy is probably:
   a. Diphenhydramine, ranitidine, corticosteroids, and epinephrine
   b. Elevation of the head of the bed, diuretics, and corticosteroids
   c. Pericardiocentesis
   d. Right-sided chest tube
   e. Right-sided thoracentesis

2. A patient with known cerebral metastases presents with an acute headache. CT scan reveals bleeding into a metastasis with surrounding edema. This patient would benefit from all of the following except:
   a. IV fluid bolus
   b. Intubation and hyperventilation
   c. Elevation of the head of the bed to 60 degrees
   d. Dexamethasone
   e. Mannitol and furosemide

3. A 52-year-old man presents with hypoxemia and tachypnea. He is afebrile and has not been coughing. He has no evidence of focal infection or pulmonary embolism. He has diffuse bilateral infiltrates on his chest radiograph and a WBC count of 134,000. Of the following, the most likely underlying disorder is:
   a. Acute lymphocytic leukemia
   b. Acute myelogenous leukemia
   c. Chronic lymphocytic leukemia
   d. AIDS
   e. Polycythemia vera

4. An 86-year-old man with prostate cancer presents with a 4-day history of worsening back pain, new urinary incontinence, and bilateral leg weakness. Physical examination is notable for midline lumbar spine tenderness, normal rectal tone, a slightly asymmetric prostate, moderate leg weakness, and decreased lower extremity deep tendon reflexes. Plain films of the lumbosacral spine are negative. The most important next study to obtain is:
   a. Voiding cystourethrogram
   b. CT of the head
   c. CT of the spine
   d. MRI of the spine
   e. Vital capacity measurement

5. Which of the following is a common complication of multiple myeloma?
   a. Obstructive uropathy
   b. Spinal cord compression
   c. Hyperviscosity syndrome
   d. Amyloidosis
   e. All of the above

6. Which of the following should not be considered as a possible treatment for hypercalcemia from malignancy?
   a. Subcutaneous calcitonin
   b. IV fluids and loop diuretics
   c. IV phosphate
   d. IV pamidronate
   e. Treatment for the underlying malignancy

7. Which of the following chemotherapeutic agents is most commonly associated with severe, dose-dependent cardiotoxicity?
   a. Bleomycin
   b. Cyclophosphamide
   c. Doxorubicin (Adriamycin)
   d. Vincristine
   e. Methotrexate

8. Common adverse effects of methotrexate administration include all of the following except:
   a. Renal toxicity
   b. Neutropenia
   c. Mucositis
   d. Rash
   e. Constipation

9. Which of the following disorders causes the vast majority of cases of the hyperviscosity syndrome?
   a. Sickle cell anemia
   b. Chronic granulocytic leukemia

c. Polycythemia vera
d. Waldenström's macroglobulinemia
e. Multiple myeloma

10. Which of the following is the most common cause of the superior vena cava syndrome?
    a. Thyroid goiters and tumors
    b. Lung cancer
    c. Thrombosis from an indwelling IV catheter
    d. Hodgkin's and non-Hodgkin's lymphoma
    e. Pulmonary and mediastinal fibrosis

11. The syndrome of inappropriate antidiuretic hormone results in:
    a. Decreased serum Na, decreased urine osmolarity
    b. Decreased serum Na, increased urine osmolarity
    c. Increased serum Na, decreased urine osmolarity
    d. Increased serum Na, increased urine osmolarity
    e. None of the above

12. The leading cause of death in patients with hematologic malignancies is:
    a. Hemorrhage
    b. Pericardial tamponade
    c. Thrombosis
    d. Respiratory insufficiency from pleural effusion
    e. Sepsis

13. Which of the following antimicrobial regimens would be inadequate as initial empiric therapy for the febrile patient with neutropenia without a source?
    a. Ceftazidime alone
    b. Gentamycin alone
    c. Ticarcillin-clavulanate and gentamycin
    d. Imipenem-cilastatin alone
    e. Ceftazidime and amikacin

14. Treatment of the tumor lysis syndrome commonly includes all of the following except:
    a. Allopurinol
    b. Aluminum hydroxide antacids
    c. Calcium chloride
    d. Potassium chloride
    e. Sodium bicarbonate

15. A 10-year-old boy develops intussusception. Once the acute process is treated, he should:
    a. Be discharged home
    b. Be admitted for observation
    c. Undergo bone marrow biopsy to exclude associated myelodysplastic syndrome
    d. Undergo abdominal CT and exploratory laparotomy to exclude associated non-Hodgkin's lymphoma
    e. Undergo exploratory laparotomy to evaluate the possibility of ischemia in the affected segment of bowel

16. Which of the following metabolic abnormalities seen in the setting of cancer tends to decrease serum calcium levels?
    a. Production of parathyroid hormone–related peptide
    b. Increased hydroxylation of 25-OH-cholecalciferol to 1,25-OH-cholecalciferol by tumor-related macrophages
    c. Increased osteoclast activity
    d. Decreased glomerular filtration rate
    e. Increased serum phosphate levels with tumor lysis

17. Typhlitis, a condition seen in neutropenic leukemics, is an inflammation of the:
    a. Perianal region
    b. Oral gingiva
    c. Cecum
    d. Cerebellum
    e. Liver

18. Symptoms and signs of cancer-related hypercalcemia include all of the following except:
    a. Constipation
    b. Lethargy
    c. Hyperreflexia
    d. Muscle weakness
    e. Polyuria

19. A 64-year-old woman with non-Hodgkin's lymphoma presents with 2 days of increasing dyspnea. Her chest radiograph demonstrates moderate bilateral interstitial edema. Her ECG is notable only for an alternating beat-to-beat variation in voltage (height of QRS complex). The most likely cause of her symptoms is:
    a. *Pneumocystis carinii* pneumonia
    b. Superior vena cava syndrome
    c. Pericardial tamponade
    d. Cardiomyopathy
    e. Cardiac conduction abnormality

20. The most common site of spinal cord compression from metastatic cancer is:
    a. Cervical spine
    b. Thoracic spine
    c. Lumbar spine
    d. Sacral spine
    e. Thoracic and lumbar spines in approximately equal proportions

Answers

1.b. The symptoms described in this case are most consistent with superior vena cava syndrome. Superior vena cava syndrome results from obstruction of the superior vena cava either from external compression or from within. Most cases result from lung cancer (typically right upper lobe lesions). Patients present with headache; visual change; edema of the face, neck, and ipsilateral arm; dyspnea; and dry cough. Physical examination may reveal edema and engorged veins. The head of the bed should be elevated; diuretics and corticosteroids can be administered in the ED before definitive therapy (most commonly chemotherapy and/or radiotherapy). Antihistamines, steroids, and epinephrine are the treatment choices for an allergic reaction, which would tend to start acutely, with bilateral symptoms and an urticarial rash. Pericardiocentesis is the treatment for a malignant pericardial effusion, which would tend to result in bilateral edema from right heart failure. A chest tube is the treatment for a pneumothorax; either a chest tube or thoracentesis is the treatment for a malignant pleural effusion. These entities, however, would not generally result in unilateral edema and tend to cause decreased breath sounds on the affected side. *(Emergency Medicine, Chapter 69, pp 693–711)*

2.a. This patient has elevated intracranial pressure from cerebral edema. Hyperventilation causes cerebral vasoconstriction, thus reducing cerebral perfusion pressure and, by extension, intracranial pressure. The $PaCO_2$ should be maintained at about 25 to 30 mm Hg. Hyperventilation, however, is only a temporizing measure prior to definitive therapy. If time permits, intubation should be performed in a manner designed to blunt the hypertensive response to laryngoscopy: Intravenous lidocaine and a defasciculating dose of a nondepolarizing neuromuscular blocking agent can be administered prior to oral rapid-sequence intubation. Most physicians avoid induction agents that tend to elevate intracranial pressure, such as ketamine, in favor of more hemodynamically neutral agents, such as etomidate. The dosage of succinylcholine should be increased slightly after a defasciculating dose of a neuromuscular blocking agent. Elevation of the head of the bed can reduce intracranial pressure through the effect of gravity. Although controversial, dexamethasone is widely used in the setting of elevated intracranial pressure in malignant brain lesions, particularly when there is cerebral edema. Diuresis with mannitol and furosemide can rapidly reduce intracranial pressure. Intravenous fluids should be limited unless there is hypotension, because excessive hydration can worsen cerebral edema. *(Emergency Medicine, Chapter 69, pp 693–711)*

3.b. The hyperleukocytic syndrome (also called the leukostasis syndrome) is a hyperviscous state from leukocytosis that results from decreased microperfusion to tissues (most commonly the lungs and central nervous system). Signs and symptoms include confusion, coma, dyspnea, pulmonary infiltrates, visual changes, retinal hemorrhages, and occasionally priapism. Acute myelogenous leukemia can result in this syndrome when WBC counts exceed 100,000/mL. Acute lymphocytic leukemia and chronic myelogenous leukemia cause this disorder less commonly, usually only at WBC counts exceeding 250,000/mL (such as blast crisis of chronic myelogenous leukemia); the more mature cells in these disorders are less "sticky." This syndrome is more common in myelogenous than lymphocytic leukemias because of the larger size of the myeloid cells. Leukapheresis is the cornerstone of management; hydroxyurea and chemotherapy can also play important roles.[1] Although *Pneumocystis carinii* pneumonia in the setting of AIDS may present in a similar way clinically, the WBC count should not be this high. Polycythemia vera causes primarily an increased hematocrit with somewhat increased platelet and WBC counts; a WBC count over 100,000/mL would be very unusual. *(Emergency Medicine, Chapter 72, pp 740–757)*

4.d. This patient's symptoms should be taken very seriously in the setting of prostate cancer as possible epidural spinal cord compression. Taken individually, back pain, urinary incontinence, and leg weakness are each somewhat nonspecific in an elderly man, but considered together they are quite worrisome. Other signs and symptoms of epidural spinal cord compression include muscle atrophy or fasciculations, gait disturbances, anesthesia, urinary retention or incontinence, and constipation. Bowel and bladder symptoms, related to autonomic dysfunction, are late symptoms that are poor prognostic indicators. Patients with malignancies that metastasize to bone (breast, lung, and prostate cancer) and hematologic malignancies (lymphoma and multiple myeloma) are at increased risk for epidural spinal cord compression. Plain films are the usual initial study and are abnormal in about 30% of cases. Magnetic resonance imaging of the spine is the radiographic study of choice for detecting epidural disease, vertebral metastases, and paraspinal masses. It provides excellent visualization to evaluate the possibility of ongoing or impending spinal cord compression. Excluding epidural spinal cord compression is one of the few true emergent indications for MRI. Computed tomography of the spine is less sensitive and specific than MRI, although this modality is sometimes used in concert with myelography in centers without access to MRI. Lower extremity weakness is occasionally a result of the Guillain-Barré syndrome; in this setting, vital capacity is followed serially to evaluate the need for ventilatory support as respiratory muscles weaken. Initial ED treatment for epidural spinal cord compression is with high-dose corticosteroids (dexamethasone 10–100 mg IV initial dose). Definitive management is most commonly with radiotherapy; surgical decompression and chemotherapy may also be considered. *(Emergency Medicine, Chapter 69, pp 693–711)*

5.e. All of the listed conditions are complications of multiple myeloma. Several forms of obstructive uropathy may occur in the setting of multiple myeloma. Hypercalcemia from bony destruction can result in calcium-containing kidney stones. In myeloma kidney, kappa and gamma light chains combine with albumin, IgG, and giant cells to form casts that obstruct the proximal and distal tubules.[2] Involvement of the vertebral column by multiple myeloma, and consequent pathologic fracture, may result in spinal cord compression. The hyperviscosity syndrome, a consequence of increased serum viscosity, results in bleeding (of mucous membranes or the retina), visual disturbances, and a wide range of neurologic complaints (from CNS ischemia). Treatment is plasmapheresis. Amyloidosis associated with multiple myeloma can result in macroglossia, hepatomegaly, nephrotic syndrome, and an infiltrative cardiomyopathy. There is no good specific treatment, although various chemotherapeutic regimens have been used. Recurrent infections and immunosuppression is another very important consequence of multiple myeloma. Pneumococcal, hemophilus, and gram-negative infections are common. *(Emergency Medicine, Chapter 72, pp 740–757)*

6.c. Therapy should begin with vigorous hydration because most patients are dehydrated. Loop diuretics for volume overload and treatment of the underlying cancer are the mainstays of therapy for hypercalcemia of malignancy. Although previously recommended, IV phosphate in hypercalcemia can result in diffuse calcium phosphate precipitation. Calcitonin (which decreases osteoclastic bone resorption and increases urinary excretion) and pamidronate (which decreases bone resorption) have demonstrated efficacy in reducing serum calcium levels but have a slow onset of action, over hours to days. Mithramycin and gallium nitrate are additional agents that are used less frequently to reduce serum calcium levels. *(Emergency Medicine, Chapter 69, pp 693–711)*

7.c. The cardiotoxicity associated with doxorubicin (Adriamycin) is usually irreversible. Doxorubicin and other related anthracyclines (e.g., daunorubicin, epirubicin, mitoxantrone) are the chemotherapeutic agents that are the most damaging to the heart. Myocardial ischemia has been well documented with 5-fluorouracil. There have been a few isolated reports of ischemia with vinca alkaloids, bleomycin, cisplatin, and interleukin-2.[2] Bleomycin causes pulmonary fibrosis; cyclophosphamide causes hemorrhagic cystitis; and vincristine causes peripheral neuropathy and mucositis. Toxicity of methotrexate is discussed in the answer to question 18. *(Emergency Medicine, Chapter 69, pp 693–711)*

8.e. Methotrexate is used in a large variety of cancers, in rheumatologic conditions, and as an abortifacient. Because it interferes with folate metabolism, it has disproportionate effects on tissues with rapid cell turnover. When methotrexate is administered in high dosages, its side effects are minimized by coadministration of leukovorin, a folate "rescue" agent. Methotrexate can cause direct injury to renal tubular cells and indirect injury by precipitation in the tubules. Hydration, urinary alkalinization, and leukovorin minimize this toxicity. Neutropenia is extremely common, usually seen about 10 days after methotrexate administration. Mucositis is also common about 4 days after methotrexate administration. An erythematous rash, normally clinically insignificant, is commonly seen after methotrexate administration. Methotrexate may cause diarrhea from sloughing of the gastrointestinal epithelium, but constipation would be an unusual side effect. *(Emergency Medicine, Chapter 69, pp 693–711)*

9.d. Although all of the mentioned disorders may cause the hyperviscosity syndrome, 85% to 90% of cases result from Waldenström's macroglobulinemia. Multiple myeloma is the second most common cause. This syndrome is manifested by hemorrhage from mucous membranes, neurologic changes, angina, CHF, and renal failure. Plasmapheresis is the cornerstone of management; small reductions in plasma protein concentration can reduce serum viscosity considerably. Fluid and red cell administration should be performed cautiously because patients may be in CHF.[3]

10.b. Although all of the listed entities can cause superior vena cava syndrome, bronchogenic carcinoma is far and away the most common cause. Lung cancer accounts for 80% of cases, whereas lymphoma accounts for 15%. Of cases related to lung cancer, 50% occur in the setting of small cell lung cancer. Other causes of superior vena cava syndrome include tuberculosis, aortic aneurysm, goiter, fibrosis, indwelling catheter, trauma, sarcoidosis, and thrombi. *(Emergency Medicine, Chapter 69, pp 693–711)*

11.b. The syndrome of inappropriate antidiuretic hormone is seen in 1% to 2% of cancer patients, especially those with small cell lung cancer. It is also seen in other patients with cancer involving the pituitary, brain, lung, adrenal, pancreas, esophagus, or prostate or after chemotherapy with cyclophosphamide or vincristine. Patients present with hyponatremia and a urine osmolarity exceeding the serum osmolarity. *(Emergency Medicine, Chapter 69, pp 693–711)*

12.e. Overwhelming sepsis is the leading cause of death in patients with hematologic malignancies. Lymphocytes and neutrophils are commonly reduced in number and function. In addition, patients with chronic lymphocytic leukemia, multiple myeloma, and non-Hodgkin's lymphoma often have abnormal immunoglobulin production. The other listed entities are all potentially lethal complications of hematologic malignancy, but none approaches the frequency of sepsis as a cause of mortality. *(Emergency Medicine, Chapter 72, pp 740–757)*

13.b. Commonly recommended initial antimicrobial regimens for the febrile neutropenic patient usually include either monotherapy or a combination of two agents. Monotherapy generally employs an antipseudomonal cephalosporin such as ceftazidime or a carbapenam such as imipenem-cilastatin. Combination therapy generally employs two of three of the following: an antipseudomonal cephalosporin, an antipseudomonal penicillin, or an aminoglycoside. Monotherapy with fluoroquinolones such as ciprofloxacin has been evaluated in several clinical trials. Results of these trials have been variable. Some concern has been raised about these agents' limited efficacy against gram-positive cocci and their association with multidrug-resistant organisms. In selected cases, consideration is given to the addition of vancomycin for additional gram-positive coverage (in patients with indwelling catheters), clindamycin or metronidazole for additional anaerobic coverage, or amphotericin B for fungal coverage. *(Emergency Medicine, Chapter 72, pp 740–757)*

14. **d.** Tumor lysis syndrome is a combination of metabolic derangements resulting from cell lysis several days after chemotherapy. The most common abnormalities are hyperkalemia, hyperphosphatemia, and hyperuricemia. The phosphate often binds to serum calcium, resulting in hypocalcemia. This syndrome is seen most commonly in high-grade lymphomas and leukemias, but it can also occur after chemotherapy for solid tumors. Clinical manifestations are mental status changes, nausea and vomiting, and oliguria. This oliguria is often caused by uric acid nephropathy. Treatment consists of hydration, diuretics as needed, and correction of electrolyte abnormalities. Hypocalcemia is treated with calcium chloride. Hyperuricemia is treated with allopurinol and bicarbonate. Hyperphosphatemia is treated with aluminum hydroxide antacids. Hyperkalemia is treated with calcium, bicarbonate, Kayexalate, and insulin with glucose. Hemodialysis is sometimes necessary. *(Emergency Medicine, Chapter 69, pp 693–711)*

15. **d.** Because intussusception is relatively uncommon in older school-age children and because it may be associated with non-Hodgkin's lymphoma, children older than 5 years who develop intussusception should undergo exploratory laparotomy to rule out non-Hodgkin's lymphoma. Although ischemia in the affected segment of bowel is possible in the setting of intussusception, routine exploratory laparotomy to evaluate for this is not recommended unless symptoms persist. *(Emergency Medicine, Chapter 35, pp 323–337)*

16. **e.** All of the listed abnormalities tend to increase serum calcium levels except for increased serum phosphate, which precipitates with serum calcium to decrease its level. *(Emergency Medicine, Chapter 69, pp 693–711)*

17. **c.** Typhlitis is an inflammatory cellulitis involving the cecum. Patients present with fever, abdominal pain, and watery diarrhea. Septicemia, usually gram-negative, is seen in 70%; mortality is 30% to 50%. Antimicrobials, hydration, nasogastric suction, and possible surgical resection are the mainstays of treatment. *(Emergency Medicine, Chapter 69, pp 693–711)*

18. **c.** Hypercalcemia is associated with hyporeflexia, not hyperreflexia. *(Emergency Medicine, Chapter 69, pp 693–711)*

19. **c.** Electrical alternans, characterized by P wave and QRS complex voltage alternation from beat to beat, is virtually pathognomonic for cardiac tamponade. It is thought to result from the heart swinging in its fluid-filled pericardium closer to and farther from the chest wall on successive beats. This electrocardiographic finding is seen in only a minority of patients with cardiac tamponade; the majority will have nonspecific abnormalities such as sinus tachycardia or ST wave changes. Some demonstrate decreased voltage. Most malignant effusions result from metastases. Neoplasms that commonly involve the pericardium include lung, breast, Hodgkin's and non-Hodgkin's lymphomas, leukemia, melanoma, gastrointestinal malignancy, and sarcoma. The majority of patients with nontraumatic pericardial tamponade present with nonspecific signs and symptoms, such as dyspnea or cough alone. Only a very small minority present with Beck's classic triad of jugular venous distention, muffled heart sounds, and hypotension. Emergency treatment is with pericardiocentesis or subxiphoid pericardotomy. *(Emergency Medicine, Chapter 69, pp 693–711)*

20. **b.** About 65% of cases of spinal cord compression from metastatic spread of cancer occur in the thoracic spine. Degenerative joint disease more commonly affects the more mobile joints in the cervical and lumbar spines, which are more likely to be subjected to acute and chronic trauma. *(Emergency Medicine, Chapter 69, pp 693–711)*

Red Blood Cell and White Blood Cell Disorders

1. Which of the following is an uncommon physical finding for the initial presentation of acute lymphocytic leukemia?
   a. Lymphadenopathy
   b. Bony tenderness
   c. Splenomegaly
   d. Papilledema
   e. Petechiae or ecchymosis

2. A 22-year-old man sustains splenic trauma in an assault and subsequently undergoes a partial splenectomy. Three weeks later, he presents to the ED with a mild upper respiratory illness. His platelet count is noted to be 1,100,000/μL. There is no suggestion of pulmonary embolism. Further investigation and treatment of this thrombocytosis should include:
   a. Bone marrow biopsy
   b. Chemotherapy with an alkylating agent
   c. Plasmapheresis
   d. Bleeding time
   e. No further investigation or therapy is necessary

3. A 5-year-old African-American girl becomes markedly jaundiced 36 hours after starting a course of trimetho-

prim-sulfamethoxazole for otitis media. She feels well and denies abdominal pain. There is no focal rash and no abdominal tenderness. Her hematocrit is 22.6%. Additional laboratory and radiographic evaluation is likely to reveal:
   a. An elevated alkaline phosphatase
   b. An elevated lactate dehydrogenase
   c. A decreased reticulocyte count
   d. An elevated haptoglobin
   e. A dilated common bile duct on right upper quadrant ultrasound

4. The most common inherited cause of a hypercoagulable state is:
   a. Antiphospholipid antibody syndrome
   b. Antithrombin III deficiency
   c. Protein C deficiency
   d. Protein S deficiency
   e. Factor V Leiden mutation

5. A 2-week-old infant has a CBC drawn as a part of a sepsis evaluation. The hematocrit is 57%. This laboratory finding should be further investigated or treated with:
   a. Bone marrow biopsy
   b. Renal ultrasound
   c. Arterial blood gas
   d. Phlebotomy
   e. No further investigation or therapy is necessary

Answers

1.d. Splenomegaly and lymphadenopathy are seen in about three fourths of cases of acute lymphocytic leukemia; hemorrhagic findings, in two thirds; hepatomegaly, in half; sternal tenderness, in one third. Evidence of elevated intracranial pressure from CNS involvement is relatively rare in early acute lymphocytic leukemia. (*Emergency Medicine, Chapter 72, pp 740-757*)

2.e. Reactive thrombocytosis is normal after any surgery but especially after splenectomy, because there is reduced ability for sequestration. In the absence of symptoms of thrombosis or hemorrhage, no additional investigation or therapy for this abnormality is indicated. After splenectomy, clinicians should have an increased index of suspicion for infection with encapsulated organisms such as *Pneumococcus, Haemophilus influenzae,* and *Neisseria* species. (*Emergency Medicine, Chapter 71, pp 725-739*)

3.b. The patient's anemia and lack of abdominal symptoms make acute hemolysis the most likely cause of jaundice. This patient may have acute hemolysis secondary to glucose-6-phosphate dehydrogenase deficiency. Seen most commonly in individuals of African, Mediterranean, and Middle Eastern heritage, glucose-6-phosphate dehydrogenase deficiency causes hemolytic anemia in the setting of certain antioxidant precipitants such as sulfonamides, antimalarials, certain antimicrobials, salicylates, dapsone, and fava beans. Laboratory abnormalities seen with hemolysis include a normocytic anemia, elevated (predominantly indirect) bilirubin, elevated lactate dehydrogenase, decreased haptoglobin, elevated urine urobilinogen, and anisocytosis and schistocytes on peripheral smear. With normal bone marrow function, reticulocytes should increase. In the setting of obstructive jaundice, alkaline phosphatase and gamma glutamyltransferase are elevated and the common bile duct may be dilated. If laboratory values are correctly interpreted in acute hemolysis, there is usually no reason to perform an abdominal ultrasound examination. (*Emergency Medicine, Chapter 72, pp 740-757*)

4.e. All the listed entities can cause a hypercoagulable state. A recently identified mutation in factor V (Factor V Leiden) is the most common known cause of hypercoagulability. This inherited mutation, which results in resistance to activated protein C, is present in 2% to 5% of the general population and about 40% of patients with venous thromboembolism. It appears to increase risk of thrombosis about fivefold to tenfold.[4] The presence of either the lupus anticoagulant or an anticardiolipin antibody can cause the antiphospholipid antibody syndrome. This syndrome is a common cause of acquired hypercoagulability. Deficiencies in antithrombin III, protein C, and protein S are inherited thrombotic disorders related to a defect in one anticoagulant factor. Of patients with thrombosis, one of these deficiencies is present in about 5% to 10%.

5.e. The normal hematocrit for a 2-week-old child is 53%. No further investigation or therapy is necessary. (*Emergency Medicine, Chapter 72, pp 740-757*)

REFERENCES

1. Flotre M: Evaluation and management of oncologic emergencies. Emerg Med Rep 1991; 12(2):1-19.
2. Holland JF, Frei E, Bast RC, et al (eds): Cancer Medicine, 3rd ed. Philadelphia, Lea & Febiger, 1993, pp 2442-2465.
3. Bell WR: Hematologic and Oncologic Emergencies. New York, Churchill Livingstone, 1993.
4. Dahlbäck B: Factor V gene mutation causing inherited resistance to activated protein C as a basis for venous thromboembolism. J Intern Med 1995; 237:221-227.

BIBLIOGRAPHY

Brookoff D: The cancer patient in the emergency department. *In* Harwood-Nuss AL, Linden CH, Luten RC, et al (eds): The Clinical Practice of Emergency Medicine, 2nd ed. Philadelphia, Lippincott-Raven, 1996, pp 922-928.

Clark M: Gastrointestinal obstruction. *In* Howell JM, Altieri M, Jagoda AS, et al (eds): Emergency Medicine. Philadelphia, WB Saunders, 1998, pp 323-337.

Coyne MA: Avoiding indecision and hesitation with hemophilia-related emergencies. Emerg Med Rep 1992; 13(22):165-176.

Edelson OW, Kleerekoper M: Hypercalcemic crisis. Med Clin North Am 1995; 79(1):79-92.

Giamarellou H. Empiric therapy for infections in the febrile, neutropenic, compromised host. Med Clin North Am 1995; 79(3):559-580.

Gilbert JA Jr, Gossett CW: Disorders of hemostasis. *In* Howell JM, Altieri M, Jagoda AS, et al (eds): Emergency Medicine. Philadelphia, WB Saunders, 1998, pp 725–739.

Handin RI, Lux SE, Stossel TP: Blood: Principles and Practice of Hematology. Philadelphia, JB Lippincott, 1995.

Pimental L, McPherson SJ: Oncologic emergencies. *In* Howell JM, Altieri M, Jagoda AS, et al (eds): Emergency Medicine. Philadelphia, WB Saunders, 1998, pp 693–711.

Ruggenenti P, Remuzzi O. The pathophysiology and management of thrombotic thrombocytopenic purpura. Eur J Haematol 1996; 56:191–207.

Sarko J, Gin-Shaw SL: Lymphoma and disorders of red and whilte blood cells. *In* Howell JM, Altieri M, Jagoda AS, et al (eds): Emergency Medicine. Philadelphia, WB Saunders, 1998, pp 740–757.

Warrell RP: Metabolic emergencies. *In* DeVita VT, Hellman S, Rosenberg SA (eds): Cancer: Principles and Practice of Oncology, 4th ed. Philadelphia, JB Lippincott, 1993, pp 2128–2141.

32 Hemoglobinopathies

THEA JAMES, MD

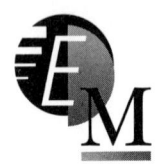

1. Most homozygous pediatric patients (HgbSS) develop painful crises before what age?
   a. 1 year
   b. 2 years
   c. 6 months
   d. 5 years

2. The evaluation of a child with sickle cell disease and fever who is younger than 5 years includes:
   a. Chest radiograph
   b. Blood cultures
   c. Broad-spectrum antimicrobials
   d. Urinalysis
   e. All of the above

3. All of the following are indications for transfusion in sickle cell patients except:
   a. Severe anemia
   b. Persistent priapism
   c. Cerebrovascular accident
   d. Hyphema
   e. Chest crisis

4. Which of the following is a characteristic of persons with sickle cell variants?
   a. Pain occurs commonly.
   b. Pain occurs under conditions of mild hypoxia.
   c. They are at risk of developing splenic sequestration into adulthood.
   d. They have the same life expectancy as homozygous sickle cell patients.

5. The pathophysiology of painful crises includes all except:
   a. Hypoxia
   b. Decreased blood viscosity
   c. Sickled erythrocytes
   d. Acidosis

6. Common precipitants of painful crises include which of the following?
   a. Infection
   b. Alcohol intoxication
   c. Menstruation
   d. Emotional stress
   e. All of the above

7. Patients with HgbSS disease are at particularly increased risk for severe infection from all of the following infectious agents except:
   a. *Haemophilus influenzae*
   b. *Staphylococcus aureus*
   c. *Streptococcus pneumoniae*
   d. *Salmonella* species

8. A 4-year-old with HgbSS disease who was recently diagnosed with a viral illness presents to the ED hypotensive, with an enlarged spleen. The most likely etiology of this presentation is:
   a. Urinary tract infection
   b. Pneumonia
   c. Unprotected exposure to high altitude
   d. Sequestration crisis
   e. Hemolytic crisis

9. A patient with HgbSS presents to the ED with a 2-hour complaint of headache and a visual field defect. The emergency physician should have a high suspicion for:
   a. Temporal arteritis
   b. Sinus infection
   c. Cerebrovascular accident
   d. Migraine headache

10. Which of the following analgesics must be used with caution in painful crises?
    a. Morphine sulfate
    b. Meperidine
    c. IM/IV ketorolac
    d. Patient-controlled analgesia

11. New forms of therapy for sickle cell disease include which of the following?
    a. Hydroxyurea
    b. Bone marrow transplantation
    c. High-dose corticosteroids
    d. All of the above

12. The most common mistake physicians make when determining the etiology of abdominal pain in a person with sickling disorders is to assume that the most likely etiology of the pain is:
    a. Cholelithiasis
    b. Complications of pregnancy
    c. Sequestration
    d. Painful crisis
    e. Intestinal obstruction

13. A mother brings in her three daughters, aged 4, 7, and 10, each of whom has sickle cell anemia. All three have been complaining of fatigue, dyspnea, and arthralgias increasing over the past 2 days. Their hematocrits range from 15% to 20%; their WBC counts range from 3 to 6; their platelet counts range from 60 to 90. All of these values are decreased compared with these children's baseline CBCs. The most likely cause of the children's acute illnesses is:
    a. Adenovirus infection
    b. Carbon monoxide poisoning
    c. Family stress
    d. Parvovirus infection
    e. Hypoxemia

14. A patient with sickle cell anemia complains of unremitting pain in the right shoulder. Plain films of the right shoulder are negative. The next step in management should be:
    a. Analgesia and reassurance
    b. Analgesia and CT of the shoulder
    c. Analgesia and MRI of the shoulder
    d. Analgesia and cervical spine films
    e. Analgesia and nerve conduction studies

15. A patient with sickle cell anemia complains of decreased vision in his right eye. Visual acuity is very poor; a small collection of blood in the anterior chamber is noted. The most worrisome complication of hyphema in sickle cell anemia is:
    a. Lens dislocation
    b. Globe rupture
    c. Iridocyclitis
    d. Keratitis
    e. Glaucoma

16. Treatment of patients with thalassemia includes all of the following except:
    a. Pain management
    b. Treatment of infections
    c. Repeated transfusions
    d. Splenectomy
    e. Iron chelation

Answers

1.a. Most homozygous (HgbSS) patients develop a crisis before 1 year of age. Dactylitis, or the hand-foot syndrome (acute painful swelling of the hands and feet), is the first manifestation of sickle cell disease in many infants. Other common symptoms are irritability and refusal to walk.

2.e. Given the markedly increased risk for sepsis and meningitis in the pediatric population with HgbSS disease and fever, nothing less than a full sepsis evaluation is appropriate. This includes CBC, blood cultures, electrolytes, urinalysis, chest radiograph, and lumbar puncture for even minimal signs of meningitis. These patients should be treated with broad-spectrum antimicrobials that are effective against *S. pneumoniae* and *H. influenzae*. In some areas of the United States, there are cephalosporin-resistant strains of *S. pneumoniae*; in these regions, vancomycin has been added to the regimen of empiric therapeutics. (*Emergency Medicine, Chapter 70, pp 713–724*)

3.d. Indications for transfusion in sickle cell patients include anemia severe enough to cause high-output cardiac failure, angina, dyspnea, postural hypotension, or cerebral dysfunction (usually hemoglobin less than 5.0 g/dL) or an acute decrease in hemoglobin concentration (acute splenic or hepatic sequestration crisis). Exchange transfusion should be considered when there is a need to improve perfusion by decreasing the proportion of sickled erythrocytes, such as acute cerebrovascular accident, multiorgan failure, acute chest syndrome with persistent hypoxemia, and priapism. Chronic exchange transfusion programs are used to maintain a hemoglobin A concentration above 50% to 70% in children with a history of cerebrovascular accident and patients with chronic CHF. Relative indications for transfusion in sickle cell anemia include intractable painful crises, leg ulcers that are refractory to all other forms of treatment, complicated pregnancy, and chronic organ failure. (*Emergency Medicine, Chapter 70, pp 713–724*)

4.c. Patients with sickle cell trait (HgbSA) generally have a normal life expectancy. Given that sickling occurs under conditions involving low oxygen tension, pain crisis is uncommon in these patients except in severe hypoxia. Spontaneous hematuria, splenic infarction, and hyphema occur in these patients with greater frequency than in normal individuals. People with HgbSC also have a near-normal life expectancy with fewer vaso-occlusive manifestations. They do have a propensity for proliferative retinopathy, avascular necrosis of the femoral head, renal disease, and acute chest syndrome. Patients with sickle cell variants are at risk of developing splenic sequestration into adulthood. (*Emergency Medicine, Chapter 70, pp 713–724*)

5.b. The pathophysiology of a painful crisis in sickle cell disease is believed to be ischemic tissue injury caused by obstruction of blood flow from sickled erythrocytes. Reduced blood flow leads to hypoxia and acidosis, which further increases sickling and ischemic injury. Hydration is important first-line therapy. Although the role of oxygen in the normoxic patient is controversial, it should be administered. (*Emergency Medicine, Chapter 70, pp 713–724*)

6.e. Hypoxia, infection, fever, acidosis, dehydration, menstruation, pregnancy, sleep apnea and obstructive snoring, cold exposure, emotional distress (including depression), changes in altitude, alcohol intoxication, and physical exhaustion may all be precipitants of painful crises in people with sickle cell disease. *(Emergency Medicine, Chapter 70, pp 713–724)*

7.b. Patients with HgbSS are essentially asplenic at an early age because of multiple splenic infarcts and splenic fibrosis. They have suboptimal humoral immunity as a result of defective alternate pathway complement activation. There is also suboptimal opsonization. This predisposes these patients to infection with encapsulated organisms (such as *H. influenzae, S. pneumoniae,* and *Salmonella* species). They have a greater than 300-fold increased risk of pneumococcal septicemia or meningitis. Prophylactic penicillin should be administered two times a day to children from ages 3 to 4 months until age 5 to decrease the risk of infection with *S. pneumoniae.* The *H. influenzae* vaccine should be administered. *(Emergency Medicine, Chapter 70, pp 713–724)*

8.d. Infants and young children who are not yet asplenic (as well as adults with sickle cell variants) can develop sudden intrasplenic pooling of large volumes of blood (sequestration crisis). This can occur from 2 months up to 3 or 4 years of age and is usually associated with viral or bacterial infections. On physical examination, the spleen is dramatically enlarged, and there may be hypotension, tachycardia, tachypnea, weakness, and pallor. There can be profound anemia and thrombocytopenia. This is a dangerous event that can result in hypovolemic shock and death. The emergency physician should maintain a high degree of suspicion, because immediate resuscitation is vital. *(Emergency Medicine, Chapter 70, pp 713–724)*

9.c. Stroke and transient ischemic attacks occur in 6% to 12% of patients with HgbSS. It is rare in persons with sickle cell variants. The most common cause of stroke is cerebral infarction, resulting from vessel narrowing from intimal and medial proliferation. Sickled cells cause endothelial damage, which serves as a nidus for platelet adhesion and further sickling of cells, resulting in thrombus formation. Hemorrhagic strokes are also more common and may present as coma, headache, and seizures. Diagnostic modalities include CT, MRI, and MR angiography. *(Emergency Medicine, Chapter 70, pp 713–724)*

10.b. Large doses of meperidine are relatively contraindicated in patients with renal dysfunction or CNS disease because its metabolite normeperidine can lower seizure threshold. *(Emergency Medicine, Chapter 70, pp 713–724)*

11.d. Hydroxyurea is a cytotoxic chemotherapeutic agent that has been shown to augment fetal hemoglobin production in HgbSS patients without serious toxicity. Fetal hemoglobin interferes with the polymerization of Hb S in solution and with the sickling of Hb SS red blood cells.[1] Bone marrow transplantation may be considered for severely affected children.[2] Use of high-dose corticosteroids in acute pain crises is controversial but may decrease the duration of pain.[3] *(Emergency Medicine, Chapter 70, pp 713–724)*

12.d. Abdominal crisis may be associated with sequestration crisis, acute cholecystitis or cholelithiasis, pyelonephritis, bowel ischemia, or obstruction. Sickle cell patients have increased risk of pigmented gallstones as a result of increased breakdown of hemoglobin. One should assume that the patient with sickling disease has a potential abdominal catastrophe until proven otherwise. *(Emergency Medicine, Chapter 70, pp 713–724)*

13.d. Parvovirus B19 is a very contagious pathogen that causes transient aplastic episodes in patients with sickle cell anemia and other erythrocyte abnormalities. Patients may present with fatigue, dyspnea, extreme confusion, or CHF. Spread of the infection within families is rapid. This agent is also responsible for hydrops fetalis in infants and fifth disease (characterized by a "slapped cheek" malar rash) in children. Treatment is supportive; most episodes are self-limited, although patients with sickle cell anemia commonly require blood products before clinical improvement is seen. *(Emergency Medicine, Chapter 70, pp 713–724)*

14.c. Unremitting pain in the shoulder or hip in a patient with sickle cell anemia is worrisome for the possibility of osteonecrosis of the humeral or femoral head from vaso-occlusion. MRI is the study of choice for early diagnosis and often will detect aseptic necrosis when plain films are unrevealing. Early diagnosis may allow for conservative management or core decompression, thus sparing the patient severe disability or need for joint replacement. *(Emergency Medicine, Chapter 70, pp 713–724)*

15.e. Even a small hyphema in sickle cell anemia is an ophthalmologic emergency that requires immediate consultation. Sickled cells are more likely to cause obstruction of the canal of Schlemm, leading to glaucoma. Intraocular pressure should be determined using tonometry because pressures over 25 mm Hg can cause retinal infarction or central retinal artery occlusion. Either of these complications can result in blindness. If intraocular pressure is high, timolol can be used initially, but anterior chamber paracentesis may also be necessary. In acute glaucoma, methazolamide (Neptazane) should be used instead of acetazolamide (which causes acidification of the fluid in the anterior chamber and increases sickling of cells). *(Emergency Medicine, Chapter 70, pp 713–724)*

16.a. The thalassemias are a group of genetic disorders of abnormal globin chain formation. The excess unbound globin chains are unstable and interfere with the functioning of red cells. This leads to hemolysis, anemia, splenomegaly, and marrow hypertrophy. Thalassemia major (homozygous beta-chain anemia) often presents as severe anemia, CHF, and splenomegaly in the first few months of life, and it is fatal if not treated. Treatment consists of monthly transfusions, iron chelation therapy with deferoxamine, splenectomy if needed, and meticulous early treatment of infection. Thalassemia minor patients present with a mild hypochromic anemia. *(Emergency Medicine, Chapter 70, pp 713–724)*

REFERENCES

1. Charache S, Tarrin ML, Moore RD, et al: Effect of hydroxyurea on the frequency of painful crises in sickle cell anemia. N Engl J Med 1995; 332(10):1317–1322.
2. Apperley JF: Bone marrow transplantation for the haemoglobinopathies: Past, present, and future. Baillieres Clin Hematol 1993; 6(1):229–325.
3. Griffin TC, McIntire D, Buchanan GR: High dose methylprednisolone therapy for pain in children and adolescents with sickle cell disease. N Engl J Med 1994; 330(11):733–737.

BIBLIOGRAPHY

Pollack CV, Pollack ES: Hemoglobinopathies. *In* Howell JM, Altieri M, Jagoda AS, et al (eds): Emergency Medicine. Philadelphia, WB Saunders, 1998, pp 713–724.

33 Disorders of Hemostasis

THEA JAMES, MD   MARK SAGARIN, MD   ROBERT J. VISSERS, MD

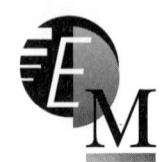

1. A patient with von Willebrand's disease who is bleeding is likely to benefit from all of the following except:
   a. Fresh frozen plasma
   b. Cryoprecipitate
   c. Factor VIII concentrate
   d. Factor IX concentrate
   e. Desmopressin

2. Initial ED therapy (first 15 minutes) for disseminated intravascular coagulation may include all of the following except:
   a. Cryoprecipitate
   b. Fresh frozen plasma
   c. Heparin
   d. Platelet transfusion
   e. Therapy directed against the underlying cause

3. Which of the following is the most efficacious therapy for thrombotic thrombocytopenic purpura?
   a. Corticosteroids
   b. Antimicrobials
   c. Platelet transfusion
   d. Plasma exchange
   e. Hemodialysis

4. Each of the following patients has a moderate to severe hemophilia A. Which of them should receive approximately 25 IU/kg of Factor VIII replacement upon presentation to the ED?
   a. A patient with hip pain, worsening over the past 36 hours
   b. A patient with a headache after being struck in the back of the head with a baseball
   c. A patient with a sense of swelling in the back of the throat with some dysphasia
   d. A patient with melena for 2 days
   e. All of the above

5. A 50-kg patient with hemophilia has nephrolithiasis associated with significant flank pain. Which of the following analgesics is appropriate initial treatment?
   a. Ketorolac, 30 mg IV
   b. Ketorolac, 30 mg IM
   c. Meperidine, 50 to 100 mg IM, with hydroxyzine 25 mg IM
   d. Morphine sulfate, 6 to 10 mg IV
   e. More than one of the above is appropriate

6. A patient with Christmas disease presents to the ED with gastrointestinal bleeding. Which of the following therapies may be helpful in achieving hemostasis?
   a. Fresh frozen plasma
   b. Cryoprecipitate
   c. Desmopressin
   d. Factor VIII replacement
   e. More than one of the above may be useful

7. An 8-year-old girl was recovering from a week-long viral illness when she gradually developed erythematous plaques on her chest and arms. Physical examination revealed multiple petechiae on her gingiva and extremities as well as a purpuric rash. There was no lymphadenopathy, organomegaly, or gastrointestinal bleeding. She has no neurologic abnormalities. Her platelet count was 7000; all other laboratory results were normal. The most likely diagnosis is:
   a. Acute lymphocytic or myelogenous leukemia
   b. Acute immune thrombocytopenic purpura
   c. Chronic immune thrombocytopenic purpura
   d. Aplastic anemia
   e. Hemolytic-uremic syndrome

8. Match the following clinical presentations to the disease.
   a. Von Willebrand's disease
   b. DIC
   c. Hemophilia A/B
   d. Thrombocytopenia

   i. Hemarthrosis, deep hematomas, delayed bleeding
   ii. Petechiae, mucosal and gastrointestinal bleeding
   iii. Prolonged bleeding after dental extractions, menorrhagia, epistaxis
   iv. Underlying disease process, purpura fulminans, diffuse oozing from venipuncture sites, acral cyanosis

9. The leading cause of death in hemophiliacs is:
   a. Retroperitoneal bleeding

b. Hemarthrosis
c. Intracranial hemorrhage
d. Gastrointestinal bleeding
e. Epistaxis

10. A patient presents to the ED with a malabsorption syndrome and a bleeding diathesis. What aspect of hemostasis is affected?
    a. Platelet number
    b. Coagulation factor inhibition
    c. Vitamin K–dependent factors
    d. Grave's factor
    e. Von Willebrand's factor

11. _____ measures the _____ and _____ coagulation pathways.
    a. PT/intrinsic/extrinsic
    b. PTT/extrinsic/common
    c. PT/intrinsic/common
    d. PTT/intrinsic/common

12. Appropriate therapy for known hemophiliacs who present to the ED with retroperitoneal, neck, or CNS bleeding is:
    a. 25 units/kg of Factor VIII
    b. 15 units/kg of Factor IX
    c. Platelets (10 units)
    d. 50 units/kg of the appropriate factor

13. All of the following are laboratory values reflective of disseminated intravascular coagulation except:
    a. Normal PT/prolonged PTT
    b. Prolonged PTT/prolonged PT
    c. Elevated fibrinogen
    d. Both a and b
    e. Both a and c

14. In thrombotic thrombocytopenic purpura and hemolytic uremic syndrome the predominant respective systemic sequelae are:
    a. Hepatic and neurologic
    b. Renal and neurologic
    c. Microangiopathic and neurologic
    d. Neurologic and renal
    e. Pulmonary and adrenal

15. All are indications for use of fresh frozen plasma except:
    a. Volume expansion
    b. Reversal of warfarin effects
    c. Use in massive blood transfusions
    d. Disseminated intravascular coagulation
    e. Treatment of thrombotic thrombocytopenic purpura

16. A 44-year-old obese female on chronic warfarin therapy for recurrent deep venous thrombosis develops acute emphysematous cholecystitis and requires immediate surgery. What preparation should be given preoperatively (most correct answer)?
    a. Platelets
    b. Vitamin K
    c. Fresh frozen plasma
    d. Cryoprecipitate

Answers

1. **d.** Von Willebrand's disease is characterized by a deficiency of von Willebrand's Factor VIII complexes and platelet dysfunction. Affected patients present with hemorrhage ranging from minor to life-threatening. Patients typically present with prolonged mucocutaneous bleeding (nosebleeds, prolonged bleeding after dental extraction, excessive menstrual bleeding). Laboratory studies reveal a prolonged PTT with a normal PT. Fresh frozen plasma, cryoprecipitate, and Factor VIII concentrate all may be beneficial because each contains Factor VIII. Desmopressin may also be helpful in mild to moderate bleeding, because it increases secretion of von Willebrand's factor by endothelial cells. Factor IX concentrate is used in Factor IX deficiency (Christmas disease). *(Emergency Medicine, Chapter 71, pp 725–739)*

2. **c.** Both cryoprecipitate and fresh frozen plasma contain clotting factors that are lost in disseminated intravascular coagulation. Severe thrombocytopenia requiring platelet transfusion may develop during disseminated intravascular coagulation, although hematologists tend to recommend platelet repletion at lower platelet counts than were recommended several years ago. Correction of the underlying cause (e.g., antimicrobials) is important, although it is unclear the extent to which such correction is likely to stop disseminated intravascular coagulation once it has begun. Optimal management of disseminated intravascular coagulation is controversial. Most agree, however, that heparin should never be employed initially before lost clotting factors have been repleted. Used too early, heparin may exacerbate hemorrhage and further deplete clotting factors. Even later in the disorder, heparin should be used cautiously after consultation with a hematologist. *(Emergency Medicine, Chapter 71, pp 725–739)*

3. **d.** Thrombotic thrombocytopenic purpura is a microangiopathic hemolytic anemia characterized by the pentad of fever, neurologic changes, hemolytic anemia, thrombocytopenia, and renal failure. The hemolytic-uremic syndrome is a closely related microangiopathy characterized by a lesser degree of neurologic change and a greater degree of renal failure. Hemolytic-uremic syndrome has been linked to infection with cytotoxin-producing *Shigella* and *Escherichia coli* in children. Plasma exchange with fresh frozen plasma has dramatically reduced mortality and is the most clearly efficacious therapy for thrombotic thrombocytopenic purpura. The benefit of corticosteroids in this disorder is unclear, although they are often used. Antimicrobials are sometimes initiated to treat infections associated with thrombotic thrombocytopenic purpura, such as *E. coli* 0157:H7 gastroenteritis, but they are unlikely to alter thrombotic thrombocytopenic purpura's natural course. Platelet transfusion often worsens the degree of thrombocytopenia and symptomatology and thus is contraindicated except in severe thrombocytopenia with hemorrhage. Hemodialysis may be considered in

cases with a severe degree of renal failure, but renal function generally improves with plasmapheresis. There are a wide range of infections, neoplasms, autoimmune diseases, drugs, and obstetric conditions that have been reported in association with thrombotic thrombocytopenic purpura and hemolytic-uremic syndrome. Unfortunately, many of these associations with thrombotic thrombocytopenic purpura and hemolytic-uremic syndrome have not been confirmed because they rely on case reports and anecdotal experience. *(Emergency Medicine, Chapter 71, pp 725–739)*

4.a. The dosage for 100% Factor VIII replacement is 50 IU/kg; 25 IU/kg provides 50% replacement (1 IU/kg = 2% replacement). Even late hemarthrosis may be treated initially with 50% replacement, but the possibility of intracranial, retropharyngeal, or gastrointestinal bleeding requires 100% factor replacement. Intracranial hemorrhage in hemophiliacs is fatal about one third of the time and is the leading cause of death among hemophiliacs. About half of those with intracranial bleeds do not recall head trauma.[1] The emergency physician, therefore, should have a low threshold for rapid, full factor replacement in the setting of head trauma or a prolonged headache of uncertain etiology. Retropharyngeal bleeding has the potential for airway compromise and should be treated aggressively with full replacement. Gastrointestinal bleeding also requires full replacement because it can become life-threatening if not controlled.

5.d. Intramuscular injections may cause painful hematomas in hemophiliacs. Nonsteroidal anti-inflammatory agents should be avoided because their antiplatelet effect may exacerbate the bleeding associated with hemophilia. An IV narcotic such as morphine is ideal for pain management. *(Emergency Medicine, Chapter 71, pp 725–739)*

6.a. Christmas disease, also known as Factor IX deficiency or hemophilia B, responds best to Factor IX concentrate. Fresh frozen plasma contains Factor IX and is useful in this disease when Factor IX concentrate is not available. Neither cryoprecipitate nor Factor VIII concentrate is a good source of Factor IX. Cryoprecipitate is richest in Factor VIII, von Willebrand's factor, and fibrinogen. Desmopressin is ineffective in raising Factor IX levels. *(Emergency Medicine, Chapter 71, pp 725–739)*

7.b. Acute immune thrombocytopenic purpura is generally seen in preschool and school-age children in the setting of a recent infectious illness. Males are affected equally as frequently as females. The chronic form of immune thrombocytopenic purpura is more common in adults, with a 3:1 female predominance. Autoantibodies bind to platelets and cause their destruction in the spleen and liver. Hemorrhagic skin and mucous membrane lesions are the most prominent physical finding. Life-threatening hemorrhage occurs rarely. The platelet count is very low and there is occasionally mild anemia. Corticosteroids and IV immunoglobulins have demonstrated efficacy in this disorder. Although acute leukemia may present with isolated thrombocytopenia, there are usually other symptoms or effects on other hematopoietic cell lines. In the above case, however, some hematologists would have performed a bone marrow biopsy to rule out malignancy and thus confirm the diagnosis of acute immune thrombocytopenic purpura. It would be difficult to make the diagnosis of aplastic anemia in the absence of anemia or at least some effect on the WBC lineage. Hemolytic-uremic syndrome is a microangiopathic hemolytic anemia characterized by fever, renal failure, thrombocytopenia, and hemolytic anemia. It is closely related to thrombotic thrombocytopenic purpura, in which there are also neurologic changes. Hemolytic-uremic syndrome is seen more commonly than thrombotic thrombocytopenic purpura in children. *(Emergency Medicine, Chapter 71, pp 725–739)*

8.a. iii; b. iv; c. i; d. ii. Von Willebrand's disease is a disorder of Factor VIII cofactor and commonly presents with epistaxis, menorrhagia, or prolonged bleeding after dental procedures (for the type 1 mild form), but it can present with hemarthrosis similar to hemophilia A (type 3). Laboratory tests reveal normal PT and thrombin time; PTT can be prolonged in severe cases. Disseminated intravascular coagulation results from activation of the clotting cascade by some event (usually sepsis, pregnancy, carcinoma, liver disease, or trauma). Activation of the clotting cascade eventually leads to depletion of clotting factors and uncontrolled bleeding. The PT, PTT, and D-dimer are elevated, and fibrinogen and platelets are decreased. Clotting (cyanosis) or bleeding (petechiae, oozing from venipuncture sites, genitourinary or gastrointestinal bleeding) may predominate. Treatment of the underlying disorder is paramount, but treatment with clotting factors or heparin may be appropriate. Patients with hemophilia A (Factor VIII deficiency) and B (Factor IX deficiency or Christmas disease) present with hemarthrosis and deep hematomas. Laboratory tests often reveal prolonged PTT. Thrombocytopenia presents with mucosal bleeding, petechiae, and epistaxis. Laboratory tests reveal normal PT, PTT, thrombin time, and increased bleeding time. *(Emergency Medicine, Chapter 71, pp 725–739)*

9.c. Intracranial hemorrhage is the leading cause of death in hemophiliacs, accounting for 33% of deaths. Up to 13% of head trauma in hemophiliacs is complicated by intracerebral bleeding. Only 50% of these patients have a history of head trauma, and neurologic signs may not present for 1 day to 1 week after trauma. Therefore, hemophiliacs with or without a history of trauma who have neurologic complaints should receive a head CT scan. The same approach should be followed in patients with acquired disorders that require Coumadin therapy. *(Emergency Medicine, Chapter 71, pp 725–739)*

10.c. Coagulation Factors II, VII, IX, and X require vitamin K and a functioning liver for proper formation. Vitamin K is absorbed in the intestine, and diseases that cause malabsorption (such as celiac sprue and ulcerative colitis) could lead to a vitamin K deficiency and nonfunctioning coagulation factors. *(Emergency Medicine, Chapter 71, pp 725–739)*

11.d. The PT and PTT measure the extrinsic and intrinsic coagulation pathways, respectively. The PTT is sensitive to Factors VIII and IX. Heparin inhibits Factor IX; hence, the PTT is a useful monitor for heparin therapy. The PT is sensitive to Factors II, VII, and X, which are vitamin K dependent and inhibited by Coumadin-like drugs. The PT is therefore used to monitor Coumadin therapy. *(Emergency Medicine, Chapter 71, pp 725–739)*

12.d. The location of bleeding in patients with congenital single-factor bleeding disorders determines the therapeutic approach. Bleeding into the neck, CNS, and retroperitoneum is life-threatening and should be addressed immediately. Appropriate therapy for bleeding in these locations is 50 IU/kg of the appropriate factor. Appropriate therapy for bleeding into joint spaces, the oral cavity, gastrointestinal tract, soft tissues, or muscles is 25 IU/kg of Factor VIII or Factor IX. *(Emergency Medicine, Chapter 71, pp 725–739)*

13.e. Patients with disseminated intravascular coagulation have prolonged PT and PTT caused by involvement of multiple coagulation factors; disseminated intravascular coagulation involves multiple coagulation factors as well as platelets and can affect multiple systems. There is constant stimulation of the clotting cascade leading to depletion of clotting factors; markedly increased activity of the fibrinolytic system and fibrinogen consumption leads to low fibrinogen levels. *(Emergency Medicine, Chapter 71, pp 725–739)*

14.d. In thrombotic thrombocytopenic purpura, neurologic abnormalities predominate and renal dysfunction is seen less often. The opposite is characteristic of hemolytic-uremic syndrome. Of patients with thrombotic thrombocytopenic purpura, 63% to 100% have neurologic dysfunction and 18% to 89% have renal dysfunction. Other systems affected are adrenals, brain, kidneys, liver, lungs, and muscle. Thrombi are composed predominantly of platelets rather than thrombin, correlating with the fact that coagulation factors are generally not depleted in thrombotic thrombocytopenic purpura as they are in disseminated intravascular coagulation. *(Emergency Medicine, Chapter 71, pp 725–739)*

15.a. Fresh frozen plasma is the fluid portion of 1 unit of human blood that has been centrifuged, separated, and frozen to $-18°C$ within 6 hours of collection. It contains all of the clotting factors. A typical unit volume is 250 to 300 mL. The indications for fresh frozen plasma are replacement of isolated factor deficiencies, reversal of warfarin effects, use in blood transfusions that are greater than one blood volume (with evidence of coagulopathy), and treatment of thrombotic thrombocytopenic purpura and disseminated intravascular coagulation. It should not be used as a volume expander. Complications of fresh frozen plasma use include infectious disease transmission (HIV, hepatitis, but not cytomegalovirus and Epstein-Barr virus, which are transmitted in the cellular portion of blood products), hemolytic transfusion reaction, alloimmunization, and rarely anaphylaxis. *(Emergency Medicine, Chapter 71, pp 725–739)*

16.c. Warfarin interferes with the synthesis of vitamin K–dependent factors (II, VII, IX, and X). Emergency surgery necessitates emergent reversal of warfarin. Of all the choices, only fresh frozen plasma contains these factors. Vitamin K would take hours to days (assuming an intact liver) to correct the coagulation defects. Cryoprecipitate and platelets do not contain the necessary factors. *(Emergency Medicine, Chapter 71, pp 725–739)*

REFERENCE

1. Coyne MA: Avoiding indecision and hesitation with hemophilia related emergencies. Emergency Medicine Reports 1992; 13(22):165–176.

BIBLIOGRAPHY

Gilbert JA, Gossett CW: Disorders of hemostasis. *In* Howell JM, Altieri M, Jagoda AS, et al (eds): Emergency Medicine. Philadelphia, WB Saunders, 1998, pp 725–739.

SECTION TEN

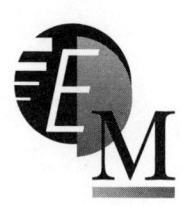

Neurologic Disorders

34 Approach to Altered Mental Status and Coma, Dizziness, and Vertigo

JOSEPH TURBAN, MD

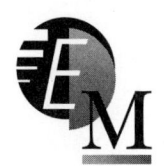

1. The initial management of a patient who presents with an altered mental status/coma (unresponsive) includes all of the following except:
   a. Obtain rapidly a D-stick or give one ampule of D_{50} IV
   b. Naloxone
   c. Thiamine, 100 mg IV
   d. Obtain history/information from EMS crew
   e. Intubation

2. Regarding assessment and management of patients with altered mental status, all of the following are correct except:
   a. The Glasgow Coma Scale score should be documented early.
   b. The ECG may be diagnostic.
   c. All patients should be placed on a cardiac monitor.
   d. Pulse oximetry accurately depicts hemoglobin saturation.
   e. Early IV access is a priority.

3. Which of the following is false?
   a. Dysarthria is slurred or difficult-to-understand speech; dysphasia is clearly spoken but meaningless language.
   b. Lesions in the lateral medulla and ventrolateral cervical spinal canal may cause an ipsilateral Horner's syndrome, but the light reflex will be preserved.
   c. Unequal pupil size is always an abnormal finding.
   d. Miosis can be from opiate poisoning or pontine lesions.
   e. Oculomotor movement that is asymmetric suggests an anatomic lesion.

4. Which of the following is false?
   a. A supranuclear pathway lesion will cause the eyes to deviate to the side of the lesion.
   b. A lesion in the brain stem will cause the eyes to deviate to the contralateral side.
   c. Skew deviation—one eye looking up and the other down—is diagnostic of a brain stem lesion.
   d. Ocular reflexes are absent in most metabolic causes of coma.
   e. A present oculovestibular (caloric) reflex indicates intact function from brain stem to eyes.

5. A 48-year-old male presents in apparent total paralysis. Vital signs are normal. The patient has no response to painful stimuli or commands. There is no extraocular movement except for vertical eye movement. Which of the following is true?
   a. The patient is probably malingering.
   b. A metabolic insult is the most likely etiologic cause.
   c. Recovery is likely.
   d. Lid elevation may be preserved in some cases in this condition.
   e. None of the above are true.

6. If a patient suffers a right-sided hemispheric lesion, you would expect all of the following except:
   a. Upgoing plantar reflex (positive Babinski's) on the left
   b. Hyperreflexia on the left
   c. Expressive aphasia
   d. Intact brain stem reflexes
   e. Normal mental status

7. A trauma patient presents to the ED in a coma. The left pupil is nonreactive and larger than the right, which reacts to light. There is an upgoing plantar reflex (positive Babinski's) on the right. Which of the following statements is false?
   a. Most likely a head CT scan would show an expansive process in the left cerebral hemisphere causing left-sided uncal herniation.
   b. You would expect the right eye to retain lateral (abduction) movement on right ear caloric testing.
   c. The left eye retains full medial movement with right ear caloric testing.
   d. The patient is at risk for brain stem herniation.
   e. In the late stages of progression without corrective measures, the clinical picture is similar to central transtentorial herniation.

8. When considering pediatric causes of altered mental status/coma, which of the following is false?
   a. The possibility of abuse must be considered.
   b. Special emphasis should be placed on metabolic and electrolyte imbalances and abnormalities.

c. Intussusception may occur without any gastrointestinal complaints.
d. A careful examination will always reveal signs of trauma or abuse.
e. Early consideration should be given to head CT and lumbar puncture.

9. A 10-year-old female presents with altered mental status. The mother states the child has been vomiting profusely since this morning. She had the flu 1 week ago. The patient is afebrile, mildly tachycardic, and tachypneic but hemodynamically stable. She does not respond to verbal stimuli and groans to pain. All of the following are true except:
    a. Rapid and copious fluid resuscitation is appropriate.
    b. Baseline laboratory testing of CBC, urinalysis, electrolytes, toxicology screen, and acetaminophen and aspirin levels should be performed.
    c. Ammonia level and liver function tests may be diagnostic.
    d. ABG and fingerstick should be performed rapidly.
    e. Hepatomegaly would be a consistent physical finding.

10. To differentiate cortical from reticular activating formation causes of decreased consciousness, which of the following is true?
    a. A hemispheric cortical lesion, if large enough, can cause decreased consciousness.
    b. Cortical lesions causing decreased consciousness are usually anatomic.
    c. Reticular activating formation lesions are usually metabolic.
    d. A supratentorial lesion causing decreased consciousness most likely involves the other hemisphere rather than the reticular activating formation.
    e. None of the above are true.

11. Regarding asymmetry of pupils, which of the following is false?
    a. It can be considered a normal finding in up to 10% of the population.
    b. It can be caused by previous surgery.
    c. It can be caused by previous unilateral application of cycloplegic drugs.
    d. It can be caused by isolated unilateral eye trauma.
    e. Intracranial causes will always result in altered mental status.

12. Which of the following is false?
    a. Dysequilibrium is the sensation of loss of balance without a rotational sensation.
    b. Sensation of an impending faint or loss of consciousness is termed *near-syncope*.
    c. A rotational sensation is termed *vertigo*.
    d. Near-syncope and syncope have different etiologic causes.
    e. *Lightheadedness* is used to describe ill-defined sensations that are not rotational, syncopal, or representing dysequilibrium.

13. Regarding vertigo, which of the following is true?
    a. Distinguishing central from peripheral vertigo is difficult in the ED.
    b. Symptoms of vertigo that recur every few hours are an ominous sign.
    c. Peripheral causes are associated with other neurologic findings.
    d. Both central and peripheral vertigo are worsened by head movement.
    e. None of the above are true.

14. Which of the following is the most ideal method for diagnosing orthostasis?
    a. A drop in systolic BP of more that 15 mm Hg.
    b. A drop in diastolic BP of more than 10 mm Hg.
    c. A rise of heart rate greater than 20.
    d. Symptoms during the test.
    e. A positive tilt-table test.

15. A 75-year-old female complains of having felt dizzy since early this morning. She denies vertigo or any other complaints and has no previous significant past medical history. Her vital signs are within normal limits. Her physical examination is unremarkable, with negative Nylen-Bárány testing. Which of the following statments is false?
    a. Complaints of dizziness are more frequent in women than in men.
    b. Complaints of dizziness increase with age.
    c. An evaluation of this patient would include blood chemistries, blood count, ECG, pulse oximetry, testing for orthostatic hypotension, and a trial of fluids.
    d. This patient is likely to respond to meclizine.
    e. This patient may be safely discharged even if symptoms persist.

16. A previously well 49-year-old female presents complaining of vertigo and ringing in her left ear. On examination, she has lateral unidirectional nystagmus, with the fast phase toward the right. She has decreased hearing in her left ear. She most probably has:
    a. Vestibular neuronitis
    b. Acute labyrinthitis
    c. Benign paroxysmal positional vertigo
    d. Schwannoma or other process involving the eighth cranial nerve
    e. Meniere's disease

17. A 36-year-old male presents with complaints of dizziness since awakening. Upon further questioning, it is revealed that he feels that "the room is spinning." He denies any tinnitus. Vital signs are normal. Hearing tests are within normal limits. Upon extraocular muscle testing, he is noted to have nystagmus toward the right horizontally, which resolves when he fixates. The rest of the cranial nerve examination is unremarkable, and he has no other neurologic findings. He most likely has:
    a. Vestibular neuronitis in the left ear
    b. Vestibular neuronitis in the right ear
    c. Acute labyrinthitis in the right ear
    d. Meniere's disease
    e. Central vertigo

18. Regarding central vertigo:
    a. Onset of vertigo is usually sudden.
    b. It is worsened by positioning and maneuvers.
    c. Hearing loss and tinnitus are frequently features.
    d. Marked nystagmus with minimal vertigo is suggestive of central etiology.
    e. It may be present without other brain stem findings.

Answers

1.e. Two of the most common and readily reversible causes of altered mental status in the ED are hypoglycemia and opiate overdose. These are easily reversible with IV dextrose and naloxone. "The routine use of thiamine is probably still warranted. . ."[1] in patients with altered mental status to treat possible Wernicke's encephalopathy and to assist with glucose metabolism in possibly nutritionally depleted patients. Often, the only sources of historical information are the EMS personnel, who may have valuable information from family and bystanders. The EMS team should be questioned before departing the ED. Intubation is indicated only if there is evidence of airway or ventilatory compromise, or trauma with rapid deterioration. *(Emergency Medicine, Chapter 73, pp 759–770)*

2.d. Regardless of etiology, certain interventions and assessments are mandatory. Intravenous access to treat potential arrhythmias or for naloxone administration is a priority. Electrocardiography may reveal conduction abnormalities such as tricyclic antidepressant overdose as well as ischemia, or it may provide clues to other causes of altered mental status, e.g., bradycardia from beta-blockade or calcium channel blocker overdose or supraventricular tachycardia from cocaine or amphetamine abuse. Early Glasgow Coma Scale score assessment can be used to gauge the patient's response to interventions or the degree of deterioration. Pulse oximetry may be falsely reassuring in carbon monoxide poisoning and methemoglobinemia, necessitating ABG analysis for Pao_2 assessment. *(Emergency Medicine, Chapter 73, pp 759–770)*

3.c. Approximately 10% of the population has anisocoria, pupil asymmetry of 1 to 2 mm. However, the larger pupil will be reactive to light. If there is enough uncal herniation to cause ipsilateral mydriasis, the patient will have significant altered mental status/coma. Unilateral prior application of mydriatics may confound the clinical picture; however, mydriasis with altered mental status must always be pursued with cranial imaging. *(Emergency Medicine, Chapter 73, pp 759–770)*

4.d. Patients with depressed mental status or altered mental status from metabolic causes will usually retain eye reflexes. The rest of the statements are true. *(Emergency Medicine, Chapter 73, pp 759–770)*

5.d. The patient suffers from "locked-in syndrome," also known as the "Count of Monte Cristo" syndrome. It is caused by hemorrhage or infarction of the ventral pons from vertebrobasilar artery thrombosis. This destroys the ventral pontine motor tracts. Lid elevation may be partially preserved because the midbrain area controlling this function may lie outside the area affected by vertebrobasilar artery thrombosis. Acute polyneuritis or severe myasthenia gravis attacks may mimic this condition with the patient seemingly unresponsive, but awake; however, these conditions do not selectively preserve vertical eye movement.[2] *(Emergency Medicine, Chapter 73, pp 759–770)*

6.c. Right hemispheric lesions will cause sensory and motor changes on the left side of the body as a result of decussation in the medulla. A left upgoing plantar reflex and hyperreflexia are signs of an upper neuron lesion and are consistent with a right hemispheric lesion. Unless the lesion is huge and causes brain stem herniation, brain stem function remains intact. It would require either bilateral hemispheric involvement or a reticular activating formation lesion to cause altered mental status. In most patients, speech control centers are in the left hemisphere and should not be affected by a right hemispheric lesion.[3] *(Emergency Medicine, Chapter 73, pp 759–770)*

7.c. The patient is in the late stages of uncal herniation, causing third cranial nerve compression from an expanding epidural or subdural hematoma in the left hemisphere. As such, the right pupil, contralateral to the lesion, retains reactivity and normal response to caloric testing. The left eye, however, shows signs of third nerve compression. It is unresponsive to light and would not move medially with caloric testing because of involvement of the left medial longitudinal fasciculus. If uncorrected, the left-sided process may continue to expand, leading to a clinical syndrome indistinguishable from central transtentorial herniation along with respiratory depression and brain death. *(Emergency Medicine, Chapter 73, pp 759–770)*

8.d. In pediatric altered mental status/coma, the possibility of abuse must always be ruled out. The lack of any physical findings on physical examination consistent with abuse does not rule abuse out, because there may be chronic subdural or subarachnoid hemorrhage or cerebral edema. A careful fundoscopic examination must always be performed to evaluate for retinal hemorrhage, a sign of shaken-baby syndrome. Infants and children also have a higher incidence of inborn errors of metabolism, initial presentation of diabetes mellitus, dehydration, and endocrine abnormalities including adrenal hyperplasia. Intussusception *can* occur without any gastrointestinal signs or symptoms. Head CT and lumbar puncture are indicated if there is no obvious explanation for altered mental status. *(Emergency Medicine, Chapter 73, pp 759–770)*

9.a. The child presents with a classic picture of Reye's syndrome, a very rare but potentially life-threatening emergency of unclear etiology characterized by hepatic dysfunction and encephalopathy. Typically, the patient has a flu-like illness, commonly influenza B or varicella, associated with aspirin use, then develops copious vomiting and altered mental status. Elevated liver function tests and ammonia levels three times normal are typical. Metabolic acidosis and respiratory alkalosis are common, as is hypoglycemia. Acetaminophen and salicylate toxicity should be excluded. Because the prognosis for Reye's syndrome patients correlates with the amount of cerebral edema, cautious fluid resuscitation is the rule. Judicious administration of IV fluids may be necessary in the hemodynamically unstable patient. Hyperventilation and mannitol are the most effective ED measures for severe Reye's syndrome patients.[2] *(Emergency Medicine, Chapter 73, pp 759–770)*

10.e. Decreased consciousness and coma are caused by involvement of either both cortices or the reticular activating formation. An isolated hemispheric lesion, regardless of size, alone cannot cause altered consciousness. Insults affecting both hemispheres are most likely metabolic, e.g., decreased glucose or hypoxia, or toxins (metabolic or toxic encephalopathy), whereas insults to the reticular activating formation are more likely structural (pontine hemorrhage or compression from uncal herniation). Typically, an expanding lesion in one hemisphere will progress to uncal herniation and then transtentorial herniation with brain stem compression.[3] *(Emergency Medicine, Chapter 73, pp 759–770)*

11.e. Although the finding of a unilateral nonreactive pupil and altered mental status is ominous, there are many other causes besides uncal herniation from a mass lesion. These include idiopathic anisocoria, previous ocular surgery, application of cycloplegic drugs, and isolated eye trauma (traumatic mydriasis). Intracranial causes other than mass lesions causing uncal herniation include an expanding aneurysm of the posterior cerebral artery compressing on the third cranial nerve, which will not present with altered mental status. *(Emergency Medicine, Chapter 73, pp 759–770)*

12.d. Syncope and near-syncope are conditions along a continuum, differing only in magnitude. Circulatory failure manifested as postural hypotension, orthostasis, hypovolemia, or reduced cardiac output is a frequent cause. Other causes include hypoxia, anemia, hypoglycemia, and cerebral arterial insufficiencies. Vertigo has either central or peripheral etiologies, which must be distinguished from one another. Lightheadedness has a myriad of causes, ranging from medication misadventures to psychiatric etiologies. *(Emergency Medicine, Chapter 78, pp 809–816)*

13.e. A detailed history and physical examination can usually discriminate central (serious) from peripheral causes. Vertigo that abates and recurs every few hours suggests a peripheral etiology. Central vertigo is characterized by gradual onset and constancy and is not positional, although central vertigo from a transient ischemic attack or cerebellar hemorrhage may be of sudden onset. The finding of a cranial nerve abnormality other than eighth cranial nerve, cerebellar findings, or blurred vision suggests a central etiology. Peripheral vertigo is characterized by nystagmus that is suppressible with fixed gaze, is horizontal or rotatory, is elicited with Nylen-Bárány maneuvers, and fatigues with repetition. Central vertigo is characterized by vertical nystagmus, is not suppressible or positional, and is not fatigable. *(Emergency Medicine, Chapter 78, pp 809–816)*

14.d. Alterations in vital signs during testing for "orthostatic hypotension" are neither sensitive nor specific for hypovolemia. They may miss more than 75% and falsely include 50% of patients who are not volume depleted. The most reliable indicator is the patient's experiencing symptoms while standing. Tilt-table testing is impractical for ED use. *(Emergency Medicine, Chapter 78, pp 809–816)*

15.e. Dizziness is a chief complaint in 1% of office visits for patients younger than 15 years and 3.7% for patients 85 years or older. Two thirds of these patients are female. Although of low yield, laboratory testing of CBC, chemistries, and electrolytes is indicated because the patient with no apparent etiology and persistent symptoms after adequate hydration would require admission and evaluation for possible transient ischemic attack or cardiac causes. Meclizine has been shown to be effective in a majority of both peripheral vertigo and nonspecific cases of dizziness. A response to meclizine is nondiagnostic. *(Emergency Medicine, Chapter 78, pp 809–816)*

16.e. Vertigo can be divided into physiologic and pathologic types. Physiologic vertigo occurs when there is a sensory mismatch from the three stabilizing sensory systems (the ocular, proprioceptive, and vestibular) or when the vestibular apparatus is subjected to unfamiliar stimuli, such as in seasickness. Pathologic vertigo is divided into visual, somatosensory, and vestibular causes. Vestibular dysfunction is the most common of the three. Benign paroxysmal positional vertigo is characterized by vertigo precipitated by recumbent head position, and it may be reproduced with Nylen-Bárány testing. Schwannoma or other slow processes of the eighth cranial nerve may present with tinnitus and hearing deficits, but usually the cerebral cortex is able to compensate for the labyrinthine dysfunction, and vertiginous symptoms are uncommon and less pronounced. Meniere's disease is characterized by tinnitus, hearing loss, and vertigo. It is caused by dysfunctional absorption of endolymph. If cochlear symptoms (hearing loss and tinnitus) are absent, vestibular neuronitis is suggested. Vertigo and hearing loss without tinnitus is characteristic of acute labyrinthitis, usually following a viral or rarely a bacterial infection.[2] *(Emergency Medicine, Chapter 78, pp 809–816)*

17.a. This patient suffers from vertigo with a lack of any neurologic findings save a horizontal nystagmus to the right. The absence of other neurologic findings along with the horizontal component points toward a peripheral etiology. Other associated features of peripheral vertigo include fatigability, inhibition by fixation, possible vomiting, diaphoresis, diarrhea, tinnitus, hearing loss, and aggravation by position or movement. Central vertigo is characterized by vertical nystagmus that is not positional or fatigable and other CNS findings such as ataxia, diplopia, dysphasia, and cranial nerve palsies. In normally functioning vestibule, movement elicits excitation of a semicircular canal that causes the eyes to look away from that canal (the vestibulo-ocular reflex, slow phase). The cortex then exerts a quick corrective movement in the opposite direction (fast phase), which causes the nystagmus. In peripheral vertigo, there is inhibition of the diseased canal. The unaffected canal causes first the slow phase away from, then the quick phase toward the "good" side; thus, in peripheral vertigo, the nystagmus moves away from the affected ear. Vestibular neuronitis is characterized by vertigo without hearing loss or tinnitus. Acute labyrinthitis causes vertigo with hearing loss. Meniere's disease is characterized by vertigo with hearing loss and tinnitus. The differential diagnosis in such a scenario includes tertiary syphilis and cerebello-pontine angle tumors. *(Emergency Medicine, Chapter 78, pp 809–816)*

18.d. Although transient ischemic attacks and stroke may bring on sudden onset of central vertigo, the onset is usually gradual. Central vertigo is caused by conditions affecting the brain stem and cerebellum and is therefore unaffected by Nylen-Bárány maneuvers and positioning that diagnose dysfunctioning vestibular apparatuses. As such, hearing loss and tinnitus are uncommon. The patient may downplay the vertigo complaints, which may be much less dramatic than peripheral vertigo. Vertical nystagmus as well as nystagmus with little or no vertigo suggests a brain stem lesion. Central vertigo is always associated with other neurologic findings, which may be subtle, including ataxia, discoordination, dysphagia, diplopia, Horner's syndrome, and other cranial nerve palsies.[2] *(Emergency Medicine, Chapter 78, pp 809–816)*

REFERENCES

1. Hoffman R, et al: The poisoned patient with altered mental status. JAMA 1995; 274:562–569.
2. Ropper AH, Martin JB: Coma and other disorders of consciousness. *In* Isselbacher KT, Braunwald E, Wilson JD, et al (eds): Harrison's Principles of Internal Medicine, 12th ed. New York, McGraw Hill, 1994, pp 146–153.
3. Sudarsky L: Pathophysiology of the Nervous System. Boston, Little Brown Publishers, 1990, pp 139–161, 183–220, 223–249.

BIBLIOGRAPHY

Herr RD: Dizziness and vertigo. *In* Howell JM, Altieri M, Jagoda AS, et al (eds): Emergency Medicine. Philadelphia, WB Saunders, 1998, pp 809–816.

Mickel HS: Approach to altered mental status and coma. *In* Howell JM, Altieri M, Jagoda AS, et al (eds): Emergency Medicine. Philadelphia, WB Saunders, 1998, pp 759–770.

35 Cerebrovascular Emergencies and Cranial Nerve Disorders

KEVIN BAUMLIN, MD   PHILLIP FAIRWEATHER, MD

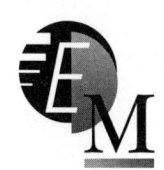

1. Prehospital treatment of patients with altered mental status and possible stroke includes all of the following except:
   a. Airway control
   b. Dextrose administration to the suspected hypoglycemic patient
   c. Naloxone administration
   d. Early recognition and treatment of hypertension
   e. Thiamine administration

2. A 59-year-old male presents with left-sided weakness of the leg greater than the arm; he is confused and the nurse reports that upon undressing the patient it was noted that he was incontinent of urine. This is a classic presentation of a:
   a. Left anterior cerebral artery infarct
   b. Right cerebellar artery infarct
   c. Right anterior cerebral infarct
   d. Right middle cerebral infarct
   e. Left middle cerebral infarct

3. All of the following statements are true concerning subarachnoid hemorrhage except:
   a. ECG changes, including ST and T wave abnormalities, are well known and should be differentiated from primary cardiac disease.
   b. Noncontrast CT is the best initial study.
   c. Patients who present with a "warning leak" or sentinel bleed usually have focal neurologic findings.
   d. The majority of acute subarachnoid hemorrhages occur with nonexertional activity.
   e. Lumbar puncture is a requirement to exclude subarachnoid hemorrhage.

4. All of the following statements are true concerning physical examination except:
   a. Miosis suggests drug overdose or pontine infarct.
   b. Mydriasis may suggests an anticholinergic effect.
   c. Third nerve palsy suggests impending transtentorial herniation.
   d. The sixth cranial nerve is the longest cranial nerve and is frequently the last nerve affected by gradually increasing intracranial pressure.
   e. Brain stem infarcts may result in gaze preference away from the side of the insult.

5. All of the following are correctly matched except:
   a. Unilateral visual loss—ophthalmic artery infarct
   b. Cortical blindness, confusion and impaired memory—posterior cerebral artery infarct
   c. 39-year-old with chronic renal insufficiency with seizure and headache—subarachnoid hemorrhage
   d. Vertigo and subtle cranial nerve deficits—vertebrobasilar insufficiency
   e. Aphasia and right hemineglect—right middle cerebral artery infarct

6. Concerning treatment of patients with stroke:
   a. Thrombolytic therapy should begin within 6 hours of symptoms.
   b. Current American Hospital Association recommendations include routine heparinization.
   c. Posterior fossa infarctions necessitate prompt neurosurgical consultation.
   d. Vitamin K therapy alone is sufficient for the correction of coagulopathies associated with Coumadin therapy.
   e. Patients should be treated prophylactically for seizures.

7. A patient presents to the ED complaining of double vision. Which of the following is inconsistent with the diagnosis of a right third nerve palsy?
   a. Inability to fully adduct the right eye
   b. Dilated right pupil
   c. Inability to fully abduct the right eye
   d. Right ptosis
   e. Intact ability to close the right eyelids against resistance

8. Which of the following statements regarding ptosis is false?
   a. Orbicularis occuli muscle weakness never results in ptosis.
   b. Ptosis with contralateral miosis and anhidrosis is characteristic of Horner's syndrome.
   c. Ptosis with ipsilateral myosis and diplopia is characteristic of third nerve palsy.
   d. Myasthenia gravis and botulism cause ptosis from direct impairment of the eyelid muscles.

e. The presence of diplopia is a distinguishing feature of Horner's syndrome and third nerve palsy.

9. Which cranial nerves have purely motor function?
   a. I, III, V
   b. VII, VIII, IX
   c. V, VII, VIII
   d. IV, VI, VII
   e. None of the above

10. A 33-year-old man presents with an acute third cranial nerve palsy. Which diagnostic test should be performed?
    a. Head CT with contrast
    b. Magnetic resonance angiography
    c. MRI
    d. Cerebral angiography
    e. Lumbar puncture

11. Which of the following statements regarding cranial nerve abnormalities is false?
    a. Corticosteroids have been proven effective in shortening the duration of facial nerve weakness in Bell's palsy.
    b. The pupillary dilation seen in third nerve palsy is reversible with instillation of 1% pilocarpine in the affected eye.
    c. Isolated fourth and sixth nerve palsy is uncommon but can be associated with diabetes mellitus and hypertension.
    d. The treatment of choice for trigeminal neuralgia is a graduating dose of carbamazepine.
    e. The 9th, 10th, 11th, and 12th cranial nerves are anatomically very closely related, so isolated lesions of only one nerve are uncommon.

Answers

1.d. Prehospital treatment of stroke includes airway control, oxygen, and naloxone to patients with suspected opiate overdose. Dextrose administration is recommended only if the patient has a low serum glucose or it is suspected. It is strongly suggested that hypertension *not* be treated in most circumstances, unless severe hypertension exists (systolic BP >220 mm Hg; diastolic BP >140 mm Hg) or evidence of other end-organ injury is present. If antihypertensive agents are used, target BP in the range of 150 to 180 mm Hg systolic/ 90 to 110 mm Hg diastolic. Another rule of thumb is to lower the systolic BP by no more than 20%. Hypertension is largely transient, and treatment may decrease cerebral perfusion, thus worsening the ischemic insult. (*Emergency Medicine, Chapter 77, pp 799–808*)

2.c. Contralateral weakness of the leg greater than the arm associated with confusion and incontinence is a classic presentation of anterior cerebral infarct. A right middle cerebral artery infarct would classically present with left arm greater than leg weakness. Middle cerebral infarcts of the dominant hemisphere (usually left) may present with aphasia, speech impairment, or difficulty understanding language. Cerebellar infarcts usually present with vertebrobasilar symptoms, including vertigo, ataxia, cranial nerve abnormalities, or dysarthria and may include features such as confusion, impaired memory, and cortical blindness. (*Emergency Medicine, Chapter 77, Table 77–3*)

3.c. Subarachnoid hemorrhage is devastating and associated with high mortality and morbidity. Patients present with headache, nausea, vomiting, photophobia, or neck stiffness and may have ECG changes. The majority of subarachnoid hemorrhages present with nonexertional activity, including during sleep (14%). Exertional activities are the setting for subarachnoid hemorrhage in less than 25% of patients. On examination, patients with sentinel bleeds usually are nonfocal neurologically. Noncontrast CT is the initial test of choice, but it is only 95% sensitive and should be followed by lumbar puncture when the diagnosis of subarachnoid hemorrhage is being considered. Once a lumbar puncture has been performed, xanthochromia may be present. This represents lysed erythrocytes in the space and usually occurs 6 to 8 hours after the acute subarachnoid hemorrhage. (*Emergency Medicine, Chapter 77, pp 799–808*)

4.d. The sixth cranial nerve is the longest cranial nerve, but it is the first nerve affected by increased intracranial pressure. Miosis suggests drug overdose or pontine infarct. Mydriasis may suggest an anticholinergic drug effect, but it more commonly is a result of third cranial nerve impairment. Third nerve palsy (nonreactive pupil, inability to direct gaze upward or medially past midline) suggests a brain stem infarct, an expanding aneurysm in the circle of Willis, or impending transtentorial herniation. Brain stem infarct usually results in gaze preference away from the side of the insult. Cerebral infarcts direct gaze toward the side of the infarct. (*Emergency Medicine, Chapter 77, pp 799–808*)

5.e. Middle cerebral artery infarcts are associated with contralateral weakness, paresthesia, and neglect. Amaurosis fugax, sudden onset of unilateral visual loss, may be secondary to acute ophthalmic artery infarct. This can be considered a warning sign, and this patient would need admission and inpatient evaluation for carotid artery disease. Posterior circulation events pose a real challenge to clinicians; they are often difficult to diagnosis and may present a more immediate threat to the patient. Vertebrobasilar events may present with vertigo, lightheadedness, syncope, ataxia, confusion or somnolence, and incontinence. Patients may give a history of difficulty standing or incoordination. Cerebellar infarcts may worsen in the early hours after onset, and patients or family may relate a history of rapid deterioration. The most important task is to maintain a high index of suspicion. It is important that the diagnosis of subarachnoid hemorrhage be considered in any patient who presents with a new headache and seizure. (*Emergency Medicine, Chapter 77, pp 799–808*)

6.c. Restoration of blood flow, via the use of thrombolytic agents within the first 3 hours of onset of symptoms, is the current recommendation for the definitive treatment of the acute ischemic stroke patient. Although commonly still used, heparin is not recommended for treatment of acute stroke. Posterior fossa events may rapidly progress and cause fourth ventricular and midbrain compression from edema; therefore, they need to be rapidly identified for acute neurosurgical intervention when indicated. In patients with hemorrhagic stroke who are receiving Coumadin, fresh frozen plasma is indicated. Seizures may occur hours to years after a stroke. Stroke is the most common cause of new seizures in patients older than 60 years. Prophylactic treatment is not recommended. *(Emergency Medicine, Chapter 77, pp 799–808)*

7.c. Abduction of the eyes is a function of the sixth cranial nerve (abducens). A third cranial nerve palsy may result in ptosis, pupillary dilation, and an inability to adduct that eye. The orbicularis oculi is innervated by the seventh cranial nerve, so eye closure remains intact. *(Emergency Medicine, Chapter 79, pp 817–826)*

8.b. Horner's syndrome is characterized by ptosis with ipsilateral miosis and anhidrosis. Ptosis arises from weakness of either the levator palpebrae (cranial nerve III) or tarsalis (fibers from the sympathetic trunk) muscles. The orbicularis oculi muscle is innervated by the facial nerve (cranial nerve VII). Weakness of the facial nerve causes difficulty closing the eye, not ptosis. All of the other statements are correct. *(Emergency Medicine, Chapter 79, pp 817–826)*

9.e. Cranial nerves IV (trochlear), VI (abducens), XI (accessory), and XII (hypoglossal) are pure motor nerves. The pure sensory cranial nerves are I (olfactory), II (optic), and VIII (acoustovestibular). The remaining cranial nerves (III, V, VII, IX, and X) have mixed functional neuronal components. *(Emergency Medicine, Chapter 79, pp 817–826)*

10.d. In patients who present with an acute third cranial nerve palsy, an evaluation to determine if cerebral aneurysm is the cause must be done. Cerebral angiography is the gold standard for evaluation of patients with suspected cerebral aneurysm. This diagnosis cannot be excluded with any of the other tests listed. A lumbar puncture is indicated if a subarachnoid bleed is suspected and CT of the head is negative or if meningitis is suspected. *(Emergency Medicine, Chapter 79, pp 817–826)*

11.a. Corticosteroids have not been proven to have benefit in the treatment of idiopathic seventh nerve palsy (Bell's palsy). Some patients are thought to have shorter periods of facial pain if therapy is begun within 48 hours of symptom onset. The current accepted steroid regimen is prednisone, 1 mg/kg per day for 5 days, then a taper over the next 5 days. *(Emergency Medicine, Chapter 79, pp 817–826)*

BIBLIOGRAPHY

Pellegrino T: Cranial nerve disorders. *In* Howell JM, Altieri M, Jagoda AS, et al (eds): Emergency Medicine. Philadelphia, WB Saunders, 1998, pp 817–826.

Younger JG, Barsam WG: Cerebrovascular emergencies *In* Howell JM, Altieri M, Jagoda AS, et al (eds): Emergency Medicine. Philadelphia, WB Saunders, 1998, pp 799–808.

36 Neuromuscular Disorders

MARY RYAN, MD

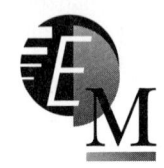

1. Match the following pattern of weakness with disease entity:
   a. Ascending paralysis
   b. Descending paralysis
   c. Proximal weakness
   d. Distal weakness
   i. Lambert-Eaton syndrome
   ii. Motor neuron disease
   iii. Guillain-Barré syndrome
   iv. Botulism

2. Answer true or false to the following regarding poliomyelitis:
   a. A symmetric pattern of weakness is typical.
   b. Sensation remains intact.
   c. Paralysis is typically rapid and progressive.
   d. Prodromal symptoms of urinary tract infection or gastrointestinal symptoms are common.
   e. The Salk vaccine has been implicated in some cases of polio.

3. All of the following statements about myasthenia gravis are true except:
   a. Reflexes are preserved.
   b. It is the most common neuromuscular junction disorder.
   c. Sensation is typically preserved.
   d. Coordination is affected early.
   e. 80% to 90% of patients have detectable serum antibodies.

4. A patient with known myasthenia gravis presents to the ED with respiratory difficulties. All of the following are appropriate in managing this patient except:
   a. ICU admission
   b. Consider giving methylprednisolone
   c. Consider plasmapheresis
   d. Increase cholinesterase inhibitor dose temporarily
   e. Intubatate if forced vital capacity is less than 10 to 12 mL/kg

5. All of the following statements about adult botulism are true except:
   a. Reflexes remain intact.
   b. Treatment is with trivalent antiserum and antibiotics.
   c. Early cranial nerve palsies occur.
   d. Presynaptic acetylcholine release is inhibited.
   e. The toxin is an exotoxin.

6. A young Asian male presents to the ED with profound weakness. Many of his family members have had similar episodic weakness. You suspect periodic paralysis. All of the following are true except:
   a. Acetazolamide is recommended in the acute setting only.
   b. Electrolytes should be checked before initiating specific treatment.
   c. Swallowing and respiration are seldom involved.
   d. Oral potassium replacement is preferred over IV replacement.
   e. Thyroid function tests may prove useful and should be performed.

7. Which of the following exerts its effect outside the neuromuscular junction?
   a. Tick paralysis
   b. Lambert-Eaton syndrome
   c. Botulism
   d. Diphtheria
   e. Myasthenia gravis

8. A 25-year-old woman presents 10 days post viral syndrome with ascending paralysis. You suspect Guillain-Barré syndrome. Which of the following is least supportive of this diagnosis?
   a. Areflexia
   b. Impaired nerve conduction velocities
   c. Autonomic disturbances
   d. CNS disturbances
   e. Albuminocytologic dissociation on lumbar puncture

9. All of the following statements about Lambert-Eaton syndrome are true except:
   a. Proximal weakness is typical.
   b. It is associated with small cell lung carcinoma.
   c. EMG studies often show "post-tetanic potentiation."
   d. Calcium channel antagonists are useful in treating this condition.
   e. Release of acetylcholine from presynaptic motor terminals is diminished.

10. Answer true or false to the following regarding the Tensilon test:
   a. A positive result is sensitive but not specific for myasthenia gravis.
   b. Brief fasciculations are common following edrophonium injection.
   c. Edrophonium chloride is relatively contraindicated in asthma and dysrhythmias.
   d. The typical dose regimen for edrophonium is 2 mg initially; 3 mg after 1 min; 5 mg after a further 3 min.
   e. Improvement in hand grip is a simple and useful end point.

Answers

1.a. iii; b. iv; c. i; d. ii. When faced with patients with weakness, the pattern of progression can give clues to the diagnosis. In Lambert-Eaton syndrome, release of acetylcholine from presynaptic motor terminals is diminished. The typical pattern of weakness seen is of proximal muscle weakness. Motor neuron disease results from the progressive degeneration of motor neurons. Muscle weakness and wasting often begins in the small muscles of the hand, giving a characteristic pattern of early distal weakness. Guillain-Barré syndrome is an acute demyelinating neuropathy. The weakness begins distally but proceeds proximally, giving an ascending picture to the weakness. Botulism is a neuromuscular junction disorder in which cranial nerve dysfunction often occurs early; hence, the paralysis appears to be descending. (*Emergency Medicine, Chapter 74, pp 771–779*)

2.a. false; b. true; c. true; d. true; e. false. Polio virus is a picornavirus. The virus damages the anterior horn cell of the spinal cord, producing a lower motor neuron lesion and a flaccid paralysis. Sensation is preserved. The clinical picture of weakness often follows prodromal urinary tract infection or gastrointestinal symptoms. An asymmetric pattern of weakness is typical. Once paralysis begins it is usually rapid and progressive. Bulbar paralysis may occur. Worldwide, there are two vaccines in existence. The first vaccine was developed by Salk. This is an inactivated vaccine and as such it is not capable of transmitting the illness. It is available in injectable form and produces good blood antibody response but does not give gut immunity. The second vaccine available is the Sabin live attenuated virus vaccine. It is administered in oral form and as such gives both blood and gut immunity. Because the vaccine is a live vaccine, some viral shedding may occur. The vaccine is considered safe. Rare cases of mild paralysis have, however, been reported after use of the vaccine worldwide. The incidence is estimated at 1 per million doses.[1] (*Emergency Medicine, Chapter 74, pp 771–779*)

3.d. Myasthenia gravis is the most common disease of neuromuscular transmission. It has a prevalence of 5 to 12.5 per 100,000 of the general population. There appears to be an autoimmune basis to the disease, with detectable antibodies against acetylcholine receptors in 80% to 90% patients. The antibodies reduce the number of available acetylcholine receptors at the neuromuscular junction. They do this by direct blockade of binding sites, acceleration of receptor degradation, and complement-mediated damage to receptors. The result is progressive failure of neuromuscular transmission that manifests clinically as weakness. Reflexes are preserved; sensation is intact; and coordination remains intact. (*Emergency Medicine, Chapter 74, pp 771–779*)

4.d. A patient with known myasthenia gravis and respiratory failure is by definition in myasthenic crisis. Priority in management is to maintain an adequate airway, support ventilation, and control secretions. Forced vital capacity measurement is consistently more sensitive than peak flow rates in following patients with respiratory insufficiency from neuromuscular dysfunction. In this group of patients, intubation is generally recommended with forced vital capacity of 10 to 12 mL/kg. Cholinesterase inhibitors play an important role in the long-term management of patients with myasthenia gravis. In the acute setting of crisis, however, withdrawal of cholinesterase inhibitors is recommended. Reintroduction of the drug several days later is associated with increased responsiveness in certain patients. Because there appears to be an autoimmune etiology in myasthenia, immune suppression with steroids and other agents is frequently used. Plasmapheresis also plays a role in the management of myasthenia gravis and is generally reserved for cases with acute deterioration or crisis. Edrophonium has no role to play in the setting of myasthenic crisis. (*Emergency Medicine, Chapter 74, pp 771–779*)

5.b. *Clostridium botulinum* is a spore-forming, anaerobic, gram-positive bacillus. The spores are ubiquitous. Food contamination with resultant spore germination and toxin formation can produce botulism. The exotoxin binds irreversibly at the neuromuscular junction, producing presynaptic blockade. Reflexes are normal. Cranial nerve abnormalities often present early (e.g., diplopia, dysphagia, dysphonia), followed by descending paralysis. Diagnosis is made by finding the organism in stool or wound or finding the toxin in serum, stool, or food samples. Treatment consists of supportive care, spore elimination, and toxin neutralization. A trivalent antitoxin exists and can help prevent further paralysis; it will not affect already involved muscle. Antimicrobials have not been shown to be helpful in treating botulism.[2] (*Emergency Medicine, Chapter 74, pp 771–779*)

6.a. This history suggests a diagnosis of periodic paralysis. Both hypokalemic and hyperkalemic varieties of the disease exist, so electrolytes should be checked to determine which variety is involved. In the hypokalemic variety, replacement of potassium may shorten the duration of weakness. Oral potassium supplements are generally recommended. Swallowing and respiration are rarely involved. Acetazolamide, 250 mg two to four times per day, is recommended both in the acute setting and in chronic management to prevent weakness. The hypokalemic variety of periodic paralysis may occur in association with hyperthyroidism. In these cases, correction of the hyperthyroidism is the most definitive care, but in the interim, beta-blockers are very useful.[3,4] *(Emergency Medicine, Chapter 74, pp 771–779)*

7.d. In diphtheria, the organism involved is *Corynebacterium diphtheriae*. It produces an exotoxin that acts on the heart and nervous system. The characteristic onset is fever and exudative pharyngitis; later, the exotoxin acts at the level of the peripheral nervous system to produce mononeuritis, mononeuritis multiplex, or polyneuritis. The other entities listed exert their effect at the level of the neuromuscular junction. In myasthenia gravis, antibodies are formed against the presynaptic acetylcholine receptors at the junction. Exotoxin formed in botulism irreversibly binds at the presynaptic terminal. In tick paralysis, the neurotoxin involved inhibits acetylcholine release at the neuromuscular junction. The Lambert-Eaton syndrome is a paraneoplastic phenomenon in which release of acetylcholine from presynaptic motor terminals is diminished. *(Emergency Medicine, Chapter 74, pp 771–779)*

8.d. Guillain-Barré syndrome is an acute idiopathic demyelinating polyneuropathy. It has an incidence of 0.7 to 2.0 per 100,000 population. Typically, there is a prodromal illness followed by an ascending paralysis, and cranial nerve involvement occurs occasionally. There are frequently complaints of sensory changes, such as paresthesia, but objective sensory findings are variable. Autonomic instability is not unusual, and BP swings and dysrhythmias can occur. Areflexia is typical and occurs early in the disease. Investigations include nerve conduction studies and lumbar puncture. Lumbar puncture typically shows increased protein without cells—this is the classic "albuminocytologic dissociation." Nerve conduction studies are impaired early and are helpful in confirming the diagnosis. Treatment is supportive care. High-dose steroids are commonly used, although they have never been proved effective. Plasmapheresis is reserved for severe or progressive symptoms and is effective especially if carried out early in the illness. Pooled gamma globulin is being considered as a treatment option. Prognosis is generally good and most patients make a full recovery. The CNS is spared in this disease process. *(Emergency Medicine, Chapter 74, pp 771–779)*

9.d. Lambert-Eaton syndrome is a paraneoplastic phenomenon, and small cell lung carcinoma is the most commonly associated malignancy. A myasthenic picture exists with diminished acetylcholine release from presynaptic motor terminals. The resultant weakness is more pronounced in proximal muscle groups, and deep tendon reflexes are reduced. EMG studies using high-frequency nerve stimulation show a characteristic post-tetanic potentiation, which is helpful in making the diagnosis. Treatment is aimed at the underlying malignancy if possible, and additional supportive measures are provided as needed. Worsening of symptoms has been reported with the use of beta-blockers, and they are considered contraindicated in this syndrome.[5] *(Emergency Medicine, Chapter 74, pp 771–779)*

10.a. false; b. false; c. true; d. true; e. false. Edrophonium administration as a diagnostic tool in myasthenia gravis constitutes the Tensilon test. Edrophonium chloride is the preferred agent because it has a rapid onset (<2 min) and short duration of action (<10 min). It is a cholinesterase inhibitor and as such it is relatively contraindicated in asthma and cardiac dysrhythmias. The test consists of identifying a single muscle that is clearly weak, administering edrophonium, observing objective evidence of improvement in muscle strength, and observing the effect fade as edrophonium's effect diminishes. The most commonly monitored sign is ptosis. Simple hand grip is not suitable because it involves more than one muscle group, and objective assessment is difficult. Improvement in muscle strength must be observed objectively to constitute a positive result. Subjective improvement alone is not sufficient. In addition, the observed effect must then be observed to fade as the effect of edrophonium diminishes. After a positive test result, the test should be repeated with a control substance, such as normal saline, to confirm that the effect was as a result of edrophonium. The usual regimen of edrophonium administration is as follows: an initial test dose of 2 mg is given, followed in about 1 min by a 3-mg dose. If necessary, a third dose of 5 mg can be given 3 min later—total 10 mg per test. The test can be repeated in 30 min if needed. A small number of people show cholinergic side effects during the Tensilon test. These effects are generally transient, but atropine can be given to counteract them if needed. Fasciculations are not usually seen in myasthenia gravis when edrophonium is administered. *(Emergency Medicine, Chapter 74, pp 771–779)*

REFERENCES

1. Timbury MC: Enterovirus infections. *In* Timbury MC (ed): Medical Virology, 9th ed. Edinburgh. Churchill Livingstone, 1991, p 67.
2. Goldfrank LR, Flomenbaum NE, Weisman RS: Botulism. *In* Goldfrank LR, Flomenbaum NE, Lewin NA, et al (eds): Goldfrank's Toxologic Emergencies, 5th ed. Norwalk, Appleton & Lange, 1994, pp 937–946.
3. Bergeron L, Sternbach G: Thyrotoxic periodic paralysis. Ann Emerg Med 1988; 17:843.
4. Cannon L, Bradford J, Jones J: Hypokalemic periodic paralysis. J Emerg Med 1986; 4:287.
5. McEvoy KM, Windebank AJ, Daube JR, Low PA: 3,4-Diaminopyridine in the treatment of Lambert-Eaton myasthenic syndrome. N Engl J Med 1989; 321:1567–1571.

BIBLIOGRAPHY

Huff JS: Neuromuscular emergencies. *In* Howell JM, Altieri M, Jagoda AS, et al (eds): Emergency Medicine. Philadelphia, WB Saunders, 1998, pp 771–779.

37 Seizures and Headaches

ANDY JAGODA, MD

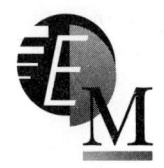

1. Which of the following suggests that a patient found with an altered mental status had a generalized tonic-clonic seizure?
   a. Hyperreflexia on initial examination that returns to normal while in the ED
   b. Extensor plantar reflex on initial examination that becomes a flexor plantar reflex while in the ED
   c. A posterior shoulder dislocation
   d. An anion gap metabolic acidosis that resolves over 1 hour
   e. All of the above

2. Which of the following regarding alcohol withdrawal seizures is true?
   a. Alcohol withdrawal seizures usually occur 5 to 7 days after serum alcohol levels drop to 0.
   b. Alcohol withdrawal seizures are usually focal seizures.
   c. Patients who have had an alcohol withdrawal seizure should be placed on phenytoin for at least 6 months.
   d. Alcohol withdrawal seizures will usually respond to IV phenytoin.
   e. Alcohol withdrawal seizures are often multiple but the events rarely recur after 12 hours from onset.

3. A 25-year-old university student with a known seizure disorder since childhood presents to the ED after a generalized event that was characteristic of his past events. His seizures have been well controlled on phenytoin, 300 mg qhs, without a change in medications for the past 5 years. His last seizure had been 2 years prior. On questioning the patient, he claims to be compliant with his medications but says that he is studying for final examinations and has not slept for over 36 hours. His physical examination is completely normal, and his phenytoin level returns at 10 µg/dL. Which of the following is the best treatment strategy in the ED?
   a. Increase his phenytoin to 400 mg qhs because his level is low therapeutically and have him follow up with his primary care provider.
   b. Add carbamazepine to his therapy regimen because polydrug therapy has been clearly shown to be superior to monodrug therapy.
   c. Counsel the patient on the importance of minimizing physical stress and send the patient home without adjusting the phenytoin dosing after discussing management with the patient's primary care provider.
   d. Give the patient 250 mg of IV phenytoin to raise his level within the midtherapeutic range and discharge him on phenytoin 200 mg twice a day.
   e. Obtain a head CT, toxicologic screen, and metabolic profile and base therapy on the findings of these tests.

4. A patient has a generalized tonic-clonic seizure that stops with 2 mg of IV lorazepam. Two hours after the seizure, the patient remains unresponsive to verbal stimuli. The patient's pupils are equal and reactive and he localizes and withdraws to pain appropriately. Which of the following is in the differential diagnosis?
   a. An intracranial bleed
   b. Hypoglycemia
   c. Postictal state
   d. Nonconvulsive status
   e. All of the above

5. A 3-year-old child experiences a generalized tonic-clonic seizure that lasts 2 minutes. The child arrives in the ED 30 minutes after the event and is found to have a rectal temperature of 38°C; otherwise, the child appears very well, is alert and playful, and has a nonfocal physical examination. There is no past medical history. Which of the following is true?
   a. Simple febrile seizures are often focal events.
   b. Simple febrile seizures generally last less than 20 minutes and occur in children between the ages of 1 year and 10 years.
   c. Parents should be advised that febrile seizures may recur in the future with febrile episodes.
   d. All patients with first-time febrile seizures should have a lumbar puncture.
   e. Children who have had a febrile seizure should be scheduled for an EEG.

6. Which of the following best explains the advantage of using lorazepam instead of diazepam as the initial drug in managing status epilepticus?

a. The anticonvulsant action of lorazepam lasts longer than diazepam's.
b. Lorazepam has fewer side effects than diazepam.
c. Lorazepam does not interfere with the pharmacokinetics of phenytoin to the same degree that diazepam does.
d. Lorazepam is metabolized faster than diazepam.
e. Lorazepam has a faster onset of anticonvulsant action than diazepam.

7. Which of the following is a true statement regarding the physiologic consequences of status epilepticus?
   a. Neuronal injury can be prevented by the early use of paralyzing agents, thus preventing acidosis and hypoxia.
   b. Seizures may cause a cerebrospinal fluid pleocytosis.
   c. In general, seizures do not cause an elevated WBC count.
   d. Nonconvulsive status epilepticus is not associated with neuronal injury.
   e. Hypothermia frequently complicates untreated status epilepticus.

8. A 61-year-old woman suffers a closed head injury while in-line skating in Manhattan. EMS reports that she had a 30-second tonic generalized seizure in the field. In the trauma center, she has a Glasgow Coma Scale score of 4 and is observed to have a brief period of stiffening with all four extremities in extension. The best initial management of this patient includes:
   a. Phenytoin loading with 18 mg/kg at 50 g/min
   b. Lorazepam, 1 mg/min until the event stops or a maximum dose of 10 mg is given
   c. Phenobarbital, 10 mg/kg at 100 mg/min
   d. Rapid-sequence intubation, hyperventilation, and mannitol
   e. Valproic acid, 10 mg/kg through a nasogastric tube

9. Which of the following is a false statement?
   a. An aura is the beginning of a seizure and usually represents the seizure's focus.
   b. Absence seizures are a primary generalized process that usually lasts less than 20 seconds.
   c. Secondary generalized seizures begin with a focus but may spread so quickly that the focus remains unrecognized.
   d. Complex partial seizures are focal events associated with altered mental status.
   e. Generalized convulsions that involve only the motor areas of the brain often do not result in altered mental status.

10. Indications for obtaining an EEG in the ED for patients in status epilepticus include all of the following except:
    a. Initiation of high-dose phenytoin
    b. Induction of pentobarbital anesthesia
    c. Suspected nonconvulsive status
    d. Use of long-acting paralyzing agents
    e. Prolonged postictal period without improving mental status

11. Which of the following is true of psychogenic seizures?
    a. They can occur concomitantly in patients with epilepsy.
    b. They are not associated with incontinence or tongue biting.
    c. They usually represent malingering.
    d. They are responsive to low-dose phenytoin.
    e. They are more often diagnosed in men than in women.

12. Which of the following tests may be helpful in distinguishing a psychogenic seizure from an epileptic event?
    a. A serum prolactin level at 20 minutes and 60 minutes after the event
    b. A serum pH and bicarbonate immediately after the event
    c. A saline infusion test
    d. An EEG performed during the event
    e. All of the above

13. In the evaluation of a patient who has had a new-onset seizure, which is a true statement?
    a. A noncontrast CT of the head is the best initial study in patients with altered mental status who have had a seizure.
    b. Hypoglycemia can be excluded as the etiology of a seizure if the patient is alert and cooperative.
    c. A lumbar puncture is indicated in the evaluation of all new-onset seizure patients.
    d. Occult hypomagnesemia frequently presents with seizures.
    e. A drug screen is indicated in all new-onset seizure patients.

14. Which of the following best characterizes the headache associated with a subarachnoid hemorrhage?
    a. Severe with nausea and cranial nerve VII or VIII involvement
    b. Slowly progressive with a throbbing quality radiating into the neck
    c. Retro-orbital with cranial nerve involvement and visual blurring
    d. Unilateral, severe with icepick quality, associated with vertigo
    e. Sudden onset, diffuse, with altered mental status and nausea

15. Which of the following is a true statement regarding migraine headaches?
    a. Migraine and tension headaches may have a common pathophysiologic mechanism.
    b. Migraine without an aura is usually a generalized, nonthrobbing headache.
    c. In migraine with aura, the headache commonly precedes the aura by 30 to 60 minutes.
    d. Complicated migraines refer to headaches that are associated with neurologic deficits that precede the headache.
    e. Basilar migraines commonly present with unilateral upper or lower extremity weakness.

16. A 40-year-old male presents with a severe, unilateral, orbital headache that is associated with lacrimation, mio-

sis, and ptosis. The headache occurred at night. He had several similar episodes 2 years ago. Which of the following is the most likely diagnosis?
a. Subarachnoid bleed
b. Ophthalmoplegic migraine
c. Cluster headache
d. Subarachnoid hemorrhage
e. Sphenoid sinusitis

17. A new-onset, diffuse headache in a 70-year-old who gives a history of worsening symptoms while eating and who has scalp tenderness on examination suggests which of the following diagnoses?
a. Complicated migraine
b. Cluster headache
c. Trigeminal neuralgia
d. Temporal arteritis
e. Pituitary adenoma

18. Which of the following statements is correct regarding the eye examination in the patient presenting with the complaint of headache?
a. A finding of decreased visual acuity that corrects with the pinhole test in a patient who does not wear glasses suggests headache due to eye strain.
b. A finding of decreased visual acuity, a fixed pupil, and corneal clouding suggests venous sinus thrombosis as the etiology of the headache.
c. Pain with eye movement and a Marcus-Gunn pupil are the classic findings in glaucoma.
d. The finding of papilledema and third cranial nerve palsy suggests that the headache is the result of an ophthalmoplegic migraine.
e. Visual field defects and loss of central vision with the preservation of color vision are the classic findings in headaches from intracranial hypertension.

19. In a patient presenting 6 hours into a "typical" migraine headache characterized by vomiting, photophobia, and severe, unilateral, throbbing headache pain, which of the following would be the best treatment?
a. Ketorolac, 60 mg orally
b. Demerol, 25 mg IV
c. Ergotamine, 1 mg sublingually every 5 minutes up to 3 mg
d. Prochlorperazine, 10 mg IV
e. Sumatriptan, 10 mg orally

20. Which of the following is true regarding headache management?
a. Cluster headaches, if treated immediately, often respond to 100% oxygen therapy.
b. Narcotics are first-line drugs in managing cluster headache.
c. Due to its potential complications, prednisone should be held in cases of suspected temporal arteritis until the diagnosis is confirmed by biopsy.
d. Because trigeminal neuralgia pain tends to be chronic, it is best managed by using a fentanyl patch.
e. The pain of trigeminal neuralgia often responds to a combination of 100% oxygen and prochlorperazine.

21. Which of the following is true regarding headache pain mechanisms?
a. Acetylcholine is the primary neurotransmitter involved in pain transmission.
b. The sixth cranial nerve transmits most pain above the tentorium.
c. Scalp pain is primarily transmitted by the fifth cranial nerve.
d. The brain parenchyma is extremely pain sensitive.
e. Serotonin receptors are involved in mediating pain in most types of headaches.

22. An 8-year-old child presents to the ED confused, with a severe left-sided headache, an expressive aphasia, and left-sided weakness. Which of the following is the most likely diagnosis?
a. Subarachnoid hemorrhage
b. Hemiplegic migraine
c. Stroke
d. Hysteria
e. Drug intoxication

Answers

1.e. All are physical and laboratory findings that have been associated with generalized tonic-clonic seizures. Hyperreflexia, including an extensor planter reflex (positive Babinski's test), is frequently found and gradually resolves during the postictal period. Posterior shoulder dislocations are rare events and highly suggestive of a seizure when other causes of trauma are absent. An anion gap acidosis from lactic acidosis occurs predictably after a tonic-clonic event but should resolve within 1 hour; otherwise, other causes of the anion gap should be sought. (*Emergency Medicine, Chapter 75, pp 780–789*)

2.e. Alcohol withdrawal seizures generally occur within 48 hours after serum alcohol levels begin to decline, but they can occur up to 7 days after alcohol cessation. The seizures can be multiple, but in more than 95% of patients they cease within 12 hours. Delirium tremens, on the other hand, characteristically occurs after the third postabstinence day. It is important to distinguish alcohol withdrawal seizures from alcohol-related seizures, the latter being due to an underlying seizure disorder that is exacerbated by alcohol. Phenytoin has been clearly shown to be ineffective in preventing or controlling alcohol withdrawal seizures. (*Emergency Medicine, Chapter 75, pp 780–789*)

3.c. The most common cause of seizure recurrence is medication noncompliance. However, physical and chemical stressors potentially exacerbate seizure disorders and when identified must be addressed if seizure control is to be gained. In this case, the patient appears to be compliant and probably does well at a low phenytoin level of 10 μg/dL; therefore, management should include minimizing stressors. Serum levels are only a guide in therapy, and multiple factors must be considered in interpreting a level. In general, antiepileptic drugs are taken to toxic levels before a second antiepileptic drug is added. Single-day dosing of phenytoin can result in peak and trough levels that vary by more than 100%; phenytoin is protein bound, so drugs and medical conditions that alter protein binding may result in elevated or decreased serum phenytoin levels. (*Emergency Medicine, Chapter 75, pp 780–789*)

4.e. A potential pitfall in the management of patients who have had a seizure is to assume that persisting altered mental status is due to the postictal state. A period of altered mental status generally follows a tonic-clonic event but should gradually resolve over several hours. Depressed sensorium from either antiepileptic drugs (benzodiazepines, phenobarbital) or drugs taken in overdose may account for prolonged altered mental status. Unrecognized hypoglycemia or an intracranial event must always be considered and assessed for when the patient's clinical picture remains unclear. Nonconvulsive status is a well-described entity in which there is ongoing seizure activity without significant motor involvement. It is estimated that nonconvulsive status accounts for up to 25% of all cases of status epilepticus. Nonconvulsive status should be considered in patients who present with an alteration in their baseline mental status, especially when they have had a preceding convulsion, even if the alteration is considered minor, such as agitation, staring, or mild confusion. (*Emergency Medicine, Chapter 75, pp 780–789*)

5.c. Febrile seizures are convulsions associated with fevers occurring in children between the ages of 6 months and 5 years. Simple febrile seizures are defined as primary generalized convulsions that last less than 15 minutes and do not recur for 24 hours. Complex febrile seizures are either focal and prolonged, lasting more than 15 minutes, or multiple during a 24-hour period. In general, diagnostic testing in children who have had a simple febrile seizure is directed by the child's history and physical examination; lumbar puncture is not indicated in well-appearing children older than age 18 months. EEGs are not predictive of future afebrile seizures. Up to 50% of children will have a second febrile seizure. (*Emergency Medicine, Chapter 75, pp 780–789*)

6.a. Overall, lorazepam and diazepam are equivocal in terminating seizures and have the same side effect profile. Both drugs are lipid soluble with short distribution half-lives and long elimination half-lives and have a moderate degree of protein binding. However, diazepam has a greater partition coefficient than lorazepam, resulting in a much greater volume of distribution of free diazepam than free lorazepam. Consequently, diazepam, which enters the CNS within 1 minute (lorazepam enters within 2 minutes), has a duration of anticonvulsant efficacy of approximately 15 minutes; lorazepam has an anticonvulsant effect for at least 2 hours. (*Emergency Medicine, Chapter 75, pp 780–789*)

7.b. The etiology of neuronal damage in status epilepticus includes the effects of excitatory amino acids, acidosis, and hypoxia. Neuronal injury occurs even when acidosis and hypoxia are controlled with paralysis, and recent studies have documented injury in cases of nonconvulsive status. Status epilepticus has been associated with a cerebrospinal fluid pleocytosis (more than 5 WBCs) in up to 18% of patients without a CNS infection; approximately 60% of patients will have a WBC count greater than 12,000 cells/mm^3; and hyperthermia is much more frequent than either euthermia or hypothermia in these patients. (*Emergency Medicine, Chapter 75, pp 780–789*)

8.d. Tonic seizures are rare and characteristically described as extension of the lower extremities and slow abduction of the upper extremities at the shoulder. Decerebrate posturing, on the other hand, is described as extension of all four extremities with internal rotation of the arms and plantar flexion of the feet. In this case, the patient's posturing is most likely due to increased intracranial pressure and not to seizure activity; therefore, management must focus on lowering the intracranial pressure. (*Emergency Medicine, Chapter 75, pp 780–789*)

9.e. Seizures are classified as partial (focal) or generalized. The clinical manifestations of a focal seizure depend on the area of the brain involved and thus can be motor, somatosensory, autonomic, or psychic. Auras are focal seizures that are often followed by secondary generalization, in which case the patient usually has a generalized tonic-clonic convulsion. Complex partial seizures are focal seizures that are associated with an altered mental status. Primary generalized seizures are convulsions in which there is no initial focal event but that instead result from diffuse involvement of both cerebral hemispheres. Absence seizures are primary generalized seizures that do not have a motor component and are characterized by a sudden onset of unresponsiveness lasting usually less than 20 seconds. All generalized motor seizures are associated with unresponsiveness; when responsiveness is retained, a diagnosis of seizures is suspect. (*Emergency Medicine, Chapter 75, pp 780–789*)

10.a. Morbidity and mortality in status epilepticus are related to length of time the patient is in status. Neuronal damage will occur when neuronal firing continues despite control of motor activity. Consequently, interventions that stop motor activity, such as use of paralyzing agents, may mask potentially damaging ongoing neuronal discharges, in which case EEG monitoring must be instituted. Patients who have prolonged postictal periods or altered mental status may be in nonconvulsive status epilepticus, which can be diagnosed with EEG monitoring. High-dose phenytoin is not necessarily an indication for emergent EEG monitoring because phenytoin does not usually alter mental status or suppress motor activity. (*Emergency Medicine, Chapter 75, pp 780–789*)

11.a. Psychogenic seizures (also referred to as pseudoseizures) are events that mimic epileptogenic seizures but are psychiatric in origin. Psychogenic seizures can be motor or nonmotor events and at times are difficult to distinguish from epileptogenic events; this is complicated by the finding that approximately 20% of patients with psychogenic seizures also have epileptic seizures. Psychogenic seizures are often the result of a conversion reaction, and as such the patient is neither in control of nor aware of the psychiatric etiology of the disorder. They occur more frequently in women and are rare after age 50 years. Self-injury and incontinence occur in up to 40% of cases of psychogenic seizures. *(Emergency Medicine, Chapter 75, pp 780–789)*

12.e. Serum prolactin levels increase under many conditions that induce physical stress, including seizures. Prolactin levels peak at 20 minutes into the postictal period in the majority of patients who experience a generalized tonic-clonic seizure and return to the patient's baseline by 60 minutes, making the timing of testing critical. An anion gap metabolic acidosis rapidly develops during epileptic convulsions but very rarely occurs as the result of a psychogenic event. Saline infusion has been reported to reproduce psychogenic seizures in more than 90% of patients, although this in not a recommended diagnostic test to be used in the ED. *(Emergency Medicine, Chapter 75, pp 780–789)*

13.a. In patients who have had a seizure and who have a persisting altered mental status, a noncontrast head CT is the neuroimaging study of choice since it is fast and will diagnose intracranial edema, mass lesions, and blood. Occult hypoglycemia has been identified as a cause of seizures in patients who have a normal examination in the ED. There is no literature to support the routine use of lumbar puncture in asymptomatic patients. Hypomagnesemia has been identified as a potentiator of seizures, but there are no clear cases in the literature of occult hypomagnesemia presenting as a seizure. Seizures have been associated with cocaine use and other drug abuse, but the literature does not support obtaining a drug screen on all patients with new-onset seizure. *(Emergency Medicine, Chapter 75, pp 780–789)*

14.e. Headaches that are severe and sudden (referred to as thunderclap) suggest a subarachnoid bleed. There is often a history of preceding, less severe, sentinel headaches. Subarachnoid bleeds can be associated with mental confusion, nausea, vomiting, pain radiating into the neck or even in a sciatic distribution, fever, and ECG dysrhythmias. There are usually no focal neurologic findings associated with subarachnoid hemorrhages; however, aneurysms may involve cranial nerves III, IV, and VI. *(Emergency Medicine, Chapter 76, pp 790–798)*

15.a. Migraine and tension headaches possibly exist on a continuum, unified by a common pathophysiologic mechanism. Migraine without aura (once referred to as common migraine) and migraine with an aura (once called classic migraine) are the two major groups of migraine headache. The headache in migraine without an aura is moderate to classically severe in intensity, throbbing, and unilateral. It can be associated with nausea, vomiting, anorexia, photophobia, phonophobia, yawning, drowsiness, and difficulty concentrating. The diagnosis requires five previous attacks. The headache in migraine with an aura is preceded by visual, sensory, or motor symptoms that do not last more than 60 minutes. Diagnosis requires at least two attacks. Complicated migraine is a term used to describe neurologic defects that persist after resolution of a migraine headache and includes hemiplegic migraines, ophthalmoplegic migraines, and migrainous infarction. Basilar migraines present with neurologic symptoms in the basilar artery distribution with symptoms that include visual field defects, dysarthria, vertigo, tinnitus, ataxia, confusion, or syncope. *(Emergency Medicine, Chapter 76, pp 790–798)*

16.c. Cluster headaches are severe, usually with unilateral orbital or maxillary pain with sudden onset that lasts up to 2 hours before terminating. Rarely, patients have bilateral symptoms. Cluster periods last 2 to 3 months, and the patient can stay in remission for several years. The headaches often demonstrate a circadian regularity, half of the time occurring at night. Attacks tend to occur in groups and are seen more frequently in men, between the third and fifth decades, though they can occur at any age. The pain is associated with lacrimation, rhinorrhea, miosis, and ptosis. *(Emergency Medicine, Chapter 76, pp 790–798)*

17.d. Temporal arteritis is a generalized arteritis that involves large and medium-sized arteries and must be suspected in any patient older than 50 years with a recent-onset headache. There is a female predominance and peak age of occurrence is in the 70s. The dominant feature is scalp tenderness, especially over the temporal artery, but any artery can be involved. Pain is often described as "needles and pins," and 65% of patients have jaw claudication. Other symptoms can include weight loss, fevers, sweats, and arthralgia. Recent-onset headache with jaw claudication and temporal artery tenderness has a 100% predictive value for this final diagnosis. Confirmation of a clinical diagnosis begins with obtaining a sedimentation rate. *(Emergency Medicine, Chapter 76, pp 790–798)*

18.a. Several headache etiologies are identified on eye examination. Decreased visual acuity can indicate headache caused by eye strain, in which case a pinhole test corrects the refractory deficit. Corneal clouding and decreased visual acuity are seen in glaucoma. Periorbital swelling occurs in cavernous sinus thrombosis. Papilledema suggests increased intracranial pressure. Visual field defects indicate optic chiasm lesions. Double vision suggests mass lesions compressing the oculomotor cranial nerves. Optic neuritis presents with pain on eye movement, loss of central vision, and loss of color vision; the hallmark is a positive afferent nerve defect identified with the swinging flashlight test. There is a high correlation between optic neuritis and multiple sclerosis. *(Emergency Medicine, Chapter 76, pp 790–798)*

19.d. The most effective migraine medications work by stabilizing vascular tone, modulating serotonin receptors, and controlling inflammatory responses; analgesics alone, such as narcotics, are not recommended. Intramuscular ketorolac effectively aborts 60% to 70% of migraine headaches, which is equal to or better than treatment with narcotics and results in significantly less drowsiness. Ergotamine tartrate is an alpha-adrenergic blocker with vasoconstrictor and with serotonergic mediation properties. Ergotamine (Cafergot) is commercially available in combination with caffeine, 100 mg administered orally, sublingually, or rectally. It is associated with nausea, vomiting, abdominal and muscle cramps, and paresthesias. It cannot be used more than twice weekly due to tolerance and a rebound effect that can actually result in worsening of headache. Ergotamine tartrate is contraindicated in hypertension, ischemic heart disease, pregnancy, sepsis, peripheral vascular disease, and renal or hepatic failure. Dihydroergotamine (DHE-45) is a venoconstrictor with a broad range of 5-HT receptor activity, including stimulation of CNS chemotactic receptors, which results in nausea and vomiting. DHE will abort migraine headaches in 60% to 70% of cases. It is contraindicated in patients with hepatic, renal, cardiovascular disease and pregnancy. Sumatriptan, a serotonin-receptor modulator, works predominantly at 5-HT 1_d receptors. Orally, it aborts 51% of migraines versus 10% with placebo. Subcutaneously, it decreases the headache in migraine in 70% to 90% without producing drowsiness, nausea, or vomiting. However, headache recurrence is common within hours of the initial treatment, requiring repeat dosing. Sumatriptan is contraindicated in the same patients as DHE. The antiemetics and phenothiazines are also 5-HT receptor modulators and consequently are effective as sole agents and as adjuncts to the other antimigraine medications. Intravenous prochlorperazine (Compazine) gives relief in up to 88% of patients with an acute migraine attack. *(Emergency Medicine, Chapter 76, pp 790–798)*

20.a. The same drugs used in the acute management of migraine are effective in cluster headaches. Both DHE and sumatriptan have been studied and are well tolerated. Seventy percent of patients with an cluster headache who were treated at headache onset have their pain relieved almost immediately with oxygen, 5 to 8 L/min. Patients with refractory cluster headache can be tried on nasal 4% lidocaine or dexamethasone, 8 mg/day for 3 to 4 days. There is no role for narcotics in the initial management of cluster headaches. The pain of trigeminal neuralgia is dramatically improved with carbamazepine (Tegretol) or phenytoin (Dilantin) used individually or in combination. Patients suspected of temporal arteritis should be started on prednisone, 60 mg a day. There should be a positive response within 48 hours; otherwise the diagnosis is reassessed. *(Emergency Medicine, Chapter 76, pp 790–798)*

21.e. The trigeminal nerve is responsible for pain reception above the tentorium and of the face and most of the scalp, whereas cranial nerves IX, X, and XII are responsible for areas below the tentorium. The brain parenchyma itself is insensitive to pain. Pain responsive areas are the dura, large blood vessels, and the periosteum. Cervical nerves 1, 2, and 3 are responsible for transmitting pain from the posterior scalp and neck, and thus pain involving these areas can represent cervical disease. The pathophysiologic mechanisms responsible for headache and its perpetuation in syndromes such as migraine are becoming better understood with the identification of serotonin-mediated pain receptors and pathways. There are at least four 5-HT receptors, 5-HT$_{1-4}$, and four subtypes of 5-HT$_1$, 1a-1d. Stimulation of 5-HT$_1$ receptors results in vasoconstriction and partially explains the effect of sumatriptan and DHE. Other serotonin receptors are involved in centrally mediated nausea and vomiting, thus the emphasis on identifying drugs that have selective receptor response. *(Emergency Medicine, Chapter 76, pp 790–798)*

22.b. Familial hemiplegic migraine has a dramatic migraine presentation in which the child presents with progressive unilateral sensory or motor symptoms that can be associated with dysarthria, aphasia, or altered mental status. When receptive aphasias are present, the child can appear confused or even psychotic. The headache is usually unilateral and on the same side as the neurologic deficit. These events begin in childhood and have been reported to last up to a week. Subarachnoid bleeds are very rare in children and do not usually present with motor deficits. Stroke is also rare in children; left-sided weakness reflects a right-sided lesion, whereas aphasia usually represents a left-sided lesion. *(Emergency Medicine, Chapter 76, pp 790–798)*

BIBLIOGRAPHY

Jagoda AS: Headache. *In* Howell JM, Altieri M, Jagoda AS, et al (eds): Emergency Medicine. Philadelphia, WB Saunders, 1998, pp 790–798.

Jagoda AS, Riggio S: Seizures. *In* Howell JM, Altieri M, Jagoda AS, et al (eds): Emergency Medicine. Philadelphia, WB Saunders, 1998, pp 780–789.

SECTION ELEVEN

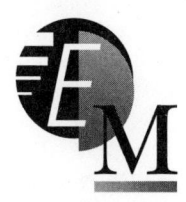

Renal, Urinary, and Male Genitourinary System Disorders

38 Renal Failure, Hematuria, Renal Insufficiency, and Urinary Tract Infection

ERNST PAUL, Jr, MD   PHILLIP FAIRWEATHER, MD   SANDRA SALLUSTIO, MD, PhD

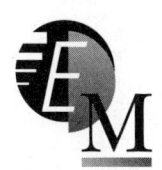

1. All of the following statements about acute renal failure caused by acute tubular necrosis are true except:
   a. Both oral and IV contrasts are common causes of acute tubular necrosis.
   b. Acute tubular necrosis is usually caused by an ischemic or nephrotoxic event.
   c. Streptomycin is the aminoglycoside most likely to cause acute tubular necrosis.
   d. Patients with diabetes and/or hypertensive renal disease develop acute tubular necrosis with minor insults.
   e. Acute tubular necrosis is the most common cause of intrinsic (renal) failure.

2. The least useful parameter in determining the cause (prerenal/renal/postrenal) of acute renal failure is:
   a. Fractional excretion of sodium
   b. BUN
   c. Creatinine
   d. Urinalysis

3. Hypertensive emergency in chronic renal failure may present as:
   a. Retinal changes
   b. Cardiac ischemia
   c. Seizure/encephalopathy
   d. CHF
   e. All of the above

4. Pericardial effusion/tamponade in patients with chronic renal failure is suggested by all of the following findings except:
   a. An enlarging cardiac silhouette, water-bottle contour of the heart, and/or a new pleural effusion on chest x-ray
   b. Right atrial and right ventricular collapse during diastole on echocardiography
   c. Alternating voltage height of the QRS complex on ECG
   d. Systolic blood pressure that increases more than 10 mm Hg during inspiration

5. A 32-year-old male with end-stage renal disease presents complaining of generalized aches, malaise, fever, and mild tenderness at the site of a temporary subclavian access. All of the following are true except:
   a. One third of patients with angioaccess infection have no symptoms.
   b. Pseudoaneurysms of synthetic vascular grafts are rarely a source of infection in end-stage renal disease.
   c. The second most common cause of morbidity and mortality in end-stage renal disease is infection.
   d. Vascular access sites are the most common sites of infection in patients undergoing hemodialysis or peritoneal dialysis.

6. Which statement is true about electrolyte abnormalities in end-stage renal disease?
   a. Hypermagnesemia causes neurologic complaints such as loss of deep tendon reflexes, lethargy, change of mental status, and paralysis.
   b. In hyperkalemia, the ECG findings consist of nonspecific ST/T changes.
   c. Patients with severe hypercalcemia (>11.5 mg/dL) are usually asymptomatic.
   d. None of the above statements is true.

7. Considering complications of dialysis catheters, which of the following is true?
   a. *Staphylococcus epidermidis* and *S. aureus* are the most common infectious agents in vascular access infection.
   b. Angiography can help differentiate a thrombotic from a mechanical obstruction of vascular access.
   c. Bleeding at vascular access sites can be caused by heparin, platelet dysfunction, frequent cannulation, or graft immaturity.
   d. All of the above statements are true.

8. All of the following are possible causes of hematuria except:
   a. Vigorous exercise
   b. Vitamin C
   c. Aspirin
   d. Sulfonamides
   e. All are associated with hematuria

9. Regarding urinalysis, which of the following statements is true?
   a. Isomorphic red blood cells seen on microscopic examination of the urine arise from the glomerulus.
   b. Abnormally shaped red blood cells generally arise from an infraglomerular source.
   c. A false-positive dipstick result may arise from contamination of the urine with povidone-iodine solution.
   d. Bacterial overgrowth in the urine container may give a false-negative dipstick result.
   e. All of the above statements are true.

10. An 18-year-old male is brought in by his mother after a fall from his bicycle with a complaint of lower back pain. The patient reports no past medical history, and his physical examination is normal except for mild tenderness over the left lower paraspinal muscles. A urinalysis done at triage reveals moderate hemoglobin, 4+ protein. Microscopic analysis shows no WBCs, few casts, and 7 RBCs per high-power field. What is the appropriate next step in this patient's care?
   a. Outpatient urologic follow-up
   b. Stat urologic consultation
   c. Stat intravenous pyelogram
   d. Plain abdominal x-rays of the kidney, ureter, and bladder
   e. BUN and creatinine and medical follow-up

11. A 32-year-old woman presents with a complaint of high fever, back pain, dysuria, and hematuria. You make the diagnosis of pyelonephritis. Which of the following diagnostic studies is not indicated in the ED?
   a. BUN/creatinine
   b. Urinalysis
   c. Urine culture
   d. Coagulation profile
   e. All of the above are indicated

12. All of the following may be appropriate courses of therapy for uncomplicated cystitis in a female patient except:
   a. Ciprofloxacin, 500 mg PO twice a day for 3 days
   b. Cefaclor, 500 mg PO every 8 hours for 3 days
   c. Tetracycline, 500 mg PO every 6 hours for 3 days
   d. Amoxicillin, 500 mg PO every 8 hours for 3 days
   e. Trimethoprim, 160 mg, Sulfamethoxazole, 800 mg (Bactrim DS), PO twice a day for 3 days

13. Urine culture collection and initiation of antimicrobial therapy in the ED are indicated in all of the following patients except:
   a. A pregnant woman with dysuria
   b. An 8-week-old baby boy with fever, irritability, lethargy, and decreased PO intake
   c. An 89-year-old female with hypertension, coronary artery disease, and asymptomatic bacteriuria
   d. An 8-year-old girl with a history of ureterovesical reflux and asymptomatic bacteriuria
   e. A 20-year-old male with lower left quadrant pain, fever, and pyuria

14. All of the following statements about xanthogranulomatous pyelonephritis are true except:
   a. The most common causative organisms reduce urinary nitrates to nitrites.
   b. Renal calculi may be associated with this entity.
   c. Histologic findings include the presence of foam cells (or lipid-laden macrophages).
   d. Radiologic differentiation of this entity from an abscess or avascular carcinoma may be difficult.
   e. All of the above are true statements.

15. Which of the following statements about the prevalence of urinary tract infections is least accurate?
   a. During the first 3 months of life, urinary tract infections are equally common in boys and girls.
   b. Among preschool children, urinary tract infections are more common in boys than in girls.
   c. Among young adults, urinary tract infections are 5 to 10 times more frequent in women than in men.
   d. In patients over the age of 65, the prevalence of urinary tract infections is slightly lower in women than in men.
   e. All of the above statements are inaccurate.

16. Nitrites are produced as a metabolic byproduct of all of the following organisms except:
   a. *Proteus mirabilis*
   b. *Enterococcus faecium*
   c. *Escherichia coli*
   d. *Klebsiella pneumoniae*
   e. *Enterobacter cloacae*

17. All of the following statements about acute bacterial prostatitis are false except:
   a. The most common etiologic agent is *Neisseria gonorrhoeae*.
   b. Acute bacterial prostatitis does not respond well to antimicrobial therapy.
   c. The presence of leukocytes in prostatic fluid is specific for diagnosis of this entity.
   d. Reported complications include bacteremia, epididymitis, and pyelonephritis.
   e. All are false statements.

18. The most common CT findings in patients with renal or perinephric abscess include all of the following except:
   a. Thickening of Gerota's fascia
   b. Renal enlargement
   c. Patchy areas of decreased density
   d. Fluid or air in and around the kidney
   e. All of the above

19. Relapse or recurrence of symptoms and bacteriuria 1 to 2 weeks after cessation of antimicrobial treatment for previous cystitis may be caused by all of the following except:
   a. Acute bacterial prostatitis
   b. Upper tract infection
   c. Structural abnormalities of the genitourinary tract
   d. Obstructing calculi
   e. All of the above

20. Which of the following is most reliable for localization of infection to a given site in the genitourinary tract?

a. Ureteral catheterization with culture
b. A thorough history and physical examination
c. Bladder washout (Fairly technique)
d. Needle biopsy of the kidney
e. Antibody-coated bacterial assays

21. All of the following are true statements except:
    a. The dipstick leukocyte esterase test is both sensitive and specific in detecting pyuria.
    b. The presence of more than 5 to 10 WBCs per high-power field in a centrifuged, clean-catch midstream urine sample is considered abnormal.
    c. The presence of at least one bacterium per high-power field in an uncentrifuged urine specimen obtained from suprapubic aspirate correlates with the presence of more than 100,000 bacteria per milliliter of urine.
    d. Optimal agents for treatment of urinary tract infections in patients with renal insufficiency include cephalosporins.
    e. All of the above are true.

Answers

1.c. Acute renal failure caused by intrinsic (parenchymal) renal disease is most commonly caused by acute tubular necrosis. Acute tubular necrosis results from either an ischemic or a nephrotoxic assault to the kidneys. Common causes are radiocontrast media, aminoglycoside antimicrobials, intrinsic pigment (hemoglobin/myoglobin), and shock states. Other causes include heat stroke, hyperosmolar nonketotic coma, third spacing, and chemotherapeutic agents. Both oral and IV contrast agents pose an increased risk of acute tubular necrosis, especially when given in a patient with advanced age, dehydration, preexisting renal disease (diabetic/hypertensive), and multiple myeloma. Neomycin is the most common aminoglycoside to cause acute tubular necrosis, followed by gentamicin, tobramycin, and amikacin. Streptomycin is least likely to cause this disorder. *(Emergency Medicine, Chapter 81, pp 833–852)*

2.b. Acute renal failure from prerenal causes presents with a fractional excretion of sodium less than 1%, suggesting high reabsorption of sodium at the renal tubules. The fractional excretion of sodium is more than 1% in patients with intrinsic renal disease. The serum creatinine can parallel fluctuations in the hemodynamic status of patients with prerenal azotemia, in contrast to its steady rise in patients with intrinsic renal disease. Urinalysis is helpful at identifying the cause of renal failure when the urinary sediment and supernatant are examined microscopically. The BUN is unreliable because of its unpredictable fluctuations and its multiplicity of origins (gastrointestinal hemorrhage, infections, trauma, and steroid therapy). *(Emergency Medicine, Chapter 81, pp 833–852)*

3.e. Hypertensive emergency is defined as an accelerated, severe type of hypertension associated with progressive end-organ damage. This can present as retinal hemorrhages or papilledema, acute change of mental status, stroke, and seizure as well as findings suggestive of cardiac ischemia or failure. The treatment of choice is dialysis, but if it is unavailable, IV labetalol, nitroprusside, and nitroglycerin are effective at reducing BP. Decreasing BP by 30% in 30 to 60 minutes and/or maintaining a mean arterial pressure above 120 mm Hg are effective therapies. *(Emergency Medicine, Chapter 81, pp 833–852)*

4.d. With a comparative chest radiograph, an increasing cardiac silhouette, a water-bottle–shaped heart, and a new pleural effusion are highly suggestive of a pericardial effusion. This can be further investigated by obtaining an ECG. The ECG finding suggestive of an effusion is electrical alternans, a varying of the QRS voltage height in all leads of the ECG. This occurs because of changes in position as the heart beats floating in a fluid-filled sac. An effusion may progress to cause a cardiac tamponade. This is marked by increased pressure by the effusion on the heart, causing increased end-diastolic pressures, decreased ventricular compliance, decreased volumes (venous return), and thus decreased output. This diagnosis can be further supported by an echocardiogram showing collapse of the right atria/ventricle in diastole. Pulsus paradoxus, although not specific to tamponade, is defined as a decrease of more than 10 mm Hg of systolic BP during inspiration. *(Emergency Medicine, Chapter 81, pp 833–852)*

5.b. In end-stage renal disease, the various sites used for vascular access and peritoneal access have a propensity toward infection. Infections of access grafts are second in frequency to cardiovascular complications of end-stage renal disease. Synthetic vascular grafts can form pseudoaneurysms, a common source of infection in chronic renal failure. *(Emergency Medicine, Chapter 81, pp 833–852)*

6.a. Hypermagnesemia in patients with end-stage renal disease most likely results from ingestion of magnesium-containing products and lithium. Increased magnesium inhibits presynaptic release of acetylcholine and norepinephrine, thus resulting in neuromuscular complications (decreased reflexes, lethargy, weakness, and paralysis). In hyperkalemia, the ECG findings are specific and progressive. With worsening hyperkalemia, T waves are increasingly peaked, progressing to distortion (widening) of the QRS complex, to an eventual sine wave. Calcium gluconate/chloride, sodium bicarbonate, insulin/glucose, and Kayexalate are the immediate therapies. Hypercalcemia above 11.5 mg/dL is usually symptomatic, causing nausea, vomiting, fatigue, malaise, and mental status changes. *(Emergency Medicine, Chapter 81, pp 833–852)*

7.d. *S. epidermidis* and *S. aureus* are the most common organisms in infection of both peritoneal and hemodialysis catheters. Other organisms to be considered are gram-negative organisms (*Escherichia coli, Pseudo-*

monas, Enterobacter) and fungi. In the patient who presents with probable occlusion of a temporary or permanent graft, look for loss of thrill/bruit or edema of the involved extremity. Probable causes are venous hyperplasia, inadvertent compression while sleeping, trauma, or dialysis (low flow state, hypercoagulability). Angiography will help identify the cause of obstruction. Bleeding at vascular access sites can result from multiple cannulation with resultant formation of pseudoaneurysms or aneurysms. These have an increased risk of rupture and bleeding. This condition is further complicated by the bleeding tendencies of dialysis patients because of platelet dysfunction and heparin use. Bleeding can also complicate immature grafts. *(Emergency Medicine, Chapter 81, pp 833–852)*

8.e. All are associated with hematuria. Hematuria can also be associated with ingestion of anticoagulants, acetaminophen, phenazopyridine, rifampin, and nitrofurantoin. *(Emergency Medicine, Chapter 80, pp 827–832)*

9.c. The urine dipstick is a readily available method of qualitatively determining the presence of RBCs, hemoglobin, or myoglobin in urine. False-positive results may result from contamination of the urine specimen with povidone-iodine cleaning agent or if bacterial overgrowth occurs. False-negative results may be obtained if the specimen container is contaminated with formaldehyde or if the patient ingests large quantities of vitamin C. If the urine dipstick is positive for blood, then a microscopic analysis is indicated. RBCs arising from the glomerulus tend to be dysmorphic, whereas those arising distal to the glomerulus are normal in shape. Microscopic analysis of the urine also enables one to determine presence of casts, crystals, and WBCs. *(Emergency Medicine, Chapter 80, pp 827–832)*

10.e. Although this patient could have sustained a renal contusion, his degree of proteinuria, relative to the red cells in the urine, suggests a glomerular disorder requiring medical evaluation. Blunt trauma patients who are hemodynamically stable and have microhematuria do not require emergent urologic evaluation. These patients can be followed as outpatients. Plain abdominal radiographs would be of little diagnostic value in this case, and an intravenous pyelogram could potentially cause severe renal damage. A renal ultrasound would be an appropriate first imaging study for this patient. *(Emergency Medicine, Chapter 80, pp 827–832)*

11.d. There is no indication for a coagulation profile in this patient unless she is taking anticoagulation therapy or is thought to have disseminated intravascular coagulation. All of the other studies are appropriate and will likely have a direct impact on her care in the ED. *(Emergency Medicine, Chapter 80, pp 827–832)*

12.d. The frequency of *E. coli* resistant to ampicillin/amoxicillin in community-acquired infections has been reported to be as high as 25% to 35%. Amoxicillin may be indicated when the identification/sensitivity profiles of the pathogen are known; as first-line agents, the aminopenicillins are less effective than the other agents listed. Tetracyclines and fluoroquinolones are best avoided in pregnancy. *(Emergency Medicine, Chapter 83, pp 859–868)*

13.c. Except for the elderly female, the consequences of untreated bacteriuria in all of the patients described may be potentially severe: the school-age girl may go on to manifest renal scarring or abnormal kidney development and, rarely, renal failure. Infants with bacteriuria may harbor congenital anomalies of the genitourinary tract and warrant further imaging studies. Bacteriuria in pregnancy often predisposes patients to the development of upper tract infection. The finding of pyuria in a patient with a clinical picture of ureteral calculus suggests a "complicated" urinary tract infection that warrants initiation of IV antimicrobial therapy and hospitalization. Asymptomatic bacteriuria should not be treated, except in pregnancy. *(Emergency Medicine, Chapter 83, pp 859–868)*

14.e. Xanthogranulomatous pyelonephritis is a rare and chronic renal parenchymal inflammatory condition characterized histologically by the presence of foamy macrophages, giant cells, and leukocytes; most often, the condition follows infection with *Proteus* sp. The diagnosis may be made by CT scan or renal biopsy. Radiologically, two major patterns may be seen: nodular changes and a localized mass. *(Emergency Medicine, Chapter 83, pp 859–868)*

15.e. Urinary tract infections are much more common in boys than girls during the first 3 months of life. Subsequently, the prevalence of urinary tract infections is greater in the female than the male patient population and ranges from a nearly 30:1 female-to-male ratio in young adults to a nearly equal female-to-male ratio in the elderly. *(Emergency Medicine, Chapter 83, pp 859–868)*

16.b. The reduction of urinary nitrate to nitrite (as detected on urine dipstick testing) is a property of most Enterobacteriaceae. Unlike the other organisms listed, *E. faecium* is a gram-positive, group D streptococcus that is an occasional etiologic agent in urinary tract infections. Gram-positive bacteria do not produce nitrite. *(Emergency Medicine, Chapter 83, pp 859–868)*

17.d. The most common pathogen isolated in the pre-antimicrobial era was *N. gonorrhoeae*. Today, gram-negative enterics are the most frequently isolated organisms. Most antimicrobials achieve bactericidal concentrations in the acutely inflamed gland, thus leading to bacteriologic cure for this condition, as long as treatment is continued for a minimum of 4 weeks. The finding of more than 15 WBCs per high-power field in prostatic fluid can be considered abnormal in the setting of simultaneous demonstration of the absence of pyuria in midstream/urethral urinary specimens. All of the complications of acute bacterial prostatitis described have been reported; additional reported complications include prostatic abscess and seminal vesiculitis. *(Emergency Medicine, Chapter 83, pp 859–868)*

18.e. Perinephric and renal abscesses are reported complications of acute pyelonephritis. Patients with either condition may present with similar symptoms: fever, chills, flank pain, and a poor response to antimicrobial therapy for acute pyelonephritis. CT scanning provides both a sensitive and a specific modality for diagnosis of these types of abscesses. On CT, the finding of gas/air within a low-density mass is pathognomonic for the presence of an abscess. Another characteristic CT finding is the so-called rind sign, or enhancement of the outer wall of the abscess by the contrast material. *(Emergency Medicine, Chapter 83, pp 859–868)*

19.a. Relapse or persistence of an organism in spite of antimicrobial therapy usually occurs because of an insufficiently long course of treatment (e.g., in patients with unsuspected renal infection who receive a short course of antimicrobials for presumed uncomplicated lower urinary tract infection) as well as because of structural and functional abnormalities of the genitourinary tract that prevent eradication of the offending pathogen. The latter include anatomic conditions such as vesicoureteral reflux and obstructive calculi. Chronic rather than acute, bacterial prostatitis is another condition that may result in relapsing urinary tract infections. In this case, the organisms persist in the prostate and intermittently seed the genitourinary tract, thereby leading to reinfection by overwhelming local host defense mechanisms. *(Emergency Medicine, Chapter 83, pp 859–868)*

20.a History and physical examination have been shown to be of little value in the differentiation of upper from lower urinary tract infection. The focal nature of pyelonephritis may yield false-negative results on renal biopsy specimens that accidentally sample uninvolved tissue. Although fairly reliable in the differentiation of upper versus lower urinary tract infection, the Fairly bladder washout procedure yields equivocal results in 10% to 20% of patients. Antibody-coated bacterial testing is insufficiently sensitive and specific. Although ureteral catheterization with quantitative cultures is the most reliable method for localizing infection to the upper or lower genitourinary tract, this technique still plays a very limited role in actual clinical practice. *(Emergency Medicine, Chapter 83, pp 859–868)*

21.e. In general, the presence of 10 to 50 WBCs per milliliter of uncentrifuged urine (equivalent to 1 to 5 WBCs per high-power field of urine after centrifugation at 2000 rpm for 5 minutes in a tabletop centrifuge) is considered abnormally high. The high sensitivity (75%–96%) and specificity (94%–98%) of the leukocyte esterase test in detecting 10 WBCs per milliliter of uncentrifuged urine render it a useful screening test for pyuria. Both penicillins and cephalosporins are concentrated to significant levels in the urine of individuals with impaired renal function. *(Emergency Medicine, Chapter 83, pp 859–868)*

BIBLIOGRAPHY

Balows A, et al: Manual of Clinical Microbiology. Washington, DC, American Society for Microbiology, 1991.

Belleza W, Browne BJ, Doherty RJ: Renal insufficiency and failure. *In* Howell JM, Altieri M, Jagoda AS, et al (eds): Emergency Medicine. Philadelphia, WB Saunders, 1998, pp 833–852.

Bolgioano EB, Naradzay JF: Approach to hematuria. *In* Howell JM, Altieri M, Jagoda AS, et al (eds): Emergency Medicine. Philadelphia, WB Saunders, 1998, pp 827–832.

Sobel JD, Kaye D: Urinary tract infections. *In* Mandell G, Bennett J, Dolin R (eds): Mandell, Douglas and Bennett's Principles and Practice of Infectious Diseases. New York, Churchill Livingstone, 1995, pp 662–690.

Stewart C: Urinary tract infections. *In* Howell JM, Altieri M, Jagoda AS, et al (eds): Emergency Medicine. Philadelphia, WB Saunders, 1998, pp 859–868.

39 Noninfectious Disorders of the Male Genital Tract; Renal and Ureteral Calculi

DOUGLAS W. FIELDS, MD

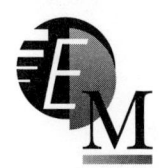

1. Patients presenting with urinary retention:
   a. Should be admitted
   b. May present with incontinence
   c. Do not need antimicrobials
   d. Should have an intravenous pyelogram
   e. All of the above

2. Chronic outlet obstruction is characterized by:
   a. Decreased force of stream
   b. Terminal dribbling
   c. Hesitancy
   d. Frequency
   e. All of the above

3. Treatment of urinary retention requiring bladder decompression may include:
   a. Catheter drainage with 14F to 18F Foley catheter
   b. Coudé catheter placement
   c. Filiforms and followers
   d. Suprapubic catheter drainage
   e. All of the above

4. Which of the following is involved in normal micturition and continence?
   a. Pons sensing a full bladder and relaxation of the external sphincter
   b. Increased alpha stimulation causing detrusor relaxation and voiding
   c. Increased parasympathetic tone causing relaxation of voluntary sphincter
   d. Inhibition of sympathetic contraction of external sphincter allowing voiding
   e. Parasympathetic activation of detrusor contraction

5. All of the following are true concerning benign prostatic hypertrophy except:
   a. It is not associated with carcinoma of the prostate.
   b. It is associated with symptoms of nocturia, dribbling, and decreased force of the urinary stream.
   c. It may cause sudden urinary retention without prior symptoms.
   d. It starts before age 40.
   e. Prostate size is related to degree of obstruction.

6. Urinary retention may be caused by all of the following neurologic disorders except:
   a. Multiple sclerosis
   b. Amyotrophic lateral sclerosis
   c. Diabetic neuropathy
   d. Anogenital herpes zoster
   e. Shy-Drager syndrome

7. True statements about testicular torsion include all of the following except:
   a. Manual detorsion should first be attempted with medial rotation of the testis.
   b. Nuclear scintigraphy may identify a "cold spot."
   c. Prehn's sign is negative.
   d. Doppler studies show decreased arterial flow.
   e. The cremasteric reflex is lost.

8. Hydroceles may be associated with:
   a. Tumors
   b. Epididymitis
   c. Trauma
   d. Patent processus vaginalis
   e. All of the above

9. Proper management of priapism includes:
   a. Prostatic massage
   b. Cold compresses
   c. Warm enemas
   d. Intracavernosal injection of vasoactive drugs
   e. All of the above

10. Which condition commonly mimics renal colic?
    a. Ruptured abdominal aortic aneurysm
    b. Retrocecal appendix
    c. Ectopic pregnancy
    d. Renal artery thrombosis
    e. All of the above

11. Ureteral obstruction may be seen in:
    a. Analgesic abuse
    b. Diabetes mellitus
    c. Chronic pyelonephritis
    d. Sickle cell disease
    e. All of the above

12. All of the following statements are true concerning the evaluation of renal colic except:
    a. The definitive diagnosis must be made before giving analgesics.
    b. Costovertebral angle tenderness may be present.
    c. A mild ileus is often present.
    d. Microscopic hematuria is often present.
    e. Pyuria necessitates an immediate intravenous pyelogram or ultrasound.

13. The following statements are true regarding nephrolithiasis and ureterolithiasis except:
    a. Plain abdominal films rarely alter patients' care.
    b. CT is useful in the diagnosis of radiolucent calculi.
    c. Intravenous pyelogram should be performed in the ED to make a definitive diagnosis.
    d. Ultrasound cannot visualize a calculus in the middle third of the ureter.
    e. Ultrasound is preferred when IV contrast agents are contraindicated.

14. All the following are typical radiographic findings of ureteral obstruction on intravenous pyelogram except:
    a. Nonvisualization of the kidney
    b. Delayed nephrogram
    c. Columning of the ureter above the point of obstruction
    d. Narrowing of the ureteral lumen distal to the obstruction
    e. Intensified nephrogram on the obstructed side

15. All of the following statements regarding ureteral obstruction are false except:
    a. Approximately 50% of stones pass spontaneously.
    b. A filling defect on IVP is synonymous with a calculus.
    c. A ureteropelvic junction obstruction may show dilation of the ureter.
    d. Ureteropelvic junction stones may cause irritative voiding symptoms.
    e. Nonvisualization of the kidney is always a sign of complete obstruction.

16. All of the following statements about nephrolithiasis and urinary extravasation are true except:
    a. Most patients require antimicrobials and admission.
    b. It is more common in males.
    c. There is less associated hydronephrosis.
    d. It does not change outcome.
    e. It is associated with larger stones.

17. All of the following statements about allergic reactions to IV contrast are true except:
    a. They are anaphylactoid reactions.
    b. Hypotension should be treated with fluids.
    c. They occur in 1 to 2 per thousand.
    d. Nonionic contrast lessens the risk of reaction.
    e. Antihistamines should be administered.

18. All of the following statements regarding nephrolithiasis and ureterolithiasis are true except:
    a. The chance of spontaneous passage of a ureteral stone is 90% if it is less than 4 mm.
    b. Patients with large proximal ureteral stones should have a urologic consult.
    c. 20% of patients with urinary calculi require urologic intervention.
    d. Extracorporeal shock-wave lithotripsy is the treatment of choice for distal ureteral stones.
    e. A ureteral stent may be placed in an obstructed ureter to relieve pain not relieved by analgesics.

19. Patients requiring admission for nephrolithiasis include all of the following except:
    a. Evidence of urinary tract infection with obstruction
    b. Uninephric patients with obstruction
    c. Pain not controlled with oral analgesics
    d. Intractable vomiting
    e. Evidence of urinary extravasation on intravenous pyelogram

Answers

1.b. Patients in urinary retention may present with overflow incontinence and should have bladder decompression. The history may be consistent with chronic outlet obstruction with hesitancy, decreased force of stream, and postvoid dribbling. If postobstructive diuresis occurs or the patient is unable to care for the catheter, admission is required. Patients with grossly contaminated urine or pyelonephritis or urosepsis require antimicrobials. (*Emergency Medicine, Chapter 122, pp 1261–1274*)

2.e. Chronic outlet obstruction may be from urethral strictures or benign prostatic hypertrophy. It is characterized by decreased force of stream, hesitancy, frequency, nocturia, and terminal dribbling. Split urinary stream may also be seen with urethral stricture. Chronic outlet obstruction may lead to bladder decompensation with massive bladder distention. (*Emergency Medicine, Chapter 122, pp 1261–1274*)

3.e. Bladder decompression should be attempted with straight Foley 14F to 18F catheters. Coudé catheters are angled and may be useful in posterior urethral obstruction from benign prostatic hypertrophy. Consultation is needed for anterior urethral stricture. Urologists may use filiforms and followers to dilate the stricture. Bladder neck contractions from transurethral prostatectomy are not easily traversed and may require placement of a suprapubic catheter. (*Emergency Medicine, Chapter 122, pp 1261–1274*)

4.e. During bladder filling, sympathetic stimulation of beta-receptors in the bladder causes bladder relaxation. Sympathetic alpha-receptor stimulation causes contraction of the internal sphincter. The frontal cortex senses a full bladder and allows for voluntary relaxation of the external sphincter. Parasympathetic activation causes detrusor contraction. The coordinated efforts of the frontal cortex, the pons, and the sacral micturition centers are required for normal urinary function. (*Emergency Medicine, Chapter 122, pp 1261–1274*)

5.e. The prostate begins to grow before 30 years of age and continues to grow throughout life. Prostate size does not always correlate with degree of obstruction. The prostate may enlarge without encroaching on the urethral diameter. Sudden onset of retention without previous symptoms is more characteristic of prostate carcinoma or may be caused by drugs such as sympathomimetics and antihistamines. *(Emergency Medicine, Chapter 122, pp 1261–1274)*

6.b. Amyotrophic lateral sclerosis is not associated with urinary retention. Diabetes is associated with a neuropathic bladder. Multiple sclerosis is associated with detrusor sphincter dyssynergy. Detrusor contraction occurs against a closed sphincter. Anogenital herpes and sacral root zoster are associated with urinary retention. Shy-Drager is a syndrome characterized by autonomic dysfunction. The autonomic dysfunction causes orthostatic hypotension, anorectal dysfunction, and urinary retention or urgency incontinence. *(Emergency Medicine, Chapter 122, pp 1261–1274)*

7.a. Manual detorsion of the testis may be attempted if surgery is delayed. The patient may be supine or standing while facing the physician, and the testis should be rotated laterally. The patient should have relief of pain. If the patient experiences increased pain, the testis is rotated medially. Urologic consult is mandatory. If the testis detorses on its own, surgery may be delayed and performed on an elective basis. Nuclear scintigraphy identifies a "cold spot" where there is no perfusion. Sensitivity and specificity are up to 100% and 97%, respectively. Doppler ultrasound is used to identify decreased blood flow to potentially ischemic testes. In testicular torsion, the testis is often high riding with a horizontal lie. There is loss of the cremasteric reflex. Prehn's sign (pain relief with elevation of the scrotum) is thought to indicate epididymitis, but slight pain relief may also be found with testicular torsion. *(Emergency Medicine, Chapter 122, pp 1261–1274)*

8.e. Hydroceles may be reactive as with tumors, trauma, or epididymitis. Trauma may also cause a hydrocele filled with blood—a hematocele. A communicating hydrocele is caused by the failure of the processus vaginalis to close. This allows peritoneal fluid to accumulate in the scrotum when standing, which may subside when supine. *(Emergency Medicine, Chapter 122, pp 1261–1274)*

9.d. Intracavernosal injection of vasoactive medications, such as phenylephrine in 200 to 400 μg aliquots, until detumescence is achieved is the treatment of choice. The corpora are sometimes irrigated with saline to remove the clotted blood before instillation of medications. Cold compresses, warm and cold enemas, and prostatic massage are generally ineffective and should not delay definite treatment. *(Emergency Medicine, Chapter 122, pp 1261–1274)*

10.e. All of these entities can mimic renal colic. Patients who present with acute back pain and are at risk for abdominal aortic aneurysm should have a definitive diagnosis made as soon as possible. Risk factors for abdominal aortic aneurysm are those for arteriosclerosis, i.e., older age, smoking, diabetes mellitus, hypercholesterolemia, and hypertension. To exclude an abdominal aortic aneurysm, an abdominal ultrasound or CT should be performed. Patients with retrocecal appendicitis may present with noncolicky flank pain and rectal tenderness. Ectopic pregnancy should be suspected in women of childbearing age who present with lower abdominal or back pain. *(Emergency Medicine, Chapter 82, pp 853–858)*

11.e. Papillary necrosis can present with flank pain and hematuria. Commonly, patients have fever and chills. Ureteral obstruction from sloughed renal papillae may be seen in patients with analgesic nephropathy, diabetes mellitus, chronic pyelonephritis, and sickle cell disease. Renal papillary necrosis is one of the etiologies of an acute deterioration of renal function in diabetic patients and patients with chronic obstruction. *(Emergency Medicine, Chapter 82, pp 853–858)*

12.a. It is not necessary to have confirmation by intravenous pyelogram or ultrasound of calculi or obstruction before giving patients analgesics. In patients who have a history suggestive of renal colic, analgesics should be offered early while performing a detailed history, physical examination, and urinalysis. The physical examination often reveals a patient writhing in pain. There may be costovertebral angle tenderness, mild lower abdominal tenderness, and decreased bowel sounds. The patient may have a mild ileus. Microscopic hematuria is present in about 80% of patients with ureteral stones. In patients who present with pyuria and symptoms of ureteral calculi, an immediate intravenous pyelogram or ultrasound should be performed to exclude complete ureteral obstruction. *(Emergency Medicine, Chapter 82, pp 853–858)*

13.a. Plain radiographs rarely add to patient management and treatment. Although approximately 75% of renal stones are radiopaque, the visualization of radiopaque stones on abdominal films may be difficult because of phleboliths, calcified lymph nodes, bony structures, and overlying stool and gas. Ultrasound is the preferred diagnostic examination when IV contrast is contraindicated. The middle third of the ureter is not visualized as well as on an intravenous pyelogram because of overlying small bowel gas. Intravenous pyelogram need not be performed emergently in the ED, unless necessary for diagnostic purposes. *(Emergency Medicine, Chapter 82, pp 853–858)*

14.a. Nonvisualization of the kidney is a sign either of a nonfunctional kidney or that the patient is uninephric. In a nonfunctional kidney, a vascular lesion should be suspected. A delayed and intensified nephrogram is seen in ureteral obstructions. There is a column of contrast material above the point of obstruction. There may appear to be narrowing of the ureter distal to the site of obstruction. *(Emergency Medicine, Chapter 82, pp 853–858)*

15.d. Ureterovesical junction obstruction is typically associated with irritative voiding symptoms of frequency and dysuria. This has been referred to as the tunnel syndrome because the stone passes through the intravesical ureteral tunnel. Approximately 80% of stones will pass spontaneously, which typically depends on the size of the stone. Stones 4 mm and smaller pass spontaneously 90% of the time. A calculus obstructing the ureteropelvic junction would cause renal pelvic dilatation. *(Emergency Medicine, Chapter 82, pp 853–858)*

16.e. Urinary extravasation is associated with smaller stones. It occurs because of increased intrarenal pressure, causing a rupture at the renal fornix. Ureteral peristalsis is reconstituted and the stone is propelled down the ureter. Thus, it is associated with greater chance of passage of calculi and less complications. *(Emergency Medicine, Chapter 82, pp 853–858)*

17.d. Nonionic contrast media do not lower the risk of allergic reactions, but they may decrease the risk of contrast-induced renal failure. Minor contrast reactions, such as pruritus and rash, should be treated by stopping the infusion and administering antihistamines. Contrast reactions are anaphylactoid reactions and are not IgE mediated. *(Emergency Medicine, Chapter 82, pp 853–858)*

18.d. Ureteroscopy with basket retrieval and laser or ultrasonic lithotripsy are the treatments of choice for distal ureteral stones that do not pass spontaneously or are very large stones. Patients with large proximal ureteral stones should have a urologic consult because the stones are unlikely to pass spontaneously. *(Emergency Medicine, Chapter 82, pp 853–858)*

19.e. Urinary extravasation is not a criterion for admission or urologic consult unless massive. Patients with a urinary tract infection and obstruction are at high risk of damage to the obstructed kidney as well as bacteremia and septicemia. Uninephric patients with high-grade obstruction need prompt intervention with either ureteral stent placement or removal of the calculi. *(Emergency Medicine, Chapter 82, pp 853–858)*

BIBLIOGRAPHY

Bossart PJ: Renal and ureteral calculi. *In* Howell JM, Altieri M, Jagoda AS, et al (eds): Emergency Medicine. Philadelphia, WB Saunders, 1998, pp 853–858.

Datner EM: Noninfectious disorders of the male genital tract. *In* Howell JM, Altieri M, Jagoda AS, et al (eds): Emergency Medicine. Philadelphia, WB Saunders, 1998, pp 1261–1274.

SECTION TWELVE

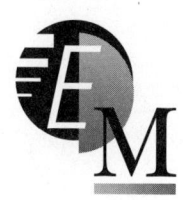

Dermatologic Disorders

40 Rashes, Dermatitis, and Skin Lesions

DAVID K. HOSHIZAKI, MD   DAVID L. LEVINE, MD

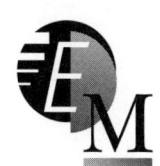

1. When prescribing a topical agent for the treatment of dermatitis, all of the following are true except:
   a. Infants and small children should be prescribed only class 6 or 7 topical steroid preparations.
   b. Lotions work well for hair-bearing areas.
   c. Persons with rashes on the face or groin should be prescribed only class 6 or 7 topical steroid preparations.
   d. In general, ointments are more potent than lotions or creams.
   e. Topical anesthetic preparations are helpful in soothing pain and irritation from rashes.

2. Which of the following best describes a bulla?
   a. An elevated skin lesion less than 0.5 cm in diameter
   b. A flat lesion with coloration different from normal surrounding skin
   c. A blister filled with clear fluid greater than 0.5 cm in diameter
   d. An elevated lesion greater than 0.5 cm in both diameter and depth
   e. A papule or plaque of dermal edema often with central pallor and an irregular border

3. All of the following regarding acne and its treatment are true except:
   a. The papules and pustules of acne are caused mainly by free fatty acids released from sebum by the organism *Propionibacterium acnes*.
   b. Excessive dryness and/or irritation are common complications of topical acne agents (benzoyl peroxide, tretinoin, and sulfur-based preparations).
   c. Isotretinoin (Accutane) is an effective agent for cystic acne and may appropriately be prescribed by the emergency physician.
   d. Common side effects of systemic antimicrobial therapy with tetracycline include photosensitivity and candidal vaginitis.
   e. Systemic agents should be reserved for deep papular or cystic acne lesions, or if there is scarring.

4. A 26-year-old man presents to the ED complaining of an itchy rash. He states that he has had a mild rash on his wrists and neck for many years. Now the rash has suddenly spread over his right arm and trunk. Examination reveals multiple small vesicles over his chest, back, and right arm as well as two lichenified plaques over the volar aspect of his wrists. The most appropriate treatment for this patient's condition would be:
   a. Acyclovir
   b. Oral antihistamines, Burow's solution compresses, and a topical steroid
   c. Tar preparations and phototherapy
   d. Antimicrobials to cover gram-positive organisms
   e. Prednisone, 20 to 40 mg PO with slow taper over 2 to 3 weeks

5. Which of the following is true of seborrheic dermatitis?
   a. When a scale is removed, bleeding points may appear (Auspitz's sign).
   b. It can vary in severity from a mild fine scaling to severe fissuring and large scaling papules.
   c. It is commonly associated with venous insufficiency.
   d. It begins with erythematous patches that spread rapidly over the entire skin surface and become edematous.
   e. It primarily affects the upper and lower extremities.

6. A 12-year-old girl presents to the ED with fever of 103°F and lethargy. Physical examination reveals skin lesions over the buttocks and lower extremities. The lesions are maculopapular, 3 to 5 mm in diameter, and do not blanch with pressure. All of the following are appropriate diagnostic tests or treatments of this condition except:
   a. CBC and coagulation studies
   b. Lumbar puncture
   c. Blood and urine culture followed by antimicrobials
   d. Stool for occult blood
   e. Topical steroids and follow-up with a dermatologist the next day

7. All of the following are true of urticarial lesions except:
   a. They often follow the natural lines of cleavage of the skin.
   b. They can occur in primigravid women, usually in the third trimester.

c. They can be associated with underlying leukemia or lymphomas.
d. They can be induced by minor physical irritation of a cutaneous lesion in a patient with mastocystosis.
e. Acute urticarial eruptions are commonly seen with food allergies.

8. A 40-year-old man presents to the ED complaining of a recurrent painful lesion on his back. He states he has had two small "lumps" on his back for a long time, but recently one has enlarged and become very painful. He saw his family doctor last week and had the lesion incised, drained, and packed. Although this provided temporary relief, the patient's symptoms had returned.
   Physical examination reveals two nodules on the patient's upper back. One nodule is 2 cm in diameter, erythematous, fluctuant, and very painful. The other measures 1 cm and is fluctuant but not inflamed and has a small punctum in the center. The most likely diagnosis for this patient is:
   a. Cystic acne
   b. Furuncles
   c. Epidermal cysts
   d. Dermatofibromas
   e. Malignant melanoma

9. Which of the following is not a potentially fatal skin disorder?
   a. Stevens-Johnson syndrome
   b. Bullous pemphigoid
   c. Petechial rash from meningococcemia
   d. Pemphigus vulgaris
   e. Toxic epidermal necrolysis

10. All of the following are true about erythema multiforme except:
    a. Etiologic associations include infections, medications, collagen vascular disease, and internal malignancy.
    b. It may have a remarkably variable appearance, including macules, papules, vesicles, bullae, urticaria, and purpura.
    c. It is thought to be an acute hypersensitivity syndrome.
    d. The classic appearance is target lesions: a macular zone of ring-like erythema with a central erythematous macule.
    e. Lesions commonly occur on the skin or pretibial region in a symmetric pattern.

11. The most common medication-related cause of erythema nodosum is
    a. Barbiturates
    b. NSAIDs
    c. Oral contraceptives
    d. Sulfonamides
    e. Thiazides

12. Which of the following is true about urticaria?
    a. It is classified as subacute, acute, and chronic.
    b. Individual lesions last longer than 24 hours.
    c. It is limited to torso and extremities.
    d. It may be painful on palms and soles.
    e. It responds to topical steroids.

13. Erythema multiforme:
    a. Often appears as iris (target) lesions
    b. Is an acute hypersensitivity syndrome with subcutaneous involvement
    c. May develop into toxic shock syndrome
    d. Is treated with dapsone
    e. Has a single etiology

14. Which of the following lesions is commonly found on flexor surface of the wrist and forearm?
    a. Lichen planus
    b. Senile purpura
    c. Leukocytotactic vasculitis
    d. Pityriasis rosea
    e. Epidermal cysts

15. Which of the following is true concerning pruritic urticarial papules and plaques of pregnancy?
    a. It usually arises in the second trimester of pregnancy.
    b. It is likely to recur with future pregnancy.
    c. Eruptions begin in the extremities and spread to the trunk and the abdomen.
    d. Papules form urticarial-type plaques and are intensely pruritic.
    e. Systemic steroids should be avoided.

16. Which of the following is true concerning erythema toxicum neonatorum?
    a. It is associated with fever.
    b. It begins on day 1 of life and lasts 2 months.
    c. It classically presents as papules.
    d. The etiology is presumed to be viral.
    e. Treatment is with corticosteroids.

Answers

1.e. Topical anesthetic preparations can cause a contact dermatitis, often making skin rashes worse. Topical corticosteroids are classified by potency, with class 1 agents being the most potent through class 7 being the least. Only class 6 or 7 steroids should be prescribed for the face, groin, axilla, or inflamed areas. Because their large surface area to volume ratio increases systemic absorption, infants and children should also be prescribed only class 6 or 7 topical corticosteroids, and only for limited periods. Lotions work well in hair-bearing areas; gels or creams are used for moist rashes; and ointments work best for dry, scaly rashes. Ointments are more potent than creams or lotions. *(Emergency Medicine, Chapter 84, Table 84–2)*

2c. A bulla is a blister measuring greater than 0.5 cm in diameter filled with clear fluid, whereas a vesicle measures less than 0.5 cm in diameter. Answer a best describes a papule; b, a macule; d, a nodule; and e, a wheal. An accurate description of a patient's rash is essential when communicating with other medical personnel and consultants. *(Emergency Medicine, Chapter 84, pp 869–871)*

3.c. Isotretinoin (Accutane) is a potent teratogenic agent with multiple side effects. Because the treatment period is usually 16 to 20 weeks, emergency physicians should not prescribe isotretinoin because they are not in a position to properly follow the patient for these side effects. Papules and pustules of acne are caused by the irritation produced by the breakdown of sebum into free fatty acids produced by *P. acnes*. Excessive skin dryness, irritation, and erythema are common problems of topical acne agents. Systemic antimicrobial agents should be reserved for severe cases of acne because of possible side effects, altering of normal host microflora, and inducing resistant strains of bacteria. Common side effects of systemic tetracycline include photosensitivity, Candidal vaginitis, nausea, heartburn, and staining of developing teeth. Tetracycline can also decrease the effectiveness of oral contraceptives. *(Emergency Medicine, Chapter 85, pp 872–876)*

4.a. Kaposi's varicelliform eruption (eczema herpeticum) is a sudden widespread vesicular eruption in an individual with atopic dermatitis caused by cutaneous spread of a herpes simplex superinfection. The correct treatment for this disorder acutely is acyclovir. *(Emergency Medicine, Chapter 85, pp 872–876)*

5.b. Seborrheic dermatitis is a chronic superficial pink or flesh-colored scaly eruption involving mainly the scalp, eyebrows, eyelids, ears, nasolabial folds, axillae, umbilicus, and groin. Mild involvement often consists of fine scaling, whereas severe involvement progresses to greasy yellow scales and fissures. Auspitz's sign, small bleeding points seen on removal of a scale, may be seen in psoriasis. Stasis dermatitis is a red-brown pigmented eruption over the legs associated with venous insufficiency. Erythematous patches that spread rapidly over the skin surface and become edematous are typical of exfoliative dermatitis. *(Emergency Medicine, Chapter 85, pp 872–876)*

6.e. The differential diagnosis for this patient includes diseases that cause palpable purpura, including leukocytoclastic vasculitis (like Henoch-Schönlein purpura), sepsis, and meningococcemia. Other causes of petechiae and purpura include thrombocytopenia, capillaritis, coagulopathies, and trauma. Because sepsis and meningococcemia are immediately life-threatening conditions, an aggressive sepsis evaluation including lumbar puncture and blood and urine cultures should be done, followed by administration of broad-spectrum antimicrobials. A CBC and coagulation studies should be done to exclude thrombocytopenia and coagulopathies as a cause. Stool should be tested for occult blood because of frequent gastrointestinal involvement in leukocytoclastic vasculitis. Steroids and outpatient follow-up are not an option when evaluating life-threatening disorders. *(Emergency Medicine, Chapter 86, pp 877–887)*

7.a. Acute urticaria lasts for less than 6 weeks. Causative factors include insect bites, food allergies, drugs, infections, and physical factors such as cold, heat, or skin trauma. Intensely itchy urticarial eruptions are seen in pruritic urticarial papules and plaques of pregnancy, usually in the third trimester of a woman's first pregnancy. Urticaria may also be a manifestation of underlying cryoglobulinemia, lymphoma, leukemia, or parasitic diseases. Darier's sign is the induction of an urticarial wheal and flare with physical irritation of lesions in a patient with mastocytosis. Pink-colored oval papules with a fine collarette scale are typical of pityriasis rosea. These lesions follow the natural lines of cleavage in the skin, producing a "Christmas tree" pattern of distribution over the trunk. *(Emergency Medicine, Chapter 86, pp 877–887)*

8.c. This patient most likely suffers from epidermal cysts, one of which has become acutely inflamed. The noninflamed lesion provides a clue to the diagnosis. It is a small, nontender, fluctuant nodule with a small punctum. Epidermal cysts can become acutely inflamed, usually by gram-positive bacteria. Treatment includes antimicrobials, intralesional steroids, and warm compresses. Although incision and drainage provide temporary relief, the cyst tends to recur unless the cyst wall or capsule is completely excised. *(Emergency Medicine, Chapter 86, pp 877–887)*

9.b. Of all the disorders listed, only bullous pemphigoid is not potentially fatal. Bullous pemphigoid is most commonly seen in the elderly and is characterized by large tense bullae, usually localized to one area of the body but sometimes becoming more generalized. Petechiae are an ominous sign in the setting of meningococcemia, a disease characterized by a rapidly progressive overwhelming sepsis. Stevens-Johnson syndrome, toxic epidermal necrolysis, and pemphigus vulgaris are all potentially fatal because large areas of denuded skin can cause hypothermia, fluid loss, electrolyte imbalance, and infection. Treatment consists of removal of offending agents and supportive care similar to that for second-degree burns. Pemphigus vulgaris is thought to be an autoimmune disorder and can be treated with corticosteroids, gold salts, immunosuppressants, and plasmapheresis. *(Emergency Medicine, Chapter 86, pp 877–887)*

10.e. See answer to question 13. All of the answers correctly describe erythema multiforme, except answer e, which better describes the lesions associated with erythema nodosum. The lesions of erythema multiforme may be found on the skin anywhere on the body, with or without superficial erosions of the mucous membrane. *(Emergency Medicine, Chapter 86, pp 877–887)*

11.c. Erythema nodosum is a characteristic tender nodule found most commonly in the pretibial region. Although the lesions are characteristic, multiple etiologies have been identified. Etiologies include infections (tuberculosis, *Streptococcus*, fungal diseases, leptospirosis), collagen vascular diseases (sarcoid), pregnancy, oncologic diseases (acute and chronic leukemia), inflammatory bowel disease, and medication. The most common medication is oral contraceptives, yet all the drugs listed may cause erythema nodosum.[1] *(Emergency Medicine, Chapter 86, pp 877–887)*

12.d. Urticaria is subclassified into acute and chronic forms. Individual lesions last for less than 24 hours. Eruptions may be localized or may become generalized. Management includes avoiding the offending agent and treatment with antihistamines and systemic steroids. Urticarial lesions are usually itchy but may be painful on the palms and soles.[1] *(Emergency Medicine, Chapter 86, pp 877–887)*

13.a. Erythema multiforme eruptions may be macular, papular, vesicular, bullous, urticarial, or purpuric. The most common appearance is target or iris-shaped lesions. Erythema multiforme involves the skin and occasionally the mucous membranes. It is managed by treating the underlying cause and by administration of antihistamines. In more severe cases (Stevens-Johnson, with severe mucous membrane involvement), treatment includes fluid replacement and skin care. There are multiple etiologies, including infections, medications, collagen vascular disease, and malignancy. Toxic shock syndrome is not related to erythema multiforme.[1] *(Emergency Medicine, Chapter 86, pp 877–887)*

14.a. The lesions of lichen planus are found on the flexor surfaces of the wrists and forearm. Senile purpura is most commonly found on the extensor surfaces. Leukoclastic vasculitis is found on the legs and feet. Pityriasis rosea is a rash consisting of pink to salmon-colored oval papules, classically described as having a fine collarette of scale. It is commonly found on the trunk, along the lines of skin cleavage in a "Christmas tree" pattern. A single "herald patch" consisting of a larger lesion that preceded the eruption may be identified. Epidermal cysts are commonly found on face, scalp, neck, and trunk. *(Emergency Medicine, Chapter 86, pp 877–887)*

15.d. Pruritic urticarial papules and plaques of pregnancy commonly occurs during the third trimester, is not likely to recur, and starts on the abdomen and spreads to the buttocks, thighs, arms, and lower legs. Treatment includes emollients, topical steroids, antihistamines, and systemic steroids. Papules form urticarial-type plaques and are very pruritic. *(Emergency Medicine, Chapter 86, pp 877–887)*

16.d. Erythema toxicum neonatorum is a rash that may have a variety of presentations, including macules, papules, pustules, and occasionally erythema. It begins on the third or fourth day of life, is not associated with fever or systemic symptoms, and resolves spontaneously. There is no specific treatment except skin care and cleansing. The etiology is presumed viral, yet no specific virus has been identified. *(Emergency Medicine, Chapter 86, pp 877–887)*

REFERENCE

1. Arnold HL Jr, Odom RB, James WD: Andrew's Diseases of the Skin: Clinical Dermatology, 8th ed. Philadelphia, WB Saunders, 1990.

BIBLIOGRAPHY

Henry J, Paganussi PJ: Approach to rashes. *In* Howell JM, Altieri M, Jagoda AS, et al (eds): Emergency Medicine. Philadelphia, WB Saunders, 1998, pp 869–871.

Henry J, Paganussi PJ: Dermatitis and eczema. *In* Howell JM, Altieri M, Jagoda AS, et al (eds): Emergency Medicine. Philadelphia, WB Saunders, 1998, pp 872–876.

Henry J, Paganussi PJ: Maculopapular, nodular, erythematous, and vesiculobullous skin lesions. *In* Howell JM, Altieri M, Jagoda AS, et al (eds): Emergency Medicine. Philadelphia, WB Saunders, 1998, pp 877–887.

41 Infections and Infestations, Skin Cancer, and Cutaneous Manifestations of Illness

DAVID L. LEVINE, MD

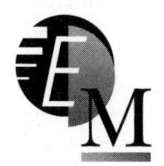

1. Hutchinson's sign is:
   a. Grouped vesicles on the nose
   b. Gray purpura
   c. A ring-like raised rash
   d. One finding associated with gonococcemia
   e. Classically located on the palms and soles

2. The causative agent of erythrasma is:
   a. *Corynebacterium minutissimum*
   b. Group A beta-hemolytic streptococcus
   c. *Pseudomonas*
   d. *Staphylococcus aureus*
   e. Viral

3. Which of the following statements is true?
   a. Pediculosis capitis affects primarily adults.
   b. Maculae ceruleae are small red macules that itch.
   c. Permethrin cream may cause renal toxicity in children.
   d. Lice in the eyelashes of children may be a sign of sexual abuse.
   e. Permethrin treatment for pediculosis capitis must be repeated in 1 week.

4. Which of the following is incorrect about Lyme disease?
   a. The etiologic agent is *Rickettsia rickettsii*.
   b. The classic manifestation is erythema chronicum migrans.
   c. Treatment of early disease is with doxycycline.
   d. It may progress to arthritis or meningitis.
   e. Constitutional symptoms may be part of early presentations.

5. The most common type of skin cancer is:
   a. Adenocarcinoma
   b. Basal cell carcinoma
   c. Melanoma
   d. Squamous cell
   e. Kaposi's sarcoma

6. Which of the following is not a risk factor for melanoma?
   a. Atypical moles
   b. Light hair
   c. Family history
   d. Previous burn or scar
   e. Sunburn during childhood

7. The single most common drug reaction is:
   a. Erythema multiforme
   b. Erythema nodosum
   c. Fixed drug eruption
   d. Lichenoid reaction
   e. Morbilliform reaction

8. Which of the following is incorrect concerning thrombotic thrombocytopenic purpura?
   a. Hemolytic anemia is a characteristic.
   b. Renal abnormalities are common.
   c. Fever is common.
   d. Physical examination often includes ecchymosis, jaundice, and pale mucous membranes.
   e. Systemic steroids is treatment of choice.

9. Erythema marginatum is the characteristic rash of:
   a. Reiter's syndrome
   b. Rheumatic fever
   c. Sarcoid
   d. Dermatomyositis
   e. Lyme disease

10. Elements of CREST syndrome include all of the following except:
    a. Cardiomegaly
    b. Raynaud's phenomenon
    c. Esophageal dysmotility
    d. Sclerodactyly
    e. Telangiectasis

11. Which of the following drugs cause a phototoxic reaction?
    a. Heparin
    b. Narcotics
    c. Penicillin
    d. Barbiturates
    e. Sulfonamides

12. Which of the following is true of Kawasaki's disease?
    a. Patients are typically between 5 and 10 years old.
    b. A serious complication is coronary artery aneurysm.
    c. Treatment includes high-dose systemic steroids.
    d. A major diagnostic criteria is thrombocytopenia.
    e. The test of choice for diagnosis is chest radiography.

13. All of the following statements about impetigo are true except:
    a. It is caused by group A beta-hemolytic streptococcus and/or *Staphylococcus aureus*.
    b. It commonly occurs on the face.
    c. Eruption begins with erythematous macules that develop into vesicles or bullae that rupture with yellow crust.
    d. Prompt treatment prevents complication of acute glomerulonephritis.
    e. It most commonly occurs in childhood.

14. All of the following are true of erysipelas except:
    a. It is an acute cellulitis involving superficial dermis.
    b. Vesiculation may be present.
    c. The most common etiologic agent is *Streptococcus pyogenes*.
    d. The face is affected most often.
    e. Treatment is with topical and systemic antimicrobials.

15. Many children complain of a pruritic rash on their trunk, buttocks, and axillae after swimming at a camp outing. Which of the following is true?
    a. They most likely have a contact dermatitis from poison ivy.
    b. Treatment consists of acetic acid compresses.
    c. Treatment consists of systemic corticosteroids.
    d. The etiologic agent is *Streptococcus*.
    e. The etiologic agent is an insect.

Answers

1.a. Hutchinson's sign is grouped vesicles on the nose. It is highly suggestive of herpes zoster of the eye from involvement of the nasociliary branch of the ophthalmic nerve. Ophthalmologic consultation is mandatory if ophthalmic involvement is suspected.[1] *(Emergency Medicine, Chapter 87, pp 888–895)*

2.a. Erythrasma is a dry brown, scaly, patchy eruption commonly found in the crural and groin region, axillae, and toe web spaces. It is caused by *Corynebacterium minutissimum*. It is usually asymptomatic, except for itching in the groin. Treatment consists of erythromycin for 1 week. *(Emergency Medicine, Chapter 87, pp 888–895)*

3.d. Pediculosis capitis primarily affects children but may affect adults. Maculae ceruleae are asymptomatic blue macular lesions thought to be caused by the saliva of fleas or lice. Lindane causes CNS toxicity in young children and should therefore be avoided. Permethrin cream is safe in children. Permethrin should be repeated in 2 weeks for pediculosis capitis (to treat the eggs that hatch after the first treatment). Lice in the eyelashes of children may be a sign of sexual abuse. It is uncommon for lice to manifest primarily in the eyelashes of children, and transmission from the genital region in a sexual encounter should be considered.[1] *(Emergency Medicine, Chapter 87, pp 888–895)*

4.a. Lyme disease is caused by the spirochete *Borrelia burgdorferi*. The vector is the deer tick *(Ixodes)*. Treatment of early disease is 3 weeks of doxycycline. Alternative agents (for children, who should not be treated with doxycycline) include amoxicillin and cefuroxime. Ceftriaxone should be used for Lyme arthritis and neurologic involvement. *(Emergency Medicine, Chapter 87, pp 888–895)*

5.b. Basal cell carcinoma is the most common type of skin cancer but is also the least invasive. Its appearance is waxy nodules with rolled-up edges, often with fine telangiectasia overlying. Squamous cell carcinoma is less common but tends to be more invasive (especially when involving the lip or arising from a burn scar, chronic ulcer, or radiation dermatitis). Its appearance is discrete, hard, red, sometimes scaly nodules or plaques that may ulcerate.[1] Malignant melanoma is the least common (although incidence is increasing) yet the most invasive. Its appearance is commonly a lesion with an irregular border and variegated color, which may bleed. *(Emergency Medicine, Chapter 88, pp 896–910)*

6.d. Risk factors for melanoma include a history of blistering sunburn during childhood; large number of melanotic nevi; atypical mole syndrome; phenotype of light hair, skin, or eye color; tendency to freckle; and family history of melanoma. Burn or scarring is not a risk factor (except for sunburn that occurs during childhood). *(Emergency Medicine, Chapter 88, pp 896–910)*

7.e. The single most common drug reaction is the morbilliform eruption. *(Emergency Medicine, Chapter 88, pp 896–910)*

8.e. Plasmapheresis is the treatment of choice for thrombotic thrombocytopenic purpura. *(Emergency Medicine, Chapter 88, pp 896–910)*

9.b. Erythema marginatum is the characteristic rash of rheumatic fever. The rash seen in Reiter's syndrome consists of cutaneous vesicles and crusted painless pustules. Erythema nodosum may be associated with sarcoid. Dermatomyositis has a heliotrope rash. Lupus erythematosus has a butterfly malar rash. Erythema chronicum migrans is the classic rash associated with Lyme disease. *((Emergency Medicine, Chapter 87, pp 888–895; Chapter 88, pp 896–910)*

10.a. CREST syndrome includes the complex of calcinosis, Raynaud's phenomenon, esophageal dysmotility, sclerodactyly, and telangiectasis. *(Emergency Medicine, Chapter 88, pp 896–910)*

11.e. Phototoxic reactions may be caused by chlorpromazine, tetracycline, griseofulvin, naproxen, and sulfonamides. The most common reactions to heparin are alopecia, pruritus, or skin necrosis. Narcotics commonly cause erythema, fixed drug eruptions, morbilliform erythema, and urticaria. Penicillin reactions include anaphylaxis, angioedema, erythema multiforme, erythema nodosum, toxic epidermal necrolysis, and urticaria. Barbiturates may cause bullous skin lesions, erythema multiforme, exfoliative lesions, Stevens-Johnson syndrome, and toxic epidermal necrolysis. *(Emergency Medicine, Chapter 86, pp 877–887; Chapter 88, pp 896–910)*

12.b. Kawasaki's disease commonly affects children from infancy to 4 years old. Treatment includes high-dose salicylates and IV gamma globulin. Major criteria include unresponsive fever, conjunctival congestion, oropharyngeal changes, hand and foot erythema, polymorphous exanthem, and cervical lymphadenopathy. Chest radiography is not helpful in making the diagnosis. *(Emergency Medicine, Chapter 88, pp 896–910)*

13.d. Treatment of impetigo does not prevent the complication of glomerulonephritis, which presents after a latent period of 18 to 21 days. *(Emergency Medicine, Chapter 87, pp 888–895)*

14.c. Erysipelas is a cellulitis involving the superficial dermis. It is characterized by a warm, erythematous rash, with a well-demarcated raised border. There may occasionally be vesicles. The most common etiologic agent of erysipelas is group A beta-hemolytic streptococcus. Treatment is with penicillin or a first-generation cephalosporin. *(Emergency Medicine, Chapter 87, pp 888–895)*

15.b. The children most likely have "hot tub" or *Pseudomonas* folliculitis. This is usually a self-limited rash, caused by *Pseudomonas* found in contaminated pools or hot tubs. Treatment usually consists of acetic acid (Burow's solution) compresses but occasionally consists of systemic antibiotics for fever, headache, and otitis media. *(Emergency Medicine, Chapter 87, pp 888–895)*

REFERENCE

1. Arnold HL Jr, Odom RB, James WD: Andrews' Diseases of the Skin: Clinical Dermatology, 8th ed. Philadelphia, WB Saunders, 1990.

BIBLIOGRAPHY

Arndt KA, LeBoit PE, Robinson JK, et al: Cutaneous Medicine and Surgery. Philadelphia, WB Saunders, 1996.

Henry J, Paganussi PJ: Maculopapular, nodular, erythematous, and vesiculobullous skin lesions. *In* Howell JM, Altieri M, Jagoda AS, et al (eds): Emergency Medicine. Philadelphia, WB Saunders, 1998, pp 877–887.

Henry J, Paganussi PJ: Skin cancer and cutaneous manifestations of disease. *In* Howell JM, Altieri M, Jagoda AS, et al (eds): Emergency Medicine. Philadelphia, WB Saunders, 1998, pp 896–910.

Henry J, Paganussi PJ: Skin infections and infestations. *In* Howell JM, Altieri M, Jagoda AS, et al (eds): Emergency Medicine. Philadelphia, WB Saunders, 1998, pp 888–895.

SECTION THIRTEEN

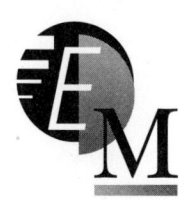

Behavioral Disorders and Substance Abuse

42 Approach to Delirium and Psychiatric Illness, Thought Disorder, and Suicide

LISA B. NAMEROW, MD   TAREG BEY, MD

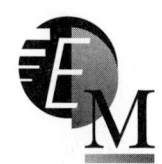

1. Psychosis may present with which of the following?
   a. Hallucinations, visual or auditory
   b. Delusions
   c. Agitation
   d. Combative behavior
   e. All of the above

2. Psychosis may be the result of all but which of the following illnesses?
   a. Schizophrenia
   b. Bipolar illness
   c. Alzheimer's dementia
   d. Parkinson's disease
   e. Cerebral palsy

3. A feature of delirium that distinguishes it from dementia is:
   a. Disorientation
   b. Its organic basis
   c. Changes in sensorium
   d. Memory loss
   e. Psychotic features

4. A combative, agitated psychiatric patient in the prehospital setting is likely to need all of the following except:
   a. A show of force by law enforcement personnel
   b. A rapid assessment of the possibility of intoxication or overdose
   c. Rapid history taken from family, friends, or neighbors
   d. Verbal redirection and limit-setting by EMS personnel
   e. Physical restraint for transport

5. Any of the following findings on a mental status exam of a schizophrenic patient would suggest the need for acute hospitalization except:
   a. Catatonia with refusal to eat or drink
   b. Extreme guardedness
   c. Command auditory hallucinations with suicidal or homicidal content
   d. Noncompliance with medications
   e. Homelessness, poor social support

6. The differential diagnosis of a 48-year-old white male with no previous psychiatric history who presents with acute onset of visual hallucinations, combative behavior, disorientation, irritability, and paranoia would include all but which of the following?
   a. Schizophrenia
   b. Toxic encephalopathy
   c. Viral encephalopathy
   d. Delirium tremens
   e. Hyperthyroidism

7. Haloperidol (Haldol) is appropriate for the control of psychotic behavior in all but which of the following presentations?
   a. Bipolar illness, manic episode
   b. Schizophrenia
   c. Cocaine overdose
   d. Tricyclic antidepressant overdose
   e. LSD intoxication

8. In an 8-year-old with chicken pox who presents with confusion and visual hallucinations, one must consider all but which of the following?
   a. Use of Caladryl (calamine and Benadryl)
   b. Antihistamine ingestion
   c. Varicella encephalitis
   d. Schizophrenia, first episode
   e. Fever delirium

9. Causes of hallucinations in children younger than 10 years old may include:
   a. Developmental language disorder
   b. Cognitive impairment
   c. Age-appropriate finding
   d. Schizophrenia
   e. All of the above

10. All of the following are antipsychotic medications except:
    a. Olanzapine (Zyprexa)
    b. Risperidone (Risperdal)
    c. Clozapine (Clozaril)
    d. Venlafaxine (Effexor)
    e. Molindone (Moban)

11. All of the following are true about the newer antipsychotic medications except:
    a. Decreased tendency to cause dyskinesia
    b. Decreased potential for orthostatic hypotension
    c. Increased potential to cause leukopenia
    d. Decreased potential for causing extrapyramidal symptoms
    e. Increased effect on reducing negative symptoms

12. All but which of the following characteristics of a patient with schizophrenia may interfere with his or her ability to give a medical history in the ED?
    a. Presence of paranoia
    b. Flat affect
    c. Presence of delusions
    d. Presence of confusion and disorientation
    e. Presence of disorganized thinking

13. An irritable mood may be characteristic of which of the following illnesses?
    a. Bipolar illness
    b. Dysthymia
    c. Major depressive disorder
    d. Hypothyroidism or hyperthyroidism
    e. All of the above

14. All of the following statments about patients with anxiety disorders are true except:
    a. They often present to the ED with numerous somatic complaints.
    b. Their anxiety is often reduced by negative medical findings and reassurance.
    c. They can present with cardiac symptoms resembling a heart attack.
    d. Their anxiety usually responds to alprazolam (Xanax) or lorazepam (Ativan) in the ED, but these should be used only if there is no previous history of substance dependence.

15. Patients with post-traumatic stress disorder or acute stress disorder may present with all but which of the following?
    a. Agitation
    b. Flashbacks
    c. Insomnia
    d. Delusions
    e. Depression

16. Patients with narcissistic, borderline, or histrionic personality disorders are often difficult to treat in the ED because of their:
    a. Desire for attention
    b. Tendency to exaggerate
    c. Tendency to devalue
    d. Tendency to become easily offended
    e. All of the above

17. Patients with narcissistic, borderline, or histrionic personality disorders are best handled in the ED by:
    a. Spending as much time as possible with them
    b. Being direct, personable, and friendly
    c. Extensively evaluating each somatic complaint
    d. Getting as many staff involved as possible
    e. Responding to their rage with minimal affect

18. Schizoid and schizotypal individuals can be differentiated from schizophrenics because of their:
    a. Ease of relatedness
    b. Lack of oddities of thought
    c. Lack of delusions and hallucinations
    d. Lack of blunted affect
    e. Less-agitated presentation

19. The best indicator of potential violence in the ED is:
    a. History of schizophrenia
    b. History of anxiety disorder
    c. History of histrionic or borderline personality disorder
    d. History of prior assaultive behavior
    e. All of the above

20. Identified risk factors for an individual's potential for suicide include:
    a. The presence of an underlying psychiatric illness
    b. A history of a prior suicide attempt
    c. Access to firearms
    d. Intoxication
    e. All of the above

21. The age group with the highest prevalence of completed suicide is:
    a. 1 to 14 years
    b. 15 to 24 years
    c. 25 to 49 years
    d. 50 to 65 years
    e. Over 65 years

22. When assessing safety in the suicidal patient, all of the following might allow disposition to home except:
    a. A verbal commitment to safety by the patient
    b. A contract between the psychiatrist and the patient for outpatient follow-up
    c. Strong family support and the ability to provide one-to-one monitoring
    d. Expression of suicidal intent while intoxicated
    e. No prior history of suicide attempt

23. All of the following statements about the management of psychotic and violent patients are true except:
    a. To safely restrain a violent and combative patient, at least three people are required.
    b. An ED needs an organized plan for dealing with violent patients.
    c. Restraining orders must be documented in writing and must indicate the length of the order and the reason the restraints were ordered.
    d. A calm, nonaggressive, and nonjudgmental approach often helps to pacify the violent patient.
    e. The restrained patient should be searched for weapons, drugs, and identification.

24. All of the following statements are true when clinically evaluating the violent and agitated patient except:

a. Some patients need early antipsychotic medication in order to facilitate adequate evaluation.
b. Normal functioning prior to the first psychotic break indicates a psychiatric rather than a medical cause.
c. Dilated pupils may indicate amphetamine, cocaine, or atropine use.
d. EMS, police, and relatives often have important clues for etiology of the psychosis, especially when the patient is uncooperative.
e. A rigid neck may be caused by meningitis, subarachnoid bleed, or extrapyramidal side effect of antipsychotic drugs.

25. Which test is the least helpful in identifying the cause of psychosis?
    a. Serum sodium, calcium, magnesium
    b. ABG
    c. WBC count
    d. Serum glucose
    e. Urine drug of abuse screen

26. Which of the following statements about delirium is true?
    a. Withdrawal of a substance of abuse can cause delirium.
    b. Delirium can be produced by infections, endocrinopathies, and metabolic disturbances.
    c. Increased age and preexisting brain damage predispose to delirium.
    d. Fluctuation of the sensorium is the hallmark of delirium.
    e. All of the above are true.

27. All of the following statements about schizophrenia are true except:
    a. Schizophrenia cannot be confirmed by laboratory or radiographic findings.
    b. Schizophrenia usually has a gradual onset.
    c. Major depression can present with psychotic features.
    d. Schizophrenia responds well to psychotherapy.
    e. Besides schizophrenia, other causes of acute psychosis include mania, bipolar disorders, and cyclothymic personality disorders.

28. Which patients are least likely to have an impaired minimental status examination?
    a. Patients on amphetamine overdose
    b. Patients with alcohol withdrawal with delirium
    c. Patients with schizophrenia and depression
    d. Patients with meningitis
    e. Patients with epidural hematoma

Answers

1.e. Psychosis is an acute disturbance of thought process resulting in a thought disorder. When thinking is impaired, a patient might present with any of the symptoms noted above as well as extreme guardedness, disorientation, magical thinking, and ideas of reference. It is an uncomfortable mental state resulting in much anxiety and can be caused by both medical and psychiatric illness. *(Emergency Medicine, Chapter 89, pp 911–916)*

2.e. Cerebral palsy is a *static* encephalopathy not prone to exacerbations or disturbances of thought. Both Alzheimer's and Parkinson's diseases may result in dementia severe enough to induce a psychosis. *(Emergency Medicine, Chapter 89, pp 911–916)*

3.c. Classically, the one feature best distinguishing dementia (a progressive deterioration of cognitive processing) from delirium is that the findings of delirium occur rapidly, usually within a 24-hour period. Dementia is usually associated with a global decrease in intellectual functioning, and there is usually no severe clouding of the sensorium. *(Emergency Medicine, Chapter 89, pp 911–916)*

4.d. Although calm, soothing verbal redirection may help some psychiatric patients, most combative psychotic patients will find verbal limit-setting threatening and become more agitated and paranoid. Minimal verbal intervention could be used along with a show of force to ensure the safety of the patient and others. *(Emergency Medicine, Chapter 89, pp 911–916)*

5.e. Although homelessness and poor social support are poor prognostic indicators overall, in the era of managed care and limited resources this is usually not an indication for acute hospitalization. Extreme guardedness (refusal to answer questions concerning safety), catatonia (especially with refusal to speak, eat or drink), and command hallucinations all indicate a danger to self or others and warrant hospitalization. *(Emergency Medicine, Chapter 89, pp 911–916)*

6.a. The lack of prior psychiatric history and the presence of more "organic" psychotic features (visual hallucinations, disorientation) would suggest an organic rather than psychiatric illness. *(Emergency Medicine, Chapter 89, pp 911–916)*

7.d. Haloperidol (Haldol) has its own anticholinergic effects and should not be used if an anticholinergic delirium is suspected. *(Emergency Medicine, Chapter 89, pp 911–916)*

8.d. Schizophrenia is extremely rare in children younger than 10 years and would present with auditory hallucinations, delusions, and agitation. *(Emergency Medicine, Chapter 89, pp 911–916)*

9.e. Hallucinations may not indicate true psychiatric illness in childhood and should be evaluated within the context of the history and mental status examination. *(Emergency Medicine, Chapter 89, pp 911–916)*

10.d. Effexor, a new non-selective sertonin-reuptake inhibitor antidepressant, is not considered an antipsychotic. The rest of the agents listed antagonize dopamine receptors, thus providing antipsychotic activity. *(Emergency Medicine, Chapters 91–93, pp 926–957)*

11.b. The new antipsychotics (clozapine [Clozaril], risperidone [Risperdal], olanzapine), which have a lower side effect profile, are being marketed as having decreased potential for tardive dyskinesia and extrapyramidal symptoms and increased potential for reducing negative symptoms. Clozapine, however, can induce leukopenia, and all can induce orthostatic hypotension and tachycardia. *(Emergency Medicine, Chapters 91–93, pp 926–957)*

12.d. Schizophrenia does not induce confusion or disorientation. If present on mental status examination, one must consider an organic psychosis or intoxication (intentional or medication related). *(Emergency Medicine, Chapters 91–93, pp 926–957)*

13.e. An irritable mood may be present in all the conditions listed. A more complete history and mental status examination as well as routine thyroid function tests will help delineate these conditions. *(Emergency Medicine, Chapters 91–93, pp 926–957)*

14.b. Negative findings and verbal reassurance rarely reduce anxiety when it is caused by a psychiatric disorder. In fact, it may send the patient "doctor shopping" until the "true cause" is determined. *(Emergency Medicine, Chapters 91–93, pp 926–957)*

15.d. Delusions are not a finding in post-traumatic stress disorder or acute stress disorder, although a traumatic event may induce a brief reactive psychosis and must be considered as part of the differential diagnosis. Rarely, patients describing flashbacks seem delusional or hallucinatory but in fact are reliving prior traumatic events. *(Emergency Medicine, Chapters 91–93, pp 926–957)*

16.e. These individuals can be extremely difficult, and their characteristic behavior needs to be recognized early and limited. *(Emergency Medicine, Chapters 91–93, pp 926–957)*

17.e. These individuals crave attention and can characteristically "split" staff if too many caretakers get involved. The best approach is to be professional and empathetic, with minimal show of affect, to help limit their chief complaint. *(Emergency Medicine, Chapters 91–93, pp 926–957)*

18.c. Although odd and often withdrawn with poor relatedness and bizarre ideas, these individuals do not show "positive" symptoms of schizophrenia, such as hallucinations or delusions. They may, like other psychotic patients, become easily agitated and paranoid. *(Emergency Medicine, Chapters 91–93, pp 926–957)*

19.d. Only a prior history of assaultive behavior is a known prognostic indicator of violent potential. Psychiatric illness per se is not a prognostic indicator. *(Emergency Medicine, Chapter 91, pp 926–937)*

20.e. Research shows all of these to be risk factors. Access to firearms and intoxication are the greatest risk factors among males; history of psychiatric illness is greatest among females; and a history of previous suicide attempt is common in both males and females. The suicide rates in elderly men are the highest. *(Emergency Medicine, Chapter 90, pp 917–925)*

21.e. Males are much more likely to complete suicide over age 65 than at any other time of life, usually selecting highly effective methods. Although there has been a significant increase in the suicide rate, especially in the 15- to 24-year-old age group, suicide is far more prevalent in elderly patients. *(Emergency Medicine, Chapter 90, pp 917–925)*

22.d. Intoxicated patients or those under the influence of drugs frequently express suicidal ideation that resolves after the effects of the intoxication disappear. Appropriate management includes securing the patient until the effects of the intoxication are negligible, at which time the patient should be reevaluated. The fact that the patient expressed suicidal thoughts while intoxicated should not be reassuring as the patient in fact may be suicidal. The tenet of managing the suicidal patient is "if in doubt, admit." Ensuring the safety of a potentially suicidal patient is one of the most important goals of initial management. Disposition to home has inherent risks that can be ameliorated to some extent by a number of factors. *(Emergency Medicine, Chapter 90, pp 917–925)*

23.a. The violent and psychotic patient is a special challenge for the ED. An organic cause including drug abuse has to be excluded in the initial assessment of any violent patient. Each ED needs an organized plan when dealing with a violent or armed patient. These patients are a potential threat to the health care personnel. In order to protect the medical staff and other patients, professional security personnel should be summoned when dealing with the threatening individual. Restraining orders require exact documentation including the vital signs. To safely restrain an agitated patient, five persons are recommended: four for the extremities and one person for the head and airway. *(Emergency Medicine, Chapter 89, pp 911–916)*

24.b. Normal functioning before the patient's first psychotic break should prompt a medical evaluation. A psychiatric diagnosis is a diagnosis of exclusion. Sympathomimetics (cocaine, amphetamines) and anticholinergics can cause psychosis and dilated pupils. A rigid neck in a psychotic patient can be caused by CNS infection or an intracranial bleed. Antipsychotic medications such as butyrophenones can also cause a stiff neck and temperature elevation. *(Emergency Medicine, Chapter 89, pp 911–916)*

25.c. Electrolyte and glucose derangements can cause psychosis. A urine drug of abuse screen is helpful in the evaluation of illicit drug abuse. Typically, the WBC is of little use in defining the cause of psychosis. *(Emergency Medicine, Chapter 89, pp 911–916)*

26.e. Fluctuation of the sensorium is the hallmark of delirium. Age and prior brain damage predispose to delirium. The underlying cause of delirium must be recognized and treated. The differential diagnosis includes infectious etiology and structural-anatomic and toxic-metabolic causes. *(Emergency Medicine, Chapter 89, pp 911–916)*

27.d. By definition, schizophrenia can be diagnosed only after all organic causes have been excluded. The onset is usually gradual, with onset during late adolescence, but late first manifestations have been described as well. Schizophrenia is not a neurotic disorder and does not respond to psychotherapy; medication, such as butyrophenones, is required to control symptoms. Major depressions can manifest with psychotic features, and it may be difficult to establish the correct diagnosis. *(Emergency Medicine, Chapter 89, pp 911–916)*

28.c. A basic mental status examination includes questions about person, time, and place; current events; and famous people (e.g., the President). Patients with infectious diseases, toxic-metabolic abnormalities, or structural diseases of the brain usually have impaired memory and poor cognition and are disoriented. The patient with schizophrenia maintains good memory and is well oriented but has fixed hallucinations and a lack of insight. *(Emergency Medicine, Chapter 89, pp 911–916)*

BIBLIOGRAPHY

Frame S: Approach to delirium and psychiatric illness. *In* Howell JM, Altieri M, Jagoda AS, et al (eds): Emergency Medicine. Philadelphia, WB Saunders, 1998, pp 911–916.

Gharda-Ward S, Charda-Ward G: *In* Howell JM, Altieri M, Jagoda AS, et al (eds): Emergency Medicine. Philadelphia, WB Saunders, 1998, pp 926–937.

Griepp AEZ, Stern R, Hubeishy K, et al: *In* Howell JM, Altieri M, Jagoda AS, et al (eds): Emergency Medicine. Philadelphia, WB Saunders, 1998, pp 947–957.

Griepp AEZ, Warren C, Williams T, et al: *In* Howell JM, Altieri M, Jagoda AS, et al (eds): Emergency Medicine. Philadelphia, WB Saunders, 1998, pp 938–946.

Lane C: Suicide. *In* Howell JM, Altieri M, Jagoda AS, et al (eds): Emergency Medicine. Philadelphia, WB Saunders, 1998, pp 917–925.

43 Substance Abuse, Addiction, and Withdrawal

LISA B. NAMEROW, MD   TAREG BEY, MD

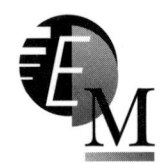

1. The following are recommended procedures in the assessment and stabilization of a patient suspected of having an alcohol or drug overdose except:
   a. Thiamine, 100 mg IV or IM
   b. Naloxone, 0.04–1.2 mg IV
   c. Restraints to facilitate the evaluation and treatment of the intoxicated patient
   d. Activated charcoal as the decontamination agent for the conscious patient
   e. A search for the cause of an abnormal level of consciousness to exclude head injury, vascular events, intoxications and metabolic etiologies

2. Which of the following statements is true concerning alcohol or drug use?
   a. Cocaine is often taken with other drugs.
   b. CAGE questions are helpful to quickly screen for occult alcohol use.
   c. A bundle is about 10 bags of heroin and a considerable habit if used daily.
   d. Being nonjudgmental in taking an alcohol/substance abuse history is more likely to elicit honest answers.
   e. All of the above are true.

3. Among the substances below, which is most highly associated with obstetric complications?
   a. Heroin
   b. Alcohol
   c. Cocaine
   d. Benzodiazepines
   e. Cannabinoids

4. Which of the following is true?
   a. Marijuana is the most commonly used illegal drug.
   b. Women are more likely to use heroin and cocaine than men.
   c. More blacks than whites use illicit drugs.
   d. Socially illicit drug use is not unrelated to poor scholastic achievement.
   e. None of the above are true.

5. Which of the following is thought to act by blocking dopamine reuptake?
   a. Benzodiazepines
   b. Cocaine
   c. Alcohol
   d. Heroin
   e. LSD

6. How long after usage can cannabis be detected in the urine?
   a. 2 to 5 days
   b. 1 to 2 days
   c. 7 to 9 days
   d. 10 to 14 days
   e. 14 to 43 days

7. Which of the following statements concerning the management of alcohol or substance abuse withdrawal is incorrect?
   a. IV benzodiazepines may be necessary for severe withdrawal from alcohol.
   b. Long-acting benzodiazepines are usually used in treating benzodiazepine withdrawal.
   c. Clonidine and guanabenz can be used for opioid withdrawal.
   d. Opioids are necessary to manage abdominal cramping in heroin withdrawal.
   e. Motrin can be used to treat the abdominal cramping associated with heroin withdrawal.

8. All of the following are true about the management of the intoxicated patient except:
   a. Patients who appear intoxicated should be asked directly about alcohol and drug abuse.
   b. Alcohol and drug abusers are at high risk for trauma.
   c. Patients may continue to consume drugs while in the ED.
   d. Unconscious patients with suspected opioid dependence should initially receive 2.0 mg naloxone as a part of the "coma cocktail."
   e. Unconscious patients should receive thiamine before dextrose when being given the "coma protocol."

9. Which of the following is not part of the "coma protocol" that is used to treat the unconscious patient?

a. Naloxone
  b. Dextrose
  c. Flumazenil
  d. Oxygen
  e. Thiamine

10. Typical clinical presentations associated with cocaine use include all of the following except:
  a. Excoriated areas of skin
  b. Chest pain
  c. Pneumothorax and pneumomediastinum
  d. Premature rupture of membranes and abruptio placentae
  e. Vertical, horizontal, and rotary nystagmus

11. All of the following are true about withdrawal except:
  a. Benzodiazepine tapering may be more difficult in alprazolam withdrawal if the drug is replaced by a longer-acting benzodiazepine.
  b. Clonidine and guanabenz are useful in the management of opioid withdrawal.
  c. Alcohol withdrawal can be life-threatening.
  d. For patients who do not participate in a methadone program, it is necessary to give at least 50 mg methadone to prevent opioid withdrawal.
  e. Cannabis intoxication or withdrawal is mild and requires no specific treatment.

12. A young patient with an altered mental status presents to the ED. Which statement concerning drug screening is incorrect?
  a. He has a positive Breathalyzer reading for alcohol; therefore, a urine toxicology screen for drugs of abuse can be omitted.
  b. Up to about 35% of patients presenting to psychiatric ED test positive for at least one substance of abuse.
  c. If the blood alcohol level is high and the patient does not seem to be very intoxicated, tolerance can be presumed.
  d. The ECG is an important tool in evaluating patients with cocaine-induced chest pain.
  e. Designer drugs and fentanyl may be missed on the routine urine toxicology screens.

13. All of the following statements are true about the management of withdrawal from alcohol and sedative-hypnotics except:
  a. IV benzodiazepines may be necessary for severe alcohol withdrawal symptoms.
  b. Although opioid withdrawal symptoms are usually life-threatening, sedative-hypnotic withdrawal is not.
  c. Indicators of high-risk alcohol withdrawal delirium include decreased serum electrolyte concentrations, elevated alanine aminotransferase, ataxia, and polyneuropathy.
  d. Phenobarbital can be used to treat both alcohol and benzodiazepine withdrawal.
  e. Beta-blockers are effective to control peripheral withdrawal symptoms but are not useful to control seizures or delirium.

14. Which of the following parts of the history should be elicited in a drug- or alcohol-dependent patient?
  a. Amounts of alcohol/drugs used
  b. Means of obtaining money for drug use
  c. Family history of drug use
  d. Past periods of abstinence
  e. All of the above

15. Treatment options for drugs of abuse include all of the following except:
  a. To treat alcohol withdrawal symptoms, it may be necessary to start with 10 to 40 mg diazepam daily.
  b. The IM absorption of diazepam is excellent.
  c. A patient in delirium tremens should be admitted to an ICU setting if physiologic symptoms do not stabilize.
  d. 50 to 200 mg chlordiazepoxide per day is an adequate starting dose for alcohol withdrawal.
  e. Doses of lorazepam of 12 mg per day or more may be needed for the initial management of severe alcohol withdrawal.

16. An unconscious 24-year-old woman is brought to the ED. Her parents state she took "a handful of unknown pills." Which of the following statements is true?
  a. After addressing the ABCs, the patient should receive dextrose, oxygen, naloxone, and thiamine (DONT protocol).
  b. The serum toxicology test should at least contain acetaminophen, aspirin, and alcohol. A pregnancy test should also be included.
  c. An ECG may be helpful in searching for a tricyclic antidepressant overdose.
  d. If all metabolic and toxicology tests remain negative, a head CT and lumbar puncture should be considered.
  e. All of the above are true.

Answers

1.c. Restraints should be used only when a patient's agitation, aggressiveness, or wandering endangers himself or others. Restraints can also allow staff to perform an expeditious medical evaluation as needed. (*Emergency Medicine, Chapter 94, pp 958–972*)

2.e. All are true. The CAGE questions screen for possible alcohol problems. They are:
  1. Have you ever felt that you ought to *C*ut down on your drinking?
  2. Have people *A*nnoyed you by criticizing your drinking?
  3. Have you ever felt *G*uilty about your drinking?
  4. Have you ever had a drink first thing in the morning as an *E*ye-opener?

A positive answer to two or more of these questions suggests an alcohol problem exists, and further evaluation should be performed. (*Emergency Medicine, Chapter 94, pp 958–972*)

3.c. Cocaine is associated with more obstetric complications than the other substances listed, including premature rupture of membranes, abruption, microcephaly, and intrauterine growth retardation. *(Emergency Medicine, Chapter 94, pp 958–972)*

4.a. Although the National Household Survey noted a general decrease in the total number of substance abusers from 1979 to 1992, hallucinogen use in high school students has increased since 1992. Marijuana is the most commonly used illicit drug. *(Emergency Medicine, Chapter 94, pp 958–972)*

5.b. Cocaine is thought to cause euphoria and paranoia alike by blocking dopamine reuptake, which may make dopamine more available at dopaminergic synapses. *(Emergency Medicine, Chapter 94, pp 958–972)*

6.e. Although it is unclear how long traces of tetrahydrocannabinol can be detected in the urine with only occasional use, frequent use can be detected for 2 to 7 weeks after discontinuing the drug. *(Emergency Medicine, Chapter 94, pp 958–972)*

7.d. Nonsteroidal anti-inflammatory medications can be used to abate the abdominal cramping that is associated with heroin withdrawal. *(Emergency Medicine, Chapter 94, pp 958–972)*

8.d. A physician should address frankly the possibility of illicit drug abuse and alcohol abuse in a patient with an altered mental status. It may be helpful to direct the diagnostic and therapeutic intervention, but the patient's history may not be accurate or complete. The ED staff should be aware of the possibility of continuous drug abuse while the patient is in the ED. Some patients or their friends may bring drugs of abuse to the hospital and consume those substances while being left alone or waiting. In an unconscious patient with suspected opioid dependence, some clinicians favor starting naloxone at doses between 0.4 mg and 1.2 mg to avoid severe withdrawal symptoms. Thiamine should be started before or immediately after dextrose to prevent Wernicke's encephalopathy. *(Emergency Medicine, Chapter 94, pp 958–972)*

9.c. The "coma protocol" is applied to patients with an altered mental status or a seizure. It consists of dextrose, oxygen, naloxone, and thiamine, also known as the DONT protocol. Thiamine should be given before dextrose. Flumazenil is not routinely recommended to reverse an altered mental status. It can precipitate a seizure in benzodiazepine-dependent patients or in patients with a mixed benzodiazepine–tricyclic antidepressant overdose. *(Emergency Medicine, Chapter 94, pp 958–972)*

10.e. Cocaine use is associated with cardiovascular and CNS stimulation. The clinical effects are numerous and are not always predictable. Cocaine has been associated with MI, pneumothorax through forceful inhalation, and multiple obstetric problems. Excoriated skin areas are a result of skin picking. Vertical, horizontal, and rotatory nystagmus is more typical for phencyclidine than for cocaine. *(Emergency Medicine, Chapter 94, pp 958–972)*

11.d. Clonidine and guanabenz are medications that prevent the sympathetic effects of opioid withdrawal. Alcohol and sedative-hypnotic withdrawal can be life-threatening and need medical treatment. Patients who are not on a methadone maintenance program seldom need more than 20 mg of methadone to prevent opioid withdrawal. *(Emergency Medicine, Chapter 94, pp 958–972)*

12.a. Even if the patient tests positive for alcohol in his blood, he may still have an altered mental status caused by another drug of abuse. The ECG is an important tool in evaluating patients with sympathomimetic drug intoxications. Chest pain, due to angina pectoris and AMI, is a frequent presenting complaint associated with the use of these drugs. Fentanyl, designer drugs, inhalants, and certain hallucinogens are not routinely tested for on urine toxicology screens for drugs of abuse. *(Emergency Medicine, Chapter 94, pp 958–972)*

13.b. Both benzodiazepines and barbiturates are commonly used to control alcohol or sedative-hypnotic withdrawal symptoms. Although alcohol or sedative-hypnotic withdrawal symptoms may be life-threatening, opioid withdrawal is usually not, the only exception being neonatal opioid withdrawal. Beta-blockers control the peripheral effects of withdrawal, such as tachycardia and tremors, but add little to the management of delirium and seizures. *(Emergency Medicine, Chapter 94, pp 958–972)*

14.e. Further questions should focus on route of administration, sequelae of drug and alcohol abuse, past treatment programs, and what types of drugs have been used. *(Emergency Medicine, Chapter 94, Table 94–2, p 960)*

15.b. Diazepam should be given either orally or IV; IM absorption is poor. On the other hand, lorazepam is well absorbed by the IM route. Physicians who treat patients for alcohol withdrawal should be familiar with the different dosing regimens of benzodiazepines and barbiturates, because different hospitals may keep different types of drugs on formulary. *(Emergency Medicine, Chapter 94, pp 958–972)*

16.e. In an unknown drug overdose, an acetaminophen and aspirin level should be determined because these are treatable coingestants that can be easily missed. All women of reproductive age, especially when unconscious, should have a pregnancy test. Although an alcohol level may help to determine whether alcohol intoxication is the reason for the change of mental status, a negative alcohol level should trigger further evaluation. In a patient with a negative metabolic-toxic evaluation, a further evaluation for structural-anatomic and infectious etiologies should be pursued. *(Emergency Medicine, Chapter 94, pp 958–972)*

BIBLIOGRAPHY

Baciewicz GJ, Griepp AEZ, Bamford KA, et al: Substance abuse. *In* Howell JM, Altieri M, Jagoda AS, et al (eds): Emergency Medicine. Philadelphia, WB Saunders, 1998, pp 958–972.

SECTION FOURTEEN

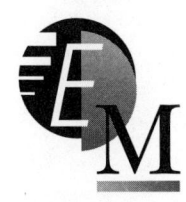

Trauma

SECTION FOURTEEN

44 Approach to Multiple Trauma and Spinal Trauma

YVETTE CALDERON, MD

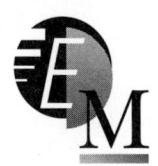

1. The Glasgow Coma Scale was designed to assess the mental status function of a patient with traumatic head injuries. The criteria used to assess this include all of the following except:
   a. Motor response
   b. Cognitive response
   c. Eye opening response
   d. Verbal response

2. The prehospital care for a hypotensive patient in a multicar accident includes all of the following except:
   a. Delay transport until IV access is secured
   b. During transport, attempt access and infuse lactated Ringer's solution
   c. Rapidly apply cervical spine immobilization prior to the transport of the patient
   d. Begin fluid resuscitation with the goal of establishing a low-normal blood pressure

3. Prehospital cervical spine immobilization:
   a. Uses a soft cervical collar and hard board for comfort and immobilization
   b. Ideally maintains cervical lordosis and alignment without rotation and distraction or compression
   c. Is adequate when each cervical level is limited to 25 degrees of motion
   d. Cannot protect spinal canal tissue from further damage

4. Military antishock trousers can be beneficial in which setting?
   a. To stabilize a pelvic fracture
   b. In a patient with a penetrating chest wound injury who is hypotensive
   c. Pulmonary contusion
   d. Stab wound to the neck with uncontrolled bleeding
   e. Suspected diaphragmatic rupture

5. All the following are true statements regarding the initial management of a patient with suspected spine trauma except:
   a. Spinal immobilization replaces compromised spinal column stability and protects spinal cord tissue from further damage.
   b. Proper immobilization requires semirigid cervical collar, sandbags, or foam blocks on each side of the head, and an entire head block unit taped to the backboard.
   c. Diagnostic studies are not indicated in patients with nonfocal neurologic exams and high-risk mechanisms.
   d. Patients with airway compromise can be intubated using rapid-sequence intubation and manual cervical immobilization.

6. A 27-year-old man presents to the ED after being involved in a high-speed motor vehicle accident. The patient has a pulse of 120, BP that is slightly decreased, and an RR of 34. The estimated amount of blood loss for this patient is:
   a. Up to 15%
   b. 15% to 30%
   c. 30% to 40%
   d. >40%
   e. <1 L

7. A 28-year-old male is brought into the ED after being ejected from his motorcycle. On primary survey, the patient was profoundly agitated and had sustained significant midface injuries. The best initial approach to managing this patient is:
   a. Placing a nasogastric tube to evaluate the abdominal injury
   b. Protecting his airway by blind nasotracheal intubation
   c. Obtaining cervical spine, chest, and pelvis films
   d. Obtaining airway control through strict in-line immobilization of the cervical spine and orotracheal intubation
   e. Giving low-flow oxygen

8. After the above patient was successfully intubated, a secondary survey was performed. During the initial resuscitation the patient was hemodynamically stable. However, before being sent to the CT scanner to evaluate a head injury, the patient became hypotensive. What is the best sequence of events?

a. Send the patient to the CT scanner
   b. Reevaluate the patient's airway and breathing
   c. Transfuse the patient with 4 units of type-specific blood
   d. Perform a diagnostic peritoneal lavage
   e. Call surgery consult

9. A 19-year-old female is brought into the ED after being struck by a car. The patient is only complaining of right lower leg pain over the site of an obvious tibia deformity. The following management decisions are acceptable except:
   a. Only a leg film is ordered because the patient has no other complaints.
   b. Routine labs, serum pregnancy test, and lactate level are sent.
   c. The patient is placed on a cardiac monitor.
   d. Urine is sent for analysis.

10. A 34-year-old male is brought into your ED after falling from a three-story building. He is hemodynamically stable but complaining of lower abdominal pain. The patient is awaiting initial radiographs. The most appropriate management course is:
    a. Place a Foley catheter prior to secondary survey.
    b. Admit to the surgical intensive care unit immediately.
    c. Perform an infraumbilical diagnostic peritoneal lavage.
    d. Obtain an orthopedic consult for immediate external fixation.
    e. Order a CT of the abdomen and pelvis.

11. The following statements about hangman's fracture are true except:
    a. Cord damage is minimal in this injury.
    b. The pedicle of C2 at the pars interarticularis is fractured.
    c. Patients may complain of occipital headaches.
    d. The mechanism associated with this injury is hyperflexion.

12. A 20-year-old male presents to the ED after sustaining a blow to the left side of his face with a piece of wood. He is complaining of diffuse C-spine pain and inability to straighten his neck and has a nonfocal exam. Your management should next consist of:
    a. Sending the patient home with muscle relaxants
    b. Forcing the patient's neck in a rigid collar
    c. Obtaining cervical spine films and oblique films
    d. Loading the patient with methylprednisolone

13. Which of the following is not an indication for CT scan in cervical spine injuries?
    a. For evaluation of persistent localized neck pain or neurologic deficits despite negative cervical films
    b. For evaluation of spinal cord parenchyma
    c. For evaluation of suspected injuries to facet joints
    d. For defining the position of fragments in relation to the spinal canal

14. A patient is brought in by EMS after jumping out of a five-story building. After initial resuscitation is completed, the patient is hypotensive, hypothermic, bradycardiac, and areflexic. The best management approach to this case initially is:
    a. Load the patient with methylprednisolone prior to any diagnostic or therapeutic intervention.
    b. Continue aggressive fluid resuscitation despite normal central venous pressure and exclusion of occult bleeding or mechanical causes for shock.
    c. Consider and eliminate all possibility of hypovolemic shock, cardiogenic shock, or mechanical causes for shock.
    d. Start dopamine immediately.

15. An 8-year-old child presents to the ED after being involved in a high-speed motor vehicle accident. The patient was a back-seat passenger who was wearing a lap seat belt. The patient is complaining of pain along the thoracolumbar area. The lateral view of the thoracolumbar radiograph demonstrates a distracted L2 spinous fracture with a wedge-shape fractured body. All of the following statements concerning this injury are true except:
    a. The degree of lumbar kyphosis has important prognostic value.
    b. This injury is the result of a severe hyperflexion insult.
    c. This injury is associated with intraperitoneal injuries.
    d. This type of injury is more common in adults.

16. EMS transports a 70-year-old female who was the front-seat passenger who was wearing her seat belt in a minor motor vehicle accident. The patient presents complaining of neck pain and distal upper extremity weakness and minimal sensory loss in that area. The following statements are true regarding this injury except:
    a. It is commonly seen in patients with spinal stenosis or cervical spondylitis.
    b. The suspected mechanism is hyperextension resulting in buckling of the ligamentum flavum into the spinal cord, causing cord compression and central microhemorrhage.
    c. Deficits are greatest at C3, the site of significant spinal canal narrowing.
    d. Treatment includes immobilization and methylprednisolone therapy.

17. A patient presenting with a loss of motor function and pain and temperature sensation below the level of the injury has the following spinal cord syndrome:
    a. Central spinal cord syndrome
    b. Brown-Séquard syndrome
    c. Anterior spinal cord syndrome
    d. Cauda equina syndrome

18. In the radiographic evaluation of the cervical spine, which of the following statements is true?
    a. The pre-dens space in an adult normally measures 5 mm or less.
    b. Stability of the spinal column depends primarily on the integrity of the anterior column.
    c. Spondylolysis is the anterior subluxation of one vertebral body on another.

d. A normal variant in pediatric cervical spine films is the appearance of C2 subluxation on C3 up to 3 mm.

Answers

1.b. The Glasgow Coma Scale was devised to assess the level of consciousness in a head injury patient. Eye opening response is used as an indicator of brain stem function. Motor response is used as a reflection of CNS function, and verbal response as a reflection of the degree of integration of CNS function. The Glasgow Coma Scale is the sum of the scores of these three areas of assessment. The highest score one can obtain is 15 and the lowest score is 3. A Glasgow Coma Scale score of 8 or less indicates a coma. Although the Glasgow Coma Scale was not designed as a prehospital tool, it is frequently used by prehospital health care providers.[1] *(Emergency Medicine, Chapter 95, pp 975–984)*

2.a. Stabilization procedures before the delivery of patients to definitive care should be minimized. Although the value of IV fluid therapy during transport for a severely hypotensive patient is still controversial, it is very clear that the patient's transfer to the hospital should never be delayed. IV access can be attempted while en route to the hospital. Cervical immobilization and splinting of obvious fractures should be done before moving the patient, if possible. *(Emergency Medicine, Chapter 95, pp 975–984)*

3.b. Spinal immobilization not only replaces compromised spinal column stability but also protects spinal cord tissue from further damage. Ideal cervical spine immobilization maintains cervical lordosis and alignment without axial distraction, rotation, or compression. For adequate immobility, each cervical level is limited to less than 5 degrees of motion. *(Emergency Medicine, Chapter 97, pp 992–1006)*

4.a. Applying military antishock trousers in a patient with suspected diaphragm injury (ruptured or paralyzed) significantly compromises the patient's respiratory status. Military antishock trousers can be used to stabilize pelvic and lower extremity fractures. They may help to control retroperitoneal hemorrhage in a severe pelvic fracture by providing retroperitoneal vascular tamponade.[1] *(Emergency Medicine, Chapter 95, pp 975–984)*

5.c. None of the commonly used semirigid cervical collars provide adequate immobilization by themselves. Patients must be transported with a semirigid cervical collar, sandbags, or foam blocks on each side of the head to prevent lateral bending, and the entire head/block unit is taped to the backboard. The goal for an emergency physician is to identify the patient with the spinal column injury and prevent spinal cord injury. Therefore, it is extremely important to take into account the mechanism of injury when evaluating a patient with a normal neurologic exam. *(Emergency Medicine, Chapter 97, pp 992–1006)*

6.c. A patient's response to blood loss is a function of the rapidity of ongoing blood loss, the degree of efficacy of compensatory mechanisms such as vasoconstriction, and the amount of prehospital resuscitation. In young healthy patients, vasoconstriction may maintain blood pressure until the patient becomes critically hypovolemic. Elderly patients, patients with hypertension or cardiovascular disease, and patients taking cardioactive medications, e.g., beta-blockers, may not be able to compensate as well for their degree of shock. These patients may also have "normal" vital signs with a significant degree of shock. *(Emergency Medicine, Chapter 95, pp 975–984)*

7.d. Any significant midface fracture is a contraindication to either nasotracheal intubation or nasogastric tube placement. These patients may have a cribriform plate fracture, and any tube placed through the nose may be inadvertently placed intracranially. Blind nasotracheal intubation may significantly increase intracranial pressure and should not be used in patients with head injury. *(Emergency Medicine, Chapter 95, pp 975–984)*

8.b. Trauma is a dynamic process and continual reassessment must be made. When a patient decompensates during a resuscitation, reassessment beginning with the primary survey is needed. The airway and breathing should be assessed first. The endotracheal tube may have gone down the right main stem bronchus, or a tension pneumothorax may have occurred. *(Emergency Medicine, Chapter 95, pp 975–984)*

9.a. The mechanism of injury helps to identify occult injuries in seemingly stable patients. Prehospital care providers should provide a description of the scene, including the estimated amount of blood loss, the force of collision, and extraction time. Evaluating cervical spine injuries or abdominal injuries can be difficult in a patient with a distracting orthopedic injury. *(Emergency Medicine, Chapter 95, pp 975–984)*

10.e. In blunt trauma, it is important to determine whether the patient has intra-abdominal or retroperitoneal bleeding. Diagnostic peritoneal lavage can determine if there is intra-abdominal bleeding. Abdominopelvic CT scan can determine intra-abdominal as well as retroperitoneal hemorrhage. False-positive diagnostic peritoneal lavage may occur in cases of pelvic fracture. If a pelvic fracture is suspected and the decision to perform a diagnostic peritoneal lavage is made, an open, supraumbilical approach should be performed. *(Emergency Medicine, Chapter 95, pp 975–984)*

11.d. A hangman's fracture is a fracture through the posterior elements of C2. These fractures have been classified as type 1, 2, or 3. Type 1 hangman's fractures are caused by hyperextension. There are fractures of the axis ring with minimal displacement of the body of the axis and a normal C2–C3 disc space. Commonly, there is no neurologic deficit. At the C2 level the spinal cord occupies only approximately a third of the

AP diameter of the canal. The second and third cervical nerves innervate the soft tissue surrounding C1 and C2 as well as the occipital scalp and can cause referred pain of an occipital headache.[2] *(Emergency Medicine, Chapter 97, pp 992–1006)*

12.c. This patient has a facet dislocation and fracture. Cervical spine films can demonstrate widening of the prevertebral soft tissue space, increased interspinous space, and oblique rotation of one segment known as the "bow tie" deformity. Use of oblique films can help evaluate patients with a high suspicion of facet dislocation. *(Emergency Medicine, Chapter 97, pp 992–1006)*

13.b. CT is an impractical screening tool for cervical spine injury because of the insensitivity and cost when used in this context. It is superior to plain films in detecting fractures in suspicious areas and is better at defining fracture. CT is inferior in detecting subluxations and dislocations and can miss 40% of subluxations and dislocations. Facet joint injury is well visualized on CT scan because the image plane is perpendicular to the articular facets.[1] *(Emergency Medicine, Chapter 97, pp 992–1006)*

14.c. Prior to making the diagnosis of spinal shock in a patient with a mechanism of injury that supports major traumatic injuries, the presence of hypovolemic, cardiogenic, and mechanical shock must be excluded. Spinal shock refers to the neurologic condition shortly after spinal injury. Spinal shock is the consequence of abruptly losing sympathetic tone. Bradycardia, hypotension, and hypothermia occur. Areflexia and flaccidity occur acutely and are later replaced with spasticity and hyperreflexia when the spinal shock resolves. *(Emergency Medicine, Chapter 97, pp 992–1006)*

15.d. The seat belt syndrome described is a thoracolumbar Chance fracture. It occurs during rapid deceleration of a motor vehicle. There is severe flexion of the upper torso across the seat belt. A Chance fracture is a horizontal fracture through the spinous process, laminae, pedicles, and transverse process with extension into the vertebral body. Because of the severe flexion, there is compression of abdominal viscera. This type of injury is more common in children. *(Emergency Medicine, Chapter 97, pp 992–1006)*

16.c. This patient is suffering from a central cord syndrome. It is described as motor impairment of the upper extremities more than the lower extremities. It is most commonly seen in elderly patients with cervical stenosis. During hyperextension, the ligamentum flavum is suspected of extending into the spinal cord, causing cord compression and central microhemorrhage. Deficits are greatest below C5, the site of significant spinal cord narrowing. *(Emergency Medicine, Chapter 97, pp 992–1006)*

17.c. Anterior cord syndrome has a similar degree of motor deficit in the upper and lower extremities. Pain and temperature sensation are lost, but there is preservation of posterior column sensation, proprioception, vibration, and touch. This can be seen with anterior vertebral injuries that compress the anterior half of the spinal cord. It also is caused by anterior spinal artery insufficiency from thrombosis, hemorrhage, or compression.[3] *(Emergency Medicine, Chapter 97, pp 992–1006)*

18.d. The pre-dens space defines the space between the posterior surface of the anterior arch of C1 and the anterior surface of the odontoid process. The pre-dens space measures less than 3 mm in the adult and less than 5 mm in children. In addition, pseudosubluxation is a normal variant in pediatric cervical spine films and is defined as a C2 subluxation on C3 up to 3 mm. The stability of the spinal column depends primarily of the integrity of the posterior column. *(Emergency Medicine, Chapter 97, pp 992–1006)*

REFERENCES

1. Marx JA: Penetrating abdominal trauma. Emerg Med Clin North Am 1993; 11(1):125–135.
2. Bauman D, Bauman DH: Quality assurance for the radiology-emergency interface. Emerg Med Clin North Am 1991; 9(4):881–884.
3. Mattox KL, Moore EE, Feliciano DV: Trauma. East Norwalk, CT, Appleton & Lange, 1988, p 256.

BIBLIOGRAPHY

Barish R, Naradzay JFX: Spinal trauma. *In* Howell JM, Altieri M, Jagoda AS, et al (eds): Emergency Medicine. Philadelphia, WB Saunders, 1998, pp 992–1006.

Scalea TM, Low RB: Approach to multiple trauma. *In* Howell JM, Altieri M, Jagoda AS, et al (eds): Emergency Medicine. Philadelphia, WB Saunders, 1998, pp 975–984.

45 Head Trauma

ADRIENNE BIRNBAUM, MD

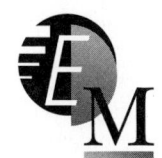

1. Which of the following is true with regard to the initial assessment and management of the patient with severe isolated head trauma?
   a. An initial bolus of crystalloid should be administered to optimize cerebral perfusion pressure.
   b. Management of the airway with endotracheal intubation should be deferred until injury to the cervical spine can be adequately ruled out with radiographs.
   c. Hyperventilation to achieve a $PaCO_2$ of 15 to 20 should be instituted.
   d. The combative patient may require emergent airway protection before cervical spine radiographs are obtained.
   e. A Glasgow Coma Scale score of less than 15 is highly suggestive of significant brain injury.

2. All of the following categories of patients should be considered to be at high risk for intracranial injury and therefore should undergo emergent head CT except:
   a. The intoxicated patient with decreasing level of consciousness
   b. The patient with a history of loss of consciousness
   c. The patient with a palpable depressed skull fracture
   d. The patient with penetrating skull injury
   e. The patient with unequal motor examination on one side of the body with regard to the other

3. All of the following are true of shaken-baby syndrome except:
   a. Intracranial injury is usually found on CT scan.
   b. The child may present with lethargy or altered mental status or appear septic.
   c. Retinal hemorrhages may be seen on examination of the fundus.
   d. Signs of external head trauma are common.
   e. Patients with suspected abuse should be admitted to allow observation of the injury and investigation of the event.

4. All of the following are examples of mechanisms of secondary brain injury except:
   a. Effect of an expanding hematoma
   b. Raised intracranial pressure
   c. Tissue hypoxia
   d. Hypotension
   e. Movement of the brain against the skull

5. Which of the following correctly describes the constellation of findings most likely to be found with uncal herniation of the temporal lobe caused by a space-occupying lesion?
   a. Ipsilateral fixed and dilated pupil and ipsilateral motor paralysis
   b. Ipsilateral fixed and dilated pupil and contralateral motor paralysis
   c. Contralateral fixed and dilated pupil and contralateral motor paralysis
   d. Contralateral fixed and dilated pupil and ipsilateral motor paralysis
   e. None of the above

6. Which of the following is true about common extra-axial lesions?
   a. Epidural hematomas generally do not cross suture lines but may cross the midline.
   b. Epidural hematomas are the most common intracranial hemorrhage to occur after head trauma.
   c. In subdural hematomas, the blood originates from the rupture of one or more arteries.
   d. An acute subdural hematoma appears on CT as a hyperdense, biconvex, or lenticular lesion.
   e. Small focal areas of hemorrhage in proximity to the third ventricle and within the white matter of the corpus callosum are indicative of subarachnoid hemorrhage.

7. All of the following are true of pediatric head trauma except:
   a. Irritability, lethargy, pallor, agitation, or poor feeding may be signs of severe head trauma.
   b. The incidence of space-occupying intracranial hematomas is greater than in adults.
   c. Diffuse cerebral edema is more common than in adults.
   d. A bulging fontanelle may indicate increased intracranial pressure.
   e. Victims of shaken-baby syndrome usually have no external signs of head trauma.

8. A patient is brought to the ED after a motor vehicle accident. Paramedics state that the patient was initially speaking coherently. A rapid repeat neurologic assessment reveals equal and reactive pupils, moaning but no use of words, eye opening in response to pain but not to verbal command, and movement of all extremities in response to pain but no purposeful pushing away of noxious stimuli. Which of the following represents the most appropriate initial management of this patient?
   a. Steroids should be administered to reduce intracranial pressure.
   b. Rapid initiation of endotracheal intubation with in-line stabilization, followed by hyperventilation, is indicated.
   c. Mannitol, 1 g/kg, should be administered IV to reduce intracranial pressure.
   d. A detailed neurologic examination should be performed.
   e. Burr hole placement should be accomplished.

9. Which of the following is considered to be diagnostic of basilar skull fracture?
   a. Blood behind the tympanic membrane
   b. Raccoon eyes
   c. Battle's sign
   d. Cerebrospinal fluid in the ear canal or nose
   e. Opacified sphenoid sinus on plain films

10. Which of the following patients can be safely discharged from the ED after head trauma?
    a. A 30-year-old alcoholic female who fell and struck her head while intoxicated. She is now awake, still appears somewhat intoxicated, and is demanding to leave.
    b. A 70-year-old female who slipped and fell, sustaining a scalp laceration. She gives a history of a recent hospital admission for atrial fibrillation and cannot remember the names of her medications. There is no history of loss of consciousness and her mental status is normal. She lives alone.
    c. A 40-year-old male involved in a motor vehicle accident, with witnessed loss of consciousness, amnesia for the event, normal head CT, and normal neurologic examination. He wishes to leave with his family.
    d. A 30-year-old male who was assaulted with a bat. There is no history of loss of consciousness and mental status has been normal since arrival. He wishes to leave with his family. On repeat examination, he is noted to have developed bilateral periorbital ecchymosis but has an otherwise normal examination.
    e. A 1-month-old brought in to the ED with a head laceration sustained when the infant rolled off a changing table, according to the parents. The laceration has been sutured, the child is awake, and the parents are anxious to leave the ED.

Answers

1. d. Treatment essentials in the management of severe head trauma include early protection of the airway, adequate oxygenation, hyperventilation, rapid CT imaging, neurosurgical consultation, and close observation for deterioration in level of consciousness. Volume administration should be minimal unless evidence of hypovolemia is present because of the danger of increased cerebral edema. Management of the airway, if indicated, should be accomplished with cervical spine stabilization and should not be deferred until radiographic evaluation of the neck can be accomplished. Overaggressive hyperventilation can lead to severe hypocapnia and result in cerebral ischemia. Blood gases must therefore be monitored carefully to ensure that the $Paco_2$ is not lowered beyond approximately 26 mm Hg. The combative patient will often require emergent airway protection before cervical spine radiographs are obtained. A Glasgow Coma Scale score of less than 9 is highly suggestive of significant brain injury. *(Emergency Medicine, Chapter 96, pp 985–991)*

2. b. The availability of CT of the head has revolutionized the management of the head-injured patient by allowing rapid and reliable diagnosis. Categories of high risk for intracranial injury include depressed level of consciousness not clearly caused by alcohol or drug use or other causes, focal neurologic signs, decreasing level of consciousness, and penetrating skull injury or palpable depressed skull fracture. The intoxicated patient presents a particular challenge in assessment and must be reassessed frequently and have CT performed immediately if deterioration in mental status occurs or if appropriate improvement fails to occur over time. The need for head CT in otherwise well patients with only a history of loss of consciousness or amnesia for the event is considerably more controversial. One recent prospective study of a consecutive series of 1382 patients with loss of consciousness or amnesia for the event after head trauma and a Glasgow Coma Scale score of 15, all of whom underwent head CT, found 6.1% to have a traumatic intracranial abnormality but only 0.2% to require surgery. Of note, of the subgroup of patients without symptoms or signs of depressed skull fracture, only 3% had an abnormal CT and no patient required surgical intervention. These investigators concluded that routine head CT in patients with a history of loss of consciousness or amnesia but no symptoms or signs of depressed skull fracture is not warranted.[1] *(Emergency Medicine, Chapter 96, pp 985–991)*

3. d. Shaken-baby syndrome is a constellation of clinical and radiographic findings that result from vigorous manual shaking of an infant. Shaking is thought to result in a whiplash-induced type of injury because of the large head and relatively weak neck muscles of the infant. It is usually seen in infants younger than 1 year of age and most frequently less than 6 months. Victims may exhibit a variety of presentations, including failure to thrive, lethargy, altered mental status, septic appearance, apnea, seizures, lethargy, bradycardia, respiratory difficulty, vomiting, coma, or death. Findings include intracranial injuries and intraocular bleeding, such as retinal or vitreous hemorrhages. A

critical point is that identification of this syndrome may be hindered by the usual lack of obvious external signs of trauma. A high index of suspicion is therefore necessary for identification of this syndrome. Cases of suspected abuse should be admitted to allow observation of the injury and investigation of the event. *(Emergency Medicine, Chapter 96, pp 985–991)*

4.e. Primary and secondary brain injury refer to sequential pathophysiologic mechanisms of injury that occur after head trauma. The concept is important because of the emphasis it places on potentially treatable phenomena that occur in the period following the initial insult that can result in ongoing damage to the brain. The outcome of the head-injured patient is related to the amount of primary and secondary brain injury sustained. Primary injury refers to the initial mechanical damage sustained, e.g., from movement of the brain against the skull or from penetrating injury. Secondary injury refers to subsequent damage caused to the brain by mechanisms such as the effects of an expanding hematoma, cerebral edema and raised intracranial pressure, tissue hypoxia, hypercarbia, hypotension, and ischemia. Secondary brain injury can be minimized by adhering to critical principles of management such as early attention to the airway to ensure adequate oxygenation and ventilation; rapid and appropriate management of increased intracranial pressure with elevation of the head, hyperventilation, and mannitol when appropriate; and close observation and immediate neurosurgical consultation if clinical or radiographic evidence of severe head injury is present. *(Emergency Medicine, Chapter 96, pp 985–991)*

5.b. Uncal brain herniation refers to a syndrome resulting from a shift of brain contents that may occur as a result of intracranial injury. Trauma that results in bleeding or swelling within the cranial vault causes an increase in intracranial pressure above the fibrous tentorium. The medial portion of the temporal lobe, the uncus, is forced downward against the tentorium, compressing ipsilateral cranial nerve III. This pressure results in loss of parasympathetic innervation to the ciliary body and an ipsilateral fixed and dilated pupil. If herniation continues, pressure on the ipsilateral cerebral peduncle can result in contralateral motor weakness because the corticospinal tract descends through this region prior to decussation. Eventually, ipsilateral motor weakness and contralateral pupillary dilation may occur as the contralateral cerebral peduncle and third cranial nerve are affected. Because a unilateral fixed and dilated pupil in a patient who is rapidly deteriorating is most suggestive of an ipsilateral epidural or subdural hematoma, burr hole placement, when necessary, is initially performed through the temporal base on the side ipsilateral to the dilated pupil. A contralateral approach is used if initial efforts are unsuccessful. *(Emergency Medicine, Chapter 96, pp 985–991)*

6.a. Epidural hematoma is a collection of blood that accumulates between the inner table of the skull and the dura. The lesion arises from rupture of arteries (most commonly from the middle meningeal or posterior meningeal) or large venous sinuses. CT demonstrates a biconvex or lenticular-shaped lesion, created by the resistance of the dura. Because the dura is anchored at the suture lines of the skull, epidural hematomas generally do not extend beyond suture lines. They may, however, extend across venous sinuses and therefore cross the midline. Subdural hematoma is a collection of blood that originates from bridging veins and dissects through the potential space located between the dura and the arachnoid membrane This injury is commonly associated with an intracerebral lesion or contralateral subdural hematoma. On CT, acute subdural hematoma typically has a hyperdense, crescent-shaped appearance, conforming to the calvarium and cortex. Due to the location beneath the dura, subdural hematomas are not bound within suture lines, in contrast to epidural hematomas. Traumatic subarachnoid hemorrhage results from tears of small subarachnoid vessels. This is the most common intracranial hemorrhage resulting from head trauma. On CT, this injury appears as increased density within the basilar cisterns, interhemispheric fissures, and sulci. Small focal areas of hemorrhage in proximity to the third ventricle and within the white matter of the corpus callosum of the internal capsule are indicative of diffuse brain injury. Diffuse brain injury represents widespread damage to axonal fibers.[2] *(Emergency Medicine, Chapter 96, pp 985–991)*

7.b. Head trauma is the leading cause of morbidity and mortality in pediatric trauma patients. Recognition of pediatric head trauma may be challenging due to the inability of the young child to communicate symptomatology and difficulty in assessing mental status in the nonverbal or uncooperative child. For this reason, a high index of suspicion is necessary as well as a recognition of the fact that nonspecific symptoms such as irritability, lethargy, pallor, agitation, or poor feeding may be signs of severe head trauma. Differences in pediatric head trauma relative to adult head trauma include a lower frequency of cerebral contusions and subdural hematomas but a greater frequency of diffuse brain swelling. The mainstay of treatment for increased intracranial pressure is hyperventilation, as it is in adults. A bulging fontanelle may indicate increased intracranial pressure from bleeding or cerebral edema in younger children. It is important to recognize that victims of shaken-baby syndrome usually have no external signs of head trauma, despite significant intracranial injury, due to the whiplash type of mechanism of the injury. *(Emergency Medicine, Chapter 96, pp 985–991)*

8.b. This patient has a Glasgow Coma Scale score of 8 and a deteriorating level of consciousness. A score less than 9 is highly suggestive of significant brain injury. The most appropriate initial management therefore involves attention to the airway with endotracheal intubation, with in-line stabilization of the cervical spine, to allow oxygenation and hyperventilation. Administration of steroids is not indicated due to a lack of evidence to suggest that this intervention is effective in reducing intracranial pressure. Although mannitol is effective in reducing or controlling intracranial pressure, management of the airway should take precedence. The Glasgow Coma Scale score of 8 and deteriorating mental status are adequate to suggest the likelihood of serious intracranial injury. The initial neurologic exam should be focused on identifying the presence of gross neurologic deficits, especially those that may suggest the need for urgent neurosurgical intervention. Performance of a detailed neurologic examination is most appropriately deferred until management of the airway, breathing, and circulation has been attended to and CT and neurosurgical consult arranged. Placement of burr holes is generally considered to be a last-ditch effort most appropriately applied in a patient who is rapidly deteriorating despite hyperventilation and mannitol and when examination findings are suggestive of impending brain herniation, e.g., when a unilateral dilated pupil and/or contralateral motor weakness are present. *(Emergency Medicine, Chapter 96, pp 985–991)*

9.d. The base of the skull is composed of the frontal, ethmoid, sphenoid, temporal, and occipital bones. Head and facial trauma may give rise to basilar skull fracture. Cerebrospinal fluid in the ear canal or nose is diagnostic of this injury. Cerebrospinal fluid leakage occurs as a result of trauma-induced communication between the subarachnoid space and the sinuses, nasopharynx, or middle ear through a tear in the dura, fractured bone, and mucosal tear. Rhinorrhea may occur from fractures into the frontal or sphenoid sinuses or through the cribriform plate into the ethmoid sinus. Cerebrospinal fluid rhinorrhea can be distinguished from nasal secretions by a higher glucose concentration in the former (approximately two thirds that of blood glucose) than in the latter (negligible glucose). Bloody nasal secretions can be distinguished from cerebrospinal fluid mixed with blood by placing a drop on filter paper or a white cloth. Cerebrospinal fluid mixed with blood will separate into a pale outer ring and darker inner ring, due to the more rapid diffusion of cerebrospinal fluid. Raccoon eyes (bilateral periorbital ecchymosis), Battle's sign (ecchymosis overlying the mastoid region), and blood behind the tympanic membranes as well as opacification of a sphenoid sinus on plain radiographs are all considered presumptive evidence of a basilar skull fracture. Treatment includes hospital admission, observation for infection, and, rarely, surgical treatment. *(Emergency Medicine, Chapter 96, pp 985–991)*

10.c. Current evidence suggests that patients with negative CT scans and normal mental status may safely be discharged home. The altered mental status of the patient described in answer a should not be assumed to be entirely attributable to intoxication. It must be assumed that this patient has a potential brain injury until proven otherwise by an appropriate improvement in condition over time or CT imaging. No patient with head trauma can safely be discharged from the ED while still under the influence of alcohol. Answer b is incorrect because the patient described is elderly and lives alone. In addition, a call to the patient's physician would reveal that the patient's medications include Coumadin, which places her at increased risk of intracranial bleeding. CT of the head and hospital admission, if appropriate home observation cannot be arranged, would be the most prudent course of action. The patient described in answer d has developed raccoon eyes, a sign suggestive of basilar skull fracture. Patients with suspected basilar skull fracture are generally admitted to the hospital for observation and supportive care and rarely require surgery. The infant described in answer e should not be allowed to leave the ED until a full evaluation can be performed to evaluate the possibility of child abuse. In this case, the fact that the mechanism of injury described does not fit the developmental capabilities of the child should alert the health care provider to the possibility of child abuse. *(Emergency Medicine, Chapter 96, pp 985–991)*

REFERENCES

1. Miller EC, Derlet RW, Kinser D: Minor head trauma: Is CT always necessary? Ann Emerg Med 1996; 27(3):290–294.
2. Harris J: The Radiology of Emergency Medicine, 3rd ed. Baltimore, Williams & Wilkins, 1993, pp 13–17.

BIBLIOGRAPHY

Olshaker J: Head trauma. *In* Howell JM, Altieri M, Jagoda AS, et al (eds): Emergency Medicine. Philadelphia, WB Saunders, 1998, pp 985–991.

46 Maxillofacial Trauma and Neck Trauma

NIELS K. RATHLEV, MD   JEREMY BROWN, MD

Maxillofacial Trauma

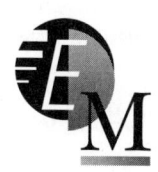

1. Which of the following statements concerning mandibular fractures is false?
   a. Multiple fractures are common.
   b. The subcondylar region is most commonly fractured.
   c. The presence of a tooth in the fracture line classifies it as an open fracture.
   d. Fractures of the condyle are easily seen on plain radiographs.
   e. A coronal CT may be required to adequately evaluate the condyles.

2. The single most informative radiograph to assess bony facial injury is:
   a. Lateral face
   b. Caldwell
   c. Waters
   d. Submentovertex
   e. Towne

3. Which of the following needs emergent repair?
   a. A human bite wound to the face
   b. A superficial 2-cm laceration to the tongue
   c. A septal hematoma
   d. A puncture wound to the cheek
   e. Clear fluid leaking from a preauricular laceration

4. Which of the following pairs is incorrectly associated?
   a. Maxillofacial fracture—inability to crack a vertically placed tongue depressor with the teeth
   b. Condylar fracture of the mandible—inability to palpate motion through the external ear canal
   c. Maxillofacial fracture—ecchymosis of the floor of the mouth
   d. Cerebrospinal fluid leak—nasal discharge positive for glucose and protein
   e. Zygoma fracture—lateral subconjunctival hematoma and flattening of the lateral facial contour

5. Which of the following is not present in simple temporomandibular joint dislocation?
   a. Trismus and spasm of the muscles of mastication
   b. Difficulty in swallowing or talking
   c. A palpable swelling below the zygomatic arch
   d. Airway compromise
   e. Anxiety and extreme discomfort

6. In dental injuries:
   a. A patient may require a chest radiograph.
   b. Primary teeth need never be replaced.
   c. An Ellis class I fracture needs urgent dental consultation.
   d. An avulsed tooth replaced after more than 2 hours has a 90% chance of being permanently retained.
   e. An Ellis class III fracture can be referred to a dentist nonemergently.

7. Which of the following features of orbital rim fractures is false?
   a. The inferior and medial walls are at greatest risk of injury.
   b. Inferior rectus entrapment is common, causing impaired downward gaze.
   c. Signs include diplopia and hypoesthesia of the ipsilateral nose, lower eyelid, and upper gum.
   d. Retrobulbar hemorrhage may be present and needs emergent surgical decompression.
   e. Hyphema may indicate injuries within the eye.

8. Which of the following statements about LeFort fractures is true?
   a. Different LeFort fracture types rarely occur together.
   b. Airway compromise is not associated with a LeFort I.
   c. A LeFort II involves craniofacial dysjunction.
   d. A LeFort fracture may involve an open skull fracture.
   e. A LeFort I fracture involves the ethmoid bones.

9. Which radiographic studies are correctly paired?
   a. Nasal fracture—emergent plain x-ray
   b. Zygoma fracture—CT scan
   c. Nasal-orbital-ethmoid fracture—CT scan
   d. Multiple facial fractures—MRI
   e. Condylar fracture—plain x-rays

10. In soft tissue injuries of the face, which of the following is incorrect?
    a. A laceration of the cheek is best anesthetized with a V2 infraorbital block.
    b. Penicillin coverage should be considered after repair of a through-and-through lip laceration.
    c. A conjunctival laceration of less than 1 cm need not be repaired.
    d. A subconjunctival hemorrhage associated with blunt facial trauma presents little concern to the physician.
    e. A laceration to the lateral forehead is best anesthetized with a supraorbital block.

Answers

1.d. Multiple fractures of the mandible are common—approximately 50% have a fracture in two or more places. Always look for a second fracture when one is detected. The subcondylar region is the most commonly fractured area, present in approximately 35% of all mandibular fractures. If a tooth lies in the fracture line, the mandibular fracture is by definition open and requires prophylactic antibiotics in addition to any definitive fixation. Condylar fractures are the most commonly missed maxillofacial fracture because they are poorly visible on plain radiographs. If there is a strong suspicion, a coronal CT scan is needed to evaluate the condyles. In bilateral parasymphyseal mandibular fractures, the genioglossus muscle (the major muscle of the tongue) may become detached, thus allowing the tongue to obstruct the airway. *(Emergency Medicine, Chapter 99, pp 1013–1026)*

2.c. The Waters view is the single most informative radiograph, providing information about the zygoma, orbital rims, nasal bones, anterior orbital floor, ethmoid air cells, and maxillary sinuses. The lateral face view is useful in mandibular fractures and demonstrates the lingual, retropharyngeal, and prevertebral soft tissues; therefore, it is helpful in the radiographic assessment of airway patency. The Caldwell projection provides the best view of the orbits, frontal bones, and frontal sinuses. The submentovertex provides a good view of the individual sphenoid sinuses, the anterior wall of the maxillary sinuses, and the zygomatic arch that may not be seen on other views. The Towne view assesses the skull base and is also helpful in assessing the condylar and subcondylars area in mandibular fractures. *(Emergency Medicine, Chapter 99, pp 1013–1026)*

3.c. An untreated septal hematoma can cause septal cartilage necrosis and a saddle deformity; it should be drained as soon as it is recognized. Human bite management is controversial, but deep bites should be treated with delayed primary closure and antibiotic coverage. Superficial tongue lacerations do not need to be repaired. Because of the possibility of damage to deeper structures, puncture wounds need careful assessment and should usually be left open. Clear fluid leaking from a wound in the preauricular region should alert the physician to the possibility of injury to the parotid gland or duct, and further exploration is required, with definitive closure performed in the operating room. *(Emergency Medicine, Chapter 99, pp 1013–1026)*

4.d. A reliable correlation has not been shown between glucose and protein found in nasal discharge and a cerebrospinal fluid leak, so a negative test does not exclude this diagnosis. All of the other signs are good markers of significant trauma, and their presence requires a thorough search for an underlying fracture. *(Emergency Medicine, Chapter 99, pp 1013–1026)*

5.d. In temporomandibular joint dislocation, trismus and spasm of the muscles of mastication prevent the condyles from sliding back over the temporal eminence, and the patient will have difficulty talking and swallowing and cannot oppose the anterior teeth. Airway compromise does not usually result from a simple temporomandibular joint dislocation. Reduction can be accomplished by infiltrating the muscles of mastication with local lidocaine or administering benzodiazepines for muscle relaxation. Gentle downward pressure with the thumbs is then applied to the occlusal surface of the molars. After reduction, the patient is cautioned not to open the mouth widely, because repeat dislocation is common. A Barton bandage may be used for chronic dislocations. *(Emergency Medicine, Chapter 99, pp 1013–1026)*

6.a. The first concern of the emergency physician is to ensure that an avulsed tooth has not been aspirated, and a chest radiograph may be necessary if the tooth cannot be accounted for. Although primary teeth do not usually need to be replaced, they may sometimes be needed to ensure correct spacing. The chances for successfully reimplanting an avulsed tooth decrease by 1% per minute. After 2 hours the chances of successful reimplantation are less than 2%. Ellis class I fractures involve only the enamel of the tooth, and treatment is to smooth the tooth and reassure the patient that cosmesis will not be affected. A class III fracture involves the enamel and pulp, is usually very painful, and appears pink with a drop of blood. Urgent referral to a dentist is required if the tooth is to be saved. *(Emergency Medicine, Chapter 99, pp 1013–1026)*

7.b. Inferior rectus entrapment is common but causes an *upward* gaze palsy. The weakest walls of the orbital rim are the medial and inferior, so they are at greatest risk of injury. Inferior orbital nerve compression may lead to diplopia and changes in skin sensation. Retrobulbar hemorrhage is rare but needs to be recognized quickly. Signs include proptosis, pain, abnormal extraocular motions, visual loss, increased intraocular pressure, and an afferent pupillary defect. Emergent surgical decompression is needed. A blowout fracture or hyphema is often associated with significant trauma to the globe. *(Emergency Medicine, Chapter 99, pp 1013–1026)*

8. d. LeFort I fractures involve only the maxilla. The LeFort II fracture is a pyramidal fracture involving the maxilla, nasal bones, and ethmoid bones. A LeFort III fracture involves craniofacial dysjunction, with the fracture involving the maxilla, zygoma, nasal bones, ethmoids, and vomer bones. Cerebrospinal fluid rhinorrhea or intracranial air may be detected and is a sign of an open skull fracture. In such a case, antimicrobial coverage with a penicillinase-resistant penicillin is recommended. A retropharyngeal hematoma occurs in virtually every case of LeFort III fractures and may not be clinically apparent. As it expands, it may occlude the airway. Two or more types of LeFort fractures are often present; for example, a LeFort II on one side with a LeFort III on the other. Although airway compromise is more commonly seen in a LeFort II and III, it can occur in any LeFort fracture, and the emergency physician should plan for its occurrence. *(Emergency Medicine, Chapter 99, pp 1013–1026)*

9. c. Nasal-orbital-ethmoid fractures are often difficult to diagnose and account for up to 40% of midline facial fractures. They are caused by severe direct trauma to the bridge of the nose and result in severe swelling. Intercanthal distance is often widened; a distance of greater than 40 mm is diagnostic. Early diagnosis is crucial, because it becomes difficult to repair nasal-orbital-ethmoid fractures after about 2 weeks. CT is the imaging modality of choice in these injuries. An isolated simple nasal fracture usually requires no emergent imaging; a nondisplaced fracture requires no treatment; and a displaced fracture should be reevaluated 7 to 10 days after the initial injury to decide whether reduction is needed. Children with suspected nasal fractures must be evaluated in 2 to 4 days because their bones heal more quickly. It is at this time that radiographs are needed. A simple zygoma fracture may be detected on plain x-rays alone and does not require prompt CT scanning. However, facial CT may be required to evaluate intraorbital injuries or complex zygomatic fractures. MRI is of little value in multiple facial fractures, because these patients are often too unstable to be transferred to the MRI scanner. CT provides more bony detail in a shorter period of time. Condylar fractures are often missed on plain radiographs but may be diagnosed by coronal CT scan. *(Emergency Medicine, Chapter 99, pp 1013–1026)*

10. d. Although most subconjunctival hemorrhages are benign and heal spontaneously, they may indicate serious ocular injury when associated with blunt or penetrating globe trauma. Conjunctival lacerations may appear as a conjunctival defect, exposure of Tenon's capsule, or orbital fat. The integrity of the underlying sclera must be evaluated to rule out globe penetration, and lacerations longer than 1 cm should be repaired by an ophthalmic surgeon. There is some controversy as to whether antimicrobial prophylaxis is needed for through-and-through oral lacerations; however, they are considered contaminated wounds. Penicillin coverage should be considered. Lacerations to the face are easily anaesthetized with blocks to branches of the facial nerve, which avoids distortion of the wound margins, allowing for better cosmesis. *(Emergency Medicine, Chapter 99, pp 1013–1026)*

Neck Trauma

1. A 45-year-old female with a self-inflicted gunshot wound to the anterior neck just below the cricoid cartilage presents in extreme respiratory distress. What is the most appropriate way to manage her airway?
   a. Awake nasotracheal intubation
   b. Orotracheal intubation
   c. Cricothyrotomy
   d. Tracheostomy
   e. Retrograde intubation

2. Which of the following is an appropriate procedure in the initial management of severe hemorrhage from a penetrating neck wound?
   a. Clamping bleeding vessels
   b. Infusing IV fluids in the ipsilateral arm in zone 1 injuries
   c. Direct pressure
   d. Reverse Trendelenburg position
   e. Probing the wound

3. Major vascular injuries from blunt neck trauma may be caused by:
   a. Direct trauma
   b. Traction injury caused by neck hyperextension
   c. Intraoral trauma
   d. Overlying fractures
   e. All of the above

4. Accurate assessment of an isolated penetrating neck wound includes evaluation of all of the following except:
   a. Violation of the platysma
   b. Zone of anterior entrance and exit wounds
   c. Anterior/posterior location
   d. Cranial nerves III through XII
   e. Presence of subcutaneous emphysema

5. Which of the following statements is true regarding esophageal injuries?
    a. Signs or symptoms indicating injury are invariably present on initial presentation.
    b. Surgical exploration will detect all injuries.
    c. Sensitivity of esophagography is greater than 95%.
    d. Delayed diagnosis results in a significantly increased rate of morbidity and mortality.
    e. Flexible endoscopy is extremely sensitive in diagnosing injury.

6. Signs and symptoms of airway injury include:
    a. Stridor
    b. Hoarseness or muffled voice
    c. Dyspnea
    d. Subcutaneous emphysema
    e. All of the above

7. A 36-year-old male presents with a zone 2 stab wound to the left anterior triangle of the neck. He has a diminished left carotid pulse and a rapidly expanding hematoma. Weakness of the right arm is noted on neurologic exam. Which of the following is true?
    a. He demonstrates signs of major vascular injury include expanding hematoma and a pulse deficit.
    b. Neurologic deficit is invariably caused by direct trauma to neurologic structures.
    c. The weakness of the right arm is most likely caused by a brachial plexus injury.
    d. Zone 2 injuries carry the highest mortality rate due to the proximity of major vascular structures.
    e. Hemorrhage is most difficult to control in zone 2.

8. Neurologic structures that may be injured directly in isolated penetrating neck trauma include all of the following except:
    a. Spinal cord
    b. Cranial nerves IX through XII
    c. Sympathetic chain
    d. Brachial plexus
    e. Pons and midbrain

9. In penetrating neck trauma, arteriography is:
    a. Indicated for all patients with zone 1 injuries
    b. Less sensitive than exploration in diagnosing major vascular injury
    c. Indicated for all victims regardless of zone of injury
    d. Used selectively based on physical examination regardless of zone of injury
    e. Indicated for all patients with zone 2 injuries

10. Which of the following statements is true regarding blunt neck injuries?
    a. Delayed manifestations of injuries can usually be predicted on initial presentation.
    b. Signs and symptoms of delayed injuries may not present for 6 months to 1 year.
    c. Large prospective trials have demonstrated the benefit of Doppler sonography in diagnosing vascular injuries.
    d. Signs and symptoms of injury are always present on initial presentation.
    e. Neurologic deficits consistent with a transient ischemic attack or stroke should be attributed to a cerebral contusion or hemorrhage.

Answers

1.d. Nasotracheal intubation is contraindicated, because it is performed blindly without direct visualization of the airway. Orotracheal intubation is performed with direct visualization of the glottis; however, the injury is located below the true vocal cords. A partial injury may be converted into a complete transection, or a "blind" passage can be created under these circumstances. Cricothyrotomy and retrograde intubation are performed through the cricothyroid membrane, which is located cephalad to the injury. Tracheostomy is the only procedure that actually bypasses the lacerated trachea. *(Emergency Medicine, Chapter 98, pp 1007–1012)*

2.c. Severe hemorrhage from a penetrating neck wound should be managed with direct pressure only. Blind attempts at clamping bleeding vessels may damage critical structures (such as nerves and other vessels) that are often located adjacent to the bleeding vessel. Probing the wound under less than ideal circumstances is also not recommended, because a partial injury can be completed with vigorous manipulation. Intravenous fluids should not be infused in the ipsilateral arm in zone 1 injuries, because the subclavian vein may have been injured. The patient should be placed supine or in slight Trendelenburg position in order to prevent air embolus.[1] *(Emergency Medicine, Chapter 98, pp 1007–1012)*

3.e. In blunt neck trauma, vascular injuries may develop as a result of direct injury to the vessel, causing intimal tearing, dissection, and thrombotic occlusion. Similar injuries can occur as a result of significant traction to the neck during blunt head or neck trauma. Intraoral injury and overlying fractures related to blunt facial trauma have been associated with injuries to the carotid arteries.[2] *(Emergency Medicine, Chapter 98, pp 1007–1012)*

4.d. All patients with an injury that penetrates the platysma should be admitted to the hospital for observation and further studies or operation, regardless of the presence or absence of signs of organ injury. The location of anterior and posterior entrance and exit wounds is important to note in order to project the track of the penetrating object. Cranial nerves VII, IX, X, XI, and XII may be injured and should be routinely examined. Cranial nerves III, IV, and VI are not affected by isolated penetrating neck trauma. Subcutaneous emphysema in the neck should immediately raise suspicion of perforation of the esophagus or airway. *(Emergency Medicine, Chapter 98, pp 1007–1012)*

5.d. Signs and symptoms of esophageal injury may not be present on initial presentation, particularly in patients with an altered mental status. Delay of more than 24 hours in diagnosing an esophageal perforation results in a high rate of morbidity and mortality. Reports have documented that this injury may be missed during operative exploration because of inadequate exposure.[3] Esophagography has a sensitivity of only 70% to 80%. Rigid esophagoscopy is more sensitive than flexible esophagoscopy, but it is also riskier because of the necessity for general anesthesia and a higher incidence of iatrogenic perforation.[4] *(Emergency Medicine, Chapter 98, pp 1007–1012)*

6.e. Stridor and a change in speech quality (such as hoarseness or a muffled voice) indicate a tracheal or laryngeal injury until proven otherwise. Acute dyspnea may result from airway obstruction due to hematoma, soft tissue swelling, and intraoral bleeding. A large expanding hematoma of the neck is an indication for prophylactic, urgent airway management including intubation, despite the fact that the patient may not currently be in extremis. The presence of subcutaneous air immediately raises the suspicion of an injured larynx, trachea, or esophagus. *(Emergency Medicine, Chapter 98, pp 1007–1012)*

7.a. Penetrating injury to the anterior neck is divided into three zones of injury, which are used for surgical management. Zone 1 is from the base of the neck to the cricoid cartilage, zone 2 is from the cricoid to the angle of the mandible, and zone 3 is above the angle to the base of the skull. Surgical exposure is the most complex for zone 1 injuries because a median sternotomy is required for adequate access to the subclavian vessels. This partly explains why the mortality rate is highest in zone 1. Conversely, bleeding is most easily controlled in zone 2 injuries because of the superficial location of the carotid arteries and jugular veins and ease of surgical exposure. Exploration of zone 3 injuries often requires subluxation of the mandible or lateral mandibulotomy for adequate exposure. Signs of major vascular injury and indications for immediate surgery include expanding, pulsatile hematoma; bruit or thrill; severe, continuous bleeding; pulse deficit; and shock. Neurologic deficit may result from direct trauma or from vascular injury, leading to ischemia of neurologic structures. *(Emergency Medicine, Chapter 98, pp 1007–1012)*

8.e. Spinal cord injuries are infrequent (but potentially devastating) in penetrating neck trauma. The brachial plexus may be injured because of its location in the posterior triangle, below and posterior to the sternocleidomastoid muscle. Injury to the sympathetic chain may lead to Horner's syndrome (miosis, anhidrosis, and ptosis). Cranial nerves VII, IX, X, XI, and XII are the most commonly injured.[1] The pons and midbrain are not affected directly by penetrating trauma isolated to the neck. *(Emergency Medicine, Chapter 98, pp 1007–1012)*

9.a. Arteriography compares favorably with operative exploration in terms of the sensitivity and specificity of detecting vascular injuries of the neck and extremities.[5] Patients presenting without signs of major vascular injury can be managed selectively based on the zone of injury and presenting signs and symptoms. Zone 1 and 3 injuries should undergo mandatory arteriography due to the inaccessibility of these regions to physical examination. Asymptomatic patients with zone 2 injuries and no signs of vascular trauma can safely be managed with serial physical examinations in the hospital without angiography.[6] *(Emergency Medicine, Chapter 98, pp 1007–1012)*

10.b. Although patients with blunt carotid artery injuries usually present with signs and symptoms within the first 24 hours, these injuries can be extremely subtle initially and may not manifest for up to 1 year. Delayed manifestations cannot always be predicted initially. Neurologic symptoms consistent with a transient ischemic attack or stroke should not automatically be assumed to be caused by blunt head trauma, e.g., contusion or hemorrhage. Distal embolization from a thrombosed carotid artery may cause a similar picture. Doppler sonography is noninvasive and less time-consuming than angiography; however, the benefit of the technique has not been demonstrated in large studies. *(Emergency Medicine, Chapter 98, pp 1007–1012)*

REFERENCES

1. Carducci B, Lowe RA, Dalsey W: Penetrating neck trauma: Consensus and controversies. Ann Emerg Med 1986; 15:208–215.
2. Pozzatti E, Giuliani G, Poppi M, et al: Blunt traumatic carotid dissection with delayed symptoms. Stroke 1989; 89:412–416.
3. Weaver AW, Sankaran S, Fromm SH, et al: The management of penetrating wounds of the neck. Surg Gynecol Obstet 1971; 133:49–52.
4. Weigelt JA, Thal ER, Snyder WH, et al: Diagnosis of penetrating cervical esophageal injuries. Am J Surg 1987; 194:619–622.
5. Richardson JD, Vitale GC, Flint LM: Penetrating arterial trauma: Analysis of missed vascular injuries. Arch Surg 1987; 122:678–683.
6. Mansour MA, Moore EE, Moore FA, et al: Validating the selective management of penetrating neck wounds. Am J Surg 1991; 162:517–521.

BIBLIOGRAPHY

Euerle B, Lottes MA: Maxillofacial trauma. *In* Howell JM, Altieri M, Jagoda AS, et al (eds): Emergency Medicine. Philadelphia, WB Saunders, 1998, pp 1013–1026.

Jolly BT: Neck trauma. *In* Howell JM, Altieri M, Jagoda AS, et al (eds): Emergency Medicine. Philadelphia, WB Saunders, 1998, pp 1007–1012.

47 Chest Trauma

SIMON ROY, MD

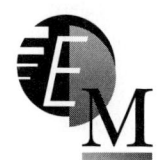

1. A 24-year-old male sustains a blunt steering wheel impact to the precordium. He has a BP of 100/60, pulse of 110. Which of the following is the most appropriate method of evaluation for possible myocardial contusion?
   a. Swan-Ganz catheter placement in the ICU
   b. Serial CPK-MB levels on telemetry
   c. Chest radiograph with detailed physical examination
   d. Echocardiography in the ED
   e. Aortography with left ventriculogram

2. The patient in question 1 presents with normal vital signs, chest radiograph, ECG, and physical examination (except for sternal tenderness). Which of the following is a true statement regarding his evaluation for possible myocardial contusion?
   a. Echocardiography should be performed in the ED.
   b. Echocardiography should be performed in the ICU.
   c. The patient should be monitored for 24 hours.
   d. Further cardiac evaluation is probably not needed.
   e. Transesophageal echocardiography will be more sensitive than transthoracic echocardiography for contusion in this setting.

3. All of the following are true statements regarding traumatic hemothorax except:
   a. It is most commonly secondary to penetrating trauma.
   b. Pleural adhesions and rib fractures increase the chances of hemothorax in blunt trauma.
   c. Pulmonary contusions are frequently associated in blunt etiologies.
   d. Thoracotomy is usually required in penetrating etiologies.
   e. Empyema and restrictive pleural disease can result from undrained hemothorax.

4. All of the following are true statements regarding flail chest except:
   a. It represents an unstable segment of the normally rigid chest wall (from multiple rib fractures) that moves independently and paradoxically to the rest of the chest wall during the respiratory cycle.
   b. It is usually caused by major blunt trauma.
   c. It is usually associated with pulmonary contusions.
   d. It often requires surgical mechanical stabilization for definitive therapy.
   e. It can be effectively managed with systemic analgesics, epidural anesthesia, and mechanical ventilation.

5. A 22-year-old male presents to the ED after sustaining an acute deceleration motor vehicle accident. His initial supine chest radiography demonstrates a widened mediastinum without other radiographic abnormalities. His initial vital signs are normal. Which of the following is the best course of action?
   a. Once axial spine has been cleared of injury, obtain an upright chest radiography. If upright chest radiography is normal, assume low probability aortic injury.
   b. Proceed to mediastinal CT.
   c. Proceed directly to aortography.
   d. Proceed directly to thoracotomy.
   e. Perform transesophageal echocardiography to exclude aortic injury.

6. The patient in question 5 has a cervical spine fracture as seen on radiography and cannot be placed in the upright position. Which of the following is the best course of action?
   a. Proceed to mediastinal CT.
   b. Proceed directly to aortography.
   c. Proceed directly to thoracotomy.
   d. Perform transesophageal echocardiography to exclude aortic injury.
   e. Perform transesophageal echocardiography to exclude aortic injury.

7. If the patient in question 5 had chest radiography findings of widened mediastinum with left apical capping, which of the following would be the best course of action?
   a. Proceed to mediastinal CT.
   b. Proceed directly to aortography.
   c. Proceed directly to thoracotomy.

d. Perform transesophageal echocardiography to exclude aortic injury.
e. Place left chest tube, then proceed to aortography.

8. All of the following are chest radiography signs suggesting aortic arch tear except:
   a. Widening of the mediastinal silhouette
   b. Left apical pleural capping
   c. Blurring of the aortic knob
   d. Multiple left upper rib fractures
   e. Deviation of the nasogastric tube in the esophagus to the left

9. All of the following are true statements regarding pneumothorax except:
   a. It can be secondary to blunt and penetrating trauma.
   b. It can be accurately quantitated by chest radiography evaluation.
   c. It always requires chest tube placement if cardiopulmonary compromise is present.
   d. It usually will resolve with either observation or chest tube placement and rarely requires thoracotomy.
   e. It can rapidly progress to tension pneumothorax in positive pressure ventilation situations.

10. Which of the following is a correct statement regarding pulmonary contusions?
    a. Systemic steroids are a useful therapeutic modality.
    b. Chest tube placement is usually required.
    c. The initially asymptomatic patient rarely develops clinically significant symptoms.
    d. They are most frequently related to massive blunt thoracic trauma.
    e. Volume resuscitation is always limited to prevent contusion edema progression.

11. A 25-year-old male sustained a penetrating left zone-1 neck wound 4 days before ED presentation. His chief complaint is shortness of breath. Vital signs are normal. Upright chest radiography reveals large left pleural effusion. A chest tube is placed and output is 300 mL of milky white fluid. Which of the following is the most appropriate course of action?
    a. Immediate thoracotomy for presumed esophageal perforation
    b. Immediate thoracotomy for presumed thoracic duct tear
    c. Observation for 48 hours in the ICU
    d. Obtain lymphocyte count on chest tube fluid, place patient on total parenteral nutrition/NPO
    e. Obtain Gastrografin swallow to exclude esophageal perforation

12. All of the following are true statements regarding traumatic diaphragmatic injury except:
    a. It can be secondary to both penetrating and blunt mechanisms.
    b. It requires an extremely high clinical index of suspicion to be diagnosed.
    c. It may be diagnosed by radiographic demonstration of abdominal contents in the chest on plain film or CT.
    d. It may present as a delayed diagnosis of bowel obstruction.
    e. In blunt trauma, it is more common on the right.

13. A patient sustains a penetrating wound to the right chest. Chest radiography reveals a large right pneumothorax. After a chest tube is placed, a massive air leak develops and the patient becomes hypoxemic. Repeat chest radiography shows failure of the lung to reexpand. All of the following are appropriate except:
    a. Place a second chest tube on the right.
    b. Perform double-lumen endotracheal intubation.
    c. Proceed to the OR for thoracotomy.
    d. Perform ED thoracotomy with right hilar cross clamping.
    e. Perform single-lumen endotracheal intubation with observation in the ICU.

14. Which of the following is a true statement regarding sternal fractures?
    a. They commonly have associated myocardial contusions.
    b. They often require operative fixation for stabilization.
    c. They have a mortality around 5%.
    d. They are usually seen on PA or AP chest radiography.
    e. They have an increased incidence in women and the elderly.

15. All of the following are true statements regarding the use of autotransfusion in thoracic trauma except:
    a. It is most commonly used in patients with a large hemothorax drained by chest tube.
    b. It requires only transient citrate anticoagulation, passage through a macrofilter, and then rapid reinfusion.
    c. It reduces the rate of blood-borne infectious disease transmission.
    d. It is safe regardless of volume reinfused.
    e. The most common complication is disseminated intravascular coagulation.

Answers

1.d. Swan-Ganz catheter readings are likely to reveal nonspecific values and to be time-consuming and invasive to obtain. Creatine phosphokinase values have been found to be of low sensitivity for contusion. Chest radiography and physical examination are of limited value, because sensitivity is low and findings are nonspecific. Echocardiography is portable, rapid, noninvasive, and sensitive/specific for clinically significant contusions. The right ventricle is hypokinetic but hypervolemic. Aortography, which evaluates left-sided structures, is of no value in this usually right ventricular event.[1] *(Emergency Medicine, Chapter 100, pp 1027–1039)*

2.d. In this setting, there are good data to suggest that further evaluation is not needed. Contusions that are hemodynamically or electrically significant are usually evident early in the patient's presentation. Occult contusions are rarely clinically significant. There is excellent prognostic value in the initial vital signs, physical examination, and ECG.[1] *(Emergency Medicine, Chapter 100, pp 1027–1039)*

3.d. Penetration is the most common mechanism, but only 15% of penetrating injuries will require surgery. The rest can be handled with simple chest tube placement. Hemothorax is uncommon with blunt trauma unless the ribs are fractured or the lung parenchyma is torn by previously existing pleural adhesions. Because of diffuse blunt forces, pulmonary contusions are commonly coexisting. Undrained pleural blood is an excellent culture medium and can also lead to pleural fibrosis, with marked impairment of lung expansion.[2] *(Emergency Medicine, Chapter 100, pp 1027–1039)*

4.d. Multiple rib fractures from blunt trauma produce the unstable chest wall segment described. Pulmonary contusions are the major cause of morbidity and mortality in this clinical situation. It is extremely uncommon for surgical stabilization to be performed, because epidural anesthesia usually results in adequate pain control and effective pulmonary toilet. In refractory cases, mechanical ventilation is the next step. *(Emergency Medicine, Chapter 100, pp 1027–1039)*

5.a. Most stable patients with isolated widened mediastinum on supine chest radiography will demonstrate no abnormality on upright chest radiography, with the widening being caused by patient position only. *(Emergency Medicine, Chapter 100, pp 1027–1039)*

6.a. In the absence of other chest radiography abnormalities, the abnormal mediastinal width is still most likely to be positional artifact. Contrast-enhanced spiral CT has excellent sensitivity (>97%) for mediastinal blood, although this finding is not specific for aortic arch injury and a positive study is usually followed by formal aortography. Direct operative intervention is not indicated at this time. Transesophageal echocardiography has good sensitivity (65% to 100% in various reported series) for arch tears but may involve unwanted neck manipulation in this patient. Its major advantage is in being a portable study modality. Transesophageal echocardiography has low sensitivity for aortic tears.[3,4] *(Emergency Medicine, Chapter 100, pp 1027–1039)*

7.b. With chest radiography findings other than isolated widened mediastinum, a mediastinal CT will rarely be normal, making further study (usually aortography) necessary. In cases with higher suspicion for aortic tear, it is more efficient and accurate to proceed directly with the gold standard in aortic imaging, aortography. Pleural capping is extrapleural blood, leaving no role for intercostal drainage. *(Emergency Medicine, Chapter 100, pp 1027–1039)*

8.e. Mediastinal widening, apical pleural capping, and blurring of the aortic knob are all nonspecific signs of mediastinal blood and are suggestive of aortic arch injury. With mediastinal hematoma formation, the esophagus and nasogastric tube become displaced to the *right*, as does the trachea. Other findings raising suspicion for aortic arch injury include downward displacement of the left main stem bronchus and obliteration of the perivertebral pleural stripe, both occurring with hematoma formation. Left upper rib fractures indicate massive arch region trauma, with increased chances of arch tearing. *(Emergency Medicine, Chapter 100, pp 1027–1039)*

9.b. Chest radiography is notoriously inaccurate for quantifying pneumothorax size. The three-dimensional aspect of a pneumothorax is misrepresented on the typical two-dimensional upright PA or AP radiograph. Pneumothorax can be caused by both penetrating and blunt trauma. Patients with any form of cardiopulmonary compromise always require chest tube placement. It is unusual for thoracotomy to be required, this being reserved for massive or persistent air leaks from damaged lung or tracheobronchial tissues. Any form of positive pressure ventilation increases pneumothorax size and is an indication for chest tube placement in the otherwise asymptomatic patient. *(Emergency Medicine, Chapter 100, pp 1027–1039)*

10.d. Massive blunt chest wall trauma is the typical mechanism leading to contused lung. Steroids have not been shown to provide improved clinical outcome. Chest tube placement may be required if pneumothorax is present, but this is not the norm. The classic presentation for pulmonary contusion is clinical deterioration over 12 to 36 hours after injury, with these patients often being initially asymptomatic. It is a major mistake in management of the trauma patient as a whole to limit volume resuscitation. Systemic perfusion restoration is always the primary goal, with fluid limitation (for pulmonary and cerebral events) being appropriate only once the primary goal has been obtained. *(Emergency Medicine, Chapter 100, pp 1027–1039)*

11.d. The most likely diagnosis is ruptured thoracic duct based on the appearance of chest tube effluent. This can easily be confirmed by increased lymphocyte count of the fluid (due to the thoracic duct's being a lymph draining conduit). Because this condition can often be managed by total parenteral nutrition/NPO (to decrease gut lymphatic flow) and chest tube drainage with spontaneous closure of the leak, immediate operation is premature. Refractory cases do require operative ligation of the duct. Esophageal perforation would probably present with profound sepsis 4 days after insult. *(Emergency Medicine, Chapter 100, pp 1027–1039)*

12.e. The liver usually prevents right-sided diaphragmatic rupture in blunt trauma. Otherwise, diaphragm injury can be from both blunt and penetrating mechanisms. A high clinical index of suspicion is the key to diagnosis because findings are subtle. Any evidence of abdominal contents in the chest (CT, chest radiography) warrants abdominal exploration. Often, radiographic appearance of the nasogastric tube in the chest is the only evidence of diaphragm injury. If the initial diagnosis is missed, patients can present with bowel obstruction caused by herniation through the diaphragmatic defect. *(Emergency Medicine, Chapter 100, pp 1027–1039)*

13.e. Positive pressure ventilation without further therapy is more likely to increase flow through the air leak into the chest tube suction system. Second chest tube placement may aid in pulmonary reexpansion, with increased chances of leak closure. Double-lumen intubation is an excellent way to provide temporary diversion of ventilation away from the injured airways on the right side. Formal operative thoracotomy is often required for repair/resection to control the leak. As a last resort in the profoundly unstable patient, right-sided ED thoracotomy may be performed with hilar clamping to decrease bronchopleural flow. *(Emergency Medicine, Chapter 25, pp 217–224)*

14.e. The elderly and women (often with osteoporosis) have an increased risk of fracture because of bone density losses. Otherwise, sternal bone is resistant to fracture. Myocardial contusions are uncommonly associated, being present in only 18% of cases in some series. Operation is required only for grossly unstable or displaced injuries. Mortality is extremely low, usually less than 1% (unless other major injuries are present). The diagnosis is most commonly made on the lateral chest radiography.[5] *(Emergency Medicine, Chapter 100, pp 1027–1039)*

15.d. Disseminated intravascular coagulation, the most common complication, is usually seen once volumes greater than 1500 mL are reinfused. Probably the most appropriate use of autotransfusion in trauma is in the hemothorax drained by chest tube. It can rapidly be accomplished by collection in a citrate-containing reservoir, passage through a macroaggregate filter, and then reinfusion. This obviously reduces blood transmission of infectious diseases. *(Emergency Medicine, Chapter 100, pp 1027–1039)*

REFERENCES

1. Cachecho R: The clinical significance of myocardial contusion. J Trauma 1992; 33(1):68–71.
2. Sabiston D: Textbook of Surgery, 13th ed. Philadelphia, WB Saunders, 1986, pp 294–330.
3. Gavant M: Blunt traumatic aortic rupture. Cardiovasc Radiol 1995; 166(4):955–961.
4. Smith M: TEE in the diagnosis of traumatic rupture of the aorta. N Engl J Med 1995; 332(6):356–362.
5. Wojcik K: Sternal fractures: The natural history. Ann Emerg Med 1988; 17:912–916.

BIBLIOGRAPHY

Carriso JC, Mileski WJ, Kaplan HS: Transfusion, autotransfusion and blood substitutes. *In* Mattox KL, Moore EE, Feliciano DV (eds): Trauma. Norwalk, CT, Appleton & Lange, 1996, pp 181–191.

Milzan DP: Chest trauma. *In* Howell JM, Altieri M, Jagoda AS, et al (eds): Emergency Medicine. Philadelphia, WB Saunders, 1998, pp 1027–1039.

O'Keefe KP, Sanson TG: Pericarditis, myocarditis, and pericardial tamponade. *In* Howell JM, Altieri M, Jagoda AS, et al (eds): Emergency Medicine. Philadelphia, WB Saunders, 1998, pp 217–224.

Shires TG, Thal ER, Jones RC: Trauma. *In* Schwartz SI (ed): Principles of Surgery, 6th ed. New York, McGraw Hill, 1994, pp 175–223.

48 Abdominal and Urogenital Trauma and Pelvic Trauma

ROBERT A. ALDOROTY, PhD, MD   DEBRA HEITMANN, MD   MARY RYAN, MD

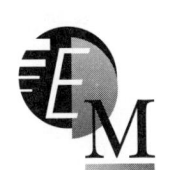

Abdominal and Urogenital Trauma

ROBERT A. ALDOROTY, PhD, MD   DEBRA HEITMANN, MD

1. Which of the following is always true regarding the number of entrance and exit wounds seen in gunshot injuries?
   a. An even number of wounds implies that there are no retained projectiles.
   b. An even number of wounds implies that there are retained projectiles.
   c. An odd number of wounds implies that there are retained projectiles.
   d. An odd number of wounds implies that there are no retained projectiles.
   e. None of the above are true.

2. Diagnostic peritoneal lavage and diagnostic laparoscopy share which of the following characteristics?
   a. Both lack acceptable sensitivity for retroperitoneal injuries.
   b. Both have adequate sensitivity for diaphragmatic injuries.
   c. Both require general anesthesia.
   d. Both can differentiate between continuing hemorrhage and hemorrhaging that has stopped.
   e. Both require the instillation of fluid into the abdominal cavity.

3. Ultrasonography used to evaluate abdominal trauma is least likely to detect:
   a. Fluid in the pouch of Douglas
   b. An injury to the spleen
   c. Fluid in the lesser sac
   d. An injury to the liver
   e. A pelvic hematoma

4. A 32-year-old man arrives in the ED with an abdominal stab wound at the level of the umbilicus in the left midclavicular line. He has a Glasgow Coma Scale score of 15. His vital signs are pulse 110, RR 12, and BP 140/80. Which of the following tests is the least sensitive for detecting the most likely injury this patient could have sustained that would require operative repair?
   a. A combination of local wound exploration and diagnostic peritoneal lavage
   b. CT scan with oral, rectal, and IV contrast
   c. Emergency ultrasonography
   d. Observation
   e. Exploratory laparotomy

5. A 55-year-old woman sustains a gunshot wound to the abdomen. She is awake and alert. Her vital signs are pulse 100, RR 10, and BP 110/60. There are two wounds, 6 inches apart, in her right upper quadrant. Of the following, which is least likely to be useful in the management of this patient?
   a. Laparotomy
   b. Diagnostic peritoneal lavage
   c. Diagnostic laparoscopy
   d. Chest radiography
   e. Abdominal radiography

6. The decision for nonoperative management of blunt hepatic and splenic injuries in an adult requires all of the following except:
   a. CT scan
   b. Admission to an ICU
   c. A grade I or II injury
   d. Angiography
   e. The absence of associated intra-abdominal injuries

7. A father and mother bring their 8-year-old son to the ED. When riding his bicycle the day before, he fell after the front of his bike struck a ditch. Although the bicycle was intact, the front wheel was in the ditch and the wheel rim was bent. He was brought home by a neighbor who had heard him crying. That night he became agitated, vomited, and had a temperature of 103.7°F. Your examination shows a child with a Glasgow Coma Scale score of 11, a pulse of 150, and a BP of 70/40. He is resuscitated with lactated Ringer's solution and after improvement of vital signs is brought for a head CT scan, which is normal. The next step would be to perform:
   a. MRI of the abdomen
   b. Endoscopic retrograde cholangiography
   c. Exploratory laparotomy

d. Gastrografin study
   e. CT scan of the abdomen

8. Which of the following associations is false?
   a. Air bags have decreased the incidence of thoracoabdominal injuries.
   b. Obesity does not change injury patterns.
   c. Seat belts are associated with small bowel injuries.
   d. Penetrating injuries are most likely associated with small bowel injuries.
   e. Lateral impacts are associated with retroperitoneal injuries.

9. In children, which of the following is false?
   a. Splenic injuries stop bleeding spontaneously less often than in adults.
   b. Injuries to the stomach are more common than in adults.
   c. Duodenal hematomas often do not have an index event.
   d. A child's abdominal musculature affords less protection than an adult's.
   e. Delayed hemorrhage occurs more frequently after liver injuries than after splenic injuries.

10. For blunt injuries a diagnostic peritoneal lavage is considered negative if:
    a. 5 mL of blood is aspirated from the peritoneal cavity
    b. 100,000 RBCs/mm^3 are found in the effluent
    c. 100 WBCs/mm^3 are found in the effluent
    e. Bilirubin is present in the effluent
    d. Amylase is present in the effluent

11. All are true of urogenital trauma except:
    a. It is most often seen after blunt trauma.
    b. Most injuries are minor in severity.
    c. It occurs in approximately 10% of patients with multisystem trauma.
    d. It usually occurs in males younger than 20 years old.
    e. It is evaluated during the secondary survey.

12. Contraindications to the placement of a Foley catheter include all except:
    a. Scrotal hematoma
    b. Blood at the urethral meatus
    c. Suspected pelvic fracture
    d. High-riding prostate on rectal examination
    e. Penile fracture with normal urinalysis

13. In the setting of multisystem trauma, urogenital evaluation should include all except:
    a. Visual inspection of the flanks, abdomen, and genitalia
    b. Urinalysis
    c. Catheter placement
    d. Monitoring of urine output
    e. Rectal examination

14. Which of the following is true of hematuria?
    a. It occurs in approximately 50% of genitourinary trauma.
    b. The degree of hematuria correlates with the severity of injury.
    c. Hematuria is always present in severe penetrating or blunt injuries to the genitourinary tract.
    d. Rhabdomyolysis can be differentiated from hematuria by microscopic analysis.
    e. Microscopic hematuria sustained during blunt trauma requires an intravenous pyelogram.

15. Risk factors for renal injury include all except:
    a. Penetrating trauma to the chest
    b. Improper seat belt use
    c. Falls from greater than 15 feet
    d. History of polycystic kidney disease
    e. Motor vehicle accident with ejection

16. Bladder or urethral injuries should be suspected in all of the following cases except:
    a. In a patient with an anterior pelvic fracture
    b. In a patient who is unable to void
    c. In a patient who sustained a straddle injury
    d. If there is blood at the urethral meatus
    e. If the testes cannot be transilluminated

17. All are true of fracture of the penis except:
    a. It can be caused by flexion beyond the elasticity of the corpus spongiosum.
    b. It can occur during intercourse, often when trying a novel position.
    c. It is followed by immediate pain.
    d. It can be diagnosed on history and examination alone.
    e. It must be operatively managed.

18. All are true of the "one-shot" intravenous pyelogram except:
    a. It is best for the unstable patient with blunt or penetrating trauma.
    b. It should be performed on the operating table so as not to delay surgery.
    c. It is restricted to patients with normal renal function prior to injury.
    d. It is fast, but yields limited information.
    e. It can show two functional kidneys.

19. On CT scan, a cleft in the renal parenchyma with contrast extravasation is a:
    a. Category I lesion
    b. Category II lesion
    c. Category III lesion
    d. Category IV lesion
    e. Category V lesion

20. Surgical exploration of the kidney is indicated in all of the following except:
    a. An expanding hematoma
    b. Large areas of "nonvisualized" parenchyma
    c. A major collecting system disruption with extravasation of urine
    d. Disruption of the renal parenchyma by a bullet
    e. Stable hematoma near a stab wound

21. All are true of posterior urethral injuries from blunt injury except:
    a. They are usually associated with pelvic fractures.
    b. They can be sustained in straddle injuries.
    c. They most commonly present with blood at the meatus.
    d. A retrograde urethrogram and a cystogram are mandatory.
    e. They can be managed solely with a cystotomy tube.

22. All are true of testicular trauma except:
    a. It is associated with a hematocele.
    b. It is suggested if examination reveals that the normal smooth contour is disrupted by a tender elevation.
    c. While the patient is standing, the injured testis commonly lies inferior to the normal one.
    d. It is best visualized by Doppler ultrasound.
    e. It is categorized according to whether the tunica has been violated.

23. Bladder trauma with rupture:
    a. Commonly occurs at the neck of the bladder
    b. Can be diagnosed only by a cystogram
    c. Is usually intraperitoneal
    d. Can be treated nonoperatively with a catheter
    e. Is rarely associated with a pelvic fracture

24. All of the following require a form of visual imaging of the renal system except:
    a. A female stabbed in the left flank in stable condition
    b. A struck motorcyclist with normal vital signs and microscopic hematuria
    c. A restrained passenger in a severe motor vehicle accident with gross hematuria in stable condition
    d. A 6-year-old male who fell one story with a pelvic fracture and microscopic hematuria
    e. A female struck in the back with an expanding flank hematoma and a normal urinalysis

25. For pediatric genitourinary injuries, all of the following are true except:
    a. Imaging studies are recommended for microscopic hematuria.
    b. Most posterior urethral injuries are through the prostatic section and not the membranous portion.
    c. The kidneys are more vulnerable to blunt injury in children.
    d. Diagnostic peritoneal lavage is the preferred diagnostic test, because most pediatric injuries cause intraperitoneal bleeding and it eliminates the risk of contrast.
    e. The bladder is predominantly an intra-abdominal organ and therefore more vulnerable.

Answers

1.c. When a bullet passes through a victim it can create two wounds, an entry wound and an exit wound. Alternatively, a bullet can be retained in the abdomen, producing only an entry wound. If only one bullet was fired the answer would be either a or c. However, if more than one bullet was fired, it is possible to have a retained projectile with an even number of wounds on the body surface. Consider the simplest case of two gunshots. If one passes through the victim and one is retained, three wounds would be observed. If, however, both were retained, there would be only two wounds on the body surface because there would be no exit wounds. It is therefore possible to have an even number of gunshot wounds on the body surface and still have retained projectiles. For gunshot wounds to the abdomen this point is largely academic because most centers perform exploratory laparotomies on all patients with gunshot wounds to the abdomen since the path of a bullet is not predictable. (*Emergency Medicine, Chapter 101, pp 1040–1050*)

2.a. Diagnostic peritoneal lavage may not detect retroperitoneal bleeding because the retroperitoneum is covered by the peritoneal lining, preventing blood from escaping into the peritoneal cavity. Examination by laparoscopy also can be inconclusive because complete examination of the retroperitoneum is often obscured by overlying viscera. As a result, neither diagnostic peritoneal lavage nor diagnostic laparoscopy is sensitive in the detection of retroperitoneal injuries. Laparoscopy has been shown to be effective in diagnosing diaphragmatic injuries. Laparoscopy also allows the physician to directly look at an injury and determine the presence of continued bleeding. Diagnostic peritoneal lavage is performed using local anesthesia. When performing laparoscopy, the abdomen is distended with CO_2, not fluid. (*Emergency Medicine, Chapter 101, pp 1040–1050*)

3.e. Ultrasonography in the ED provides a means to rapidly assess the traumatized patient for the presence of "free" fluid in the abdominal cavity. The anatomic spaces that are examined are the hepatorenal space (Morison's pouch), the rectovesicular or rectouterine space (pouch of Douglas), the splenorenal recess, the subphrenic spaces, the subhepatic space, and occasionally the colic gutters. Blood from significant hepatic or splenic injuries can be detected as fluid in these spaces. A pelvic hematoma is not in the abdominal cavity and is less likely to be detected. Although accuracy remains operator dependent, ultrasound appears to be comparable to diagnostic peritoneal lavage with regard to accuracy. (*Emergency Medicine, Chapter 101, pp 1040–1050*)

4.b. The organ most likely injured by penetrating injuries of the abdomen is the bowel. CT scan is notoriously insensitive in detecting bowel injuries, with a sensitivity of only 50%. Exploratory laparotomy is the gold standard to which all other diagnostic procedures are compared. The false-negative rate for diagnostic peritoneal lavage ranges from approximately 1%, if 10,000 RBCs/mm[3] is used as a cutoff point, to approximately 11%, if 100,000 RBCs/mm[3] is used.[1] Selective laparotomy based on observation has been advocated.[2] Only 4.8% of the patients who were observed required surgery, without a significant increase in either morbidity or mortality. *(Emergency Medicine, Chapter 101, pp 1040–1050)*

5.b. The scenario suggests a tangential gunshot wound to a patient who is hemodynamically "stable" at presentation. Laparotomy is both highly sensitive and specific for the evaluation of abdominal gunshot wounds. Laparoscopy is also highly sensitive in determining peritoneal penetration. Both chest and abdominal radiographs are considered to be routine in the care of such a patient. Diagnostic peritoneal lavage has a false-negative rate of 25% for abdominal gunshot wounds. *(Emergency Medicine, Chapter 101, pp 1040–1050)*

6.d. Angiography is the only test or condition not required to decide on the nonoperative management of an isolated hepatic or splenic injury. The choice of nonoperative management requires that there not be any associated intra-abdominal injuries that require a laparotomy, that the injury be accurately and anatomically graded by CT scan, that the injury be of a low grade, and that the patient can be admitted to a monitored bed and examined frequently. The most important condition is that the patient be hemodynamically stable. *(Emergency Medicine, Chapter 101, pp 1040–1050)*

7.c. This is a classic scenario for a "pediatric bicycle handlebar injury." Typically, the bicycle suddenly stops and the child continues forward, striking his or her abdomen against the handlebars. The prototypical injuries are fracture of the pancreas, duodenal rupture, and duodenal hematoma. This patient is presenting late, as is often the case. The hemodynamic data are consistent with sepsis or sepsis syndrome, suggesting a perforated duodenum or a severe pancreatic injury. Although any of the tests would be a reasonable choice, an exploratory laparotomy would be both diagnostic and therapeutic and is the preferred test in this patient because of his signs of sepsis from duodenal perforation. An MRI may be accurate for pancreatic injuries. Endoscopic retrograde cholangiopancreatography is rarely required but is highly specific, especially for major duct injuries. A Gastrografin study of the duodenum is positive in 50% of patients with this injury. Also, 50% of patients with a duodenal injury will have evidence of retroperitoneal air on an abdominal plain film. An isolated duodenal hematoma would present with vomiting but not septic physiology. Remember that these structures are retroperitoneal, and diagnostic peritoneal lavage may be negative. *(Emergency Medicine, Chapter 101, pp 1040–1050)*

8.b. In fact, obesity does change injury patterns. It appears that obese patients have fewer head injuries relative to torso injuries. Further, their viscera tend to be spared more than nonobese people's. Seat belts have been associated with small bowel, colon, and vertebral injuries. Lateral impacts are associated with retroperitoneal injuries that result from the transfer of energy from a direct impact. *(Emergency Medicine, Chapter 101, pp 1040–1050)*

9.a. Splenic injuries are more likely to stop bleeding spontaneously in children than in adults. Children have a thinner abdominal wall and higher costal margins than adults, affording less protection from impact. Children are known to have more gastric injuries than adults and more isolated duodenal hematomas than adults. It is often difficult to determine the incident that precipitated the abdominal injury. As with any unexplained childhood injury, child abuse should always be a consideration. *(Emergency Medicine, Chapter 101, pp 1040–1050)*

10.c. A positive peritoneal lavage with respect to WBC count is one with greater than or equal to 500 cells/mm^3, with one caveat: for bowel injuries, the WBC count reaches 500 cells/mm^3 only after 3 hours. For blunt injuries, the positive criteria are any of the following: 5 mL or more of aspirated nonclotting blood; greater than 100,000 RBCs/mm^3; greater than 500 WBCs/mm^3; amylase greater than 175 IU/dL; or the presence of bile, bacteria, or particulate matter in the effluent. The negative criteria are the following: no blood is aspirated; less than 50,000 RBCs/mm^3, less than 100 WBCs/mm^3, amylase less than 75 IU/dL, and the absence of bile, bacteria, or particulate matter in the effluent. Determination of alkaline phosphatase levels in the effluent has been suggested as a test for small bowel injuries.[3] *(Emergency Medicine, Chapter 101, pp 1040–1050)*

11.d. Urogenital injuries are seen in approximately 10% of patients who sustain multisystem trauma and usually are minor in severity. Males under 40 years old are most often affected. Evaluation takes place during the secondary survey. *(Emergency Medicine, Chapter 103, pp 1062–1072)*

12.e. Placement of a Foley catheter is contraindicated if there are findings suggestive of urethral or bladder injury, including blood at the meatus, a scrotal hematoma, a high-riding prostate, or a pelvic fracture. Placement is also contraindicated after straddle injuries, which are often associated with these injuries. *(Emergency Medicine, Chapter 103, pp 1062–1072)*

13.c. As discussed above, a catheter is placed only when the urethra or bladder is thought to be intact. *(Emergency Medicine, Chapter 103, pp 1062–1072)*

14.d. Hematuria is the presence of nonhemolyzed RBCs in the urine. It is present in 95% of cases of genitourinary trauma. It must be distinguished from rhabdomyolysis by a microscopic analysis confirming the presence of RBCs. It is noteworthy that the severity of genitourinary injury cannot be predicted from the degree of hematuria. A CT scan is required to evaluate penetrating trauma. Blunt trauma with microscopic hematuria can be managed with observation and good follow-up. A normal-appearing urine can be obtained even with severe genitourinary injury, such as a complete ureteral tear. *(Emergency Medicine, Chapter 103, pp 1062–1072)*

15. b. Injury to the kidney is more likely to occur after severe motor vehicle accidents, motor vehicle accidents with ejection or requiring extraction, falls greater than 15 feet, or direct blows to the kidney. Underlying kidney disease increases the kidney's vulnerability to injury. Penetrating trauma of the abdomen, chest, flank, or back and posterior rib fractures all increase the risk of injury. (*Emergency Medicine, Chapter 103, pp 1062–1072*)

16. e. Bladder and urethral injuries are most often associated with pelvic fractures. Patients usually complain of lower abdominal pain and difficulty voiding. Straddle injuries produce anterior urethral trauma. Failure to transilluminate the testes suggests the presence of a hematocele, a manifestation of testicular rupture. (*Emergency Medicine, Chapter 103, pp 1062–1072*)

17. a. Penile fracture is a rupture of the corpus cavernosum. (*Emergency Medicine, Chapter 103, pp 1062–1072*)

18. c. The one-shot intravenous pyelogram is reserved for the severely injured patient who may not tolerate a more time-consuming diagnostic test because of the need for immediate operative management. Given the life-threatening situation, determination of renal function is not necessary before a one-shot intravenous pyelogram. (*Emergency Medicine, Chapter 103, pp 1062–1072*)

19. b. Category II lesions, by definition, are injuries that extend into the collecting system and potentially cause extravasation. (*Emergency Medicine, Chapter 103, pp 1062–1072*)

20. e. Stable hematomas of the kidney caused by a stab wound can be managed conservatively with close observation, provided that no active bleeding or extravasation is seen on CT scan. (*Emergency Medicine, Chapter 103, pp 1062–1072*)

21. b. Straddle injuries lead to anterior urethral damage as a result of the bulbous urethra's being forced against the ischial rami. (*Emergency Medicine, Chapter 103, pp 1062–1072*)

22. c. The testes are best examined as the patient is standing but are often swollen after trauma and may lie in any position depending on the type of injury. (*Emergency Medicine, Chapter 103, pp 1062–1072*)

23. d. Bladder trauma is commonly associated with major pelvic trauma, occurring two thirds of the time after pelvic fracture. Bladder injuries can be detected using intravenous pyelography, CT scan, or cystography. Only a quarter of major bladder injuries result in intraperitoneal bladder rupture. Extraperitoneal bladder rupture can be managed nonoperatively with simple catheter drainage. (*Emergency Medicine, Chapter 103, pp 1062–1072*)

24. b. Microscopic hematuria in a stable patient can be managed with observation and good follow-up. Either a CT scan or operative exploration is required to determine the degree of injury in a patient with penetrating trauma, a pelvic fracture, or gross hematuria or a patient who has evidence of an evolving process. (*Emergency Medicine, Chapter 103, pp 1062–1072*)

25. d. Pediatric patients are more susceptible to soft tissue injuries. The threshold to order diagnostic testing should be lower than in adults and should include the finding of microscopic hematuria. The diagnostic test of choice is a CT scan with contrast. (*Emergency Medicine, Chapter 103, pp 1062–1072*)

Pelvic Trauma

MARY RYAN, MD

1. Acceptable methods of managing hemorrhage in the prehospital setting include all of the following except:
   a. Administration of IV isotonic crystalloids
   b. Application of a pneumatic antishock garment
   c. Removal of penetrating foreign body and immediate application of direct pressure
   d. Splinting long bone injuries
   e. "Scoop and run"

2. The leading cause of death after multiple blunt trauma is:
   a. Thoracic aortic disruption
   b. Transection of cervical spinal cord
   c. Major intracranial injury
   d. Exsanguination from hepatosplenic injury
   e. Sepsis

3. A 20-year-old pedestrian struck by a car is brought to the ED by EMS. She is cooperative but appears intoxicated. She admits to alcohol use and states that she is 3 months pregnant. She complains of pelvic discomfort but on examination has no localized tenderness. Which of the following statements is true?
   a. First-trimester pregnancy is a contraindication to performing pelvic radiography.

b. No pelvic radiography is needed, because the patient is cooperative and has no tenderness on examination.
c. Biplanar radiographs of the pelvis are indicated.
d. A one-view radiograph of the pelvis is sufficient to exclude pelvic fracture and will limit exposure of the fetus to radiation.
e. None of the above are true.

4. Digital rectal examination is considered contraindicated in which of the following settings?
   a. Blood at the urethral meatus
   b. Blood at the anus
   c. Perianal laceration
   d. Presence of priapism
   e. None of the above

5. A 37-year-old male is noted to have blood at the urethra after a blunt traumatic injury. Retrograde urethrography shows deformity of the bladder suggestive of an extraperitoneal hematoma. Regarding diagnostic peritoneal lavage in this patient, which of the following is true?
   a. Diagnostic peritoneal lavage is now contraindicated.
   b. Diagnostic peritoneal lavage may be performed, but a closed infraumbilical route is favored.
   c. Diagnostic peritoneal lavage may be performed, but an open infraumbilical route is favored.
   d. Diagnostic peritoneal lavage may be performed, but a closed supraumbilical route is favored.
   e. Diagnostic peritoneal lavage may be performed, but an open supraumbilical route is favored.

6. Which of the following is considered an indication for retrograde urethrography?
   a. i, iii
   b. ii, iv
   c. iv
   d. None
   e. i, ii, iii, iv

   i. Any patient with a significant straddle injury
   ii. Male patients with a major pelvic fracture
   iii. Female patients with blood at urethral meatus after blunt trauma
   iv. Male patients with blood at the urethral meatus after blunt trauma

7. All of the following are common sites for avulsion fractures except:
   a. Anterior superior iliac spine
   b. Coccyx
   c. Anterior inferior iliac spine
   d. Ischial tuberosity
   e. Iliac crest

8. In the Young classification system of pelvic ring disruptions, anteroposterior compression (APC) injuries with sacroiliac widening indicate:
   a. APC I
   b. APC II
   c. APC III
   d. APC IV
   e. None of the above

9. All are true of angiography in pelvic trauma except:
   a. It plays a useful role as both a diagnostic and a therapeutic intervention.
   b. It is equally effective in blunt and penetrating trauma.
   c. It is indicated for persistent blood requirement after pelvic stabilization.
   d. It is primarily useful for arterial, not venous injury.
   e. The procedure itself carries a low risk for major complications.

10. Which of the following are considered to be "major" pelvic fractures?
    a. i, iii
    b. ii, iv
    c. iv
    d. None
    e. i, ii, iii, iv

    i. Sacral fractures
    ii. Transverse iliac wing fractures
    iii. Acetabular fractures
    iv. Vertical iliac wing fractures

Answers

1.c. Retained impaled objects or stabbing instruments should be removed in the OR, never in the field. Ideally, foreign bodies should be stabilized to prevent further injury caused by movement. External hemorrhage should be controlled by direct pressure. Intravenous access should be obtained en route using large-bore IVs, and isotonic crystalloids infused (normal saline or lactated Ringer's). Although some studies suggest that it may be beneficial to keep IV fluids at "KVO" until the patient reaches the OR, the current standard of care is to administer up to 2 L of IV fluid en route to the hospital. For control of internal hemorrhage from fractures in the prehospital setting, splinting of the pelvis and long bone fractures may decrease blood loss. Pneumatic antishock garments can be used for pelvic stabilization, especially if prolonged transport time is anticipated. Although simple splinting of long bone fractures is also helpful, if lumbar or pelvic fracture is clinically suspected, the application of prefabricated "traction" splints for the femur is contraindicated. Because of the time required to perform these stabilizing maneuvers, some authorities have advocated "scoop and run" as the initial management of victims of severe trauma in the urban setting. *(Emergency Medicine, Chapter 102, pp 1051–1061)*

2.c. In multiple blunt trauma, many organ systems can be involved. Although solid organ injury, vascular injury, and fractures result in significant morbidity and mortality, they are not the leading cause of death in this group of patients. Although survivors of multiple blunt trauma are subject to the complications of multiorgan system failure and sepsis, the leading cause of mortality for patients with blunt trauma is major intracranial injury. This is in contrast to victims of penetrating trauma, in whom most deaths, and all immediate mortality, are the result of major vascular injury. *(Emergency Medicine, Chapter 102, pp 1051–1061)*

3.c. Pregnancy is never a contraindication to obtaining indicated radiographic studies. Clinical examination, history, and clinical suspicion are all important in identifying which studies are needed. Although the patient in this scenario is said to be cooperative and has no pelvic tenderness on examination, she admits to alcohol use and appears "intoxicated," so the absence of tenderness on examination is not reliable. Pelvic radiography is indicated because of the mechanism of injury, her complaint of pain, and her intoxication, all of which raise the suspicion of injury. Biplanar (AP and lateral) radiographs are needed to exclude fracture. In the unstable patient, the "one-view AP pelvis" has a role as an initial screening examination to exclude major pelvic injury, but it needs to be followed up with additional studies if injury is suspected, because one view is not sufficient to exclude a fracture. *(Emergency Medicine, Chapter 102, pp 1051–1061)*

4.c. The digital rectal examination plays an important role in the evaluation of any trauma patient. The presence of blood from the urethral meatus suggests a urethral injury or disruption. A rectal examination can provide information, especially in male patients, regarding the urethra. Abnormalities in the position, mobility, and consistency of the prostate suggest the presence of a surrounding hematoma and may indicate an associated urethral disruption. If blood is present at the anus, the rectal examination can help delineate the extent of bleeding and identify an associated injury (e.g., a sacrococcygeal fracture). Assessment of sphincter tone is important if history or sensorimotor examination suggests spinal cord injury. Important clues to this diagnosis are priapism and the loss of sphincter tone. The one circumstance in which a digital rectal examination should not be performed is if a perianal laceration is present, because the examination would be likely to further contaminate the wound. Management of these injuries involves operative exploration and possible diverting colostomy. *(Emergency Medicine, Chapter 102, pp 1051–1061)*

5.e. The usual criteria for performing a diagnostic peritoneal lavage apply. A diagnostic peritoneal lavage can be performed when the suspicion of an extraperitoneal hematoma is high. The indications for using the open supraumbilical technique are the presence of either an extraperitoneal hematoma or a pelvic ring disruption. The other techniques should be avoided with either of these injuries, because the introduction of a needle or catheter into an otherwise contained hematoma could have disastrous hemodynamic consequences. *(Emergency Medicine, Chapter 102, pp 1051–1061)*

6.b. Urethral injury in women is rare. Even if an injury is present, urethrography is often not helpful in making the diagnosis. Because of this, unless a catheter cannot be passed easily into the bladder, retrograde urethrography is not usually indicated in women. In contrast, injury to the male urethra is much more common and the threshold for performing retrograde urethrography much lower. The difference between the sexes is explained by the longer length of the male urethra and its anatomic course. The findings of blood at the urethral meatus or a high-riding prostate on rectal examination are suggestive of urethral disruption. If urethral injury is suspected, a Foley catheter should not be passed in the male patient, because passage can worsen an existing injury, converting a partial tear into a complete one. Further evaluation by means of a retrograde urethrogram is indicated. Urethrography is performed by inserting a 16-gauge Foley catheter 2.5 cm beyond the urethral meatus, inflating the balloon with about 1 mL of water, and injecting 30 mL of dye, while holding the penis obliquely, and obtaining a radiograph. This study outlines the anatomy of the urethra and bladder, and extravasation of contrast indicates tears. Indications for performing a retrograde urethrogram in the male patient following blunt pelvic trauma include blood at the urethral meatus, major pelvic fractures, or suspicion of a significant straddle injury. *(Emergency Medicine, Chapter 102, pp 1051–1061)*

7.b. Avulsion fractures of the pelvis result from the sudden, powerful contraction of the muscles attached to the pelvis, causing detachment of bony fragments from apophyseal sites. The most common sites for pelvic avulsion fractures are the anterior superior iliac spine, the anterior inferior iliac spine, the iliac crest, and the ischial tuberosity. Typically, these fractures occur in young athletic patients who complain of localized pain following exertion. Tenderness may be elicited at the origin of the muscles involved. Avulsion fractures are considered "minor" pelvic fractures. Treatment consists of rest and analgesia. Fractures of the coccyx result from direct force applied to the coccyx, most commonly after a fall in the sitting position. The complaint is of immediate and persistent pain. Diagnosis is established by finding marked local tenderness or mobility of the coccyx on rectal examination. Treatment is rest and analgesia, and stool softeners and sitz baths may provide symptomatic relief. *(Emergency Medicine, Chapter 102, pp 1051–1061)*

8.b. The Young classification system of pelvic ring disruption relates injury patterns to three perpendicular force vectors: anteroposterior, vertical, and lateral. Each has a characteristic radiographic pattern that provides clues to associated injuries. Anteroposterior compression injuries are subdivided into three, not four, groups:
- APC I has the radiographic finding of a symphyseal diastasis of less than 2 cm and involves injury to the symphysis and only minimal sacroiliac ligament damage
- APC II has findings of a widened sacroiliac joint, indicating disruption of anterior sacroiliac, sacrotuberous, and sacrospinous ligaments
- APC III, in which one hemipelvis appears to "float" from the sacrum, includes the features of APC II and, in addition, disruption of the posterior sacroiliac ligaments, resulting in the floating appearance because one hemipelvis can now move away from the sacrum.

Vertical shear injuries show radiologic findings similar to those of APC III, but have vertical, usually rostral, displacement of the hemipelvis.

Lateral compression (LC) injuries all involve fractures, either transverse or coronal, through the pubic ramus. Lateral compression injuries are subdivided according to their posterior component:
- LC I, sacral compression
- LC II, internal rotation of an anterior ring hinged on a fracture near an ipsilateral sacroiliac joint
- LC III, ipsilateral internal rotation and contralateral external rotation, giving the appearance of a "windswept" pelvis on radiography

(Emergency Medicine, Chapter 102, pp 1051–1061)

9.b. Angiography is indicated in any patient with pelvic injuries who has persistent blood loss after stabilization of the pelvis by external skeletal fixation. Stabilizing the pelvis helps limit ongoing venous bleeding through both fracture stabilization and a tamponade effect. Ongoing hemorrhage despite stabilization of the pelvis suggests the presence of an arterial injury. Angiography can be both diagnostic, by identifying the source of bleeding, and therapeutic, through embolization of the injured vessels. The procedure itself carries a low risk of major complications. Although angiography has played a significant role in the management of persistent hemorrhage after blunt trauma, to date, embolization of bleeding vessels after penetrating trauma has been reported only anecdotally. ***(Emergency Medicine, Chapter 102, pp 1051–1061)***

10.b Pelvic fractures are classified as either major or minor. Major fractures result from high-energy mechanisms and often have significant associated visceral injuries. Included in this group are iliac wing fractures, either transverse or vertical; all open fractures of the pelvis; all pelvic ring disruptions; traumatic hemipelvectomies; and displaced acetabular fractures. Acetabular fractures that are not displaced are considered minor, as are avulsion, stress, coccygeal, and sacral fractures. ***(Emergency Medicine, Chapter 102, pp 1051–1061)***

REFERENCES

1. Merlotti GJ, Marcet E, Sheaff CM, et al: Use of peritoneal lavage to evaluate abdominal penetration. J Trauma 1985; 25:228–231.
2. Nance FC, Wennar MH, Johnson LW, et al: Surgical judgment in the management of penetrating wounds of the abdomen: Experience with 2212 patients. Ann Surg 1974; 179:639–646.
3. Jaffin JH, Ochsner MG, Cole FJ, et al: Alkaline phosphatase levels in diagnostic peritoneal lavage as a predictor of hollow viscous injury. J Trauma 1993; 34:829–833.

BIBLIOGRAPHY

Milzman DP: Abdominal trauma. *In* Howell JM, Altieri M, Jagoda AS, et al (eds): Emergency Medicine. Philadelphia, WB Saunders, 1998, pp 1040–1050.

Swartz D, Harwood-Nuss AL: Urogenital trauma. *In* Howell JM, Altieri M, Jagoda AS, et al (eds): Emergency Medicine. Philadelphia, WB Saunders, 1998, pp 1062–1072.

Wightman JM: Pelvic trauma. *In* Howell JM, Altieri M, Jagoda AS, et al (eds): Emergency Medicine. Philadelphia, WB Saunders, 1998, pp 1051–1061.

49 Extremity Trauma

ELIZABETH L. MITCHELL, MD

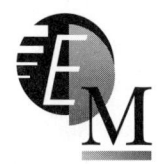

1. External extremity hemorrhage can be controlled most safely using which of the following techniques?
   a. Tourniquets proximal to the bleeding site
   b. Tourniquets distal to the bleeding site
   c. Direct pressure over the bleeding site
   d. Elevation of the bleeding extremity
   e. Clamping or ligation of any arterial injuries

2. Hard signs of vascular compromise in extremity trauma include all of the following except?
   a. A bruit or thrill over the injury
   b. An expanding pulsatile hematoma
   c. Absent or diminished pulses
   d. Distal pallor
   e. Ankle brachial index less than 1.0

3. A patient presents ambulatory to the ED with a gunshot wound to the right thigh. On physical examination you note a single entrance wound to the medial mid thigh. There is no exit wound. There are no pulsatile masses or bruits, and he has an ankle brachial index of 0.6. Which are the next appropriate actions to be taken?
   a. i, iii
   b. ii, iv
   c. i, ii, iii
   d. i, iv
   e. iv

   i. Radiographs of the femur, pelvis, and tibia/fibula
   ii. Local exploration
   iii. Angiography
   iv. Surgical exploration

4. A patient presents to the ED 24 hours after being stabbed in the right calf. He complains of severe right lower extremity pain. His leg is markedly swollen and tense. He has excruciating pain with dorsiflexion of the ankle and great toe. He has numbness along the lateral foot. Which statement is true?
   a. His compartment pressure will probably be around 15 mm Hg.
   b. He needs emergent angiography.
   c. He probably has an anterior compartment syndrome.
   d. He probably has a posterior compartment syndrome.
   e. He needs emergent fasciotomy in the ED.

5. Vascular injuries are less common in blunt trauma than in penetrating trauma.
   True or False

6. Vascular injuries caused by blunt trauma have a much better prognosis than those caused by penetrating injuries.
   True or False

Answers

1.c. Hemorrhage from an extremity should be controlled by direct pressure over the bleeding site. External hemorrhage is usually self-limited and rarely life-threatening. Tourniquets distal to a bleeding site will not help. Tourniquets proximal to bleeding will stop the bleeding but can result in ischemic injury to the entire distal extremity. Tourniquets should be used only in the rare life-threatening arterial bleed that is otherwise uncontrolled. Elevation of the bleeding extremity is helpful but as a single therapeutic intervention is rarely adequate. Elevation along with direct pressure is probably the best method. Finally, clamping or ligation of arterial injuries should not be attempted in the field and should be attempted in the ED only if the vessel is clearly a skin vessel or if all other attempts at hemorrhage control have failed. *(Emergency Medicine, Chapter 104, pp 1073–1083)*

2.e. Hard signs of extremity vascular injury are usually predictive of vascular injury. Hard signs include absent or diminished pulses, active pulsatile hemorrhage, expanding large or pulsatile hematoma, bruit or thrill, and distal ischemia (pain, pallor, paralysis, paresthesia, coolness). The soft signs of vascular injury are helpful in directing the evaluation but are poorly predictive of vascular injury. Soft signs include small, stable injury, related neurologic deficit, unexplained hypotension, history of extensive or pulsatile bleeding, and ankle or wrist brachial index less than 1.0. *(Emergency Medicine, Chapter 104, pp 1073–1083)*

3.a. This patient presents with soft findings of arterial injury (ankle brachial index <1.0). There are no hard signs of vascular injury; therefore, immediate surgical intervention is not indicated. Because of the unknown location of the bullet, radiographs should be done to try to locate the bullet, determine the bullet's path, and exclude any fractures. After radiography, the patient should be sent for angiography based on the abnormal ankle brachial index. Local exploration would be indicated only in a patient who has no evidence of orthopedic or arterial injury and will be treated as an outpatient. *(Emergency Medicine, Chapter 104, pp 1073–1083)*

4.d. There are seven P's associated with compartment syndrome:
  1. Pain disproportionate to primary diagnosis
  2. Pain worsened by passive stretch
  3. Increased pressure palpable over the compartment (the area is tense to palpation)
  4. Paresis of the affected muscle
  5. Paresthesias in the distribution of affected nerves
  6. Pallor (a late finding)
  7. Pulselessness (a very late finding)

This patient has three of the P's already: pain with passive stretch, paresthesias, and pressure over the compartment. One must assume that he has a compartment syndrome. The measured pressure in a compartment syndrome is usually greater than 30 mm Hg, with a normal pressure being less than 20 mm Hg. Assuming that this patient has a compartment syndrome, he does not need angiography. The time lost at angiography would only extend the damage to vital structures in the compartment (such as nerves and muscle tissue) and increase the risk of limb loss. The patient needs emergent fasciotomy in the operating room with as little delay as possible. The correct answer, d, can be determined by the physical examination signs that were given. Dorsiflexion of the ankle and great toe and lateral foot numbness are all signs of posterior compartment syndrome (posterior tibial nerve and sural nerve). *(Emergency Medicine, Chapter 104, pp 1073–1083)*

5. True. See answer to question 6. *(Emergency Medicine, Chapter 104, pp 1073–1083)*

6. False. Vascular injuries in blunt trauma occur with less frequency than in penetrating trauma. However, when they do occur in blunt trauma, the prognosis is much worse. This is because of the greater soft tissue injuries and other associated injuries present in blunt trauma. *(Emergency Medicine, Chapter 104, pp 1073–1083)*

BIBLIOGRAPHY

Frykberg ER: Advances in the diagnosis and treatment of extremity vascular trauma. Surg Clin North Am 1995; 75:207–223.

Mabee JR, Bostwick TL: Pathophysiology and mechanisms of compartment syndrome. Orthop Rev 1993; 22:175–181.

McGee DL, Dalsey WC: The mangled extremity: Compartment syndrome and amputations (Review). Emerg Med Clin North Am 1992; 10:783–800.

Modrall JG, Weaver FA, Yellin AE: Vascular considerations in extremity trauma. Orthop Clin North Am 1993; 24:557–563.

Silbergleit R: Extremity trauma. *In* Howell JM, Altieri M, Jagoda AS, et al (eds): Emergency Medicine. Philadelphia, WB Saunders, 1998, pp 1073–1084.

50. Trauma in Special Populations: Pediatric and Pregnant Patients

TAREG BEY, MD

Pediatric Trauma

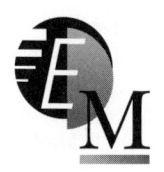

1. A 6-year-old trauma victim is brought to the ED by EMTs after a high-speed automobile accident. Initial assessment reveals an unconscious child with a heart rate of 140 and BP 90/60. Appropriate fluid management would be to start two large-bore IVs and administer:
   a. Normal saline at maintenance
   b. 10-mL/kg bolus of normal saline, reassess, and if inadequate response administer a second bolus of 10 mL/kg
   c. 20-mL/kg bolus of Ringer's lactate
   d. 30-mL/kg bolus of normal saline
   e. 30-mL/kg Ringer's lactate over 60 minutes

2. All of the following statements about pediatric shock are true except:
   a. The increased physiologic reserve of children may allow the maintenance of nearly normal blood pressure in the presence of impending shock.
   b. Hypotension in the traumatized child indicates severe blood loss and inadequate resuscitation.
   c. The child's normal systolic pressure should be 60 plus twice the age in mm Hg.
   d. Tachycardia in children can be caused by shock, fear, pain, and psychological stress.
   e. No urine output in a comatose and pale child suggests uncompensated shock with more than 45% blood volume loss.

3. All of the following are true about the pediatric airway except:
   a. As in adults, an oral airway should not be used in the conscious child.
   b. The smallest area of the airway of a child is the vocal cords.
   c. After the endotracheal tube is placed, both hemithoraces should be auscultated at the axillae.
   d. For mechanical ventilation, 7 to 10 mL/kg tidal volume is adequate to ventilate both infants and children.
   e. In small children, needle cricothyroidotomy with jet ventilation is preferred over surgical cricothyroidotomy.

4. A 3-year-old child presents to the ED in hemorrhagic shock. Which is the least beneficial action?
   a. Clear and maintain the airway.
   b. Give supplemental oxygen.
   c. If peripheral (antecubital) venous cannulation fails after several attempts, femoral venous access should be attempted next.
   d. If after a total of 40 mL/kg crystalloids fluid resuscitation, the vital signs continue to deteriorate, O-negative RBCs should be given.
   e. The bolus amount for RBCs in children is 10 mL/kg.

5. Which of the following statements about IO access in children is true?
   a. Complications of IO access include epiphysial injury, cellulitis, fracture, and joint infusion.
   b. The preferred insertion site of an IO needle is the proximal tibia below the level of the tuberosity.
   c. In skilled hands, IO access can be achieved faster than a venous cutdown.
   d. Effective fluid resuscitation can be accomplished by an IO access.
   e. All of the above are true.

6. All of the following statements about pediatric trauma are true except:
   a. In children, multisystem trauma is the rule rather than the exception.
   b. Small children are prone to hypothermia because of their high ratio of body surface to body mass.
   c. In small children, rib fractures are common after blunt trauma.
   d. All types of drugs can be infused through a functioning IO needle.
   e. If a child sustains multiple rib fractures, it usually implies a high-energy transfer, and other organ system injuries should be suspected.

7. All of the following drugs can be given via the endotracheal tube except:
   a. Epinephrine
   b. Atropine
   c. NaHCO$_3$
   d. Lidocaine
   e. Naloxone

8. All of the following statements about pediatric head trauma are true except:
   a. A patient with head trauma and a Glasgow Coma Scale score of 8 should be intubated.
   b. Children recover better from head injuries than adults.
   c. Children are not very susceptible to secondary brain injury because of their small size.
   d. A bulging fontanelle after head trauma could signify an expanding intracranial hematoma.
   e. Recurrent seizures after significant head injury is an indication for head CT.

9. All of the following statements about pediatric spinal injuries are true except:
   a. Up to 40% of children younger than 6 years of age can show an anterior pseudosubluxation between C2–C3 on the lateral cervical spine radiograph.
   b. If a young child has a normal cervical spine radiograph and a normal spine CT, a spinal cord injury can be excluded.
   c. Spinal cord injuries in children are relatively rare.
   d. The facet joints of the spine are flatter in children than in adults.
   e. In younger children the vertebral bodies of the spine are anteriorly wedged.

10. Which of the following injuries should prompt a further investigation for child abuse?
    a. Retinal hemorrhage
    b. Trauma to the genital and perineal area
    c. Multiple subdural hematomas
    d. A long bone fracture in a child younger than 3 years of age
    e. All of the above

Answers

1.c. The child is in impending shock with significant tachycardia and a marginal blood pressure. Fluid resuscitation is indicated. After establishing venous access, the child should be given a rapid bolus of crystalloid solution. The appropriate volume is 20 mL/kg. After the bolus, the child should be reevaluated. *(Emergency Medicine, Chapter 106, pp 1091–1100)*

2.c. The normal systolic BP in children is 80 mm Hg plus twice the age. In association with cold extremities, tachycardia and a systolic BP of more than 70 mm Hg indicates evolving shock. Tachycardia alone is not an indicator of shock and can be evaluated only in the context of mental status, skin color, and urinary output. *(Emergency Medicine, Chapter 106, pp 1091–1100)*

3.b. A conscious patient should not receive an oral airway because of the risk of aspiration. The smallest area of the child's airway is the subglottic or cricoid area and not the vocal cords, as in adults. In small children, surgical cricothyroidotomy is seldom indicated. This procedure carries a high risk of significant morbidity because of both the close proximity of adjacent vital structures and the long-term sequelae of the procedure. Needle cricothyroidotomy is an appropriate temporizing measure that can be used before a tracheostomy is placed under controlled conditions. *(Emergency Medicine, Chapter 106, pp 1091–1100)*

4.c. After airway and breathing, the circulation should be addressed. If percutaneous access is unsuccessful after the second attempt, then IO access should be attempted. In small children, there is considerable risk of venous thrombosis and ischemic limb loss after femoral vein cannulation. If after RBC transfusion the child is still hemodynamically unstable, operative intervention should be considered. *(Emergency Medicine, Chapter 106, pp 1091–1100)*

5.e. The IO needle should be inserted into an uninjured proximal tibia, just below the growth plate. In skilled hands, IO access can be achieved faster than access through any central line or cutdown. An IO line can be used to infuse crystalloid, blood products, and all resuscitation medications. *(Emergency Medicine, Chapter 106, pp 1091–1100)*

6.c. A small child injured by a high-impact blow to the chest usually does not sustain rib fractures. The pliable cartilaginous ribs usually bend, and most of the energy is absorbed in the underlying lung tissue. Pulmonary contusion and pulmonary hemorrhage are therefore common after blunt chest trauma in children. All types of drugs can be infused through an IO needle. *(Emergency Medicine, Chapter 106, pp 1091–1100)*

7.c. The mnemonic for endotracheal medications is NAVEL:
N = Naloxone
A = atropine
V = Valium
E = epinephrine
L = lidocaine
Recently, Valium has been removed and has been replaced by the more water-soluble Versed (midazolam). $NaHCO_3$ should not be given by the ET tube. *(Emergency Medicine, Chapter 106, pp 1091–1100)*

8.c. Children recover better from head injuries than adults. The outcome after head injuries is worse in children less than 3 months old than in the older age group. Secondary brain injury can occur through hypoglycemia; hypoxia; inadequate head, neck and body positioning; and uncontrolled seizure. A bulging fontanelle after pediatric head trauma needs to be evaluated further because the open fontanelle indicates the presence of a fairly significant potential space that can be filled through either hemorrhage or edema accumulation. *(Emergency Medicine, Chapter 106, pp 1091–1100)*

9.b. Children frequently show a "physiologic" C2–C3 anterior pseudosubluxation on the lateral cervical spine radiograph, which, once identified, requires no further investigation. Neurologic status should be carefully monitored and any deficit addressed, even if cervical spine studies are negative, because spinal cord injuries can be present even without any radiographically demonstrable injury (either plain film or CT scan). This entity has been called "spinal cord injury without radiologic abnormality" (SCIWORA). Although spinal cord injuries are rare in the pediatric population, any child with evidence of spinal cord involvement should be evaluated by a specialist. *(Emergency Medicine, Chapter 106, pp 1091–1100)*

10.e. All of the listed injuries should prompt a further investigation for possible child abuse. Other injuries to look for are evidence of a ruptured internal organ that is unexplained by history; presence of multiple healing fractures on radiography; multiple bruises at different stages of healing, especially if in unusual locations or in patterns; and bizarre injuries such as cigarette or rope burns. *(Emergency Medicine, Chapter 106, pp 1091–1100)*

The Pregnant Patient

1. All of the following statements about management of a traumatized pregnant woman are true except:
   a. Airway management and cervical spine immobilization are performed as in the nonpregnant woman.
   b. All traumatized pregnant women should receive high-flow supplemental oxygen.
   c. At 12 weeks' gestation, the gravid uterus may cause pressure on the inferior vena cava in the supine position.
   d. In traumatized pregnant women, the fetus may develop distress without evidence of maternal hypoxia.
   e. The abdominal compartment of military antishock trousers should not be used in pregnant women.

2. All of the statements about the normal physiologic changes found in a pregnant woman are true except:
   a. Mild tachycardia, decreased BP, and anemia are normal in the late stages of pregnancy.
   b. Patients in the third trimester of pregnancy have decreased functional residual capacity of the lung because of increased limitation of diaphragmatic excursion.
   c. Normal vital signs in the traumatized pregnant patient guarantee a good fetal outcome.
   d. In maternal shock, epinephrine and norepinephrine should be avoided.
   e. Patients in their third trimester tend to regurgitate faster because of increased gastric distention.

3. All of the following statements regarding the evaluation of the pregnant trauma patient are true except:
   a. Peritoneal irritation is difficult to assess in the third trimester.
   b. Any post-traumatic vaginal bleeding requires immediate evaluation by full vaginal examination.
   c. Fetal movement should be assessed after an accident.
   d. A standard trauma series (cervical spine, chest, and pelvis) should not be withheld when evaluating the pregnant trauma patient.
   e. A supraumbilical diagnostic peritoneal lavage in a late-term pregnant woman is a useful diagnostic tool.

4. Which diagnostic tests may be used to evaluate the third-trimester pregnant trauma patient?
   a. Radiographs of cervical spine, chest, and pelvis
   b. Coagulation studies and Rh determination
   c. CT of the abdomen with contrast
   d. Fetal monitoring
   e. All of the above

5. A pregnant trauma patient requires an antimicrobial. Which of the following medications should not be given during pregnancy?
   a. Penicillin
   b. Ceftriaxone
   c. Ampicillin
   d. Clindamycin
   e. Gentamicin

6. All of the following statements about treating the pregnant trauma patient are true except:
   a. RhoGAM (300 μg) should be given after the twelfth week of gestation if fetal-maternal transfusion is suspected.
   b. If a surgical procedure is required and the fetus is well, a normal delivery at a later date is preferred.
   c. If the patient has never been immunized against tetanus, 250 mg of tetanus immune globulin should be given along with tetanus toxoid, at different sites.
   d. Silver sulfadiazine for the treatment of a burned patient does not impose a risk to the fetus.
   e. If open chest massage is done in a pregnant woman, the aorta should not be cross clamped.

7. All of the following statements about medications in pregnant women are true except:
   a. Seizures should be treated with benzodiazepines.
   b. Benzodiazepines cross the placenta and can cause fetal respiratory depression after delivery.
   c. The loading dose of magnesium for the eclamptic patient is 0.75 g IV.
   d. NSAIDs for pain management pose a fetal risk.
   e. Opioids for maternal pain management cross the placenta and can suppress the neonatal respiratory drive.

8. When making a disposition for the pregnant trauma patient, the physician has to consider:
   a. Patients with multiple trauma injuries must be admitted.
   b. A patient admitted to the surgical service should have at least 4 hours of cardiotocographic monitoring.
   c. Cardiotocographic monitoring should be extended to 24 hours if abnormalities were present.
   d. Even after minor trauma, a viable fetus of 24 weeks' gestation must be monitored for 4 hours before the pregnant patient is discharged.
   e. All of the above must be considered.

9. All of the following are true about trauma in pregnancy except:
   a. Blunt trauma is more common than penetrating injuries.
   b. Stab wounds are more common than gunshot wounds.
   c. After trauma the fetus is at increased risk for premature labor, abruptio placentae, fetal-maternal transfusion, and stillbirth.
   d. Shock and hypoxia are poor prognostic indicators for both mother and fetus.
   e. After 20 weeks of gestation, the cardiac output can decrease 25% because of the vena cava compression syndrome in supine position.

10. All of the following statements are true about pregnancy except:
    a. The classic signs for abruptio placentae are abdominal pain, vaginal bleeding, amniotic fluid leakage, and a tender uterus.
    b. A retroplacental hematoma can contain several liters of blood that may not pass per vagina.
    c. Smoking, cocaine, and multiparity are all risk factors for abruptio placentae.
    d. The fetus usually has a good chance of survival if not more than 55% of the placenta is abrupted.
    e. The traumatic release of thromboplastin by the placenta can lead to a severe maternal coagulopathy.

Answers

1.c. The initial management of a pregnant trauma patient is the same as for any other trauma patient: secure Airway, establish Breathing, ensure Circulation. All trauma victims, including the pregnant patient, should receive supplemental oxygen. In patients greater than 20 weeks of gestation the gravid uterus may compress the inferior vena cava in the supine position. The abdominal compartment of the military antishock trousers should never be inflated in pregnant women. *(Emergency Medicine, Chapter 105, pp 1085–1090)*

2.c. Mild tachycardia and decreased BP can be normal in the late stages of pregnancy. On the other hand, significant maternal blood loss can go unrecognized both because of the normal volume expansion that occurs in pregnancy and because of the potential to shunt blood flow away from the placenta, while the fetus may already be in distress. Normal vital signs in a pregnant woman are no guarantee of fetal well-being. The diaphragm is higher and gastric emptying is delayed during pregnancy. Although epinephrine and norepinephrine may increase maternal BP, they adversely affect fetal survival because of decreased uterine perfusion. *(Emergency Medicine, Chapter 105, pp 1085–1090)*

3.b. Peritoneal irritation can be very difficult to assess in a pregnant women. The abdominal wall may be stretched too taut to permit an accurate manual examination. Speculum and definitely bimanual examination are contraindicated in the bleeding trauma victim during the second and third trimesters of pregnancy. The examination may itself worsen an already critical situation if abruptio placentae or placenta previa is present. A peritoneal lavage during pregnancy, using a supraumbilical approach, may be indicated but will miss retroperitoneal bleeding. *(Emergency Medicine, Chapter 105, pp 1085–1090)*

4.e. All of these tests may be used to evaluate the traumatized pregnant patient. An abdominal CT is a useful diagnostic tool and should not be omitted because of risk of radiation. In the first trimester, the fetus can be shielded because most information gained is obtained by scanning the upper abdomen. Abdominal CT will also detect retroperitoneal bleeding. *(Emergency Medicine, Chapter 105, pp 1085–1090)*

5.e. Penicillin, cephalosporins, and clindamycin are not teratogenic. Risk to the fetus may arise from tetracyclines, aminoglycosides, sulfonamides, and chloramphenicol. *(Emergency Medicine, Chapter 105, pp 1085–1090)*

6.d. RhoGAM, 300 μg IM, is recommended for fetal-maternal transfusion after the twelfth week of gestation. Aggressive tetanus management is indicated because the incubation period of disease appears to be shorter and its course more virulent during pregnancy. Silver sulfadiazine can lead to kernicterus of the fetus. *(Emergency Medicine, Chapter 105, pp 1085–1090)*

7.c. Seizures in a pregnant woman may be caused by eclampsia, head trauma, an underlying disease, or preexisting seizure disorder. Seizures must be stopped immediately. If eclampsia is suspected, magnesium is administered at a loading IV dose of 2 to 4 g followed by maintenance at 2 g/hour. Magnesium is used to treat eclampsia and to decrease uterine irritability. NSAIDs are not indicated for pain management of the pregnant patient, because they may induce premature closure of the ductus arteriosus. *(Emergency Medicine, Chapter 105, pp 1085–1090)*

8.e. Pregnant patients with trauma should have at least a 4-hour period of cardiotocographic monitoring. Even minor trauma is associated with a higher risk of miscarriage. *(Emergency Medicine, Chapter 105, pp 1085–1090)*

9.b. Blunt trauma is more common than penetrating trauma, but gunshot wounds are more common than stab wounds. The vena cava compression syndrome of the gravid uterus occurs in supine position after 20 weeks of gestation and is caused by decreased venous return to the heart. *(Emergency Medicine, Chapter 105, pp 1085–1090)*

10.d. A retroplacental hematoma can produce hemorrhagic shock with minimal vaginal bleeding. If less than 25% of the placenta is abrupted the fetal survival is usually good, but with more than 50% abruption, the fetus rarely survives. Besides smoking, cocaine use, and multiparity, diabetes, preeclampsia, and increased maternal age constitute a risk for abruptio placentae. The traumatic release of placental thromboplastin may initiate disseminated intravascular coagulation. *(Emergency Medicine, Chapter 105, pp 1085–1090)*

BIBLIOGRAPHY

Mayer TA: Pediatric multiple trauma. *In* Howell JM, Altieri M, Jagoda AS, et al (eds): Emergency Medicine. Philadelphia, WB Saunders, 1998, pp 1091–1100.

Talbot-Stern J: Trauma in pregnancy. *In* Howell JM, Altieri M, Jagoda AS, et al (eds): Emergency Medicine. Philadelphia, WB Saunders, 1998, pp 1085–1090.

51 Wound Management, Burns, and Blast Injuries

ANDREW ULRICH, MD   JEFF GALVIN, MD

Wounds

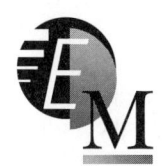

1. All of the following suture materials and indications for use are appropriate except:
   a. Silk: perioral laceration repair
   b. Nylon: any skin laceration repair
   c. Prolene: subcutaneous laceration repair
   d. Mersilene: tendon repair
   e. Dexon: mucous membrane laceration repair

2. All of the following suture materials are nonabsorbable except:
   a. Silk
   b. Chromic
   c. Nylon
   d. Prolene
   e. Mersilene

3. Closed-fist injuries are exceptionally prone to which of the following conditions?
   a. Cellulitis
   b. Septic arthritis
   c. Tenosynovitis
   d. Osteomyelitis
   e. All of the above

4. Regarding the use of tetanus immunization, all of the following are true except:
   a. For non–tetanus-prone wounds, individuals fully immunized and who have received a booster within the past 10 years do not require additional prophylaxis.
   b. For non–tetanus-prone wounds, individuals who have been fully immunized but have not received a booster within the past 10 years require only tetanus toxoid.
   c. For tetanus-prone wounds, individuals fully immunized but without a booster for 10 years require tetanus toxoid and tetanus immune globulin.
   d. For tetanus-prone wounds, individuals with incomplete immunization require both tetanus toxoid and tetanus immune globulin.

5. Which of the following medications is/are safe to use on a patient with an allergy to procaine?
   a. Bupivacaine
   b. Tetracaine
   c. Lidocaine
   d. Benzocaine
   e. Bupivacaine and lidocaine

6. The use of a tetracaine, adrenaline, cocaine solution is appropriate for the repair of all of the following except:
   a. A 2-cm superficial forehead laceration on a 2-year-old patient
   b. A through-and-through laceration to the upper lip of an 8-year-old patient
   c. A 5-cm laceration to the forearm of a 13-year-old patient
   d. A deep knee laceration on a 70-year-old patient
   e. An eyebrow laceration on a pregnant 19-year-old patient

7. Which of the following choices best represents an appropriate interval between wound repair and suture removal?
   a. 10 days for a laceration to the nasal bridge
   b. 3 to 5 days for a laceration to the patella area
   c. 3 to 4 days for a forehead laceration
   d. 10 days for an intraoral laceration
   e. None of the above

8. Lidocaine with epinephrine for local anesthesia is contraindicated in all of the following situations except:
   a. Repair of a 2-cm superficial laceration on the penis of a 12-year-old patient
   b. Repair of a deep laceration on the head of an 80-year-old patient
   c. Repair of a small nasal tip laceration on a 9-month-old patient
   d. Repair of a heavily bleeding laceration on the thumb of a 19-year-old patient
   e. Repair of a superficial laceration on the first toe of a 5-year-old patient

9. All of the following are true regarding the use of lidocaine with epinephrine for local anesthesia except:
   a. The duration of action is prolonged when compared to lidocaine alone.
   b. It may reduce bleeding from small surrounding vessels.

277

c. It reduces the risk of postrepair infection.
d. Its use should be limited to areas not supplied by end arteries.
e. The maximum suggested dose for a single injection is 7.0 mg/kg.

Answers

1.c. Suture material is categorized as absorbable or nonabsorbable. Absorbable material, such as Dexon (polyglycolic acid), is used for deep sutures and repair of mucous membranes. Nonabsorbable sutures are used for repair of skin lacerations. Monofilament materials such as nylon and Prolene cause less tissue reactivity and thus result in better wound healing. Mersilene is ideal for tendon repair because of its excellent tensile strength. Silk is best suited for repair of perioral or nasal regions. *(Emergency Medicine, Chapter 109, pp 1117–1124)*

2.b. Nonabsorbable materials such as silk, nylon, Prolene, and Mersilene have differing degrees of tissue reactivity and tensile strength. Absorbable material such as chromic, Dexon, and Vicryl (polyglactin 910) differ in the rate at which they are absorbed; slower absorption allows for increased wound strength. *(Emergency Medicine, Chapter 109, pp 1117–1124)*

3.e. Hand injuries require special attention because bones, ligaments, tendons, and neurovascular bundles are near the skin surface. Closed-fist injuries occur when a fist strikes someone's teeth, resulting in contaminated puncture wound to the extensor surface. Rapid development of cellulitis and tenosynovitis can occur. Violation of the joint capsule may result in septic arthritis and, in the long term, in osteomyelitis. All closed-fist bite injuries require irrigation, splinting, and antimicrobials. Those with signs of infection often require admission. These wounds should be left open. *(Emergency Medicine, Chapter 109, pp 1117–1124)*

4.c. Tetanus immune globulin and tetanus toxoid confer passive and active immunization, respectively. A complete immunization series consists of a three-shot series. Patients with incomplete immunization require both immune globulin and toxoid, whereas those who completed the three-shot series need only boosters every 7 to 10 years. Wounds considered tetanus prone are of longer duration, grossly contaminated, or already infected and those in which appropriate cleaning is impossible (e.g., puncture wounds). *(Emergency Medicine, Chapter 109, pp 1117–1124)*

5.e. Many patients report a history of allergy or reaction to local anesthetic agents. Although it is rare, some patients do have allergies to the ester class of agents (e.g., benzocaine, procaine, tetracaine). Allergies of the amide class (e.g., lidocaine, bupivacaine) are exceedingly rare. They are almost always due to the preservative used in multidose vials and can be avoided by using single-dose vials. If a known allergy exists, use of local anesthetic agents should be limited to those from the other class. Subcutaneous diphenhydramine may be used if the patient believes he or she is allergic to both classes. *(Emergency Medicine, Chapter 109, pp 1117–1124)*

6.b. The most commonly used topical anesthetic solution is a combination of tetracaine, adrenaline, and cocaine. Gauze soaked in the solution is applied to the wound area for 10 to 30 minutes. Blanching of the surrounding skin is evidence of adequate anesthesia. Areas that are highly vascularized are more easily anesthetized. Mucous membranes are to be avoided because of enhanced absorption and increased systemic effects. *(Emergency Medicine, Chapter 109, pp 1117–1124)*

7.c. The interval until removal of suture is determined by anatomic location, healing properties of the patient, and degree of tension across the wound. An easy rule to remember is, "The farther the wound is from the face, the longer the stitches should remain." Facial sutures should be removed in 3 to 5 days to prevent scarring. Sutures across joints and on extremities should remain in place 10 to 14 days to ensure sufficient healing and wound strength. Sutures left beyond 14 days are more likely to cause scarring. Intraoral lacerations should be repaired using absorbable material, which does not require removal. *(Emergency Medicine, Chapter 109, pp 1117–1124)*

8.b. Epinephrine is a potent vasoconstrictor. The addition to lidocaine extends the duration of anesthesia and often reduces bleeding. However, ischemia and subsequent tissue necrosis can occur when used in areas supplied by end arteries, for example, ears, nose, fingers, toes, and penis. *(Emergency Medicine, Chapter 109, pp 1117–1124)*

9.c. Lidocaine is the most widely used local anesthetic agent. Addition of epinephrine extends its duration and decreases bleeding from small surrounding vessels. As a vasoconstrictor, epinephrine is contraindicated in areas supplied by end arteries (see answer to question 8). As a result of decreased blood flow, lidocaine with epinephrine may have adverse effects on wound healing. Maximum suggested dose for a single injection of lidocaine with epinephrine is 7.0 mg/kg. The maximum dose for lidocaine without epinephrine is 4.5 mg/kg. *(Emergency Medicine, Chapter 109, pp 1117–1124)*

Burns

1. All of the following statements regarding burns are true except:
   a. Burn mortality is directly proportional to the extent of the burn.
   b. Mortality is greatest in the young and elderly.
   c. Mortality is more dependent on body surface area involved than on associated injury.
   d. Approximately 2% of burns in children result from abuse.
   e. Burns are the second leading cause of death in children less than 12 years.

2. Absence of the classic cherry-red skin and mucous membranes of carbon monoxide poisoning is evidence of a blood level less than:
   a. 15%
   b. 20%
   c. 30%
   d. 40%
   e. None of the above

3. Which of the following statements is true regarding the use of hyperbaric oxygen therapy for carbon monoxide poisoning?
   a. Hyperbaric oxygen therapy at 3 atm decreases the half-life by 50% when compared to room air at sea level.
   b. Hyperbaric oxygen therapy is contraindicated in the pediatric population.
   c. The decision to initiate hyperbaric oxygen therapy is based on symptoms and not on measured carbon monoxide hemoglobin levels.
   d. Hyperbaric oxygen therapy is contraindicated in the third trimester of pregnancy.
   e. Treatment with 100% oxygen is equally effective in decreasing the half-life of carbon monoxide.

4. Which of the following signs and symptoms is appropriately matched with an expected carboxyhemoglobin level?
   a. Severe headache, fatigue: 30% to 40%
   b. Coma, seizures: 40% to 50%
   c. Severe headache, vomiting, incoordination: 30% to 40%
   d. Syncope, obtundation: 10% to 20%
   e. Hypotension, pulmonary edema: 20% to 30%

5. When using the rule of nines, a patient with burns covering both legs, both arms, and the perineum has what percent of body surface area involved?
   a. 40%
   b. 45%
   c. 50%
   d. 55%
   e. 60%

6. All of the following are true of partial-thickness burns except:
   a. They are painless.
   b. They involve both the epidermis and the dermis.
   c. They classically present with blisters and bullae.
   d. The surrounding skin is often edematous.
   e. They may result from scalding liquid or flame.

Answers

1.c. There are reportedly greater than 1.5 million patients annually who are treated for burns. The young and the elderly account for greater than 80% of all patients with major burns, and the morbidity and mortality are highest in these age groups. Burns are the second leading cause of death in children less than 12 years of age. An estimated 2% of burns in children are the result of abuse. Although mortality is directly proportional to the extent of body surface involved, the presence of an inhalation injury or associated trauma has a *greater* effect on survival. **(Emergency Medicine, Chapter 107, pp 1101–1110)**

2.e. The classic description of cherry-red skin or mucous membranes may be found when blood levels of carbon monoxide hemoglobin exceed 40%. However, this finding is rarely evidenced. Typically, patients are noted to have pale or cyanotic skin. Other dermatologic findings may include bullae formation, edema, and erythematous patches. **(Emergency Medicine, Chapter 107, pp 1101–1110)**

3.c. Carbon monoxide has a higher affinity for hemoglobin and therefore displaces oxygen. Eventually, as carboxyhemoglobin levels increase, serum oxygen-carrying capacity becomes inadequate and tissue hypoxia occurs. Hyperbaric oxygen therapy increases the partial pressure of oxygen and displaces carbon monoxide molecules from hemoglobin. The half-life of carboxyhemoglobin at ambient pressure is 4.5 hours. One hundred percent oxygen reduces this to 80 minutes. Hyperbaric oxygen at 3 atm further reduces this time to 23 minutes. Indications for hyperbaric oxygen therapy include an absolute level greater than 30%, a history of syncope, neurologic impairment, chest pain, or ECG changes indicative of ischemia or cardiac dysrhythmias. Hyperbaric oxygen therapy should be initiated earlier in pregnant or pediatric patients because they are more susceptible to permanent damage from significant exposure. **(Emergency Medicine, Chapter 107, pp 1101–1110)**

4.b. The clinical manifestations of carbon monoxide poisoning vary from mild headache to coma and cardiovascular collapse. Because measured carbon monoxide bound to hemoglobin and symptoms are a reflection of carbon monoxide in the tissue, there is a loose association between level and symptoms. In addition, development of symptoms is associated with an individual's preexisting health status. As a rule of thumb, levels below 10% are asymptomatic. Levels between 10% and 20% produce mild headache, fatigue, and lightheadedness. Levels of 20% to 30% result in incoordination, impaired judgment, and nausea and vomiting. Levels of 30% to 40% result in syncope, obtundation, tachypnea, and tachycardia. Levels between 40% and 50% produce seizures and coma. Levels greater than 50% are associated with hypotension, pulmonary edema, and death. The end point of treatment is resolution of symptoms, not a normal laboratory study. *(Emergency Medicine, Chapter 107, pp 1101–1110)*

5.d. In adults, the rule of nines gives a good approximation of body surface area. The head and arms account for 9% each; the front and back of the torso, 18% each; the legs, 18% each; and the perineum, 1% (Figs. 51–1 and 51–2). *(Emergency Medicine, Chapter 107, pp 1101–1110)*

6.a. Burns are classified according to depth of injury. First-degree burns involve only the epidermis and result in red and painful skin. Partial-thickness burns, or second-degree burns, involve both the epidermis and the dermis. These burns are hypersensitive, painful, edematous, and classically covered with fragile fluid-filled blisters or bullae. Partial-thickness burns often result from exposure to flames or scalding liquids. Third-degree or full-thickness burns result in complete destruction of all skin layers. The remaining skin is dry, leathery to the touch, and painless. *(Emergency Medicine, Chapter 107, pp 1101–1110)*

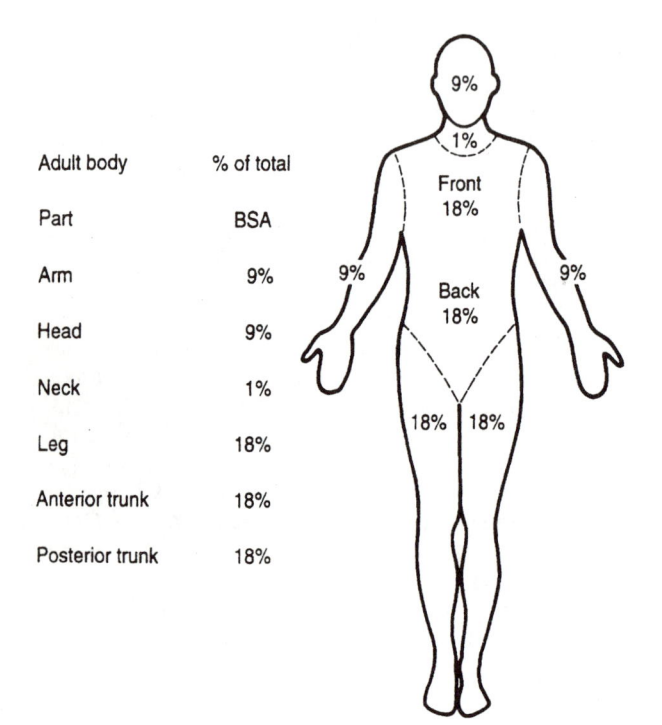

Adult body Part	% of total BSA
Arm	9%
Head	9%
Neck	1%
Leg	18%
Anterior trunk	18%
Posterior trunk	18%

FIGURE 51–1. Adult figure of nines. (From Herndon DN: Total Burn Care. London, WB Saunders, 1996, p 35.)

WOUND MANAGEMENT, BURNS, AND BLAST INJURIES **281**

Age	0–1	1–4	5–9	10–14	15
A – 1/2 of head	9 1/2%	8 1/2%	6 1/2%	5 1/2%	4 1/2%
B – 1/2 of one thigh	2 3/4%	3 1/4%	4%	4 1/4%	4 1/2%
C – 1/2 of one leg	2 1/2%	2 1/2%	2 3/4%	3%	3 1/4%

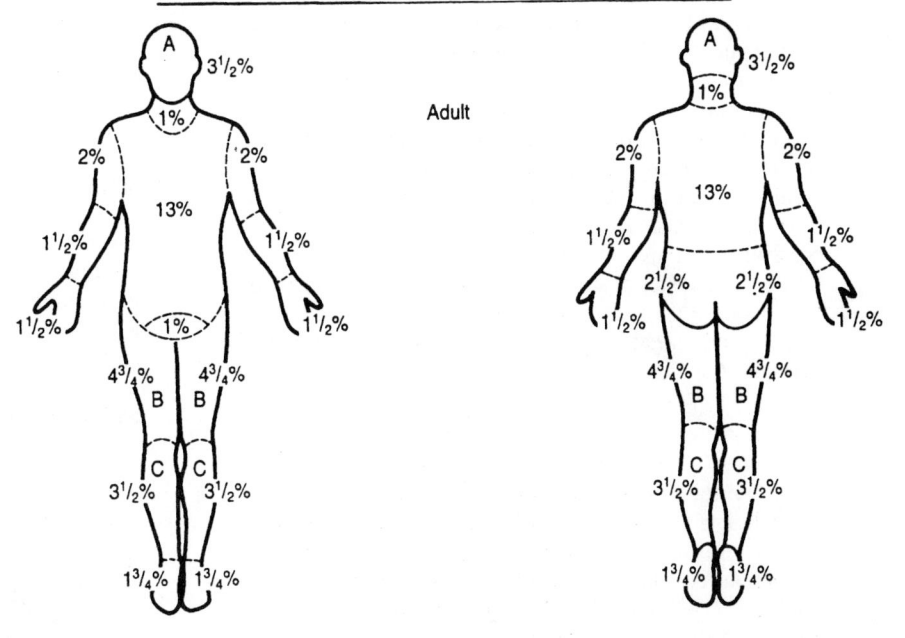

FIGURE 51–2. Lund and Browder chart. (From Herndon DN: Total Burn Care. London, WB Saunders, 1996, p 36.)

Blast Injuries

1. All of the following are important considerations in blast injury triage except:
   a. Nonambulatory injured persons should be moved to a designated clearing area for evaluation.
   b. Primary blast injury may be present despite little evidence of external trauma.
   c. Injuries from underwater blasts tend to occur at greater distances and be more severe than those on land.
   d. Emergency personnel should be prevented from entering a blast scene until after the bomb squad has cleared the area.
   e. Victims caught in the open when an explosive device goes off are less likely to suffer secondary blast injury than those who are under cover.

2. Which of the following are characteristics of blast lung?
   a. Intra-alveolar hemorrhage
   b. Pulmonary findings that may be delayed for hours
   c. Pneumothorax
   d. Fatal air embolism associated with the use of high PEEP settings
   e. All of the above

3. All of the following statements are true of blast injury except:
   a. Simple clothing may be protective against secondary blast effects.
   b. Flash burns from an explosion may cause respiratory compromise.
   c. Building collapse, large projectiles, and whole-body acceleration/deceleration are all causes of blast-related blunt trauma.
   d. Head trauma is the leading cause of blast death.
   e. All lacerations should be considered heavily contaminated and left to close by secondary intention.

4. You are the physician on the scene after a terrorist explosion. All of the following aspects of the blast are important to patient triage except:
   a. Whether the explosion occurred in a confined space
   b. The concomitant use of other agents (nuclear/chemical/biologic) in the attack
   c. The type of conventional explosive used
   d. The presence of nasopharyngeal petechiae
   e. Victims' distance from the explosive device

Answers

1. e. Blast sites must be cleared by the bomb squad before emergency team entrance because of the possibility of a second explosive device designed to ignite when rescuers arrive. Moving patients to a central clearing area for evaluation is standard procedure in disaster scene management. Secondary blast injury is caused by debris (glass, rock, metal) accelerated into flying projectiles by the blast wind. Those caught in the open are at much greater risk of injury than those under cover. The medium through which a blast wave moves plays a significant role in determining the severity of possible injuries. Because water is denser and relatively incompressible compared to air, underwater blast waves travel farther and faster than identical shock waves on land. Victims of underwater explosions are more likely to suffer abdominal injuries. *(Emergency Medicine, Chapter 108, pp 1111–1115)*

2. e. The pressure wave of an explosive blast disrupts the alveolar-venous interface and may damage the visceral pleura. Intra-alveolar hemorrhage, pneumothorax, and air emboli may result. This alveolar-venous communication can result in massive air embolism, especially if the patient is ventilated with high PEEP settings. Survivors are at risk of developing delayed progressive respiratory insufficiency and an ARDS-like syndrome caused by pulmonary edema and hemorrhage. Pulmonary damage may be delayed for hours, so victims should be constantly reassessed. *(Emergency Medicine, Chapter 108, pp 1111–1115)*

3. b. Flash burns are caused by the initial release of thermal energy from an explosive device; they are generally superficial and do not cause respiratory compromise. Huge amounts of energy, in the form of pressure and heat, are released instantaneously when an explosive is detonated. A powerful shock wave, or blast wave, propagates radially outward from the explosion, subjecting everything in its path to an overpressure wave that is often several hundred pounds per square inch. As the hot gases in the explosion's center move outward, they displace air and cause it to move very rapidly. This blast wind can transiently reach velocities greater than 1000 miles per hour. Primary blast injury results from the direct effect of a blast wave on the human body. Compressible gas-filled organs are most susceptible to injury. Lungs, ears, CNS, and the gastointestinal tract are the most common organ systems affected. Secondary blast injury is caused by the acceleration of debris by the blast wind. Simple clothing is often enough to prevent injury from smaller projectiles. Lacerations caused by larger pieces of flying debris are likely to be heavily inoculated with foreign material. When possible, these should be left to close by secondary intention. Tertiary blast injury results from the victim's being thrown by the blast wind and striking another object. Head injury is very common and is the leading cause of death. Further injuries may be caused by sequelae of the initial blast, for example, building collapse, inhalation of dust or toxic gases, thermal burns from secondary fires, or radiation exposure. *(Emergency Medicine, Chapter 108, pp 1111–1115)*

4. c. Information that the physician should consider when treating blast victims includes where the blast occurred, the distance of victims from the blast, and the release of any other toxic substances. Injuries from blasts in a confined space increase the likelihood of inhalation injuries from toxic gases, smoke, and dust and therefore tend to be worse than those occurring in the open. Proximity to the blast is an important triage consideration, because the overpressure wave created by an explosion dissipates rapidly. A blast that kills a victim at 10 feet may cause only minor injuries at 100 feet. The presence of nonconventional (nuclear/chemical/biologic) agents presents rescue and hospital personnel with added hazards. These patients require thorough decontamination before transport. The specific type of explosive does not enter into triage decisions, because most conventional explosives cause similar injury patterns. Physical findings (besides the obvious evaluation of the ABCs) that can assist in triage include nasopharyngeal petechiae and tympanic membrane rupture. The presence of nasopharyngeal petechiae has been correlated with the development of blast lung. Tympanic membrane rupture indicates a higher probability of primary blast trauma. *(Emergency Medicine, Chapter 108, pp 1111–1115)*

BIBLIOGRAPHY

Chisolm CD: Blast injuries. *In* Howell JM, Altieri M, Jagoda AS, et al (eds): Emergency Medicine. Philadelphia, WB Saunders, 1998, pp 1111–1115.

Pigman EC: Wound management. *In* Howell JM, Altieri M, Jagoda AS, et al (eds): Emergency Medicine. Philadelphia, WB Saunders, 1998, pp 1117–1124.

Smith J: Burns. *In* Howell JM, Altieri M, Jagoda AS, et al (eds): Emergency Medicine. Philadelphia, WB Saunders, 1998, pp 1101–1110.

SECTION FIFTEEN

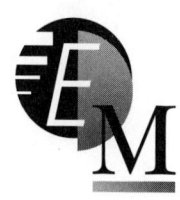

Musculoskeletal Injuries

52 Upper Extremity: Shoulder, Humerus, Elbow, Forearm, Wrist, and Hand

CAROL LEAH BARSKY, MD   PAUL BUCKLEY, MD, PhD   KATHRYN CRAIG, MD

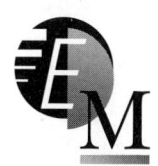

1. The direction of humeral head dislocation can often be ascertained by noting the position of the injured arm on presentation. Which of the following descriptions is correctly paired with the type of glenohumeral dislocation?
   a. Anterior—abduction and internal rotation
   b. Posterior—adduction and external rotation
   c. Inferior—abduction and external rotation
   d. All of the above are correctly paired

2. A 25-year-old bicycle messenger presents with an isolated shoulder dislocation. A Hill-Sachs deformity is evident on his postreduction films. Which is the most likely reason for its absence on the prereduction radiographs?
   a. He had a posterior dislocation.
   b. The deformity occurred during reduction.
   c. He was unable to internally rotate his arm for the technologist.
   d. The glenoid rim is obscured by the displaced humeral head.
   e. The patient did not have a transscapular Y-view radiograph.

3. Acceptable methods of reduction for anterior shoulder dislocations include all of the following except:
   a. Elevation with external rotation
   b. Adduction with full external rotation, then bringing the forearm and the elbow across the chest
   c. Scapular manipulation while prone
   d. Two-person traction-countertraction
   e. The Stimson method

4. Which of the following injuries requires orthopedic consultation in the ED?
   a. Biceps tendon rupture
   b. Middle clavicle fracture
   c. Proximal humeral epiphysis separation
   d. Proximal humeral fracture with 5-mm displacement
   e. Acromioclavicular joint separation

5. All of the following statements about clavicular fractures are true except:
   a. Proximal and distal clavicular fractures account for only 5% of clavicular fractures.
   b. Proximal and distal clavicular fractures are best evaluated with sternoclavicular views.
   c. Fractures of the middle third of the clavicle are the most common of the clavicular fractures.
   d. Treatment of fractures of the middle third of the clavicle is use of a sling, or sling and swathe.
   e. In children, acromioclavicular separations are far more common than clavicle fractures.

6. A 45-year-old male smoker presents to the ED with complaints of intermittent left burning shoulder pain. The patient believes the pain began after painting the outside of his house yesterday. The most important next step is to:
   a. Obtain an ECG.
   b. Give the patient NSAIDs.
   c. Have the patient raise his arms over his head.
   d. Call the orthopedic consultant.
   e. Test for the painful arc sign and perform a Neer test.

7. All of the following statements are true of proximal humerus fractures except:
   a. Significant displacement is defined as more than 2 cm of displacement of any segment or angulation greater than 45 degrees.
   b. Most proximal humerus fractures can be immobilized with a sling.
   c. Displaced greater tuberosity fractures are associated with rotator cuff tears.
   d. Avascular necrosis is a complication of mid–humeral shaft fractures.
   e. The typical patient is an elderly person who has fallen on an outstretched hand.

8. A 14-year-old boy fell on his outstretched right arm while skateboarding. He complains of pain at the elbow and can make a fist and supinate the forearm. After reduction of his fracture, he complains of pain in the hand; a decreased radial pulse is noted. What is the best next step in management?

a. Open surgical exploration
b. Splint pronated and flexed 70 degrees before repeat x-ray
c. CT to identify median nerve entrapment
d. Angiography of brachial artery

9. What is the best method to achieve stabilization of an isolated midshaft fracture of the ulna with 6 mm of displacement and 20 degrees of angulation?
   a. Sugar-tong splint with forearm in neutral position
   b. Long arm splint with elbow at 90 degrees of flexion
   c. Open reduction and internal fixation
   d. Short arm cast with forearm in supination

10. A 7-year-old boy fell from a jungle gym, striking his left forearm on a bar during the fall. He complains of pain near the elbow and can neither flex the elbow nor extend the fingers and thumb. What radiographic abnormality should be anticipated?
    a. Distal displacement of the ulna in a lateral view of the wrist
    b. Anterior subluxation of the radial head in a lateral view of the elbow
    c. Posterior subluxation of the radial head in a medial oblique view of the elbow
    d. Median nerve entrapment at the elbow by CT

11. A 40-year-old female factory worker presents with the first occurrence of a painful fluctuant bulge posterior to the olecranon process without overlying erythema. She is able to extend her forearm without difficulty. ED management should include which of the following?
    a. Corticosteroid injection of medial elbow
    b. Admission for IV antimicrobials covering *Staphylococcus aureus*
    c. Incision, drainage, and packing before discharge with cephalexin
    d. Joint aspiration, compressive dressing, and discharge with NSAIDs

12. Which of the following unintentional traumatic elbow injuries may be referred to an orthopedic surgeon within 24 to 48 hours after immobilization in the ED?
    a. An epicondylar fracture in a 6-year-old girl
    b. A paired radius-ulna fracture in a 10-year-old boy
    c. A Galeazzi fracture in a 17-year-old male
    d. A type I condylar fracture in a 40-year-old male

13. What is the appropriate management of extensor tendon lacerations at the level of the metacarpophalangeal joint?
    a. Immediate consultation with hand specialist for open exploration
    b. Copious irrigation followed by consultation with a hand surgeon
    c. Approximation with nonabsorbable simple interrupted sutures
    d. Splinting in hyperextension

14. A 23-year-old right-handed machine-shop worker sustained a puncture injury to his distal left long finger while working with a high-pressure air gun. What is the most appropriate disposition?
    a. Discharge with oral cephalexin and wound care instructions
    b. Exploration in the ED under wrist-block anesthesia
    c. Immediate hand consultation for open irrigation and admission
    d. 6-hour observation for appearance of occult injury

15. A 35-year-old tattoo artist presents with 3 days of progressive right index finger swelling and pain. The finger is flexed and passive extension is limited by severe pain. What is the most appropriate management?
    a. Immediate consultation for admission and IV antimicrobials
    b. Ice, elevation, and outpatient NSAID therapy
    c. Incision and drainage under digital-block anesthesia in the ED
    d. Tetanus prophylaxis and outpatient antistaphylococcal antimicrobial therapy

16. Which of the following injuries requires immediate consultation with a hand specialist?
    a. Extensor tendon laceration over the first distal interphalangeal joint
    b. Fracture at the base of the second middle phalanx, involving 20% of the articular surface
    c. Nondisplaced midshaft fracture of the third metacarpal
    d. Fracture of the fourth metacarpal with 200 degrees of rotation

17. Which of the following is an *absolute* contraindication to the replantation of an amputated finger?
    a. Total ischemia time greater than 8 hours
    b. Position at time of injury
    c. Anatomic level of transection
    d. Severe soft tissue damage from crush injury

18. Radiographically, what is the upper limit of the normal separation between the scaphoid and lunate in millimeters?
    a. Two
    b. Three
    c. Four
    d. Five

19. A tear of the triangular fibrocartilaginous complex of the wrist is associated with which of the following physical findings?
    a. Pointer finger paresthesia with 60 seconds of wrist flexion
    b. Wrist pain with axial loading of the thumb
    c. Pain exacerbated by ulnar wrist deviation with the thumb flexed
    d. Midwrist pain with extension in both pronation and supination

20. A 45-year-old male complains of pain in the ulnar volar right wrist 2 days after his baseball bat struck a post in midswing. A PA x-ray of the wrist does not demonstrate a fracture. Which carpal bone fracture should be suspected?
    a. Lunate
    b. Triquetrum

c. Hamate
   d. Pisiform

21. A chip of bone is identified on a lateral x-ray of a tender wrist after a fall. Which carpal bone is fractured?
    a. Lunate
    b. Triquetrum
    c. Trapezium
    d. Pisiform

Answers

1.c. Luxatio erecta, wherein the humeral head lies inferior to the glenoid fossa, presents with the hand held behind the head with the inferiorly displaced humeral head against the thorax and the shaft in extreme abduction and external rotation. The patient with the common anterior dislocation supports the injured side at the wrist with the arm in 45 degrees of external rotation. The patient with a posterior dislocation holds the injured arm against the torso, in adduction and internal rotation. (*Emergency Medicine, Chapter 111, pp 1145–1151*)

2.c. The Hill-Sachs deformity, a compression fracture of the humeral head, is more easily identified with the humerus in internal rotation. The most likely dislocation is anterior, which presents with the humerus in slight abduction and external rotation. One third of anterior dislocations have this associated fracture. The axillary lateral view shows the position of the humeral head within the glenoid fossa. It is also the view used to demonstrate lesions of the humeral head, the glenoid rim, and the coracoid process. A Bankart deformity is a fracture of the rim of the glenoid and would be evident on prereduction films; it may also occur during leverage reduction. (*Emergency Medicine, Chapter 111, pp 1145–1151*)

3.b. The Kocher method involves adduction of the fully externally rotated arm. Then the forearm and elbow are brought across the chest. This technique is commonly associated with spiral humerus fractures and other soft tissue injuries. The Milch method (a) is safe and effective. The modified Stimson method (c) uses gravity and may be the least traumatic if the patient can tolerate the prone position. The traction-countertraction method (d), using bedsheets to provide the force while avoiding the axillary injuries of the Hippocratic method, is also reliable. (*Emergency Medicine, Chapter 111, pp 1145–1151*)

4.c. Many injuries of the shoulder and proximal humerus can be treated with a sling, ice, analgesia, and orthopedic follow-up. Pediatric epiphyseal separation may require prompt pinning for repair. Biceps tendon rupture may or may not need surgical repair, and immediate operative fixation is not necessary. The common middle clavicle fracture is treated with a sling; in compound or proximal fractures an orthopedist should be consulted for admission. Most proximal humeral fractures are minimally displaced (less than 1 cm) and can be treated with a sling. (*Emergency Medicine, Chapter 111, pp 1145–1151*)

5.e. Fractures of the middle third of the clavicle constitute 80% of clavicular fractures; generally they are not visible on the standard trauma series. A two-view clavicular series is useful in identifying midshaft fractures. Fractures of the proximal and distal clavicle are best evaluated with sternoclavicular joint views, which are also used to evaluate sternoclavicular dislocations. Figure-of-eight clavicular splints are no longer recommended. Treatment consists of sling or sling and swathe with adequate analgesia. Patients may generally begin mild exercise in 2 or 3 weeks and return to normal activity in 6 to 8 weeks. Children are much more likely to fracture the clavicle than to sustain separation of the acromioclavicular joint. (*Emergency Medicine, Chapter 111, pp 1145–1151*)

6.a. As always, the potentially life-threatening diagnosis must be excluded first, in this case myocardial ischemia. The physician must also consider other extrinsic sources of shoulder pain such as apical lung tumors, cervical spine abnormalities, and any other process that may irritate the diaphragm. With impingement syndromes, the patient describes pain in the shoulder during overhead motion, such as reaching for a high shelf or serving a tennis ball. The painful arc sign (pain and inability to lift the arm over the head) and Neer test (pain on passive elevation of the patient's arm in front of the body while immobilizing the scapula) assess nerve impingement and rotator cuff damage. (*Emergency Medicine, Chapter 111, pp 1145–1151*)

7.d. Significant displacement of proximal humerus fractures is defined as more than 1 cm of displacement of any segment or angulation of greater than 45 degrees. Displaced greater tuberosity fractures require orthopedic consultation for open reduction and repair of the rotator cuff. Avascular necrosis is associated with fractures of the surgical neck of the humerus that present with significant angulation or displacement. (*Emergency Medicine, Chapter 111, pp 1145–1151*)

8.a. Supracondylar fractures have a relatively high incidence of neurovascular injury. If a neurologic deficit is present before reduction it is generally caused by a neurapraxia of the anterior osseous branch of the median nerve; the patient has weakness of the flexor digitorum profundus and the flexor pollicis longus. Deficits that are present only after reduction require acute surgical exploration. The most common vascular injury is to the brachial artery. Angiography is diagnostic and may be useful when pulse deficits are noted in the absence of profound ischemia but will delay definitive treatment. (*Emergency Medicine, Chapter 112, pp 1152–1171*)

9.b. Most isolated midshaft fractures of the ulna (nightstick fractures) can be treated in a sugar-tong splint or a split long arm cast with the elbow in 90 degrees of flexion and the forearm in the neutral position. The exceptions are fractures angulated more than 10 degrees or displaced more than 5 mm and all fractures of the proximal third of the ulna. These fractures need to be treated with open reduction and internal fixation. *(Emergency Medicine, Chapter 112, pp 1152–1171)*

10.b. Because of the ring relationship of the bones of the forearm, forearm injuries often occur in pairs; a recent study demonstrated a 96% frequency of double injury.[1] The second injury may involve bony or ligamentous structures. A Monteggia fracture is a fracture of the ulnar shaft with an associated dislocation of the radial head. The most common is type I, anterior dislocation of the radial head with anterior angulation of the ulnar shaft fracture. The posterior interosseous branch of the radial nerve is at risk in this injury. The anterior interosseous branch of the median nerve controls the hand flexors. The medial oblique is the best view to assess the coronoid process. The distal ulna is subluxed dorsally in a Galeazzi fracture of the radial shaft and does not limit elbow flexion. *(Emergency Medicine, Chapter 112, pp 1152–1171)*

11.d. This patient has a traumatic olecranon bursitis caused by repeated trauma. Infected bursitis may be discharged after incision and drainage unless lymphangitis or systemic illness is present. Steroids are reserved for recurrent disease with failure of repeat aspiration. *(Emergency Medicine, Chapter 112, pp 1152–1171)*

12.b. Only nondisplaced epicondylar fractures in persons older than 7 years may be discharged without orthopedic consultation in the ED. All displaced type I condylar fractures, all type II condylar fractures, all Galeazzi (and Monteggia) fractures, and all adult both-bone forearm fractures require orthopedic referral at the time of presentation. *(Emergency Medicine, Chapter 112, pp 1152–1171)*

13.b. Lacerations over the metacarpophalangeal joint are assumed to be contaminated, generally from a human bite during a closed fist injury. A consultant may recommend an intervening period of antimicrobials before closure. These are zone V extensor tendon injuries. Extensor tendon injuries are classified according to their location. Zone I (over the distal phalanx) injuries are treated with a full extension splint. Extensor tendon lacerations in zones II (over the middle phalanx), IV (over the proximal phalanx), and VI (over the metacarpals) may be safely treated in the ED. Lacerations over the proximal interphalangeal joint, zone III, also require consultation with a hand specialist. *(Emergency Medicine, Chapter 114, pp 1183–1189)*

14.c. This patient must be assumed to have an injection injury. These injuries have a high potential for occult injury; it is difficult to ascertain the path taken by the injected substance during initial physical examination in the ED. For this reason, they are generally managed with surgical exploration, open irrigation, and IV antimicrobials. *(Emergency Medicine, Chapter 114, pp 1183–1189)*

15.a. Kanavel's four cardinal signs of a purulent tendon sheath infection (purulent tenosynovitis) are a digit held in a partially flexed position, swollen digit, pain with passive extension of the finger, and tenderness over the flexor tendon sheaths. Intravenous antimicrobials need to be started in the ED with early consultation with a hand surgeon for intraoperative incision and drainage.[2] *(Emergency Medicine, Chapter 114, pp 1183–1189)*

16.c. Any fracture of the second or third metacarpal requires consultation because of the importance of recovery of rotational movement. Proximal interphalangeal joint extensor injuries require consultation; distal interphalangeal joint extensor injuries may be splinted in extension. Fourth and fifth metacarpal fractures need reduction only if there is more than 300 degrees of angulation. Middle phalanx fractures are splinted in partial flexion as long as less than 25% of the proximal interphalangeal joint articular surface is involved and there is less than 2 to 3 mm dislocation. *(Emergency Medicine, Chapter 114, pp 1183–1189)*

17.d. The absolute contraindications to finger reimplantation are the following: associated life-threatening injuries, severe avulsion or crush of tissues, segmental amputations, debilitating systemic illness, prior injury to extremity, and extreme contamination. Relative contraindications are active psychiatric diagnosis, single-digit amputation, and warm ischemia time of more than 12 hours. *(Emergency Medicine, Chapter 114, pp 1183–1189)*

18.a. Below 2 mm is considered normal. Above 4 mm is abnormal. Between 2 and 4 mm is suspicious for dissociation. When making a diagnosis of wrist sprain, it is important to evaluate this area. Greater than 2 mm of distance may indicate scapholunate instability, which should have orthopedic follow-up. *(Emergency Medicine, Chapter 113, pp 1172–1181)*

19.d. Triangular fibrocartilaginous complex injury is associated with radioulnar strain and is easily overlooked in the ED. Permanent disability may result if the patient is not properly splinted in the ED and referred to a hand surgeon. Triangular fibrocartilaginous complex injury should be suspected if there is pain on direct pressure over the distal radioulnar joint and pain on wrist extension in pronation and supination. Carpal tunnel syndrome is identified by Phalen's test (holding of the wrist in flexion for 60 seconds). Navicular fractures are associated with pain on axial loading of the thumb. Finkelstein's test, performed by asking the patient to flex the thumb while being held by the other fingers, identifies deQuervain's tenosynovitis of the thumb. *(Emergency Medicine, Chapter 113, pp 1172–1181)*

20.c. Hamate fractures are rarely identified on radiography but the history is suggestive. Navicular and hook of the hamate fractures may not be seen on radiographs. They should be suspected by mechanism of injury and physical findings. The navicular bone is the most commonly fractured carpal bone. The typical mechanism of injury is a fall onto an outstretched hand in dorsiflexion. Physical examination findings include snuffbox tenderness and pain on axial loading of the thumb. Hook of the hamate fractures occur when the patient is holding an object, such as a baseball bat, and hits it against an immovable object. There is pain and tenderness at the base of the hypothenar eminence. *(Emergency Medicine, Chapter 113, pp 1172–1181)*

21.b. Triquetrum fractures are usually only identified on the lateral view as an irregularity or chip on the dorsal wrist. On physical examination there will be tenderness just distal to the ulnar styloid. *(Emergency Medicine, Chapter 113, pp 1172–1181)*

REFERENCES

1. Goldberg HD, Young JWR, Reiner BI, et al: Double injuries of the forearm: A common occurrence. Radiology 1992; 185:223–227.
2. American Society for Surgery of the Hand: The Hand: Examination and Diagnosis, 2nd ed. New York, Churchill Livingstone, 1983.

BIBLIOGRAPHY

Beeson MS: Hand injuries. *In* Howell JM, Altieri M, Jagoda AS, et al (eds): Emergency Medicine. Philadelphia, WB Saunders, 1998, pp 1183–1189.

Beeson MS: Wrist injuries. *In* Howell JM, Altieri M, Jagoda AS, et al (eds): Emergency Medicine. Philadelphia, WB Saunders, 1998, pp 1172–1181.

Foley K: Shoulder and humerus injuries. *In* Howell JM, Altieri M, Jagoda AS, et al (eds): Emergency Medicine. Philadelphia, WB Saunders, 1998, pp 1145–1151.

Veenema KR: Elbow and forearm injuries. *In* Howell JM, Altieri M, Jagoda AS, et al (eds): Emergency Medicine. Philadelphia, WB Saunders, 1998, pp 1152–1171.

53 Lower Extremity: Leg, Knee, Ankle, and Foot

CAROL LEAH BARSKY, MD   PAUL BUCKLEY, MD, PhD

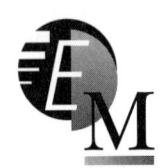

1. All of the following are goals of splinting midshaft femur fractures except:
   a. Minimize blood loss
   b. Minimize soft tissue injury
   c. Reduce pain
   d. Reduce the incidence of fat embolism

2. Traction splinting is indicated for which of the following femur fractures?
   a. Distal fracture with knee effusion
   b. Angulated fracture with decreased pulses
   c. Proximal fracture with exposed bone
   d. Midshaft fracture without angulation

3. Which of the following statements regarding patella injuries is true?
   a. Patella dislocations generally occur medially.
   b. If a spontaneously reduced patella dislocation is suspected by history, pushing the patella laterally while the knee is held in 20 to 30 degrees of flexion will elicit pain and resistance to further movement.
   c. Spontaneously reduced patella dislocations do not present with an effusion.
   d. Patella fractures associated with less than 5 mm of displacement may be treated nonoperatively.
   e. When a patella fracture is suspected but not visible on standard radiographs, a sunrise view is not helpful.

4. Knee dislocations rarely occur in isolation. Which of the following is true regarding injuries associated with knee dislocations?
   a. The absence of an effusion rules out a dislocation.
   b. Popliteal artery injuries occur in one third to one half of cases.
   c. Diminished capillary refill is a reliable predictor of popliteal artery injury.
   d. Posterior dislocations are most common.
   e. Cruciate ligaments are generally intact.

5. Clinically significant knee injuries are evident in what percentage of radiographs?
   a. 15%
   b. 30%
   c. 45%
   d. 60%

6. The most common organisms implicated in plantar puncture infections are:
   a. Gram-negative rods
   b. Gram-positive cocci
   c. *Pseudomonas aeruginosa*
   d. Fungi
   e. Anaerobes

7. Which of the following statements regarding fifth metatarsal fractures is true?
   a. It is the most commonly fractured metatarsal.
   b. The Jones fracture is more common than the pseudo-Jones.
   c. 90% of Jones fractures will require fixation.
   d. Jones fractures occur in the proximal 1 cm of the fifth metatarsal.

8. Which of the following foot fractures does not require internal fixation?
   a. Lisfranc's
   b. First metatarsal
   c. Interarticular fractures of the calcaneus
   d. Tuberosity of the fifth metatarsal

9. All of the following foot injuries may be initially diagnosed as acute sprain except:
   a. Lisfranc's
   b. Posterior talar process fracture
   c. Transchondral talar dome injury
   d. Midfoot avulsion in children

10. The Ottawa rules for evaluating for midfoot fractures include all of the following elements except:
    a. Point tenderness at the navicular
    b. Point tenderness at the base of the fifth metatarsal
    c. Ecchymosis at the base of the medial metatarsals
    d. Inability to walk four steps at the scene and in the ED

11. In the "position: force-vector" classification of ankle fractures described by Lauge-Hansen, the progression

of injury is graded by the number of anatomic sites sequentially disrupted. All of the following pairs correctly identify the initial fracture except:
   a. Supination-adduction—transverse fracture of the lateral malleolus
   b. Pronation-abduction—avulsion of the medial malleolus
   c. Supination-eversion—fibular fracture at the syndesmosis
   d. Pronation-eversion—medial malleolus

12. A useful classification of ankle fractures in the ED simply identifies the disrupted elements. Which of the following definitions is correct?
   a. Bimalleolar—medial malleolus and posterior tibia
   b. Pilon—fibula at the syndesmosis
   c. Trimalleolar—lateral malleolus, medial malleolus, and posterior tibia
   d. Maisonneuve—proximal fibula and lateral malleolus

13. The lateral ligament complex of the ankle is composed of three ligaments that incorporate all of the following bony elements except:
   a. Talus
   b. Fibula
   c. Calcaneus
   d. Navicular

14. According to the currently verified Ottawa rules for ankle injuries, radiography may safely be deferred in which of the following patients with perimalleolar pain?
   a. 13-year-old female jogger who twisted her foot on a curb and limps into the ED
   b. 18-year-old male who stumbled after drinking alcohol but was walking at the scene
   c. 20-year-old male complaining of ankle and arm pain; he is holding his right arm abducted 110 degrees after a fall on in-line skates
   d. 22-year-old female with lateral ankle swelling but without focal tenderness

15. All of the following statements regarding pediatric ankle injuries are true except:
   a. They are comparable to adult ankle injuries after the growth plates close at age 15 or 16.
   b. Radiographs may be normal in Salter-Harris type I fractures.
   c. The most common injury is a Salter-Harris type II of the distal tibia.
   d. The Tillaux fracture, a Salter-Harris type III injury, is treated with open reduction and internal fixation.

Answers

1.a. Splinting also helps to minimize spasm. Splinting is not effective in ameliorating the significant blood loss expected from midshaft femur fractures. Midshaft femur fractures may be associated with up to 3 units of acute blood loss. All patients with a midshaft femur fracture require placement of a large-bore IV, and blood sent for type and crossmatch. A high-energy force is required to produce a midshaft femur fracture; all such fractures mandate a search for associated injuries. *(Emergency Medicine, Chapter 117, pp 1208–1227)*

2.d. A traction splint is appropriate only for midshaft fractures. Distal femur fractures occur proximal to major blood vessels; traction may lead to vascular injury. The splinting of open fractures may cause retraction of exposed bone into the wound, increasing the possibility of wound infection. *(Emergency Medicine, Chapter 117, pp 1208–1227)*

3.b. Most patella dislocations occur laterally. The patient presents with the knee in flexion and the patella is visible and palpable in a position lateral to its normal location. If the dislocation has spontaneously reduced, there may be an effusion, and there is tenderness to palpation at the posterolateral border of the patella. When the patella is fractured, operative treatment is indicated for all fractures with more than 2 mm of displacement. A sunrise or axial view may be helpful if a suspected fracture is not seen on the standard views. The sunrise view shows the medial and lateral facets of the patella and its relation to the femoral condyles. *(Emergency Medicine, Chapter 117, pp 1208–1227)*

4.b. Knee dislocations are a true orthopedic emergency. The diagnosis may be made based on history alone; an effusion may be absent if the joint capsule is ruptured. Fractures and popliteal artery injuries occur in up to 60% of knee dislocations. Arteriography is indicated even in the absence of signs or symptoms of vascular injury. Generally, the cruciates and one or both collateral ligaments are ruptured. The most common type of dislocation is anterior. *(Emergency Medicine, Chapter 117, pp 1208–1227)*

5.a. Many injuries involve soft tissue and may require MRI for accurate diagnosis. Importantly, fractures, such as tibial plateau and tibial spine, may not be apparent on standard views and are frequently missed in the ED. *(Emergency Medicine, Chapter 117, pp 1208–1227)*

6.b. Wound infections from plantar puncture injuries are common, generally presenting 1 to 2 days after injury. *Staphylococcus* and *Streptococcus* are the dominant organisms in all plantar puncture infections. In puncture wounds through athletic footwear, *Pseudomonas aeruginosa* may be the etiologic organism. Anaerobic infection, such as tetanus, is now rare but may be seen in diabetic patients. Empiric choices of antimicrobial therapy must include reliable coverage of gram-positive organisms; a quinolone alone is insufficient. *(Emergency Medicine, Chapter 119, pp 1237–1246)*

7.a. The fifth metatarsal is the most common site of midfoot fractures. Jones fractures occur 1.5 to 3 cm distal to the proximal tuberosity and are much less common than avulsion, or pseudo-Jones, fractures. Thirty-five percent to 50% of Jones fractures will fail a course of conservative therapy (no weight bearing; immobilization) and require bone grafting and fixation. Any weight bearing increases the risk of nonunion. *(Emergency Medicine, Chapter 119, pp 1237–1246)*

8.d. The pseudo-Jones fracture can be treated conservatively and for this reason must be carefully distinguished from a Jones fracture, which requires absolute non–weight bearing and early orthopedic referral for possible internal fixation. Failure to obtain early orthopedic consultation for operative repair often results in long-term morbidity in the patient with Lisfranc's, calcaneal, and first metatarsal fractures. Lisfranc's fractures occur through the bony arch connecting the first through third cuneiforms with the first through third metatarsals. Approximately 20% are either misdiagnosed or missed on initial ED presentation. The interarticular fracture of the calcaneus is the most common calcaneal fracture and is best visualized on the lateral radiograph of the foot. The first metatarsal is the least commonly fractured metatarsal. Minimally or nondisplaced fractures are casted in a short leg cast for 6 weeks. Displaced fractures treated conservatively often result in long-term gait disturbances. *(Emergency Medicine, Chapter 119, pp 1237–1246)*

9.b. Fracture of the posterior process of the talus or the os trigonum rarely presents acutely but may appear as a nonhealing sprain. The remaining injuries occur in the context of acute injury and are difficult to diagnose radiographically or to distinguish from ligamentous sprain at the time of presentation. *(Emergency Medicine, Chapter 119, pp 1237–1246)*

10.c. The Ottawa ankle rules serve as clinical predictors of the need for radiographic assessment of midfoot and ankle injuries. No radiograph is required if the patient does not exhibit one of the following: point tenderness over the base of the fifth metatarsal, point tenderness over the navicular, or the inability to take four steps in the ED. *(Emergency Medicine, Chapter 119, pp 1237–1246)*

11.d. The first fracture in a pronation-eversion type of injury occurs at the fibula above the syndesmosis. This is followed in order by rupture of the deltoid ligament or medial malleolus, the anterior tibiofibular and intraosseous ligaments, and the posterior tibiofibular ligament. The correct mechanism-injury associations are:
Supination-adduction: transverse fracture of the lateral malleolus
Pronation-abduction: avulsion of the medial malleolus
Supination-eversion: fibular fracture at the syndesmosis
Pronation-eversion: fibula fracture above the syndesmosis
(Emergency Medicine, Chapter 118, pp 1228–1235)

12.c. The correct naming convention is as follows:
Bimalleolar: lateral malleolus and medial malleolus
Pilon: intra-articular
Trimalleolar: lateral malleolus, medial malleolus, and posterior tibia
Maisonneuve: proximal fibula and medial malleolus
(Emergency Medicine, Chapter 118, pp 1228–1235)

13.d. The complex comprises the anterior and posterior talofibular ligaments and the calcaneofibular ligament, whose names describe their origin and insertion. The navicular is an attachment for the superficial fibers of the deltoid ligament. *(Emergency Medicine, Chapter 118, pp 1228–1235)*

14.d. The Ottawa rules only apply to patients 18 years or older who do not have distracting injuries or impaired mental status. Radiographic assessment is recommended when perimalleolar pain is accompanied by point tenderness at the posterior edge or tip of either malleolus, if the patient was unable to bear weight at the scene, or if the pateint is unable to ambulate in the ED. Patient c likely has a posterior shoulder dislocation in addition to his ankle injury. In patient a, the Tillaux fracture, a Salter-Harris type III injury, is usually treated with open reduction and fixation. *(Emergency Medicine, Chapter 118, pp 1228–1235)*

15.d. Although most type III fractures require open reduction and fixation, the Tillaux fracture, a minimally displaced fracture through the growth plate of the lateral malleolus when it is the last remaining growth plate in the ankle, may be treated with closed reduction. Closed reduction using an internal rotation force followed by placement of a non–weight-bearing long leg cast is used. *(Emergency Medicine, Chapter 118, pp 1228–1235)*

BIBLIOGRAPHY

Michael JA: Ankle injuries. *In* Howell JM, Altieri M, Jagoda AS, et al (eds): Emergency Medicine. Philadelphia, WB Saunders, 1998, pp 1228–1235.

Silbergleit R, Haywood Y: *In* Howell JM, Altieri M, Jagoda AS, et al (eds): Emergency Medicine. Philadelphia, WB Saunders, 1998, pp 1237–1246.

Singletary EM: Leg injuries. *In* Howell JM, Altieri M, Jagoda AS, et al (eds): Emergency Medicine. Philadelphia, WB Saunders, 1998, pp 1208–1227.

54 Pediatric Orthopedic Emergencies, Joint and Bone Inflammation and Infection, Hip Injuries, and Disorders of the Spine

CAROL LEAH BARSKY, MD   PAUL BUCKLEY, MD, PhD   KATHRYN CRAIG, MD

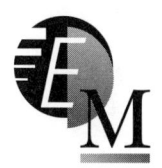

1. A child is brought into the ED with a backboard and cervical collar in place after an automobile accident. The child has no neurologic deficits on examination; however, the emergency physician becomes concerned after noting anterior displacement of C2 on C3 while reviewing the child's cervical spine films. Which of the following statements regarding this entity is true?
   a. A physiologic anterior displacement of C2 on C3 is seen when viewing the radiograph.
   b. The child is usually younger than 8 years of age.
   c. This is a normal or variant finding often misinterpreted as an acute injury.
   d. Prevertebral soft tissue swelling may be misdiagnosed if the child's neck is held in flexion during the radiograph or if the film is taken during expiration.
   e. All of the above statements are true.

2. All of the following statements regarding spinal cord injury without radiographic abnormality are true except:
   a. Although most cases develop immediately after trauma, delayed, severe defects may develop.
   b. Patients with persistent or transient neurologic deficits should have MRI or CT.
   c. Less than 25% of patients with spinal cord injury without radiographic abnormality have complete loss of spinal cord function.
   d. Activity should be limited for 3 months in children with spinal cord injury without radiographic abnormality.
   e. Imaging studies should extend two levels above and below the clinical level of injury.

3. Historical parameters and radiographic findings consistent with child abuse include:
   a. Any fracture in a child younger than 1 year of age
   b. An injury inconsistent with the history
   c. A family history of financial strain
   d. An injury improbable for the age of the child
   e. All of the above

4. The most common intrathoracic injuries associated with the pediatric trauma patient are:
   a. Subclavian artery laceration and pulmonary contusion
   b. Rib fractures and pulmonary contusion
   c. Cardiac tamponade and aortic dissection
   d. Cardiac contusion and rib fractures
   e. Tension pneumothorax and cardiac tamponade

5. All of the following are common areas for missed Salter-Harris type I injuries except:
   a. The proximal radius
   b. The distal radius
   c. The distal femur
   d. The ankle

6. Choose the inappropriately paired Salter-Harris stage with its classification.
   a. Salter V—the growth plate is crushed and the germinal matrix obliterated
   b. Salter III—an intra-articular fracture that traverses the epiphysis, epiphyseal plate, and metaphysis
   c. Salter II—a triangular fragment of metaphysis separates with a variable length of epiphyseal plate
   d. Salter I—metaphysis and epiphysis are separated without associated bony fracture

7. All of the following statements regarding elbow fractures in children are true except:
   a. Supracondylar humeral fractures are associated with the development of Volkmann's ischemic contractures.
   b. Fractures involving the medial and lateral epicondyles rarely require surgical fixation.
   c. Supracondylar humeral fractures are the result of a fall on an outstretched arm.
   d. A posterior fat pad sign is indicative of a fracture even if not radiographically apparent.
   e. Volkmann's ischemic contracture is the result of injury to the brachial artery by a bony fragment.

8. All of the following statements regarding nursemaid's elbow are true except:
   a. There may be a history of the child's caretaker pulling the child's arm.
   b. The upper extremity is kept hanging in pronation at the child's side.

c. Radiographic assessment is generally unnecessary before reduction unless bony tenderness is present.
d. During reduction, the hand is supinated fully and the elbow is flexed in a continuous motion.
e. If the child is still not using the affected hand 10 to 15 minutes after a reduction click is felt, reduction may be attempted again before radiographic assessment.

9. Radiographic assessment divides Legg-Calvé-Perthes disease into four stages. During which stage does the child usually present?
   a. First stage
   b. Second stage
   c. Third stage
   d. Fourth stage

10. Legg-Calvé-Perthes disease is characterized by all of the following except:
    a. Pain with movement of the hip or an abnormal gait
    b. Limited motion of the hip, especially with abduction and internal rotation
    c. Atrophy of the affected thigh and buttock
    d. Occasional muscle spasm in the affected hip and possible hip contracture
    e. An abnormally high WBC count and ESR

11. All of the following statements regarding transient synovitis are true except:
    a. The cause of transient synovitis is known to be viral.
    b. In transient synovitis, the WBC count and ESR are normal or slightly elevated.
    c. The child usually presents with a limp or refusal to walk for 1 to 2 days, and the hip may be positioned in abduction and external rotation on examination.
    d. Hip aspiration of an effusion will reveal yellow synovial fluid, with a WBC count of less than 20,000/mm^3.
    e. After transient synovitis is diagnosed, the child may be sent home with instructions for bed rest and antiinflammatory agents for pain control.

12. An obese 15-year-old boy in otherwise good health presents with intermittent right hip and thigh pain that is worsened by activity. The pain initially started 3 weeks ago. Laboratory data reveal a normal ESR and a WBC count of less than 15,000/mm^3. The most likely diagnosis is:
    a. Septic arthritis
    b. Transient synovitis
    c. Osgood-Schlatter disease
    d. Slipped capital femoral epiphysis
    e. None of the above

13. Systemic viral infections are often associated with acute arthritis. True statements about this entity include all of the following except:
    a. The arthritis is transient and generally does not last more than a few days.
    b. Hepatitis B and rubella are the most common etiologic agents.
    c. The diagnosis is assisted by noting concomitant or preceding fever, rash, and regional lymphadenopathy.
    d. The arthritis may precede the clinical manifestations of hepatitis in patients with hepatitis B.
    e. Arthritis caused by rubella is often insidious in onset, is monoarticular, and may involve a single large joint, mimicking gonococcal arthritis.

14. The differential diagnosis of acute monoarticular arthritis includes all of the following except:
    a. Gout
    b. Pseudogout
    c. *Staphylococcus aureus* infection
    d. Gonococcal arthritis
    e. Psoriasis

15. Select the single incorrect characteristic of gonococcal arthritis:
    a. It begins with migratory polyarthralgias in most patients.
    b. Approximately 50% of patients have positive blood cultures, even when no organism is identified in the synovial fluid.
    c. Joint fluid cultures are positive in 25% of patients.
    d. Most patients have evidence of tenosynovitis.
    e. An associated rash is common.

16. Which of the following statements regarding hip dislocations is true?
    a. PO or IV analgesia may be given during transport of patients with hip dislocations.
    b. Hip dislocations are associated with other serious injuries in up to 75% of cases.
    c. Most posterior hip dislocations result from motor vehicle crashes; most anterior dislocations are caused by forced extension during sporting events.
    d. A single attempt at relocation may be attempted during prehospital transport when the extremity is pulseless.
    e. The femoral vessels are particularly prone to injury after a posterior dislocation.

17. All of the following are true of hip fractures except:
    a. The classic physical findings of a shortened, abducted, externally rotated extremity may be absent if an ipsilateral femoral shaft fracture is also present.
    b. A pelvic film should be obtained on all patients with suspected hip fractures.
    c. Internal rotation of the affected hip provides optimal projection of the proximal femur on AP radiographs of the pelvis.
    d. When a fracture of the acetabulum is suspected, Judet views may be useful.
    e. MRI is not a useful modality for the identification of occult fractures of the proximal femur.

18. Complications of hip fractures may develop in the perioperative period or may occur years after repair. All of the following are true except:
    a. Deep vein thrombosis is diagnosed in up to 10% of patients with proximal femur fractures.

b. The most important long-term complication of femoral neck fractures is posterior hip dislocation.
c. Femoral neck fractures are associated with a higher rate of long-term complications than are intertrochanteric fractures.
d. Reduction techniques for arthroplasty dislocations are the same as those for dislocations of normal hips.
e. Dislocation of a hip arthroplasty may require operative repair.

19. A 12-year-old track star presents with severe hip pain after repeated, forceful sprinting during practice. All of the following are true of her likely injuries except:
    a. The gluteus medius muscle inserts at the greater trochanter; forceful contraction during hip flexion may cause isolated bony avulsion.
    b. Orthopedic consultants generally treat isolated trochanteric fractures operatively.
    c. Avulsion of the lesser trochanter at the epiphysis is most common in adolescents.
    d. Athletic injuries are the major cause of traumatic hip dislocations in children.
    e. The iliopsoas inserts on the lesser trochanter; powerful contraction may cause avulsion at the epiphysis.

20. A 13-year-old boy presents with knee pain after a basketball game. His examination is suspicious for a slipped capital femoral epiphysis. Which statement most correctly describes appropriate ED management?
    a. Ask the patient to refrain from weight bearing in the ED. If all radiographs are negative, reassure his parents that he most likely has a ligamentous strain. No further diagnostic evaluation is necessary.
    b. If the child has disease in one hip, advise the parents that involvement of the other hip is very unlikely.
    c. Ask the patient to refrain from weight bearing in the ED, order an AP of the pelvis, and treat with ice, elevation, and no weight bearing for 3 weeks if the film is negative.
    d. Advise no weight bearing, order a "frog-leg" radiograph, and be alert for subtle differences in epiphyseal alignment.

21. Plain-film x-rays are the most appropriate imaging modality for which of the following patients presenting with lower back pain?
    a. 65-year-old male with a history of prostate cancer, decreased rectal sphincter tone, and urinary retention
    b. 55-year-old female with pain for 2 weeks
    c. 45-year-old female with severe pain radiating down her right thigh
    d. 35-year-old male with 4 weeks of pain

22. What percentage of patients with uncomplicated lower back pain will have resolution of symptoms within 1 week?
    a. 25%
    b. 50%
    c. 75%
    d. 95%

23. Which of the following is most likely to cause a unilateral motor deficit with a contralateral loss of pain and temperature sensation localized to a thoracic spinal level?
    a. Abdominal aortic aneurysm
    b. Metastatic prostate cancer
    c. Multiple sclerosis
    d. Intervertebral disc herniation

24. Which of the following conditions is most likely to be the cause of sclerotogenous radiation of lower back pain to the buttock?
    a. Spinal metastasis
    b. Herniated disc
    c. Facet arthritis
    d. Osteoporosis

25. A 6-year-old girl presents with severe, localized lower back pain that developed over 1 day. She has a low-grade fever. Plain-film x-rays of the spine are normal. What is the most likely diagnosis?
    a. Ankylosing spondylitis
    b. Leukemic infiltration
    c. Infectious discitis
    d. Herniated disc

Answers

1. e. Pseudosubluxation is a normal or variant finding often misinterpreted as acute injury. Pseudosubluxation at C2–C3 results from the physiologic anterior displacement of C2 on C3. It is seen in 24% of patients younger than 8 years of age. The normal prevertebral soft tissues may be misdiagnosed as prevertebral soft tissue swelling if the film is taken with the child's neck flexed or during expiration. Children have a laxity of the prevertebral soft tissue; a repeat film should be taken during inspiration. *(Emergency Medicine, Chapter 110, pp 1125–1144)*

2. c. Of the pediatric patients with spinal cord injury without radiographic abnormality, 75% have complete loss of spinal cord function. Thirty percent of spinal injuries in children younger than 8 years of age and 10% of spinal injuries in children between 9 and 16 years old are caused by this entity. Any pediatric patient with transient or persistent neurologic complaints or ongoing neck pain should have additional imaging studies performed after negative plain films; either CT or MRI is acceptable. Imaging studies should include two vertebral levels above and below the clinical level of injury. For patients with spinal cord injury without radiographic abnormality, activity should be limited for 3 months. *(Emergency Medicine, Chapter 110, pp 1125–1144)*

3. e. Certain historical features raise a clinician's index of suspicion for child abuse. These include injury inconsistent with the history, a mechanism more advanced than the developmental age of the child, delay in seeking care, estrangement of the parents from the child, familial domestic violence, familial drug or alco-

hol abuse, and any fracture in a child younger than 1 year of age or in one who is not yet ambulatory. The most concerning radiographic findings are fractures, especially multiple fractures, in various stages of healing. *(Emergency Medicine, Chapter 110, pp 1125–1144)*

4.b. Of those children sustaining thoracic trauma, the most common thoracic injuries are pulmonary contusions and rib fractures (48% and 32%, respectively). Clinicians must be aware, however, that severe intrathoracic trauma can occur in children without any external evidence of trauma. Clavicular fractures are also common and may be missed in children complaining of shoulder pain. *(Emergency Medicine, Chapter 110, pp 1125–1144)*

5.a. The ankle, distal femur, and distal radius are the most common areas for misdiagnosed Salter type I fractures. Salter type I fractures involve a fracture through the growth plate that may not result in radiographic abnormality if nondisplaced. Careful physical examination is mandatory; any child who is tender over the growth plate should be completely immobilized and have close orthopedic follow-up. *(Emergency Medicine, Chapter 110, pp 1125–1144)*

6.b. Salter type IV injuries are associated with an intraarticular fracture that traverses the epiphysis, epiphyseal plate, and metaphysis. Salter type III injuries occur when a fracture of the epiphysis extends into the joint. *(Emergency Medicine, Chapter 110, pp 1125–1144)*

7.b. Supracondylar humeral fractures are the most common fractures around the elbow in children and are generally the result of a fall on an outstretched arm. Although rare, brachial artery injury may occur from a bony fragment, resulting in Volkmann's ischemic contracture. Fractures involving the medial and lateral epicondyles often require surgical fixation because of nonunion of the fragments. A posterior fat pad sign is caused by fluid in the elbow joint. It is indicative of a fracture, although one may not be radiographically apparent. *(Emergency Medicine, Chapter 110, pp 1125–1144)*

8.e. Radial head subluxation, or nursemaid's elbow, usually results from a caretaker's pulling on a child's arm. The upper extremity is usually kept hanging in pronation at the side with minimal elbow flexion. A child with no bony tenderness is unlikely to have a fracture; reduction can be attempted without radiographic assessment. A click is usually felt during full flexion of the elbow, indicating that reduction has been successful. If the click is not felt, another reduction may be attempted. If the child is unable to move his or her arm within 10 to 15 minutes after a reduction click is felt, further manipulation should be avoided until radiographs are obtained. *(Emergency Medicine, Chapter 110, pp 1125–1144)*

9.b. Most children present during the second stage of the disease, characterized by increased density in all or part of the femoral head. There may be radiolucent or radiodense areas seen on radiography. Stage 1 corresponds to the first month of the disease, during which there may be no radiographic manifestations of the disease, or plain films may demonstrate a slight widening of the joint space with lateral displacement of the femoral head. Stage 3 is characterized by increasing areas of radiolucency with new growth at the edges of the epiphysis. The fourth stage occurs during healing; the acetabulum appears relatively normal with continued widening of the femoral neck and epiphysis. *(Emergency Medicine, Chapter 110, pp 1125–1144)*

10.e. Legg-Calvé-Perthes disease results from avascular necrosis of the femoral head. It manifests as pain with movement of the hip, a limp, or an abnormal gait. Physical examination will typically demonstrate some limited range of hip motion, particularly abduction and internal rotation. The affected side may reveal atrophy of the buttock and hip during examination. Muscle spasm in the hip is not uncommon, and a flexion contracture may be present. A CBC and ESR are normal and helpful only in excluding other causes such as septic arthritis. *(Emergency Medicine, Chapter 110, pp 1125–1144)*

11.a. The cause of transient synovitis is unknown but may be infectious, traumatic, or allergic. It is commonly associated with an upper respiratory infection, concurrently or in the preceding 10 days. Typically, the children are between the ages of 3 and 8 years and present with a limp or refusal to walk for 1 to 2 days. On examination, the child may hold the hip preferentially in abduction and external rotation. The WBC count and ESR are usually normal or mildly elevated. If the possibility of a pyogenic arthritis is present and a hip effusion is demonstrated on ultrasonography, hip aspiration is required. Normal synovial fluid is yellow and nonpurulent and has a WBC count of less than 20,000/mm^3. After pyogenic arthritis and osteomyelitis have been excluded, the child may be sent home on bed rest with an anti-inflammatory agent for pain control. *(Emergency Medicine, Chapter 110, pp 1125–1144)*

12.d. Slipped capital femoral epiphysis typically occurs in children between 10 and 15 years of age, and it is associated with obesity, recurrent trauma, and a weakened proximal femoral epiphysis: Boys are twice as likely to be affected as girls. Although slipped capital femoral epiphysis is usually bilateral, symptoms may be present on one side only. The history may include pain or a limp that started weeks or months before presentation. In children with slipped capital femoral epiphysis, intermittent hip or thigh pain is usually worsened with activity. In septic arthritis, a CBC generally reveals a WBC count of greater than 15,000/mm^3 and an ESR that is significantly elevated. Osgood-Schlatter disease commonly occurs in children between ages 9 and 13 and usually resolves by age

15, when complete ossification of the tibial tuberosity has occurred. Osgood-Schlatter disease is also more common in males than females and exacerbated by activity; however, it typically causes knee pain that localizes to the tibial tuberosity. *(Emergency Medicine, Chapter 110, pp 1125–1144)*

13.e. The most common viral infections associated with arthritis are hepatitis B and rubella. The diagnosis is usually considered when there is a history of exposure and there is an associated viral syndrome. Up to 33% of patients with hepatitis B experience an episode of arthritis. The arthritis, fever, rash, and lymphadenopathy may precede the hepatitis for days to weeks. The arthritis associated with rubella is sudden in onset, is polyarticular in distribution, and involves small- and medium-sized joints. It may also occur after vaccination. *(Emergency Medicine, Chapter 110, pp 1125–1144)*

14.e. Crystalline arthritis and acute bacterial arthritis generally first present with an acute monoarticular arthritis. Arthritis associated with disseminated gonococcal infection is polyarticular in more than 50% of patients but must be considered in any infectious arthritis. Psoriatic arthritis is polyarticular and may involve the small joints of the hands, large peripheral joints, or the spine. *(Emergency Medicine, Chapter 120, pp 1247–1253)*

15.b. Disseminated gonococcal infection occurs in about 1% to 3% of patients infected with gonococci. The rash occurs during the bacteremia phase. The skin lesions can be petechial, pustular, papular, or hemorrhagic. They typically occur on the distal extremities. During this phase the patient also may have fever, polyarthralgias, and tenosynovitis. Gonococcal arthritis follows the untreated bacteremic phase. Blood cultures are positive in less than 10% of patients with gonococcal arthritis. The arthritis is typically monoarticular (occasionally polyarticular), usually involving the knees, ankles, or wrists.[1] *(Emergency Medicine, Chapter 120, pp 1247–1253)*

16.d. Hip dislocations are true orthopedic emergencies and must be recognized and treated early. If reduction is delayed 24 hours after injury, avascular necrosis of the femoral head and post-traumatic arthritis are more likely to occur. Because emergent surgery may be required, avoid PO analgesia. Hip dislocations are an important marker for multisystem trauma; associated serious injuries occur in 95% of cases. The most common cause of both anterior and posterior hip dislocations is a motor vehicle crash. Posterior dislocations occur when a flexed knee contacts the dashboard under high speed. Anterior dislocations result when the hip is abducted and externally rotated on impact. Femoral vessels are most at risk during an anterior dislocation. *(Emergency Medicine, Chapter 116, pp 1201–1207)*

17.e. In the elderly, hip fractures most often occur after a seemingly trivial mechanism such as a fall from the patient's own height. In younger people, greater force is required. Radiographic assessment of suspected hip fractures begins with an AP view of the pelvis; the entire pelvis, both hips, and the proximal third of both femurs should be seen to allow optimal comparison of both hips. Internal rotation of the femur moves the head of the femur out of the acetabulum, assisting in fracture identification. Judet views are oblique projections that help visualize the acetabulum. MRI is the recommended modality for suspected fractures of the proximal femur that are not apparent on initial plain films. *(Emergency Medicine, Chapter 116, pp 1201–1207)*

18.b. Because of the nature of the blood supply to the femoral neck, these fractures are most often complicated by fracture nonunion and avascular necrosis. Intertrochanteric fractures occur through bone with a rich blood supply and are, therefore, associated with fewer complications. Although most dislocations of hip prostheses present within 30 days of surgery, many occur later and commonly present to EDs. A variety of treatment options are available, including operative and nonoperative (spica cast or knee immobilizer) modalities. Always be sure to consult an orthopedic surgeon to develop a long-term treatment plan when treating these dislocations. *(Emergency Medicine, Chapter 116, pp 1201–1207)*

19.b. Children sustain isolated fractures of the femoral trochanters much more frequently than adults do. The most common mechanism is a forceful muscular contraction, which causes avulsion at the epiphyses. *(Emergency Medicine, Chapter 116, pp 1201–1207)*

20.c. It is important for the emergency physician to be alert to the often subtle presentation of a slipped capital femoral epiphysis in adolescents. It is most often seen between the ages of 10 and 16. The process is bilateral in 20% of patients. The frog-leg radiograph is useful in identifying the condition. However, if it is negative but the child is still in pain, pediatric orthopedic referral is necessary. *(Emergency Medicine, Chapter 116, pp 1201–1207)*

21.b. It is often recommended that those patients older than 50 years without neurologic deficit or suspected malignancy or infection should have plain films. MRI is the study of choice in the context of potentially metastatic malignancy. Severe pain or focal tenderness strongly suggests a spinal fracture that is best observed on CT. Otherwise healthy individuals with fewer than 6 weeks of mechanical lower back pain do not need imaging studies. *(Emergency Medicine, Chapter 115, pp 1191–1200)*

22.b. Fifty percent of cases resolve within 1 week, 80% within 2 weeks, and 90% within 2 months. Treatment of uncomplicated mechanical back pain includes pain relief and rest from exacerbating activities. *(Emergency Medicine, Chapter 115, pp 1191–1200)*

23. b. Hemi-cord syndrome (Brown-Séquard) is most likely caused by mass or penetrating trauma. Lateral compression from a mass causes ipsilateral motor loss and loss of vibration and position sense at the level of the lesion. There are contralateral pain and temperature loss beginning two levels below the lesion. An abdominal aortic aneurysm may cause anterior cord syndrome with spinal artery involvement. Multiple sclerosis typically causes a transverse myelitis with variable motor and sensory deficits. Disc herniation may cause an anterior cord syndrome or nerve root compression and is more likely to be lumbar than thoracic. *(Emergency Medicine, Chapter 115, pp 1191–1200)*

24. c. Degenerative joint disease and facet joint disease may cause sclerotogenous radiation to the buttock or thigh. Sciatica is most likely produced by a herniated disc in otherwise well young individuals. Osteoporosis and metastatic lesions may predispose to compression fractures and are more likely to cause midline pain and spinal cord or root compression symptoms. *(Emergency Medicine, Chapter 115, pp 1191–1200)*

25. c. Children younger than 8 years are at risk for infectious discitis because their intervertebral discs are well vascularized. Plain films may be normal during the first 2 to 4 weeks of infection. MRI is the more sensitive study; it will also reveal concomitant osteomyelitis. Discitis can, on rare occasions, be associated with epidural abscess. Ankylosing spondylitis and leukemic infiltration are subacute conditions. The pain of ankylosing spondylitis is diffuse and occurs more at night. Herniated discs are rare in children; they are caused by trauma in 50% of cases and are associated with radicular symptoms. *(Emergency Medicine, Chapter 115, pp 1191–1200)*

REFERENCE

1. Reese RE, Douglas RG: A Practical Approach to Infectious Diseases. Boston, Little, Brown, 1986, pp 359–365.

BIBLIOGRAPHY

Burg J, Moldovan G: Pediatric orthopedic emergencies. *In* Howell JM, Altieri M, Jagoda AS, et al (eds): Emergency Medicine. Philadelphia, WB Saunders, 1998, pp 1125–1155.

Garvey JL, Gibbs M: Hip injuries. *In* Howell JM, Altieri M, Jagoda AS, et al (eds): Emergency Medicine. Philadelphia, WB Saunders, 1998, pp 1201–1207.

Lucas RH: Disorders of the spine. *In* Howell JM, Altieri M, Jagoda AS, et al (eds): Emergency Medicine. Philadelphia, WB Saunders, 1998, pp 1191–1200.

Lucchesi M: Joint and bone inflammation and infection. *In* Howell JM, Altieri M, Jagoda AS, et al (eds): Emergency Medicine. Philadelphia, WB Saunders, 1998, pp 1247–1253.

SECTION SIXTEEN

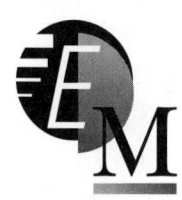

Obstetric and Gynecologic Disorders

55 Pregnancy, Labor, and Delivery

CARL K. HSU, MD

Normal Labor and Delivery

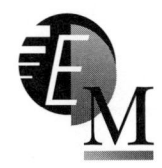

1. When faced with an imminent delivery in the ED, all of the following are critical points in the patient's history except:
   a. Complications of previous deliveries
   b. Last menstrual period
   c. Previous RhoGAM administration
   d. Vaginal bleeding, "broken water," and frequency of contractions
   e. Gravida and parity

2. Treatment essentials before imminent delivery include all of the following except:
   a. Placement of the patient in the left lateral decubitus position
   b. Supplemental oxygen
   c. IV access
   d. A vaginal examination, particularly if bleeding is present
   e. No attempt to stop delivery

3. Which statement regarding episiotomy is false?
   a. It should be completed early before the appearance of the head to facilitate passage.
   b. It may not be necessary in multiparous patients.
   c. It is performed to prevent perineal laceration.
   d. It may be achieved in either a mediolateral or midline fashion.
   e. The incision may be completed without anesthesia.

4. In making the incision for an episiotomy, the following are true except:
   a. Local anesthesia may be achieved with 1% lidocaine along the expected trajectory of the incision.
   b. Two fingers are used to pull the perineal body away from the emerging head.
   c. An incision can be made with a Mayo scissors in the mediolateral direction, toward the left thigh.
   d. An incision can be made with a Mayo scissors in the midline through the rectal tissue.
   e. A simple episiotomy incision may be closed with absorbable suture material.

5. After delivery, which of the following is false?
   a. The mother may bear down to expel the placenta if it does not deliver spontaneously.
   b. Firm downward pressure on the fundus with traction on the cord may be used to help expel the placenta.
   c. Once delivered, the placenta should be examined for completeness and the cord for two arteries and a vein.
   d. Cervical lacerations occur most frequently at the 3 and 9 o'clock positions.
   e. Oxytocin may be given after delivery of the placenta.

6. All of the following are components of the Apgar score except:
   a. Heart rate
   b. Eye opening
   c. Muscle tone
   d. Respiratory rate
   e. Color

Answers

1.c. Although Rh immunoprophylaxis is important in the management of Rh-negative mothers, it is not a critical point in a history taken before imminent delivery. RhoGAM may given up to 72 hours after maternal exposure to Rh-positive blood. *(Emergency Medicine, Chapter 124, pp 1287–1294)*

2.d. No vaginal examination should be performed if there is vaginal bleeding in the second half of pregnancy. The most serious causes of vaginal bleeding in the third trimester include placenta previa and abruptio placentae. Placenta previa is usually painless, whereas abruptio placentae usually presents with a tender, hard uterus. A bimanual examination may worsen the hemorrhaging by disrupting the placenta previa. *(Emergency Medicine, Chapter 126, pp 1307–1318)*

3.a. Episiotomy should be completed when the head is visible to a diameter of 3 to 4 cm during contraction. An episiotomy done earlier may precipitate more bleeding. An episiotomy performed later may result in more stretching of the muscles of the perineal floor and risks a possible tear if not done in time. *(Emergency Medicine, Chapter 124, pp 1287–1294)*

4.d. The Mayo scissors are used to make an incision in the midline, stopping before rectal tissue is reached. The objective is to create an easily reparable incision that facilitates delivery while preventing a traumatic tear to the rectal mucosa and surrounding structures. *(Emergency Medicine, Chapter 124, pp 1287–1294)*

5.b. Firm upward pressure is applied to the uterus with gentle traction on the cord to facilitate delivery of the placenta. This maneuver lessens the chance of pulling the uterus into the vaginal vault and causing a life-threatening uterine inversion. *(Emergency Medicine, Chapter 124, pp 1287–1294)*

6.b. The Apgar score is used to describe the health of the newborn. It is recorded at 1 and 5 minutes. The five components are heart rate, respiratory rate, muscle tone, reflex irritability, and color. The maximum score is 10. *(Emergency Medicine, Chapter 124, Table 124–3, p 1290)*

Complications of Early Pregnancy

1. In a 22-year-old female, pregnancy can be effectively ruled out by:
   a. A history of reliable use of appropriate birth control
   b. A history of tubal ligation
   c. Negative pelvic ultrasound
   d. Not being sexually active with men
   e. None of the above

2. All of the following statistics regarding ectopic pregnancy are true except:
   a. The triad of vaginal bleeding, abdominal pain, and a missed period occurs in the majority of ectopic pregnancies.
   b. 90% of patients complain of abdominal pain.
   c. 75% of patients complain of vaginal bleeding.
   d. 15% of women with ectopic pregnancies report a normal period within the previous 4 weeks.
   e. The existence of an ectopic pregnancy with a normal intrauterine pregnancy (heterotopic) is 1 in 30,000.

3. Which of the following statements about the risk of ectopic pregnancy is false?
   a. The risk is increased with a history of pelvic inflammatory disease.
   b. The risk is increased with a history of tubal ligation.
   c. The risk is increased with use of an intrauterine device.
   d. The risk is increased with use of fertility drugs.
   e. Most patients with ectopic pregnancy have at least one risk factor.

4. All of the following are true of ultrasound except:
   a. Ultrasound has replaced culdocentesis because it is less invasive and can be used to both locate a pregnancy and evaluate for fluid in the cul-de-sac.
   b. Endovaginal ultrasound is more sensitive that transabdominal ultrasound.
   c. Both endovaginal and transabdominal ultrasound require a full bladder.
   d. In normal pregnancies, ultrasound correlates well with the quantitative beta human chorionic gonadotropin (hCG) and gestational age.
   e. Transabdominal ultrasound may visualize pathology outside of the pelvis better than endovaginal studies.

5. All are true regarding ultrasound findings in early pregnancy except:
   a. A "double decidual sign" may define an early intrauterine pregnancy.
   b. A pseudogestational sac of ectopic pregnancy may mimic the "double decidual sign."
   c. Ultrasound findings may not correlate with quantitative beta hCG because of fluctuations in the first trimester.
   d. The finding on ultrasound of a fetal heartbeat in an extrauterine location is proof of an ectopic pregnancy.
   e. The beta hCG discriminatory zone for transabdominal ultrasound is 6500 mIU and for endovaginal ultrasound is 2000 mIU.

6. Which of the following statements regarding ectopic pregnancies is false?
   a. Most ectopic pregnancies are managed surgically.
   b. Medical management may be used with chemotherapy to terminate the ectopic pregnancy.
   c. Under certain circumstances, an ectopic pregnancy can be treated expectantly, with close follow-up using ultrasonography and serial beta hCGs.
   d. Some ectopic pregnancies may never be diagnosed because they may undergo involution and reabsorption.
   e. Doubling of the beta hCG rules out ectopic pregnancy.

7. The diagnosis of a completed abortion is consistent with all of the following except:
   a. The fetus and the placenta have been expelled from the uterus.
   b. The os is closed.
   c. Bleeding and cramping have stopped.
   d. The products of conception are verified.
   e. Pelvic ultrasound reveals a dilated, empty uterus.

8. For the threatened abortion, which the following is true:
   a. The os is opened.
   b. The ultrasound must show an intrauterine pregnancy.
   c. The risk of losing the pregnancy with an ultrasound finding of no fetal heart rate approaches 100%.

d. The risk of losing the pregnancy with an ultrasound finding of documented fetal heart rate is 5%.
e. Bed rest (pelvic rest) has been shown to improve the chance of sustaining the pregnancy to delivery.

9. All of the following are consistent with a molar pregnancy except:
   a. Molar pregnancy should be included in the differential diagnosis of first-trimester vaginal bleeding.
   b. A molar pregnancy is highly associated with choriocarcinoma and chorioadenoma.
   c. Grape-like vesicles may be seen at the cervical os or in the vagina with molar pregnancy.
   d. A very high beta hCG and a "snowstorm" appearance on ultrasound are highly suggestive of molar pregnancy.
   e. Molar pregnancy occurs in 1 in 2000 pregnancies.

10. Which of the following statements about hyperemesis gravidarum is false?
    a. Hyperemesis is associated with molar pregnancies and multiple gestations.
    b. The onset and severity of hyperemesis is clearly associated with elevated beta hCG, estradiol, and progesterone levels.
    c. Women who do not have morning sickness are at higher risk of spontaneous abortion.
    d. Younger primiparous women who are 25% heavier than their ideal body weight are at increased risk for hyperemesis.
    e. Patients with intractable vomiting should be evaluated for cholecystitis, gastritis, bowel obstruction, and urinary tract infections.

11. Which of the following statements regarding ectopic pregnancies is false?
    a. Ectopic pregnancies in the ampulla of the fallopian tube comprise 60% of all ectopic pregnancies.
    b. 3% of ectopic pregnancies occur in the interstitial portion of the tube and may appear under ultrasound as normal intrauterine pregnancies.
    c. Rupture of an ectopic pregnancy may be precipitated by the minimal trauma of sexual intercourse or an overzealous pelvic examination.
    d. A "tubal abortion" occurs when the embryo outgrows its limited blood supply in the fallopian tube and dies. The abortus is subsequently reabsorbed or sloughed into the peritoneum.
    e. 1% of ectopic pregnancies implant in the cervix and may be managed expectantly because of the close proximity of the os.

Answers

1.e. Nothing can rule out a pregnancy except a negative pregnancy test. Even the improved urine pregnancy tests currently in use, which have a sensitivity such that they will be positive by the time a patient misses her first period (2 days after implantation), are subject to false negatives (<1%). Urine pregnancy tests detect beta hCG levels greater than 25 to 50 mIU/mL IRP (International Reference Preparation), and serum pregnancy tests detect beta hCG levels of 5 to 10 IRP. *(Emergency Medicine, Chapter 125, pp 1295–1306)*

2.a. The triad occurs in only 14% of ectopic pregnancies. Although it has been previously estimated that heterotopic pregnancies occur in 1 of 30,000 pregnancies, recent literature suggests a rate as high as 1 in 3000. Increased incidence is noted in patients with a history of pelvic inflammatory disease, who use an intrauterine device, and who are on fertility medications. *(Emergency Medicine, Chapter 125, pp 1295–1306)*

3.e. Only 50% of the women with ectopic pregnancies will have had a risk factor. Risk factors include previous ectopic pregnancy, pelvic inflammatory disease, tubal ligation (especially the coagulation method), fertility drug treatment, history of infertility, recent or multiple abortions, older age, and intrauterine device implantation. *(Emergency Medicine, Chapter 125, pp 1295–1306)*

4.c. Transabdominal ultrasound requires a full bladder for an "acoustic window" to visualize the uterus and its contents. An endovaginal study is improved by a near-empty bladder, because a full bladder may distort otherwise normal anatomy. The studies complement each other, and sonographers will often begin with a transabdominal study, then will have the patient urinate for an endovaginal study. The patient who is going for ultrasonography should be well hydrated before the study, either orally if the patient is able to drink and tolerate fluids or intravenously if the patient cannot or should not drink. *(Emergency Medicine, Chapter 125, pp 1295–1306)*

5.c. Ultrasound findings must be correlated with the quantitative beta hCG level, as defined by the discriminatory zone for either endovaginal of transabdominal ultrasound. During the first trimester, the beta hCG doubles every 48 hours in 85% of normal pregnancies. An increase of less than 65% in 48 hours is defined as abnormal. *(Emergency Medicine, Chapter 125, pp 1295–1306)*

6.e. Expectant therapy is rare because of the risk and the need for close follow-up. The use of medical therapy with methotrexate has been increasing. Methotrexate therapy may be appropriate for patients who are hemodynamically stable, are at less than 6 weeks estimated gestational age, have no evidence of free fluid (or minimal free fluid) on ultrasound, and are at less than 4 cm without a heartbeat. Failure of the beta hCG to double in 48 hours is consistent with an ectopic pregnancy, but doubling of the beta hCG does not exclude it. *(Emergency Medicine, Chapter 125, pp 1295–1306)*

7.e. With the four other choices being true, ultrasound need not be done. However, if completed at that time, an ultrasound would probably show an empty *contracted* uterus. *(Emergency Medicine, Chapter 125, pp 1295–1306)*

8.d. Without a fetal heart rate documented on ultrasound, the risk of miscarriage is 50%. The risk drops to 5% if there is a documented fetal heart rate. Ultrasound may not show an intrauterine pregnancy if the beta hCG is below the discriminatory zone. Bed rest or "pelvic" rest, although commonly recommended, has no proven efficacy. (*Emergency Medicine, Chapter 125, pp 1295–1306*)

9.b. Eighty percent of molar pregnancies are benign. Twenty percent are associated with a choriocarcinoma or chorioadenoma. (*Emergency Medicine, Chapter 125, pp 1295–1306*)

10.b. Although hyperemesis is common during first-trimester pregnancy, its onset and severity are not associated with the rise of any particular hormone level. Hyperemesis resolves after the first trimester. (*Emergency Medicine, Chapter 125, pp 1295–1306*)

11.e. Sixty percent of ectopic pregnancies occur in the ampulla of the fallopian tube, 15% in the isthmus, 3% in the interstitial portion of the tube, and 1% in the cervix. Other less common locations include the ovaries and abdominal and pelvic cavities. Implantations in the cervix often present as massive bleeding and require hysterectomy to stop the hemorrhaging. Once a cervical ectopic pregnancy is suspected, a full evaluation and definitive treatment plan should be formulated. (*Emergency Medicine, Chapter 125, pp 1295–1306*)

Complications of Late Pregnancy

1. A 22-year-old 37-week primigravida presents to the ED after a low-velocity motor vehicle accident in which she was a belted back seat passenger. She is brought in on a backboard and a cervical collar is in place. She is awake and alert and has a complaint of neck pain. After assessment of her airway, breathing, and circulation, you note that her vital signs are BP 80/40, heart rate 100, RR 18, and O$_2$ saturation 96%. Your first intervention would be:
    a. Start two large-bore IVs for fluid resuscitation.
    b. Complete the primary survey with regard to deficits and exposure.
    c. Order a CBC, chemistry panel, and pregnancy test.
    d. Initiate fetal heart monitoring and obtain a stat ultrasound.
    e. Elevate the board and the patient with the right-side up.

2. Which of the following is false regarding preeclampsia and eclampsia?
    a. The diagnostic triad of preeclampsia is hypertension, proteinuria, and edema.
    b. Preeclampsia with seizures is characteristic of eclampsia.
    c. The HELLP syndrome is a more severe form of preeclampsia.
    d. Seizures are treated with phenytoin as a first agent.
    e. Magnesium sulfate may be used to treat both preeclampsia and eclampsia.

3. All are true of vaginal bleeding in the third trimester except:
    a. It may be associated with abrutio placentae, uterine rupture, placenta previa, vaginal polyps, or preterm labor.
    b. Vaginal bleeding may be caused by untreated hypertension, cocaine use, or trauma.
    c. A careful pelvic and speculum examination should be performed in the ED.
    d. A Kleihauer-Betke test may be helpful.
    e. Ultrasound may visualize placenta previa but is unreliable in ruling out abruptio placentae.

4. A 24-year-old female presents to the ED with pain after feeling a popping sensation in her abdomen while doing deep knee bends earlier in the morning. She is sexually active and uses condoms and recalls her last period to be 4 weeks earlier. She denies all other significant past medical history. She is diaphoretic and hypotensive and in extreme pain. She has a positive pregnancy test. An emergency bedside sonogram of the abdomen (Fig. 55–1) reveals:

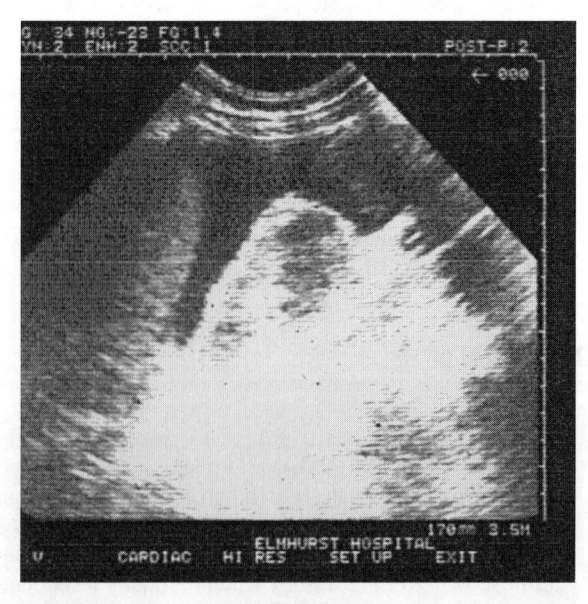

FIGURE 55–1A

a. Intrauterine pregnancy
b. Ectopic pregnancy
c. Placenta previa
d. Abruptio placentae
e. Fluid in Morison's pouch

5. Premature labor is associated with all of the following except:
   a. Spontaneous rupture of membranes
   b. Fetal death
   c. Abruptio placentae and placenta previa
   d. Urinary tract infections
   e. Structural vaginal abnormalities.

6. Contraindications for tocolysis include all the following except:
   a. Fetal abnormalities or fetal death
   b. Fetal gestational age of less than 37 weeks
   c. Preeclampsia or eclampsia
   d. Maternal hypertension
   e. Cervical dilation greater than 5 cm

7. Which of the following regarding postpartum hemorrhage is false?
   a. It can result from an undetected genital tract laceration.
   b. It can result from uterine rupture or inversion.
   c. It can be treated with methylergonovine maleate (Methergine) 0.2 mg IV bolus.
   d. It can be treated with oxytocin 20 units IV bolus.
   e. It can result from retained placental fragments.

8. All of the following are normal physiologic changes in pregnancy except:
   a. Respiratory alkalosis
   b. Leukopenia
   c. Decreased peritoneal signs
   d. Decreases systemic vascular resistance
   e. Dilation of the ureters and kidneys

Answers

1.e. Use of the left lateral position even when the patient is boarded and collared will decrease aortocaval compression by the uterus and increase blood return to the heart and maternal blood pressure. The uterus may also be displaced manually to the left side. With the exception of the pregnancy test, all other choices may be appropriate in the patient's evaluation. *(Emergency Medicine, Chapter 126, pp 1307–1318)*

2.d. Preeclampsia is diagnosed when the triad of hypertension, proteinuria, and edema is present. Preeclampsia commonly occurs after the 20th gestational week, up to 48 hours after delivery. If it occurs before the 20th week, multiple gestation or molar pregnancy should be considered. Eclampsia is characterized by seizures. Seizures are treated with magnesium sulfate as a first agent, and other agents are added if magnesium fails. The drug of choice to treat hypertension is hydralazine. The HELLP syndrome is an acronym for hemo-lysis, elevated liver enzymes, and low platelets. It is associated with increased maternal morbidity. Other associated complications include abruptio placentae, intracerebral bleed, and ruptured capsular hematoma of the liver. Definitive treatment of eclampsia is delivery of the viable fetus. *(Emergency Medicine, Chapter 126, pp 1307–1318)*

3.c. The most worrisome causes of vaginal bleeding in the third trimester include abruptio placentae and placenta previa. Abruption is characterized by a tender, firm uterus, whereas placenta previa is usually painless. In a late-trimester pregnancy with vaginal bleeding, a bimanual or speculum examination should not be performed until ultrasound has ruled out a placenta previa. The manual and speculum examination should be carried out by an obstetric consultant in the operating room, with the patient prepared for possible cesarean section should massive hemorrhage occur (the "double set-up"). *(Emergency Medicine, Chapter 126, pp 1307–1318)*

4.e. Morison's pouch is a potential space not normally seen by ultrasound. It is formed by Gerota's fascia of the kidney and Glisson's capsule of the liver. When detected by ultrasound, the "fluid" is from ascites, peritoneal dialysis, or blood from any source in the peritoneum. Given the patient's history, her findings would be consistent with a ruptured ectopic pregnancy. This patient had 2 L of blood evacuated from her peritoneum in the operating room. *(Emergency Medicine, Chapter 126, pp 1307–1318)*

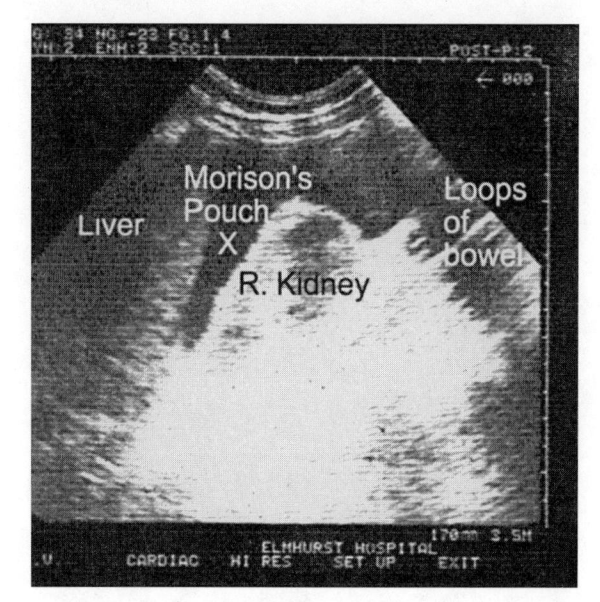

FIGURE 55–1B

5.e. Whereas uterine abnormalities are associated with premature labor, structural vaginal abnormalities have not been reported as a cause of premature labor. All of the other conditions described are associated with premature labor. Asymptomatic urinary tract infections should be treated during pregnancy because such infections are associated with an increased incidence of premature labor and fetal wastage. *(Emergency Medicine, Chapter 127, pp 1319–1330)*

6.b. Contraindications to tocolysis include vaginal bleeding, fetal distress, chorioamnionitis, preeclampsia and eclampsia, fetal death, severe fetal growth retardation, and maternal hypotension. Relative contraindications include maternal hypertension, stable placenta previa, maternal cardiac disease, mild abruption, and cervical dilation greater than 5 cm. Fetal gestation less than 37 weeks is a reason for tocolysis, not a contraindication. *(Emergency Medicine, Chapter 127, pp 1319–1330)*

7.d. An oxytocin bolus may cause hypotension, life-threatening arrhythmia, or cardiac arrest. Oxytocin should be given by diluting 20 to 40 mg in 1 L of normal saline and the solution administered at a rate of 200 to 500 mL/hr. *(Emergency Medicine, Chapter 127, pp 1319–1330)*

8.b. Many physiologic changes that occur in pregnancy have implications for special considerations in the treatment of pregnant women. A progesterone-induced, centrally mediated hyperventilation causes a respiratory alkalosis, with a compensatory increase in renal bicarbonate excretion. This decreases the buffering capacity and increases susceptibility to metabolic acidosis. Progesterone also causes a decrease in gastrointestinal motility, increasing the risk of aspiration. Stretching of the peritoneum causes decreased sensitivity to peritoneal irritation, and disease such as appendicitis and cholecystitis may present more subtly. Cardiovascular changes include increased plasma volume, decreased systemic vascular resistance, and decreased BP. The gravid uterus decreases venous return to the heart by compressing the vena cava. There is a relative *leukocytosis* that occurs in the second and third trimesters. There is a relative anemia, because the increase in red cell mass lags behind the increase in plasma volume. The levels of fibrinogen and clotting factors increase while fibrinolytic activity is decreased, therefore predisposing the pregnant woman to thromboembolic disease. *(Emergency Medicine, Chapter 128, pp 1331–1339)*

BIBLIOGRAPHY

Doan-Wiggins L: Medical illness in the pregnant patient. *In* Howell JM, Altieri M, Jagoda AS, et al (eds): Emergency Medicine. Philadelphia, WB Saunders, 1998, pp 1331–1339.

Dugan EM: Complications of labor and delivery. *In* Howell JM, Altieri M, Jagoda AS, et al (eds): Emergency Medicine. Philadelphia, WB Saunders, 1998, pp 1319–1330.

Dugan EM: Uncomplicated pregnancy, labor, and delivery. *In* Howell JM, Altieri M, Jagoda AS, et al (eds): Emergency Medicine. Philadelphia, WB Saunders, 1998, pp 1287–1294.

Hemphill RR, Santen SA, Dugan EM: Complications of late pregnancy. *In* Howell JM, Altieri M, Jagoda AS, et al (eds): Emergency Medicine. Philadelphia, WB Saunders, 1998, pp 1307–1318.

Santen SA, Dugan EM: Complications of early pregnancy. *In* Howell JM, Altieri M, Jagoda AS, et al (eds): Emergency Medicine. Philadelphia, WB Saunders, 1998, pp 1295–1306.

56 Approach to Pelvic Pain and Infectious and Noninfectious Disorders

DANIEL M. JOYCE, MD   CARL K. HSU, MD

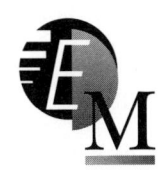

1. A 20-year-old female who denies sexual activity presents complaining of vulvovaginal pruritus. The abdominal examination is unremarkable. Examination of the external genitalia reveals mild erythema surrounding the vaginal introitus. Pregnancy test, KOH prep, wet prep, and Gram's stain are all negative. The most appropriate next step is:
   a. Reassurance and discharge
   b. Referral to a gynecologist
   c. Investigation of environmental exposures
   d. Broad-spectrum antimicrobial coverage
   e. Discontinuation of oral contraceptives

2. A patient complains of vaginal fullness and pressure. A speculum examination does not reveal any masses or a foreign body. The most appropriate next step is:
   a. Referral for a laparoscopy
   b. CT scan of pelvis
   c. Valsalva maneuver
   d. Culture of endocervical canal
   e. ESR

3. Clinical indicators of excessive vaginal bleeding include:
   a. Bleeding exceeds more than one soaked pad per hour
   b. Orthostatic hypotension that is not easily corrected by fluid administration
   c. A drop in the hematocrit (greater than 10 units) after hydration
   d. An initial hematocrit less than 30 with no baseline known
   e. All of the above

4. A 40-year-old woman presents with dysfunctional uterine bleeding. Evaluation in the ED reveals normal vital signs, a normal physical examination, and a negative beta human chorionic gonadotropin. The most appropriate treatment is:
   a. Conjugated estrogen (Premarin)
   b. VDRL or rapid plasma reagin testing
   c. Short course of any combination oral contraceptive
   d. Medroxyprogesterone, 10 mg PO daily for 10 days
   e. Endometrial biopsy

5. Oral contraceptives as "morning after" pills are effective when used within what period of time after coitus?
   a. 24 hours
   b. 48 hours
   c. 72 hours
   d. 5 days
   e. 7 days

6. The least useful modality to evaluate a child with a suspected vaginal foreign body is:
   a. Digital rectal examination
   b. Plain radiographs
   c. Vaginoscopy
   d. Mother's assistance
   e. Cotton swabs as a speculum and forceps

7. Risk factors for pelvic inflammatory disease include all of the following except:
   a. Intrauterine device
   b. Late age at first intercourse
   c. Multiple sexual partners
   d. Recent gynecologic instrumentation
   e. Vaginal douching

8. Pelvic inflammatory disease is estimated to cause infertility in what percentage of patients?
   a. 2%
   b. 5%
   c. 12%
   d. 20%
   e. 25%

9. A patient with pelvic inflammatory disease has associated right upper quadrant pain. The most likely etiology is:
   a. Tubo-ovarian abscess
   b. Acalculous cholecystitis
   c. Right lower lobe pneumonia
   d. Fitz-Hugh–Curtis syndrome
   e. Generalized peritonitis

10. A patient presents with dyspareunia and a clear mucoid discharge. Vaginal examination demonstrates tender ves-

icles and ulcers on the cervix. Painful vesicles are also noted on the labia. The most appropriate treatment is:
   a. Ceftriaxone, 125 mg IM
   b. Doxycycline, 100 mg PO BID × 10 days
   c. Erythromycin, 500 mg PO QID × 7 days
   d. Benzathine penicillin G, 2.4 million units IM
   e. Acyclovir, 200 mg PO 5 × per day × 10 days

11. Ulcerative genital lesions are found in all of the following except:
    a. Erythrasma
    b. Syphilis
    c. Chancroid
    d. Lymphogranuloma venereum
    e. Herpes

12. A patient presents with complaints of malodorous, thin, grayish vaginal discharge. Wet prep demonstrates vaginal mucosal cells with a speckled appearance and irregular cell margins. The normally rod-shaped vaginal flora has been replaced by coccobacilli. The most likely diagnosis is:
    a. Bacterial vaginosis
    b. Trichomoniasis
    c. Candidiasis
    d. Chlamydia
    e. Herpes simplex

13. A 22-year-old sexually active female presents with 4 days of worsening lower abdominal pain. She has had previous urinary tract infections but says her present symptoms are different. She denies pain or blood on urination. Vital signs are BP 70/40, temperature 99°F, pulse 120, RR 14. Her abdominal examination is significant for bilateral lower abdominal tenderness without rebound. A pelvic examination reveals scant yellowish discharge without blood in the vaginal vault. All of the following would be appropriate initial management except:
    a. Two large-bore IVs
    b. CBC, electrolytes, and type and crossmatch
    c. Pregnancy test
    d. Pelvic examination with cultures
    e. CT of the pelvis

14. The complaint of vaginal itch may be associated with all of the following except:
    a. Lice
    b. Herpes
    c. Atrophic vaginitis
    d. Use of lanolin-containing lotions
    e. Foreign body

15. All of the following are true of dysfunctional uterine bleeding except:
    a. Dysfunctional uterine bleeding is most frequently seen at the beginning or the end of the reproductive years.
    b. It is associated with inadequate function of the corpus luteum.
    c. It can be confused with endometrial carcinoma.
    d. To control hemorrhage, treatment with hormone therapy should be initiated immediately.
    e. Bleeding can be controlled with conjugated estrogens or a combination of oral contraceptives.

16. All are true of pelvic inflammatory disease except:
    a. Pelvic inflammatory disease is a disease of sexually active young women.
    b. The majority of patients with pelvic inflammatory disease are multiparous.
    c. Pelvic inflammatory disease may lead to infertility.
    d. *Neisseria gonorrhea* and *Chlamydia* are the two most common organisms responsible for pelvic inflammatory disease.
    e. Pus from the fallopian tubes may cause peritonitis, perihepatitis, or abscesses.

17. The true statement regarding the etiologic associations of pelvic inflammatory disease is:
    a. *Neisseria* infection is not menses dependent.
    b. *Chlamydia* infection is menses dependent.
    c. The use of an intrauterine device is not associated with pelvic inflammatory disease.
    d. Recent gynecologic instrumentation is not associated with pelvic inflammatory disease.
    e. Pelvic inflammatory disease is rare during pregnancy because of the early formation of a cervical mucus plug.

18. All are true of Fitz-Hugh–Curtis syndrome except:
    a. It is an inflammation of the liver capsule.
    b. Organisms are most frequently spread by the lymphatics.
    c. It may present with right upper quadrant pain with radiation to the shoulder.
    d. Diagnosis can be made with either ultrasound or laparotomy.
    e. It can be confused with cholecystitis, pyelonephritis, and pancreatitis.

19. A 15-year-old 10-week primigravida presents with her husband to the ED. She has a telegram from her primary physician indicating that she had a positive test for chlamydia. You should:
    a. Not treat and refer back to her private doctor.
    b. Treat with doxycycline, 100 mg BID for 7 days.
    c. Treat with one dose ceftriaxone, 125 mg IM only.
    d. Treat with trimethoprim-sulfamethoxazole double-strength tablets for 5 days.
    e. Treat with erythromycin, 500 mg tablets QID for 7 days.

20. All of the following are associated with *Trichomonas vaginalis* except:
    a. Pain, pruritus, or dysuria
    b. Oval to round cells (clue cells) on microscopy
    c. White, yellow, or greenish vaginal discharge
    d. Wet mount examination reveals a pear-shaped organism with a swimming motion
    e. Metronidazole, 500 mg BID for 7 days

21. A 24-year-old female with a 36-week pregnancy presents with an acute asthma attack. Management may include all except:
    a. Nebulized beta-agonist
    b. Discharge if peak expiratory flow is greater than 70% predicted after treatment
    c. Prednisone, 40 mg PO
    d. Terbutaline sulfate
    e. All of the above may be appropriate

22. Of the following, which antimicrobial should not be used during pregnancy?
    a. Penicillin
    b. Macrolides
    c. Cephalosporins
    d. Quinolones
    e. Amoxicillin

23. The following are appropriately matched except:
    a. Genital warts—condylomata lata
    b. *Gardnerella vaginalis*—amine "fishy" odor
    c. Granuloma inguinale—Donovan bodies
    d. *Candida vaginalis*—cottage cheese appearance
    e. Herpes simplex—positive Tzanck smear

24. An ill-appearing 20-year-old female presents with fever, a desquamating rash, and an injected conjunctiva. She denies any past significant history and, although sexually active, says she is not pregnant because her period began 4 days ago. She is hypotensive and tachycardic. Her O_2 saturation is 95% and her lungs are clear. There are no heart murmurs on examination, and there are positive bowel sounds without tenderness or lymphadenopathy. She refuses a pelvic examination because she is using a tampon. Her skin is warm and moist to the touch. There are no petechiae. The most likely organism responsible for her condition is:
    a. *Streptococcus viridans*
    b. *Calymmatobacterium granulomatis*
    c. *Haemophilus ducreyi*
    d. *Staphylococcus aureus*
    e. *Pneumocystis carinii*

25. All of the following may be treated with erythromycin except:
    a. Syphilis
    b. Chancroid
    c. Granuloma inguinale
    d. Lymphogranuloma venereum
    e. All of the above may be treated

26. Which is false regarding appendicitis and pregnancy?
    a. Because of the gravid uterus, the pain may be felt in the right upper quadrant.
    b. There is an increase in incidence during pregnancy.
    c. Poor outcome usually results from a delay in diagnosis.
    d. Ultrasound may be helpful to evaluate right upper quadrant pain.
    e. It may be confused with ectopic pregnancy.

27. All of the following are true of toxic shock syndrome except:
    a. It is a multisystem disease.
    b. Definitive treatment is with IV antimicrobials.
    c. The incidence of the disease has dropped since publicized in the early 1980s.
    d. It has been associated with nasal packing and packing of surgical wounds.
    e. Although initially described with tampon use, it can be seen with the use of intrauterine devices, burns, septic abortions, and sinusitis.

28. A 16-year-old female presents with low abdominal pain and is diagnosed with pelvic inflammatory disease in the ED. All of the following are indications for admission to the hospital except:
    a. Multiple previous episodes
    b. Her age
    c. Temperature above 38.5°C
    d. Suspected tubo-ovarian abscess
    e. Questionable compliance

Answers

1.c. In the absence of a vaginal discharge, inflammatory contact dermatitis caused by soaps, shampoos, fabric softeners, detergents, perfumes, lotions, and lubricants should be suspected. Advise the patient to discontinue all home remedies and other over-the-counter treatments. Lanolin (a common skin irritant) and other salves frequently exacerbate the inflammation. Recovery will be hastened by the addition of an antipruritic (e.g., an antihistamine). H_2-blockers have been used and offer a nonsedating advantage. NSAIDs can be effective for inflammation. Weak topical nonhalogenated steroids (1% hydrocortisone) can safely be used for 2 to 3 days. A short course of systemic steroids is reserved for the most difficult cases and used only after consultation. Reassurance and gynecologic referral are appropriate while waiting for the culture results. (*Emergency Medicine, Chapter 130, pp 1350–1356*)

2.c. Vaginal fullness or pressure suggests a retained foreign body (tampon), carcinoma, cystocele, rectocele, enterocele, or uterine prolapse. If the speculum examination is unrevealing and there is no obvious intrusion from the vaginal walls, withdraw the speculum and have the patient bear down, perform the Valsalva maneuver, or cough. Abnormal inward bulging of the vaginal wall suggests a possible cystocele, rectocele, or enterocele. Although early or mild uterine prolapse can present like this, it usually presents as a mass in the vagina or with the entire uterus projecting out through the introitus between the patient's legs. Uterine prolapse is more common in multiparous women and is also associated with spina bifida, pelvic tumors, obesity, and chronic pulmonary problems. (*Emergency Medicine, Chapter 130, pp 1350–1356*)

3.e. The ED complaint of abnormal vaginal bleeding is most commonly related to either pregnancy (ectopic or threatened abortion) or pregnancy avoidance (breakthrough bleeding caused by an attempt to extend a diminished supply of estrogen pills). Abnormal vaginal bleeding can also result from uterine abnormalities (fibroids), menstrual cycle irregularities, trauma, infection, or malignancy. Rarely is uterine bleeding the presenting symptom of infection or coagulopathy. When the clinical indicators of excessive vaginal bleeding are present, consultation with a gynecologist and admission to elucidate the etiology of the bleeding are appropriate. *(Emergency Medicine, Chapter 130, pp 1350–1356)*

4.e. Irregular and sometimes heavy menses can result from anovulatory cycles and endometrial buildup, usually occurring at the beginning or end of the reproductive years. Mature women can have excessive bleeding because of inadequate function of the corpus luteum or the presence of endometrial cancer. Women over age 35 are at increased risk for uterine cancer. Hormonal therapy is strongly discouraged until uterine pathology is excluded, because progesterone- or estrogen-containing compounds may invalidate a subsequent endometrial biopsy. Young women in their teens or early 20s may benefit from any combination oral contraceptive prescribed QID for 5 to 7 days. Because heavy withdrawal bleeding associated with severe cramping may take place about 1 week after the last tablet is taken, follow-up with a gynecologist should be arranged. *(Emergency Medicine, Chapter 130, pp 1350–1356)*

5.c. Oral contraceptives are effective in preventing pregnancy if used within the first 72 hours (i.e., before implantation). It is important to obtain a negative pregnancy test before prescribing a contraceptive medication. Either 2 tablets of Ovral or 4 tablets of Lo/Ovral given orally and repeated in 12 hours is effective. Warn the patient about the possibility of severe nausea, cramping, and bleeding irregularities. Promethazine, 25 mg, given before each dose should lessen the associated nausea. Patients should be instructed to follow up with their gynecologist if no menstrual period occurs in 4 weeks, because failures can occur. *(Emergency Medicine, Chapter 130, pp 1350–1356)*

6.b. Vaginal foreign bodies can present with complaints of vulvovaginitis. Poorly recognizable pieces of tissue paper are commonly found. A digital rectal examination may help identify larger solid objects. Radiographs are not usually helpful because the object is usually not radiopaque. Moistened cotton swabs may be used as a speculum and for specimen collection. Exploration with a warmed bayonet forceps or irrigation with a warmed fluid can also be useful. Examination can be facilitated by positioning the child in a seated position between her mother's legs, with the parent gently supporting the child's open legs next to her own. All of these patients should be referred for vaginoscopy to confirm the removal of all foreign material. *(Emergency Medicine, Chapter 130, pp 1350–1356)*

7.b. Pelvic inflammatory disease usually presents as lower abdominal pain described as dull, aching, and bilateral. The pain ranges from mild and intermittent to severe and constant, frequently beginning or worsening during menstruation. Risk factors for pelvic inflammatory disease include nonbarrier contraception such as an intrauterine device, young age at first intercourse, multiple sexual partners, recent exposure to sexually transmitted diseases, previous history of pelvic inflammatory disease, recent gynecologic instrumentation, vaginal douching, and bacterial vaginosis. *(Emergency Medicine, Chapter 131, pp 1357–1366)*

8.c. Pelvic inflammatory disease is estimated to cause infertility in 12% of patients, with the risk increasing with each episode. It is primarily a disease of sexually active young women. The peak incidence of pelvic inflammatory disease occurs in the 15- to 24-year age group. Patients with a history of pelvic inflammatory disease often are nulliparous or give a history of difficulty becoming pregnant. The high frequency of pelvic inflammatory disease–associated infertility is of particular concern because it affects patients in their prime reproductive years. Because pelvic inflammatory disease may cause severe pathologic changes with minimal clinical manifestations, treatment must be based on clinical grounds with a bias toward overdiagnosis. *(Emergency Medicine, Chapter 131, pp 1357–1366)*

9.d. Fitz-Hugh–Curtis syndrome, or perihepatitis, is inflammation of the liver capsule complicating pelvic inflammatory disease. Symptomatic perihepatitis occurs in 5% to 10% of patients with pelvic inflammatory disease. Although gonorrhea and *Chlamydia* usually spread transperitoneally, *Chlamydia* may also disseminate hematogenously or via the lymphatics. A purulent and fibrinous exudate develops on the liver capsule with eventual formation of adhesions between the capsule and the parietal peritoneum. The onset of upper abdominal pain is usually concurrent with the onset of lower abdominal pain, but it may occur either before or after it. Laparoscopy is the preferred study to confirm the diagnosis. Tubo-ovarian abscess is a complication of pelvic inflammatory disease. Abscess rupture is associated with peritoneal findings usually localized to the lower quadrants. Peritonitis may complicate pelvic inflammatory disease, but it is generalized, not localized to the right upper quadrant. Pneumonia and cholecystitis, although in the differential of right upper quadrant pain, are not associated with pelvic inflammatory disease. *(Emergency Medicine, Chapter 131, pp 1357–1366)*

10.e. Herpes simplex may cause both infectious cervicitis and vulvar-vaginal disease. Herpes produces painful vesicles or ulcerative lesions. The initial episode of herpes may include low-grade fever, headache, malaise, and inguinal adenopathy. The incubation period is from 5 to 10 days. The lesions are infectious until the ulcers crust over, which usually takes 12 to 14 days. Herpes is a recurrent disease that may be precipitated by menses, intercurrent illness, or other stress.

Recurrent episodes are often preceded by a prodrome of pain or pruritus and are of shorter duration than the primary episode. Of note, viral shedding may occur during asymptomatic periods. Multinucleated giant cells may be seen on Tzanck smear, but definitive diagnosis requires viral cultures. The primary episode can be treated by acyclovir, 200 mg, given orally 5 times a day for 10 days. Newer antiviral agents are also effective. Intravenous acyclovir may be required for immunocompromised patients or in those patients who have a severe primary episode. The other antimicrobial choices offered are used in the treatment of gonorrhea, chlamydia, and syphilis. *(Emergency Medicine, Chapter 131, pp 1357–1366)*

11.a. Erythrasma is caused by *Corynebacterium minutissimum* and presents with a mildly erythematous rash in the vulvovaginal region. The rash is similar to that of tinea corporis and is responsive to erythromycin. The other choices offered are all well-known causes of genital ulcers. Of these, herpes is the most common cause, with a prevalence of 30 million cases in the United States alone. Syphilis is caused by the spirochete *Treponema pallidum*. The hallmark of primary syphilis is the chancre, characterized by a single painless ulcer with a raised rounded border and an indurated clean base. Chancroid is uncommon in the United States. The causative organism is *Haemophilus ducreyi*, a gram-negative rod. Coinfection by herpes or syphilis is found in 10% of patients with chancroid. The ulcer is painful and shallow and surrounded by an erythematous ring. Lymphogranuloma venereum is caused by serotypes of *Chlamydia trachomatis* and is rare in the United States. The disease initially presents as a painless papule or vesicle, which may then ulcerate. Inguinal lymphadenopathy represents the second stage, occurring 1 to 4 weeks after the primary lesion, followed by the anogenitorectal syndrome, the third stage of infection. *(Emergency Medicine, Chapter 131, pp 1357–1366)*

12.a. The coccobacillus *Gardnerella vaginalis* is the predominant organism in bacterial vaginosis. The discharge, although often uncharacteristic, is described as thin and grayish, with small bubbles and a "fishy" odor. Examination of the discharge usually reveals a pH above 4.5, a positive amine odor, and "clue cells," which are vaginal mucosal cells with adherent coccobacilli, giving the cells a speckled appearance. Coccobacilli replace the normal rod-shaped vaginal flora. Bacterial vaginosis has been implicated in salpingitis, post-hysterectomy infections, premature labor, and postpartum endometritis. Treatment is with oral or intravaginal metronidazole or clindamycin. A grossly purulent cervical discharge suggests a coexistent gonorrhea or chlamydia infection. *(Emergency Medicine, Chapter 131, pp 1357–1366)*

13.e. A young sexually active female who presents to the ED with lower abdominal pain and unstable vital signs must be assumed to have a ruptured ectopic pregnancy until proven otherwise. All menstruating females who present with abdominal pain should have a pregnancy test. Given the patient's presentation, initial management would include vigorous fluid resuscitation with two large-bore IVs. A CT scan would not be part of the initial evaluation, because of the need to first stabilize the patient. With a positive pregnancy test, ultrasound (particularly if available at bedside) would be useful to determine if there is an intrauterine pregnancy. *(Emergency Medicine, Chapter 129, pp 1341–1349)*

14.b. All the pathogens listed cause vaginal itching except herpes, which usually causes burning and not pruritus. Although vaginal itch may be treated with H_1- and H_2-blockers and NSAIDs, the use of lanolin-containing lotions (a common component of lotions and soaps) can itself be the cause of vaginal pruritus. Although patients will frequently initiate treatment of a vaginal irritation with lotions, they should, in fact, be advised to stop the use of products containing lanolin or any other possible irritant. *(Emergency Medicine, Chapter 130, pp 1350–1356; Chapter 131, pp 1357–1366)*

15.d. Conjugated estrogens or a combination of oral contraceptives may be used to treat dysfunctional uterine bleeding in women under 35 years of age. Women over the age of 35 should have an endometrial biopsy before beginning treatment because of the increased risk of endometrial cancer. *(Emergency Medicine, Chapter 130, pp 1350–1356)*

16.b. The majority of patients with pelvic inflammatory disease are nulliparous. Other risk factors for pelvic inflammatory disease include use of nonbarrier contraception (intrauterine device), young age at first intercourse, multiple sexual partners, previous history of pelvic inflammatory disease, vaginal douching, recent gynecologic instrumentation, bacterial vaginosis, and the presence of sexually transmitted diseases. *(Emergency Medicine, Chapter 131, pp 1357–1366)*

17.e. Flare-up of *Neisseria gonorrhoeae* infections is menses dependent, occurring 5 to 7 days after menstruation. This is thought to occur because of reflux from the uterus through the fallopian tubes into the peritoneum during menses. Chlamydia infection is not associated with menses. The use of an intrauterine device is associated with pelvic inflammatory disease, as is recent gynecologic instrumentation. Although it has been said that pelvic inflammatory disease is "impossible" during pregnancy because of the mucus plug that forms, it is possible during pregnancy, though rare. *(Emergency Medicine, Chapter 131, pp 1357–1366)*

18.b. Organisms associated with Fitz-Hugh–Curtis syndrome are most frequently spread by direct contact of pus in the peritoneum, not by lymphatic or hematogenous spread. *(Emergency Medicine, Chapter 131, pp 1357–1366)*

19.e. The tetracyclines and fluoroquinolones are contraindicated in pregnancy. Bactrim does not treat chlamydia.

The use of sulfonamides (Bactrim) in pregnancy is controversial, but they may be used safely in the first and second trimesters. They should not be used in the third trimester, because they can cause fetal kernicterus. Ceftriaxone may be considered if the patient has not already been treated for gonococcal infection. Erythromycin can be used for chlamydia. Avoid the use of the estolate form of erythromycin, which has been associated with maternal cholestatic hepatitis. *(Emergency Medicine, Chapter 131, pp 1357–1366)*

20.b. *Trichomonas* should be evaluated with a specimen taken from the posterior fornix of the vagina. On wet mount, parasites can be seen attached to the surface of vaginal epithelial cells. Under light microscopy, a swimming motion of the pear-shaped protozoa as well as a lashing movement of their flagella can be seen. The protozoa die very quickly on drying of the specimen. In heavy infestations, the protozoa may be incidentally seen under microscopic examination of the urine. Clue cells are associated with *Gardnerella vaginalis*, a gram-negative coccobacillus. *(Emergency Medicine, Chapter 131, pp 1357–1366)*

21.e. All the medications listed can be used to treat asthma in pregnancy. In third-trimester pregnancy, evaluation should include an assessment of fetal heart tones. *(Emergency Medicine, Chapter 128, pp 1331–1340)*

22.d. Quinolones are contraindicated during pregnancy because of the potential for fetal injury, unless antimicrobial resistance requires the use of a quinolone. Although human studies are limited, fluoroquinolones have been associated with irreversible arthropathy in immature dogs.[1] *(Emergency Medicine, Chapter 128, pp 1331–1339; Chapter 131, pp 1357–1366)*

23.a. Condyloma latum is a skin finding of secondary syphilis that has the appearance of nontender flat warts. Genital warts are associated with condyloma acuminatum from human papovavirus and have the appearance of pedunculated growths. *(Emergency Medicine, Chapter 131, pp 1357–1366)*

24.d. This patient who is menstruating, hypotensive, and febrile most likely has toxic shock syndrome, which has been associated with *Staphylococcus aureus*. Antimicrobials are generally used, but there is little evidence that antimicrobial treatment is helpful. Because there is no history of the patient's being immunocompromised, *Pneumocystis carinii* pneumonia and endocarditis should be lower on the differential diagnosis. *Calymmatobacterium granulomatis* is the causative agent of granuloma inguinale (donovanosis). *Haemophilus ducreyi* (chancroid) and granuloma inguinale are not likely to cause the patient's toxic appearance. *(Emergency Medicine, Chapter 131, pp 1357–1366)*

25.e. All can be treated with erythromycin. *(Emergency Medicine, Chapter 131, pp 1357–1366)*

26.b. Although the incidence of acute appendicitis during pregnancy is not increased, its "atypical" presentation in the pregnant patient complicates the diagnosis. As the gravid uterus causes the peritoneum to stretch in the course of a normal pregnancy, peritoneal signs may be decreased, thus masking an appendicitis. As the abdominal contents, including the appendix, are pushed upward by the expanding gravid uterus, appendicitis may present with tenderness over the right upper quadrant. Cholecystitis, which also presents with right upper quadrant pain, has an increased incidence during pregnancy. In any patient with unexplained abdominal pain, ectopic pregnancy should also be considered. *(Emergency Medicine, Chapter 129, pp 1341–1349)*

27.b. Treatment is supportive and includes removal of the offending agent (tampon or intrauterine device) or source of toxin production. Although antimicrobials are generally used, there is little evidence that outcome is improved by their use. *(Emergency Medicine, Chapter 87, pp 888–895; Chapter 131, pp 1357–1366)*

28.a. Although most cases of pelvic inflammatory disease are treated on an outpatient basis, guidelines for admission include first episode of pelvic inflammatory disease, adolescence, pregnancy, intrauterine device, peritonitis, suspected tubo-ovarian abscess, diagnostic uncertainty, and failure to respond to outpatient therapy in 48 to 72 hours. *(Emergency Medicine, Chapter 131, pp 1357–1366)*

REFERENCE

1. Drugs and medications during pregnancy. *In* Cunningham FG, MacDonald PC, Leveno KJ, et al (eds): Williams Obstetrics, ed 19. Norwalk, CT, Appleton & Lange, 1993, pp 959–980.

BIBLIOGRAPHY

Davis TE, Anderson GV Jr: Noninfectious pelvic disorders. *In* Howell JM, Altieri M, Jagoda AS, et al (eds): Emergency Medicine. Philadelphia, WB Saunders, 1998, pp 1350–1356.

Doan-Wiggins L: Medical illness in the pregnant patient. *In* Howell JM, Altieri M, Jagoda AS, et al (eds): Emergency Medicine. Philadelphia, WB Saunders, 1998, pp 1331–1339.

Glasier A: Emergency postcoital contraception. N Engl J Med 1997; 337(15):1058–1064.

Henry J, Paganussi PJ: Skin infections and infestations. *In* Howell JM, Altieri M, Jagoda AS, et al (eds): Emergency Medicine. Philadelphia, WB Saunders, 1998, pp 888–895.

McCormack WM: Pelvic inflammatory disease. N Engl J Med 1996; 330(2):115–119.

Otsuki JA, Anderson GV Jr: Inflammation and infection of the female genital tract. *In* Howell JM, Altieri M, Jagoda AS, et al (eds): Emergency Medicine. Philadelphia, WB Saunders, 1998, pp 1357–1366.

Pepe SA Jr, Anderson GV Jr: Approach to pelvic pain. *In* Howell JM, Altieri M, Jagoda AS, et al (eds): Emergency Medicine. Philadelphia, WB Saunders, 1998, pp 1341–1349.

57 Breast Disorders

DONALD BARTON, MD   DANIEL M. JOYCE, MD

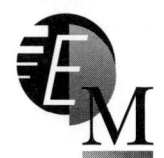

1. All of the following are true of traumatic breast injuries except:
   a. Breast implants can rupture after even minor trauma.
   b. The incidence of traumatic breast injuries has increased.
   c. Traumatic breast injuries can present as a mass.
   d. Traumatic breast injuries may mask serious underlying injuries.
   e. Most patients presenting with post-traumatic fat necrosis give a history of injury.

2. Which of the following statements about infections of the breast is incorrect?
   a. Although patients with breast abscesses must be referred for follow-up management, patients with mastitis need not be.
   b. Antimicrobial coverage should be with either a beta-lactamase–resistant penicillin or a first-generation cephalosporin.
   c. A breast abscess can be differentiated from mastitis using ultrasound.
   d. A patient with a breast abscess can continue to breast feed.
   e. Periareolar abscesses should be referred to a surgeon for drainage.

3. A 58-year-old postmenopausal woman presents to the ED with a complaint of a lump in her breast. She is accompanied by her two daughters who are 21 and 19 years old. She is particularly concerned because her mother died of breast cancer at age 65. She has non–insulin-dependent diabetes that is fairly well controlled. On examination, she is found to be a well-appearing obese woman whose only significant finding is a 1½ × 1½ cm tender mass in her left breast, lateral to the nipple. Findings that suggest the diagnosis of breast cancer include all the following except:
   a. Family history of breast cancer
   b. Obesity
   c. Multiparity
   d. Late age of first birth
   e. Advancing age

4. Mondor's disease is characterized by which of the following?
   a. Fat necrosis secondary to trauma
   b. Superficial phlebitis of the chest wall along the lateral breast
   c. Mamillary fistula associated with an abscess
   d. Cyclic mastodynia
   e. Rupture of breast implant

5. A young female presents 2 days postpartum with complaints of a swollen, painful left breast. Examination reveals a temperature of 38.4°C and a diffusely tender breast without erythema or fluctuance. The most likely diagnosis is:
   a. Mastitis
   b. Mamillary fistula
   c. Postpartum breast engorgement
   d. Fibroadenoma
   e. Breast abscess

6. The appropriate treatment of postpartum mastitis includes all of the following except:
   a. Local ultrasound if abscess is suspected
   b. Lactation suppression in women who bottle feed
   c. Antimicrobial coverage against staphylococci
   d. Cessation of breast feeding
   e. Breast drainage by pumping if necessary

Answers

1.e. Breast implants have been known to rupture after even minor trauma; treatment is operative. The incidence of traumatic injuries to the breast has increased because of the increased use of three-point seat belts. Compression injury of breast tissue causes crushed tissue and hemorrhage, followed by an inflammatory response, and resulting in a firm nodular mass, whose shape and texture is similar to that of carcinoma but that histologically is fat necrosis. Only 44% of patients found to have these lesions on biopsy give a definite history of trauma. Injuries of the ribs, cervical spine, diaphragm, or myocardium can refer to the breast and may be missed in the presence of a significant injury to the breast. *(Emergency Medicine, Chapter 133, pp 1372–1375)*

2.a. Both mastitis and breast abscesses in nonlactating or postmenopausal women should be presumed to be breast cancer until proven otherwise. Either beta-lactamase–resistant penicillin or first-generation cephalosporins cover *Staphylococcus aureus*, the most common cause of these infections. Ultrasound, performed either in the ED or by radiology, is a rapid and convenient method of discriminating mastitis from an abscess. Patients with postpartum mastitis or a breast abscess can continue to breast feed provided the antimicrobial chosen is safe for the infant, although patients with a breast abscess should not feed with the affected breast. Although peripheral abscesses usually respond to incision and drainage, periareolar and retromammary abscesses, which tend to be complex and therefore more difficult to drain, may require general anesthesia and should be referred to a surgeon. *(Emergency Medicine, Chapter 133, pp 1372–1375)*

3.c. Risk factors for breast cancer include a family history of breast cancer, obesity, nulliparity, late age at first birth, and, most importantly, advancing age. However, 80% of women with breast cancer have *none* of these risk factors. One woman in nine will develop breast cancer. Most breast masses are not malignant, fibroadenomas being the most common benign tumor of the breast. This patient is multiparous. *(Emergency Medicine, Chapter 133, pp 1372–1375)*

4.b. Mondor's disease is a rare superficial phlebitis of the chest wall that presents as a fibrous cord along the lateral breast, involving the lateral thoracic or thoracoepigastric vein. The exact cause of Mondor's disease is unknown, but it is benign and disappears with time. If there is a mass present, one must consider the diagnosis of carcinoma. *(Emergency Medicine, Chapter 133, pp 1372–1375)*

5.c. Simple postpartum breast engorgement characteristically occurs 48 to 72 hours postpartum and may be accompanied by a brief temperature elevation, rarely exceeding 39°C. The breast will be swollen, firm, and tender, but not erythematous. Postpartum patients with breast engorgement (milk stasis) may be treated with continued breast emptying, warm compresses, and analgesics. Mastitis would present with erythema, fever, and a wedge-shaped area of localized induration. The presence of palpable fluctuance would indicate an abscess. Fibroadenomas are painless, well circumscribed, mobile, and hormonally responsive, increasing in size at the end of each menstrual cycle. *(Emergency Medicine, Chapter 133, pp 1372–1375)*

6.d. When signs of infection are present, as with mastitis, one must provide coverage against staphylococci with a semisynthetic penicillin such as dicloxacillin or a first-generation cephalosporin such as cephalexin. These drugs are safe during lactation because they are not excreted in milk. Erythromycin may be used in the penicillin-allergic patient. Breast feeding need not be interrupted unless there is a concurrent abscess, but frequent feedings followed by pumping if necessary should be advised. Lactation suppression should be instituted in women who prefer to bottle feed. The distinction between mastitis and abscess may be difficult and can be aided by ultrasound. Of note, mastitis in a nonlactating or postmenopausal patient should be presumed to be cancer until proved otherwise. *(Emergency Medicine, Chapter 133, pp 1372–1375)*

BIBLIOGRAPHY

Haywood Y: Breast disorders. *In* Howell JM, Altieri M, Jagoda AS, et al (eds): Emergency Medicine. Philadelphia, WB Saunders, 1998, pp 1372–1375.

SECTION SEVENTEEN

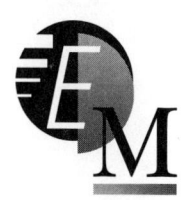

Toxicologic Emergencies

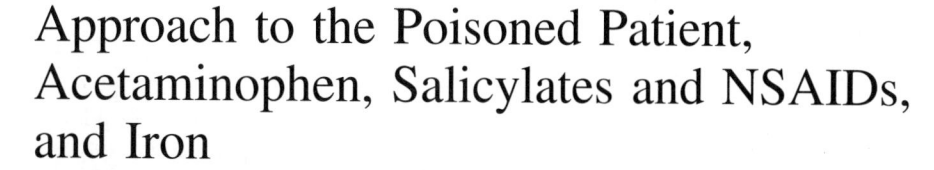

58 Approach to the Poisoned Patient, Acetaminophen, Salicylates and NSAIDs, and Iron

RICHARD J. HAMILTON, MD   OLIVER HUNG, MD   MARY PALMER, MD
RAMA B. RAO, MD

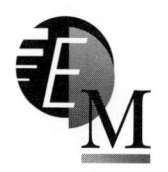

1. A serum level is most important in:
   a. Identification of opioid ingestion in the comatose patient
   b. Identification of salicylate overdose
   c. Identification of acetaminophen overdose
   d. Identification of ethylene glycol overdose
   e. Identification of tricyclic antidepressant overdose

2. All of the following are true about syrup of ipecac except:
   a. Cardiotoxicity may be produced with chronic abuse.
   b. The dose is 30 mL in adults and 15 mL in children.
   c. It is from a plant and contains the alkaloids cephaeline and emetine that act on the stomach and CNS to induce emesis.
   d. If used within an hour, approximately 80% of the ingested toxin can be removed.
   e. Persistent ipecac-induced emesis may limit the usefulness of activated charcoal.

3. All of the following patients can be considered for discharge if asymptomatic after 6 hours except:
   a. Ativan overdose patients
   b. Tricyclic antidepressant overdose patients
   c. Diabinese overdose patients
   d. Benadryl overdose patients
   e. Isopropyl alcohol overdose patients

4. Which of the following is true in the management of salicylate toxicity?
   a. Acetazolamide is a useful alkalinization therapy alternative to sodium bicarbonate.
   b. Alkalinization restores oxidative phosphorylation by changing binding to cytochromes.
   c. Alkalization causes "ion trapping" of salicylates in the urine and promotes movement of ions out of the CNS.
   d. Hyperkalemia is a common problem that complicates the management of toxicity.
   e. The Done nomogram should be used to guide management if salicylate levels are drawn at 6 hours after ingestion.

5. Indications for dialysis include all of the following except:
   a. Salicylate level at 95 mg/dL in an acute overdose
   b. Salicylate level of 70 mg/dL in a chronic overdose
   c. Tinnitus and tachycardia in acute or chronic overdose
   d. Seizures and hyperthermia in acute or chronic overdose
   e. Pulmonary edema

6. The following is true regarding salicylate poisoning:
   a. Children develop hyperglycemia and adults develop hypoglycemia.
   b. Children do not develop hyperpyrexia like adults.
   c. Children do not develop hypokalemia like adults.
   d. Children develop acidosis more rapidly than adults.
   e. Children develop hemodialysis at lower drug serum levels.

7. Salicylate toxicity manifests in all of the following ways except:
   a. Uncoupled oxidative phosphorylation
   b. Increased lipolysis and production of ketones
   c. Increased respiration
   d. Anion gap acidosis secondary to production of organic acids
   e. Hyperthermia as a consequence of direct CNS stimulation

8. Which of the following two NSAID agents are most commonly associated with serious toxicity:
   a. Ibuprofen and piroxicam
   b. Naproxen and indomethacin
   c. Piroxicam and ketoprofen
   d. Phenylbutazone and mefenamic acid
   e. Ketorolac and sulindac

9. A loading dose of N-acetylcysteine (NAC) after an acetaminophen overdose:
   a. Should be administered before obtaining a postingestion 4-hour level
   b. Can be delayed if the results from a 4-hour level will be available within 8 hours after ingestion

c. Should be administered for any postingestion level that is greater than 150 ug/mL
d. Is ineffective when administered after 8 hours
e. Must always be followed by a complete 72-hour course of NAC

10. Acetaminophen:
    a. Undergoes sulfation and glucoronidation only at toxic levels
    b. Undergoes hydroxylation to a toxic metabolite
    c. Hepatotoxicity is enhanced by inhibition of cytochrome P450
    d. Hepatotoxicity is enhanced by elevated glutathione levels
    e. Is a hepatotoxin in its unmetabolized form

11. Signs and symptoms of acetaminophen toxicity include all of the following except:
    a. Elevated ALT and AST
    b. Encephalopathy
    c. Renal failure
    d. Coagulopathy
    e. Rhabdomyolysis

12. Hepatotoxic acetaminophen overdoses should be considered for transplant:
    a. Only after the arterial pH has fallen below 7.1
    b. If the patient has a grade I hepatic encephalopathy
    c. If the patient has a serum creatinine of 1.8
    d. PT greater than 1.3 times control
    e. If the patient has a factor VIII to V ratio greater than 30

13. Charcoal interacts with NAC in the following way:
    a. Reduces NAC levels, thus requiring higher doses of the antidote
    b. Produces deleterious side effects
    c. Enhances NAC's absorption
    d. Reduces NAC's availability without adversely affecting its effectiveness
    e. Increases the amount of acetaminophen absorbed without affecting NAC levels

14. What statement concerning iron poisoning is true?
    a. Activated charcoal is an effective means of gastrointestinal decontamination.
    b. Ingestion of 30 mg/kg of elemental iron is associated with severe toxicity.
    c. Early gastrointestinal symptoms and signs such as severe nausea and vomiting are indicative of serious iron poisoning and indicate the need for the use of deferoxamine.
    d. A positive deferoxamine challenge test indicates serious iron toxicity in the setting of acute overdose.
    e. Liquid and chewable iron preparations are usually detectable by plain abdominal radiographs.

15. What laboratory test best correlates with acute iron toxicity?
    a. WBC and serum glucose
    b. Total iron-binding capacity
    c. Serum iron
    d. Serum iron/total iron-binding capacity ratio
    e. PT/PTT

16. A 20-year-old pregnant female presents to the ED after ingestion of 100 tablets of 325-mg $FeSO_4$ 2 hours ago. She reports six episodes of nausea and vomiting. Plain radiographs of the abdomen reveal numerous radiopaque tablets. What would be the most appropriate method of gastrointestinal decontamination for this patient?
    a. Syrup of ipecac
    b. Activated charcoal
    c. Gastric lavage
    d. Whole-bowel irrigation
    e. Bicarbonate or phosphate buffer

Answers

1.c. Patients with acetaminophen overdose often present with minimal or no symptoms. Acetaminophen is a common co-ingestant in suicide attempts that is easily overlooked without serum levels. There is a reliable nomogram that requires a single level drawn 4 to 24 hours after ingestion, and NAC is a safe and effective antidote. On the other hand, identifying most toxic ingestions requires clinical diagnosis initially. Their management should not await results of serum levels. For instance, opioid ingestions present classically with pinpoint pupils, mild depression of vital signs, and a depressed sensorium. In pure ingestions, signs and symptoms reverse with naloxone. Salicylism is also a clinical diagnosis based on early findings of tinnitus, vomiting, hyperventilation, or tachycardia. Diagnosis is best aided by finding respiratory alkalosis and metabolic acidosis on an ABG. Salicylate levels are important for confirmation of the diagnosis and patient management. Although laboratory diagnosis of ethylene glycol is extremely useful, most laboratories do not return results for days. When other diagnoses have been excluded in the setting of profound or worsening metabolic acidosis with an anion gap, therapy will need to be initiated without benefit of laboratory confirmation. Life-threatening tricyclic antidepressant ingestions are best screened by serial ECGs to determine if the QRS interval is widened. *(Emergency Medicine, Chapter 134, pp 1379–1386)*

2.d. Spontaneous vomiting, ipecac-induced vomiting, and gastric lavage all remove approximately 30% of toxic contents. Ipecac may be considered in patients presenting within 1 hour after ingestion. It may be useful in potentially life-threatening ingestions that do not adhere to activated charcoal and may be too large to fit through an orogastric tube. Contraindications to the use of ipecac include caustic ingestions, age younger than 6 months, battery or foreign body ingestions, ingestions in which immediate gastrointestinal decontamination is required, and altered mental status or potential altered mental status. *(Emergency Medicine, Chapter 134, pp 1379–1386)*

3.c. Most ingestions manifest symptoms within 4 to 6 hours, but there are exceptions. Common ingestions that can manifest signs and symptoms after 6 hours are oral hypoglycemics, methanol, calcium channel blockers, Lomotil (in children), and sustained-released medications. *(Emergency Medicine, Chapter 134, pp 1379–1386)*

4.c. Use of bicarbonate helps enhance salicylate elimination if urine pH is kept between 7.5 and 8.0. This also promotes movement of ionized salicylates out of the CNS because of the trapping of salicylates in the urine. Acetazolamide should not be used to alkalinize the urine because it produces an acidemia that can worsen CNS toxicity. Hypokalemia often occurs with salicylate toxicity. Because hydrogen ions are secreted in the renal tubule cells in exchange for potassium, hypokalemia often can render alkalinization ineffective. It is therefore important to correct hypokalemia. Alkalinization does not reverse the inhibition of oxidative phosphorylation. The Done nomogram was based on acute pediatric ingestions and underestimates the severity of illness. It is no longer used in the management of salicylate toxicity. *(Emergency Medicine, Chapter 156, pp 1525–1531)*

5.c. Tinnitus can occur in the upper range of therapeutic dosing and occurs in mild overdoses as well as serious ones requiring dialysis. It is not an appropriate criterion for dialysis. Indications for hemodialysis also include neurologic dysfunction, pulmonary edema, clinical deterioration despite decontamination and urine alkalinization, inability to alkalinize the urine, and renal failure. *(Emergency Medicine, Chapter 156, pp 1525–1531)*

6.d. Children may not develop the respiratory alkalosis found in adults because they are less able to proportionately increase their minute ventilation. This leads to an earlier acidosis. They also develop hypoglycemia to a greater extent than adults, presumably because they have smaller stores of hepatic glycogen. *(Emergency Medicine, Chapter 156, pp 1525–1531)*

7.e. Salicylates uncouple oxidative phosphorylation (which stimulates anaerobic metabolism), produce organic acids, and promote lipolysis with production of ketones. Uncoupling of oxidative phosphorylation also results in the production of heat, resulting in fever. Respiration, not temperature, increases as a direct CNS effect of salicylates. *(Emergency Medicine, Chapter 156, pp 1525–1531)*

8.d. NSAID ingestions rarely produce serious signs and symptoms unless NSAIDs are taken in massive overdose. It is worth remembering two exceptions that can produce toxicity in modest overdose: phenylbutazone and mefenamic acid. Phenylbutazone can produce metabolic acidosis, seizure, coma, and hypotension and is associated with gastrointestinal bleeding and blood dyscrasia such as aplastic anemia. Mefenamic acid is associated with muscle twitching and a high rate of seizures (approximately 40% of patients). Overdose with these agents deserves more aggressive gastrointestinal decontamination on presentation than with the other NSAIDs. *(Emergency Medicine, Chapter 156, pp 1525–1531)*

9.b. The goal is to determine toxicity based on the Rumack-Matthews nomogram and initiate NAC therapy within 8 hours after ingestion. Ideally, levels should be obtained after 4 hours (earlier may catch redistribution peaks) and therapy initiated after the level is obtained. If the level is nontoxic, therapy can be discontinued. If the nomogram cannot be used because more than 24 hours have passed, any evidence of transaminitis should prompt initiation of NAC. *(Emergency Medicine, Chapter 135, pp 1387–1393)*

10.b. When sulfation and glucoronidation are overwhelmed by unmetabolized acetaminophen, hydroxylation occurs by cytochrome P450 enzymes to produce N-acetyl-p-benzoquinoneimine (NAPQ1). Pretreatment with inhibitors of P450 such as cimetidine appear to prevent toxicity in animal experiments. *(Emergency Medicine, Chapter 135, pp 1387–1393)*

11.e. N-acetyl-p-benzoquinoneimine is produced by hydroxylation of acetaminophen in all organs with P450 activity. These include liver, kidney, brain, and placenta. Signs and symptoms of acetaminophen toxicity reflect injury to these organs. *(Emergency Medicine, Chapter 135, pp 1387–1393)*

12.e. Because factor VIII is produced by the endothelium and factor V is produced exclusively by the liver, this ratio is particularly sensitive for predicting poor outcome and the need for transplant consideration. Grade 3 or 4 encephalopathy, creatinine greater than 3.3, PT greater than 1.8 times control, and pH less than 7.3 are also useful predictors. Perhaps the most significant determinant is a pH less than 7.3 despite adequate rehydration. *(Emergency Medicine, Chapter 156, pp 1525–1531)*

13.d. NAC doses are as effective for an acetaminophen level of 150 µg/mL as a level of 600 µg/mL. Although NAC is adsorbed to charcoal, the quantities given are still sufficient to treat all toxic levels. *(Emergency Medicine, Chapter 135, pp 1387–1393)*

14.c. Activated charcoal is not recommended in isolated iron poisoning because it does not bind well to iron. Ingestion of less than 20 mg/kg of elemental iron results in minimal toxicity. Ingestion of 20 to 40 mg/kg usually produces mild toxicity. Ingestion of greater than 40 mg/kg has the potential for serious toxicity. Lethal doses are usually greater than 60 mg/kg. A positive deferoxamine challenge test may indicate free iron in the blood, but it does not necessarily indicate serious iron toxicity. Liquid or chewable iron may not be apparent on abdominal radiographs. Early gastrointestinal symptoms such as severe nausea and vomiting are indicative of serious iron toxicity. *(Emergency Medicine, Chapter 147, pp 1460–1464)*

15.c. Serum glucose and WBC are not sensitive and should not guide decisions in managing iron poisoning. The total iron-binding capacity is falsely elevated in iron toxicity because of the effects of excess free iron on the laboratory test. For this reason, the serum iron/total iron-binding capacity ratio is no longer used. Coagulopathy has been reported from the early effect of iron on iron proteases and as a late manifestation of direct hepatotoxicity. Early PT elevations may also result from iron interference with the assay. Peak serum iron levels correlate with clinical toxicity, and levels above 500 μg/dL should be treated with deferoxamine. *(Emergency Medicine, Chapter 147, pp 1460–1464)*

16.d. If radiopaque tablets persist after initial emesis or lavage, whole-bowel irrigation is recommended. Ipecac is not recommended in patients who have already vomited. There is no evidence to support decontamination with bicarbonate or phosphate buffer solutions. Because serious iron toxicity invariably results in vomiting, additional gastric emptying with lavage is unlikely to remove these tablets and would be contraindicated in pregnancy. *(Emergency Medicine, Chapter 147, pp 1460–1464)*

BIBLIOGRAPHY

Akhtar J, Burkhart K: Iron. *In* Howell JM, Altieri M, Jagoda AS, et al (eds): Emergency Medicine. Philadelphia, WB Saunders, 1998, pp 1460–1464.

Kerns W II: Salicylate and nonsteroidal anti-inflammatory drug poisoning. *In* Howell JM, Altieri M, Jagoda AS, et al (eds): Emergency Medicine. Philadelphia, WB Saunders, 1998, pp 1525–1531.

Rose SR: Acetaminophen. *In* Howell JM, Altieri M, Jagoda AS, et al (eds): Emergency Medicine. Philadelphia, WB Saunders, 1998, pp 1387–1393.

Stork C, Hoffman RS: Approach to the poisoned patient. *In* Howell JM, Altieri M, Jagoda AS, et al (eds): Emergency Medicine. Philadelphia, WB Saunders, 1998, pp 1379–1386.

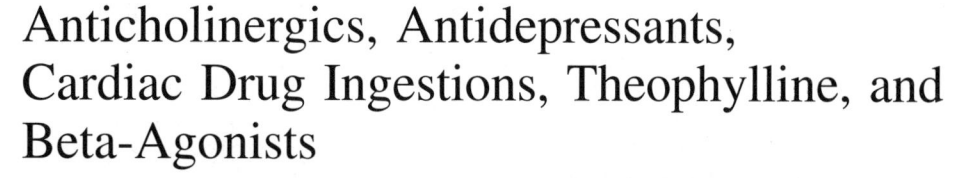

59 Anticholinergics, Antidepressants, Cardiac Drug Ingestions, Theophylline, and Beta-Agonists

RICHARD J. HAMILTON, MD   OLIVER HUNG, MD   MARY PALMER, MD
RAMA B. RAO, MD

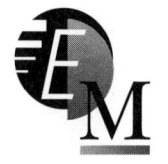

1. Physostigmine:
   a. Is ineffective in the central anticholinergic syndrome
   b. Is contraindicated in *Datura stramonium* poisoning
   c. Is effective in reversing tricyclic antidepressant cardiotoxicity
   d. Is obtained from the Calabar bean
   e. Is a competitive antagonist of the acetylcholine receptor

2. The anticholinergic toxidrome includes all of the following except:
   a. Diminished bowel sounds and flushed skin
   b. Bizarre behavior and tachycardia
   c. Dilated pupils and decreased peristalsis
   d. Bladder distention and seizures
   e. Elevated temperature and diaphoresis

3. Decreased gastrointestinal motility after anticholinergic poisoning:
   a. Excludes the possibility of acetaminophen toxicity
   b. Is inconsistent with the anticholinergic toxidrome
   c. May render gastric lavage an effective procedure for hours
   d. Is a contraindication to cathartic administration
   e. Is of no concern when administering sequential doses of charcoal

4. Which of the following antidepressants and their associated toxicologic effects is incorrect?
   a. Lithium—tremors, hyperreflexia, clonus
   b. Cyclic antidepressants—lethargy, tachycardia, seizures, arrhythmias
   c. Monoamine oxidase inhibitor overdose—rapid onset of hypotension, tachycardia, and neurologic dysfunction, followed by hypertension and bradycardia
   d. Monoamine oxidase inhibitor–tyramine interaction—early onset of headache, vomiting, hypertension, and tachycardia
   e. Serotonin-reuptake inhibitors—somnolence, lethargy

5. What is the most appropriate treatment of cyclic antidepressant–induced seizures?
   a. Phenytoin
   b. Diazepam
   c. Physostigmine
   d. Glucose
   e. Carbamazepine

6. What is the most appropriate treatment of cyclic antidepressant–induced cardiac dysrhythmias?
   a. Sodium bicarbonate
   b. Lidocaine
   c. Phenytoin
   d. Quinidine
   e. Propranolol

7. Which of the following statements concerning cyclic antidepressant toxicity is true?
   a. Serum cyclic antidepressant levels are useful in predicting toxicity.
   b. Prolongation of the QRS interval greater than 100 msec and 160 msec is associated with the increased risk of seizures and tachydysrhythmias, respectively.
   c. Manifestations of cyclic antidepressant toxicity include a leftward terminal vector of the QRS complex (S wave in lead aV_R).
   d. Cyclic antidepressants possess cholinergic properties.
   e. Coma is an unusual finding in cyclic antidepressant overdose.

8. A 68-year-old female with CHF and hypertension is brought into the ED by ambulance after having syncope at home. Her husband died last week. She is unclear about her medicines. Her vital signs are heart rate 39, BP 80/40, and RR 15, and she is afebrile. Her ECG shows a third-degree AV block. Her initial management should include:
   a. Calcium gluconate
   b. Calcium chloride
   c. Lidocaine
   d. Digoxin-specific antibody fragments
   e. Sodium bicarbonate
   f. Withholding treatment until her stat labs return and have internal pacemaker at the bedside

9. A 3-year-old female presents with drowsiness and pinpoint pupils. She has spent the day with her grandmother, who has hypertension. Her blood pressure was high in triage 40 minutes ago. She does not respond to 2 mg of naloxone. All of the following are appropriate except:
   a. Increase the amount of naloxone.
   b. Observe for 8 hours and discharge if she improves.
   c. Give the child activated charcoal.
   d. Admit the child for 24 hours of observation.
   e. Give fluids and vasopressors if hypotension develops.

10. All of the following ECG changes can occur in digoxin poisoning except:
    a. Premature ventricular contractions
    b. Atrial tachycardia with block
    c. Atrial fibrillation with rapid ventricular response
    d. Bradycardia
    e. Ventricular tachycardia

11. A 2-year-old male ingested one pill of his father's atenolol 2 hours prior to arrival. His mental status, vital signs, and laboratory values are normal. His father presents a bottle of regular-release formulation that is missing only one tablet. The most appropriate management approach includes which of the following?
    a. Administer ipecac.
    b. Give activated charcoal; toxicity is unlikely if the patient remains stable for at least 6 hours.
    c. Give whole-bowel irrigation and admit for 24 hours of observation.
    d. Start a glucagon drip now.
    e. Give whole-bowel irrigation and discharge if the patient remains stable after 24 hours.

12. A 35-year-old male presents with vomiting. He takes no medicines except that he has ingested a hard rock-like substance to enhance his sexual performance. His alternative medicine source told him it is derived from toad venom and that it had been a successful aphrodisiac for all of his male customers. On arrival, he begins to manifest a wide-complex bradycardia. The most appropriate management includes which of the following?
    a. Give fluids and an antiemetic, and observe.
    b. Give calcium, and if this fails, glucagon.
    c. Give naloxone and start a drip if this is effective.
    d. Send a toxicologic screen and observe.
    e. Give digoxin-specific antibody fragment.

13. Chronic theophylline toxicity occurs:
    a. At lower serum levels than with acute toxicity
    b. At higher serum levels than with acute toxicity
    c. At the same serum levels as with acute toxicity
    d. Without any relationship to the serum level
    e. Before serum levels begin to rise

14. Which of the following is not an effect of theophylline?
    a. Adenosine antagonism
    b. Increased levels of plasma catecholamines
    c. Hypoglycemia
    d. Increased intracellular levels of cyclic AMP
    e. Phosphodiesterase inhibition

15. Beta-agonist toxicity differs from theophylline toxicity in that it rarely produces:
    a. Tremor
    b. Seizures
    c. Hypokalemia
    d. Hyperglycemia
    e. Tachycardia

16. Which of the following scenarios least requires extracorporeal removal of theophylline?
    a. Age 30, acute overdose, level 80
    b. Age 60, chronic overdose, level 75
    c. Age 3, chronic overdose, level 70
    d. Age 40, chronic overdose, level 100
    e. Age 60, acute overdose, level 90

17. All of the following are useful therapeutic measures in theophylline toxicity except:
    a. Hemodialysis and verapamil
    b. Hemoperfusion and IV fluid replacement
    c. Adenosine and ethylene glycol solution
    d. Polyethylene glycol solution and propranolol
    e. Multiple dose–activated charcoal and benzodiazepines

Answers

1.d. Physostigmine, originally derived from the Calabar bean, is indicated for peripheral and central signs of anticholinergic toxicity from medications and plants (such as *Datura stramonium* [jimsonweed]) with the exception of tricyclic antidepressants. Clinical experience shows that while physostigmine will reverse the anticholinergic effects of tricyclic antidepressants, it will exacerbate the cardiac toxicity. It works by inhibiting acetylcholinesterase. *(Emergency Medicine, Chapter 136, pp 1394–1398)*

2.e. The anticholinergic effects of drugs like atropine, scopolamine, and certain antihistamines can be remembered by the mnemonic "Hot as Hades, dry as a bone, mad as a hatter, red as a beet, fast as a rabbit" or "Atropine man: can't see, can't spit, can't pee, can't [defecate]." Whatever works! *(Emergency Medicine, Chapter 136, pp 1394–1398)*

3.c. Decreased gastrointestinal motility may render gastric emptying a viable option later than in other ingestions. Cathartic administration is important to promote motility. To prevent charcoal bezoars, repeated doses of charcoal should be used only when some bowel sounds are present. Many over-the-counter cold medications are combined with analgesics such as acetaminophen. *(Emergency Medicine, Chapter 136, pp 1394–1398)*

4.c. Monoamine oxidase inhibitor overdose is associated with delayed onset of symptoms. When toxicity occurs, patients first manifest hypertension and tachycardia along with a range of neurologic signs and symptoms. In later stages, bradycardia and hypotension can occur as the result of catecholamine depletion. *(Emergency Medicine, Chapter 140, pp 1418–1424)*

5.b. Seizures from cyclic antidepressants are best treated with benzodiazepines. *(Emergency Medicine, Chapter 140, pp 1418–1424)*

6.a. Sodium bicarbonate infusions should be used to treat cyclic antidepressant–induced cardiac dysrhythmias. Alkalinization to a serum pH of 7.45 to 7.55 is the goal. The use of type 1A antidysrhythmics such as quinidine should be discouraged because these agents may exacerbate cardiotoxicity. *(Emergency Medicine, Chapter 140, pp 1418–1424)*

7.b. Quantitative serum levels are not helpful because there is a poor correlation between serum levels and toxicity. The limb lead QRS duration has proven value in predicting seizures and dysrhythmias from cyclic antidepressants. In one study, no patients demonstrated significant toxicity with a maximal limb QRS less than 100 msec. Seizures occurred in one third of patients with QRS duration 100 msec or more, and dysrhythmias occurred in half of patients with a QRS duration 160 msec or more. Patients with cyclic antidepressant poisoning have a rightward terminal 40 msec frontal plane QRS vector seen as a deep S in I and an R in aV_R. Cyclic antidepressants possess anticholinergic properties. Coma is a typical finding in cyclic antidepressant overdose. *(Emergency Medicine, Chapter 140, pp 1418–1424)*

8.d. In this patient, it is important to expect the worse—an overdose of a calcium channel blocker, beta-blocker, digoxin, or any combination. Although calcium is a good choice for a calcium channel blocker overdose, increased intracellular calcium can exacerbate digoxin toxicity. In a patient in shock or with a serious dysrhythmia and who may be on digoxin, treat with digoxin-specific antibody fragments as soon as possible. If the patient's course does not improve after 30 minutes, treat with calcium and/or glucagon. Complications arising from reversal of digoxin therapy are rare and can be managed with other drugs. Digoxin levels and other laboratory results may take too long to withhold treatment until they arrive. Internal pacemakers can cause ventricular arrhythmias in the setting of digoxin toxicity. *(Emergency Medicine, Chapter 142, pp 1431–1437)*

9.b. Clonidine ingestion, even of only one pill, can be fatal in a child and mandates 24 hours of observation for a potentially unpredictable course. The patient may present briefly with hypertension as clonidine first stimulates the peripheral alpha$_2$-receptors. This is invariably followed by hypotension and bradycardia when central alpha$_2$-receptors are stimulated. Only 50% of these patients respond to naloxone, but it is reasonable to give up to 10 to 20 mg and to start a drip if it is successful. Activated charcoal is a good choice for gastrointestinal decontamination, and ipecac should be avoided in the drowsy patient. Treating hypotension with fluids and vasopressors may be necessary in some overdoses. *(Emergency Medicine, Chapter 142, pp 1431–1437)*

10.c. Cardiac toxicity from digoxin overdose results from two mechanisms: increase in vagal tone and increased automaticity. Therefore, bradydysrhythmias or tachydysrhythmias often accompany digoxin poisoning, but there will be no supraventricular tachycardia without a concurrent block. *(Emergency Medicine, Chapter 142, pp 1431–1437)*

11.b. Once it is confidently established that the formulation is regular release, toxicity is unlikely if the patient remains asymptomatic for 6 hours. Prolonged toxicity is expected after ingestion of sustained-released beta-blockers and calcium channel blockers in a child. Although a good choice for beta-blocker toxicity, glucagon treatment is unnecessary unless the patient becomes hypotensive or bradycardic. Whole-bowel irrigation is a good choice to diminish gastrointestinal absorption in the setting of *sustained-release* ingestions. Ipecac is unlikely to provide benefit 2 hours after ingestion. *(Emergency Medicine, Chapter 142, pp 1431–1437)*

12.e. Cardiac glycosides exist in many plants and in toad venom. This alternative medicine ingestion may not be recognized as equivalent to an acute digoxin overdose. Without immediate digoxin-specific antibody fragment, the stable patient can rapidly deteriorate to dysrhythmia and asystole. Nausea, vomiting, and hyperkalemia are some clues to the nature of the toxin. Hyperkalemia results from acute poisoning of Na-K ATPase. *(Emergency Medicine, Chapter 142, pp 1431–1437)*

13.a. In chronic theophylline toxicity, serum levels may be relatively low, but tissues are saturated with drug. In acute toxicity, much of the drug is in the serum when levels are obtained and insufficient time has passed to allow tissue saturation. Because toxicity is determined by the amount of drug in target tissues (brain, heart, muscle, etc.), the chronic patient appears disproportionately ill for the serum level. The total body burden of drug is higher in chronic toxicity. *(Emergency Medicine, Chapter 157, pp 1532–1538)*

14.c. Methylxanthines are secretogogues and cause catecholamine release from the adrenals. The subsequent stimulation of beta-receptors increases cyclic AMP and causes hypokalemia and hyperglycemia. *(Emergency Medicine, Chapter 157, pp 1532–1538)*

15.b. The beta-agonists and theophylline share many similarities in toxicity. In beta-agonist overdoses, the predominant symptoms are tachycardia and tremor; nausea and vomiting are not as predominant as in theophylline overdoses. However, the beta-agonists rarely produce seizures or fatal dysrhythmias and have very low mortality. There have been reports of myocardial infarction and rhabdomyolysis with renal failure in beta-agonist overdoses. *(Emergency Medicine, Chapter 157, pp 1532–1538)*

16.a. In general, extremes of age and chronic overdoses lower the threshold for extracorporeal removal. Charcoal hemoperfusion is the optimal means of extracorporeal removal of theophylline because of theophylline's affinity for charcoal. Peritoneal dialysis and plasmapheresis are not effective. *(Emergency Medicine, Chapter 157, pp 1532–1538)*

17.c. Adenosine has a half-life that is too short, and it competes poorly with the antagonistic effects of theophylline. Ethylene glycol is a toxic alcohol. Polyethylene glycol solution is used for whole-bowel irrigation. *(Emergency Medicine, Chapter 157, pp 1532–1538)*

BIBLIOGRAPHY

Frenia M: Cardiac drug ingestions. *In* Howell JM, Altieri M, Jagoda AS, et al (eds): Emergency Medicine. Philadelphia, WB Saunders, 1998, pp 1431–1437.

Hamilton RJ, Hoffman RS: Theophylline and beta-agonists. *In* Howell JM, Altieri M, Jagoda AS, et al (eds): Emergency Medicine. Philadelphia, WB Saunders, 1998, pp 1532–1538.

McFarland AK III: Anticholinergics. *In* Howell JM, Altieri M, Jagoda AS, et al (eds): Emergency Medicine. Philadelphia, WB Saunders, 1998, pp 1394–1398.

Perrone J, Hoffman RS: Antidepressants. *In* Howell JM, Altieri M, Jagoda AS, et al (eds): Emergency Medicine. Philadelphia, WB Saunders, 1998, pp 1418–1424.

60 Ethanol, Toxic Alcohols, Benzodiazepines, and Anticonvulsants

RICHARD J. HAMILTON, MD   OLIVER HUNG, MD   MARY PALMER, MD
RAMA B. RAO, MD

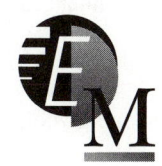

1. The metabolism of ethanol:
   a. Requires glucose
   b. Is not affected by thiamine deficiency
   c. Always produces ketoacidosis
   d. Occurs at 50 mg/dL per hour
   e. Is not affected by supplemental dextrose and fluids

2. Phenytoin is used:
   a. To prevent alcohol withdrawal seizures
   b. To treat an underlying seizure disorder
   c. As an adjunct to diazepam in delirium tremens–induced seizures
   d. To hasten metabolism of ethanol
   e. To prevent recurrent alcohol withdrawal seizures

3. Which of the following statements is incorrect?
   a. Blindness is a major complication of methanol toxicity.
   b. Renal failure is a major complication of ethylene glycol toxicity.
   c. Isopropanol is associated with an anion gap acidosis and serum ketones.
   d. Ethanol is the preferred initial treatment of methanol and ethylene glycol toxicity.
   e. Ingestions of less than 1 teaspoon of 100% methanol may be associated with serious toxicity.

4. A 22-year-old male presents after ingesting an unknown quantity of methanol. He is awake and alert and is without complaint. Laboratory studies reveal normal electrolytes (no anion gap is present) and an osmol gap of −2. A methanol level has been sent and will not be available for several hours. Which of the following statements is correct?
   a. A normal anion gap rules out significant methanol toxicity.
   b. A normal osmolal gap rules out significant methanol toxicity.
   c. If the patient remains asymptomatic for 4 to 6 hours, he can safely be medically cleared.
   d. Early gastrointestinal decontamination is effective in preventing methanol absorption.
   e. The patient should be observed. The subsequent development of metabolic acidosis or anion gap may indicate detectable methanol toxicity and the need for ethanol infusion.

5. Ethylene glycol poisoning is associated with all of the following except:
   a. Urinary calcium oxalate crystals
   b. Hypocalcemia
   c. Urine ketones
   d. Fluorescent urine or gastric contents caused by fluorescein dye additive
   e. Anion and osmol gaps

6. A 40-year-old male presents after ingestion of a bottle of ethylene glycol. Laboratory values are Na 140 mEq/L, BUN 28 mg/dL, glucose 90 mg/dL, ethanol 46 mg/dL, and serum osmolarity 330. What is the osmol gap?
   a. −10
   b. 0
   c. 15
   d. 20
   e. 25

7. All of the following statements concerning the treatment of toxic alcohol poisoning are true except:
   a. Fomepizole prevents methanol and ethylene glycol toxicity by competing for alcohol dehydrogenase and blocking methanol and ethylene glycol metabolism.
   b. A serum ethanol level of 100 mg/dL should be maintained during ethanol infusion.
   c. Hemodialysis should be considered for methanol or ethylene glycol levels greater than 25 mg/dL.
   d. Other treatment modalities include folate for methanol poisoning and thiamine and pyridoxine for ethylene glycol poisoning.
   e. Fomepizole therapy is the treatment of choice in cases of severe isopropanol toxicity.

8. Oral overdoses of benzodiazepines are associated with all of the following except:
   a. Sleepiness
   b. Apnea
   c. Ataxia
   d. Slurred speech
   e. Aspiration pneumonia

9. Which of the following statements is false concerning flumazenil?
   a. Flumazenil should be used to rapidly reverse apnea or respiratory depression in unknown overdoses.
   b. The administration of flumazenil is associated with seizures.
   c. Flumazenil is associated with adverse effects in patients with cyclic antidepressant toxicity and patients who are chemically dependent on benzodiazepines.
   d. Flumazenil should be used judiciously in the treatment of the benzodiazepine-poisoned patient.
   e. Flumazenil reverses respiratory depression from benzodiazepines.

10. Which of the following statements is most appropriate concerning the treatment of benzodiazepine poisoning?
    a. Benzodiazepine serum concentrations are clinically useful in guiding effective therapy.
    b. Mixed benzodiazepine/ethanol overdoses often require hemodialysis.
    c. Ipecac should be administered in cases of benzodiazepine overdose.
    d. A negative urine toxicology screen for benzodiazepines excludes the possibility of benzodiazepine ingestion.
    e. The presence of profound respiratory depression in an acute oral benzodiazepine overdose suggests the presence of co-intoxicants.

11. All of the following statements are true concerning benzodiazepine withdrawal except:
    a. The onset of a withdrawal reaction is variable and dependent on the elimination half-life of the parent compound and its active metabolite.
    b. Anxiety and agitation are the major manifestations of withdrawal.
    c. Severe withdrawal manifestations are more likely to occur with patients on high doses for a prolonged period of time.
    d. Benzodiazepine withdrawal seizures should be treated with phenytoin.
    e. Mild manifestations of withdrawal can be treated with oral benzodiazepine replacement.

12. Seizures are a common form of neurologic toxicity in patients with serious ingestions of:
    a. Primidone
    b. Phenobarbital
    c. Valproic acid
    d. Carbamazepine
    e. All of the above

13. Which of the following statements regarding anticonvulsant toxicity is true?
    a. Wide-complex tachycardia in carbamazepine overdose should be treated with sodium bicarbonate.
    b. Carbamazepine has traditionally been used to treat dysrhythmias from digoxin toxicity.
    c. Ataxia and tinnitus are common features of all anticonvulsants.
    d. Patients with toxic phenytoin ingestion should be on a cardiac monitor, because the drug is a type Ib antiarrhythmic.
    e. Elevated ammonia levels are pathognomonic for acute valproic acid overdose.

14. A patient with a seizure history admits to taking a full bottle of his pills. After improving over a 24-hour period he becomes somnolent again. The best explanation for his clinical status is the following:
    a. Multiple-dose activated charcoal results in enhanced absorption of anticonvulsants.
    b. Phenobarbital metabolites cause a delayed CNS depression.
    c. Phenytoin capsules are mixed with propylene glycol, which causes waxing and waning mental status.
    d. Carbamazepine has been associated with cyclic coma.
    e. Valproic acid elevates ammonia levels, causing intermittent hepatic encephalopathy.

15. Alkalinization of the urine can enhance elimination of which of the following anticonvulsants?
    a. Carbamazepine
    b. Valproic acid
    c. Phenobarbital
    d. Phenytoin
    e. All of the above

16. Loading phenytoin is best achieved by the following:
    a. Given PO to avoid hypotension
    b. Given PO to prevent cardiac toxicity
    c. Given half PO and half IV to prevent ataxia
    d. Given IV at a rate not to exceed 75 mg/min if drug levels are subtherapeutic
    e. Given IV at a rate not to exceed 50 mg/min if drug levels are subtherapeutic

Answers

1.e. The metabolism of ethanol produces ketoacidosis when glucose stores are low. This is exacerbated by thiamine deficiency. However, metabolism still proceeds, normally at a rate between 8 and 32 mg/dL per hour. Supplemental dextrose can resolve this ketoacidosis (if present) as well as prevent its development. **(Emergency Medicine, Chapter 137, pp 1399–1405)**

2.b. Although many alcoholics are on phenytoin, it is not a useful drug to treat any seizures related to the alcohol withdrawal state. Its use is in alcoholic patients who have epilepsy as an idiopathic condition or as a result of head trauma or cerebrovascular accident. **(Emergency Medicine, Chapter 137, pp 1399–1405)**

3.c. Blindness and renal failure are major complications of methanol and ethylene glycol toxicity, respectively. Ethanol is the preferred initial treatment of methanol and ethylene glycol poisoning. Exposure to small amounts of methanol may be associated with serious toxicity. Isopropyl alcohol is associated with serum

4.e. Normal anion and osmol gaps do not rule out significant methanol toxicity. Complications of methanol and ethylene glycol may be delayed by 12 or more hours. During this period, the patient may be asymptomatic or present with nonspecific complaints. Early gastrointestinal decontamination is not usually helpful because alcohols are rapidly absorbed by the gastrointestinal tract. The subsequent development of acidosis or anion gap may indicate detectable methanol toxicity and the need for ethanol infusion. *(Emergency Medicine, Chapter 138, pp 1406–1412)*

5.c. Ethylene glycol poisoning is associated with urinary calcium oxalate crystals, anion and osmol gaps, and hypocalcemia. Wood's lamp illumination of the urine or gastric contents may show fluorescence caused by fluorescein dye additives of antifreeze. Urine ketones are seen in isopropanol ingestions. *(Emergency Medicine, Chapter 138, pp 1406–1412)*

6.e. The osmol gap is the difference between the measured osmolality and the calculated osmolarity. The formula for calculating serum osmolarity is $2(Na) + glucose/18 + BUN/2.8 + ethanol/4.6$. The normal range for the osmol gap is -2 ± 12 mOsm. *(Emergency Medicine, Chapter 138, pp 1406–1412)*

7.e. Fomepizole prevents methanol and ethylene glycol toxicity by inhibiting alcohol dehydrogenase and blocking metabolism. Clinical experience has demonstrated that an ethanol level of 100 mg/dL adequately blocks the metabolism of methanol and ethylene glycol. Hemodialysis should be considered for methanol or ethylene glycol levels greater than 25 mg/dL. Folate therapy for methanol poisoning and thiamine and pyridoxine therapy for ethylene glycol poisoning may also be beneficial. The treatment of isopropanol poisoning is largely supportive. Hemodialysis has been suggested for isopropanol levels in excess of 400 to 500 mg/dL. *(Emergency Medicine, Chapter 138, pp 1406–1412)*

8.b. The remarkable safety profile and efficacy of benzodiazepines has made them one of the most frequently prescribed class of drugs worldwide. Dosages up to 100 times the recommended therapeutic dose have resulted in only mild depression. Lethal intoxications involving benzodiazepines have been recorded; however, they are largely the result of mixed overdoses. *(Emergency Medicine, Chapter 141, pp 1425–1430)*

9.a. The use of flumazenil should not be considered an innocuous maneuver. Seizures temporally related to the administration of flumazenil have occurred. The most serious adverse effects have been associated with serious cyclic antidepressant toxicity and with patients who have become physically dependent on benzodiazepines. Although flumazenil has been used as a diagnostic tool for those cases with unclear histories, it cannot be relied upon to rapidly and completely reverse apnea or respiratory depression. *(Emergency Medicine, Chapter 141, pp 1425–1430)*

10.e. Benzodiazepine serum concentrations are not clinically useful and do not correlate with any pharmacologic or toxicologic effects or clinical outcome. Ipecac is not recommended. Other substances such as Visine, hand soap, Drano, and bleach can induce a false-negative urinalysis for benzodiazepines. Routine toxicologic testing will fail to detect some benzodiazepines including flunitrazepam (Rohypnol), a drug often used to perpetrate date rape. Profound respiratory depression in an oral benzodiazepine overdose suggests the presence of co-intoxicants. *(Emergency Medicine, Chapter 141, pp 1425–1430)*

11.d. Patients presenting with benzodiazepine withdrawal–induced seizures should be treated with benzodiazepines. *(Emergency Medicine, Chapter 141, pp 1425–1430)*

12.d. Carbamazepine toxicity typically manifests as seizures, possibly because it is an adenosine antagonist at high concentrations. Phenobarbital, primidone (a barbiturate), and valproic acid do not cause seizures. Phenytoin can causes seizures in patients with an underlying seizure disorder. *(Emergency Medicine, Chapter 139, pp 1413–1417)*

13.a. Carbamazepine resembles tricyclic antidepressants in structure. Although rare, cardiac toxicity from carbamazepine resembles that of a tricyclic antidepressant overdose, and it is likewise responsive to sodium bicarbonate. Phenytoin is the anticonvulsant that has been traditionally used to treat digoxin-induced arrhythmias. Ataxia, not tinnitus, is the hallmark sign of supratherapeutic drug levels of phenytoin, phenobarbital, carbamazepine, and valproic acid. Although phenytoin is a type Ib antiarrhythmic, patients with overdoses of oral preparations of this drug do not need to be on a cardiac monitor. Cardiac toxicity is associated only with the IV form (from the propylene glycol diluent). Elevated ammonia levels can occur with acute or chronic valproic acid use but are not pathognomonic for that overdose. *(Emergency Medicine, Chapter 139, pp 1413–1417)*

14.d. Cyclic coma from carbamazepine is occasionally reported and poorly understood. It appears to occur as levels approach normal. Multiple-dose activated charcoal is associated with decreased half-lives of the drugs. Coma with phenobarbital is prolonged because fatty tissues act as a reservoir. Propylene glycol is the diluent used in IV phenytoin. It is associated with hypotension and cardiac depression if given too rapidly. A new formulation without propylene glycol, fosphenytoin, has been recently released. Valproic acid has been associated with elevated ammonia levels in chronic use, but this does not cause intermittent hepatic encephalopathy. *(Emergency Medicine, Chapter 139, pp 1413–1417)*

15.c. Phenobarbital is the only barbiturate and anticonvulsant for which alkalinization of the urine has been demonstrated to enhance elimination of the drug. Although it is an acid, at least 99% of valproic acid is eliminated by the liver, so enhancing urinary elimination would not significantly improve detoxification. *(Emergency Medicine, Chapter 139, pp 1413–1417)*

16.e. The diluent in IV phenytoin, propylene glycol, is responsible for the cardiodepressant effects of rapid IV infusion. Although giving oral phenytoin obviates problems with propylene glycol, this route of administration does not reliably achieve therapeutic drug levels. Therapeutic drug levels are best achieved by IV administration at a rate not to exceed 50 mg/min (or 25 mg/min in patients at risk for hypotension) while constantly monitoring BP. *(Emergency Medicine, Chapter 139, pp 1413–1417)*

BIBLIOGRAPHY

Hodgman MJ, Benitez JG: The toxic alcohols. *In* Howell JM, Altieri M, Jagoda AS, et al (eds): Emergency Medicine. Philadelphia, WB Saunders, 1998, pp 1406–1412.

McFarland AK: Anticonvulsants. *In* Howell JM, Altieri M, Jagoda AS, et al (eds): Emergency Medicine. Philadelphia, WB Saunders, 1998, pp 1413–1417.

Morgan BW, Ford MD: Ethanol. *In* Howell JM, Altieri M, Jagoda AS, et al (eds): Emergency Medicine. Philadelphia, WB Saunders, 1998, pp 1399–1405.

Schauben JL: Benzodiazepines. *In* Howell JM, Altieri M, Jagoda AS, et al (eds): Emergency Medicine. Philadelphia, WB Saunders, 1998, pp 1425–1430.

61

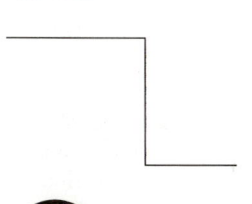

Cocaine and Stimulants, Hallucinogens, Mushrooms and Toxic Vegetations, Opioids, Pesticides, Phenothiazines, and Other Neuroleptics

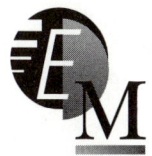

RICHARD J. HAMILTON, MD   OLIVER HUNG, MD   MARY PALMER, MD
RAMA B. RAO, MD

1. The classic toxidrome of opioid overdose includes all of the following except:
   a. Miosis
   b. Hypotension
   c. Respiratory depression
   d. Altered mental status
   e. Hypoxia

2. Fatalities from opioid overdose are usually the result of:
   a. Seizures
   b. Respiratory depression
   c. Hypotension
   d. Dysrhythmias
   e. Hypothermia

3. Which opioid is associated with the development of seizures and cardiac conduction abnormalities?
   a. Morphine
   b. Heroin
   c. Codeine
   d. Methadone
   e. Propoxyphene

4. Which statement concerning the use of naloxone in opioid overdose is false?
   a. Naloxone doses of up to 10 mg may be necessary to reverse fentanyl-induced respiratory depression.
   b. Large doses of naloxone may result in acute opioid withdrawal in opioid-addicted patients.
   c. Naloxone is a pure competitive antagonist at the mu, kappa, and delta opioid receptor sites.
   d. Patients who demonstrate a clinical response to naloxone require no further observation and may be safely discharged.
   e. History of vomiting after pentazocine use may predict naloxone-precipitated withdrawal.

5. The drug of choice for hypertension, tachycardia, and agitation in cocaine intoxication is:
   a. A mixed alpha-beta-blocker
   b. A beta-blocker
   c. A calcium channel blocker
   d. A benzodiazepine
   e. Nitroglycerin

6. The most frequent single complaint among patients who have used cocaine is:
   a. Palpitations
   b. Dyspnea
   c. Chest pain
   d. Anxiety
   e. Headache

7. A sympathomimetic toxidrome can often be distinguished from an anticholinergic toxidrome based on which of the following?
   a. Tachycardia and mydriasis
   b. Mydriasis and seizures
   c. Diaphoresis and active bowel sounds
   d. Hyperthermia alone
   e. Diaphoresis and hyperthermia

8. Species of the genus *Cortinarius* produce orellanine and orelline, which are structurally related to:
   a. Hepatic cells
   b. Paraquat
   c. Amatoxin
   d. Muscimol
   e. Acetaminophen

9. Which of the following toxicities does not correspond to the toxin listed:
   a. Liver failure—amatoxin
   b. Renal failure—orellanine
   c. Seizures—gyrometrin
   d. Disulfiram-like reactions—coprine
   e. Pulmonary failure—psilocybin

10. All of the following describe the possible effects of LSD except:
    a. Vomiting and diaphoresis
    b. Hallucinations and precipitation of psychosis
    c. Mydriasis and tachycardia
    d. Anxiety and bizarre perceptual sensations
    e. Alertness and orientation to person, place, and time

11. Phencyclidine toxicity manifests clinically in all of the following ways except:
    a. Wild behavior and nystagmus
    b. Hyperthermia and tachycardia

330 TOXICOLOGIC EMERGENCIES

    c. Prolonged QRS and formed visual hallucinations
    d. Increased pain tolerance and hyperactivity
    e. Seizures and death

12. Muscarinic symptoms of organophosphate poisoning include all of the following except:
    a. Bronchospasm and urination
    b. Weakness and fasciculations
    c. Miosis and bradycardia
    d. Bronchorrhea and increased gastrointestinal motility
    e. Lacrimation and salivation

13. Treatment of symptoms of organophosphate poisoning includes, all of the following except:
    a. Atropine
    b. Pralidoxime
    c. Benzodiazepine
    d. Pyridostigmine
    e. Airway management

14. All of the following are symptoms of pyrethrin toxicity except:
    a. Seizures and obtundation
    b. Rhinitis and bronchospasm
    c. Dysesthesias and dermatitis
    d. Urinary retention and dry skin
    e. Anaphylaxis and respiratory arrest

15. When used in superwarfarin rodenticide poisoning, vitamin K_1 (phytonadione):
    a. Cannot be given intravenously
    b. Is ineffective when given orally
    c. Is an essential cofactor for factors II, VII, IX, and X
    d. May cause renal failure if given intravenously
    e. Is best used prophylactically

16. Neuroleptic malignant syndrome features hyperthermia, altered mental status, and:
    a. Areflexia
    b. Painful flaccidity
    c. Muscle rigidity
    d. Nystagmus
    e. Abdominal distention

17. All of the following are useful for treating dystonia except:
    a. Benztropine
    b. Diazepam
    c. Diphenhydramine
    d. Amantadine
    e. Haloperidol

Answers

1.b. The classic toxidrome of opioid overdose includes respiratory depression, CNS depression, and miosis. Hypotension may occur with opioid overdose but is not a prominent finding. Normal or dilated pupils can occur with ingestions of morphine, meperidine, Lomotil, pentazocine, and propoxyphene or with a co-ingestion. (*Emergency Medicine, Chapter 152, pp 1494–1498*)

2.b. Respiratory depression is the most serious complication of opioid toxicity. (*Emergency Medicine, Chapter 152, pp 1494–1498*)

3.e. Seizures and quinidine-like cardiac conduction abnormalities can be seen in the first few hours after propoxyphene overdose. These effects have been attributed to the propoxyphene metabolite, norpropoxyphene. Meperidine's metabolite, normeperidine, has also been associated with seizures. (*Emergency Medicine, Chapter 152, pp 1494–1498*)

4.d. Naloxone is a pure opioid antagonist and is used to reverse opioid toxicity. Doses of up to 10 mg may be necessary to reverse the effects of synthetic opioids such as fentanyl. Large doses of naloxone may result in acute opioid withdrawal in the opioid-dependent patient. Most opioids have a duration of effect longer than that of naloxone. Patients who demonstrate a clinical response to naloxone should be observed for recurrence of symptoms and pulmonary edema. Many opioid-addicted patients will experience withdrawal with mixed agonist-antagonists such as pentazocine (Talwin) (*Emergency Medicine, Chapter 152, pp 1494–1498*)

5.d. Benzodiazepines are the drugs of choice for cocaine-induced hypertension, tachycardia, and agitation. They decrease the sympathetic outflow from the CNS by acting on inhibitory neurons, thus improving all aspects of acute cocaine intoxication. Mixed agents such as labetalol are largely beta-blockers, and these are contraindicated in cocaine use because they allow alpha stimulation to continue unopposed. (*Emergency Medicine, Chapter 144, pp 1443–1449*)

6.c. Chest pain is the most frequent complaint after cocaine use and can be a diagnostic challenge. In general, the clinician is wise to consider all complaints seriously and perform a thorough investigation. (*Emergency Medicine, Chapter 144, pp 1443–1449*)

7.c. Anticholinergic and sympathomimetic toxidromes share tachycardia, mydriasis, and fever. However, diaphoresis and active bowel sounds are features present in sympathomimetic toxidrome. An anticholinergic patient will have dry, flushed skin; decreased bowel sounds; and urinary retention. (*Emergency Medicine, Chapter 144, pp 1443–1449*)

8.b. Orellanine and orelline are structurally related to paraquat. Patients who eat mushrooms from the *Cortinarius* genus can have delayed onset of myalgias, fever, gastritis, thirst, and potentially oliguric renal failure (a feature present in paraquat poisoning). (*Emergency Medicine, Chapter 150, pp 1476–1488*)

9.e. Amatoxin classically causes liver failure, and orellanine, renal failure. Gyromitra mushrooms produce gyrometrin, which is similar in structure and function to isoniazid. It thereby can precipitate seizures by inhibition of pyridoxal phosphate metabolism. The *Coprinus* species of mushroom produces coprine, which can cause disulfiram-like reactions. Psilocybin produces hallucinations, not pulmonary failure. *(Emergency Medicine, Chapter 150, pp 1476–1488)*

10.a. LSD produces its hallucinogenic effect from stimulation of serotonin receptors. Although the hallucinations are often robust, the systemic manifestations of toxicity are generally mild. *(Emergency Medicine, Chapter 145, pp 1450–1454)*

11.c. Phencyclidine is an *N*-methyl-D-aspartate receptor agonist that results in sympathomimetic effects, seizures, and agitation. It does not cause prolonged QRS, and the hallucinations are more often disorganized and delusional. *(Emergency Medicine, Chapter 145, pp 1450–1454)*

12.b. Muscarinic subtype of acetylcholine receptors are found throughout the parasympathetic autonomic system. Muscarinic symptoms are described by the mnemonic SLUDGE—salivation, lacrimation, urination, defecation, gastrointestinal distress, emesis. Other muscarinic symptoms include miosis, bronchorrhea, bradycardia, and bronchospasm. Nicotinic receptors are found largely on the muscle motor end plate as well as the ganglionic fibers that stimulate the sympathetic nervous system. These receptors are largely at the motor end plates and are responsible for the weakness and fasciculations of organophosphate poisoning. Nicotinic receptors are also responsible for tachycardia, but this symptom is usually a result of catecholamine release. *(Emergency Medicine, Chapter 153, pp 1499–1506)*

13.d. Pyridostigmine is used as a pretreatment for nerve agent poisoning because it is a reversible inhibitor of acetylcholinesterase and occupies the enzyme during the time of potential exposure. When the pyridostigmine is metabolized, the protected acetylcholinesterase is freed, and some function may be restored despite the presence of nerve agent bound to the remaining acetylcholinesterase. If this agent is administered after exposure to organophosphates, it will temporarily exacerbate toxicity. *(Emergency Medicine, Chapter 153, pp 1499–1506)*

14.d. Pyrethrins are plant-derived insecticides that produce allergic reactions, including severe anaphylaxis with respiratory arrest, coma, seizures, etc. Pyrethrins do not produce anticholinergic symptoms. *(Emergency Medicine, Chapter 153, pp 1499–1506)*

15.c. Factors II, VII, IX, and X are the vitamin K–dependent coagulation factors. Vitamin K$_1$ (phytonadione) can be given by any route. Rapid IV infusion can cause a rate-related risk of anaphylactoid reaction. It should be used only when elevated INRs of the PT and PTT confirm toxicity, since superwarfarin agents may require vitamin K$_1$ (phytonadione) replacement for months. *(Emergency Medicine, Chapter 153, pp 1499–1506)*

16.c. Neuroleptic malignant syndrome is a potentially life-threatening syndrome that consists of muscle rigidity, tachycardia, autonomic instability, altered mental status, and hyperthermia. Current theories suggest that escalating doses of dopaminergic antagonists interfere with appropriate dopamine activity, causing neuroleptic malignant syndrome. Too little dopamine (excessive receptor antagonism or depletion of neurotransmitters) causes disorders of increased tone (parkinsonism, rigidity, dystonias); too much dopaminergic stimulation causes disorders of movement (choreoathetosis, hyperactivity, Tourette's syndrome). *(Emergency Medicine, Chapter 151, pp 1489–1493)*

17.e. Dystonia occurs from insufficient dopaminergic stimulation. Benztropine and diphenhydramine are potent dopamine-uptake inhibitors and overcome the dopaminergic antagonism of haloperidol. Amantadine has a similar effect but mostly increases dopamine release. Benzodiazepines are used because they inhibit CNS neuronal discharges and produce a muscle relaxation that is beneficial. Haloperidol is often the culprit in neuroleptic-induced dystonias. *(Emergency Medicine, Chapter 151, pp 1489–1493)*

BIBLIOGRAPHY

Gude W, Shepherd S: Pesticides. *In* Howell JM, Altieri M, Jagoda AS, et al (eds): Emergency Medicine. Philadelphia, WB Saunders, 1998, pp 1499–1506.

Hollander JE, Hoffman RS: Cocaine and stimulants. *In* Howell JM, Altieri M, Jagoda AS, et al (eds): Emergency Medicine. Philadelphia, WB Saunders, 1998, pp 1443–1449.

Hopkins P, Shepherd S: Hallucinogens. *In* Howell JM, Altieri M, Jagoda AS, et al (eds): Emergency Medicine. Philadelphia, WB Saunders, 1998, pp 1450–1454.

Mason TL, Ford MD: Opioids. *In* Howell JM, Altieri M, Jagoda AS, et al (eds): Emergency Medicine. Philadelphia, WB Saunders, 1998, pp 1494–1498.

McIntosh M, Shepherd S: Mushroom and toxic vegetations. *In* Howell JM, Altieri M, Jagoda AS, et al (eds): Emergency Medicine. Philadelphia, WB Saunders, 1998, pp 1476–1488.

Meggs WJ, Hoffman RS: Phenothiazines and other neuroleptics. *In* Howell JM, Altieri M, Jagoda AS, et al (eds): Emergency Medicine. Philadelphia, WB Saunders, 1998, pp 1489–1493.

62

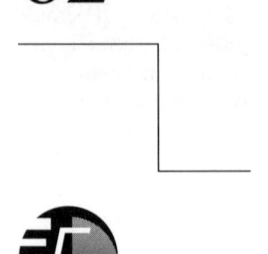

Caustic Ingestions, Hydrocarbon Ingestions, Physical and Chemical Irritants and Asphyxiants, Methemoglobinemia, and Lead

RICHARD J. HAMILTON, MD   OLIVER HUNG, MD   MARY PALMER, MD
RAMA B. RAO, MD

1. All of the following are true about caustic ingestions except:
   a. Stridor, vomiting, and drooling indicate a high likelihood for serious esophageal injury.
   b. Oropharyngeal burns correlate well with esophageal burns.
   c. Steroids may prevent stricture formation in certain types of burns.
   d. Ipecac, lavage, and charcoal are contraindicated.
   e. Household bleach generally does not produce significant esophageal injuries.

2. Which of the following is true?
   a. Asymptomatic patients with miniature button batteries beyond the pylorus on abdominal radiograph can be observed as outpatients.
   b. Glucagon is a useful adjunct for treatment of patients with miniature button batteries in the cervical esophagus.
   c. Ipecac is indicated for gastric emptying of miniature button batteries when administered within 15 minutes of ingestion.
   d. Miniature button batteries in the esophagus do not cause complications.
   e. Miniature button batteries are radiolucent.

3. Pulse oximetry is:
   a. Falsely low in carbon monoxide toxicity
   b. Falsely low in cyanide toxicity
   c. Falsely low in hydrogen sulfide toxicity
   d. Falsely normal in carbon monoxide toxicity
   e. Falsely elevated in cyanide toxicity

4. All of the following can cause toxicity in a delayed fashion except:
   a. Dermal exposure to low concentrations of hydrofluoric acid
   b. Respiratory exposure to low levels of chlorine gas
   c. Respiratory exposure to low levels of phosgene
   d. Respiratory exposure to zinc fumes from welding
   e. Respiratory exposure to hydrofluoric acid fumes

5. Respiratory exposure to hydrofluoric acid leads to all of the following except:
   a. Hypocalcemia
   b. Hypomagnesemia
   c. Hyperkalemia
   d. Cardiac dysrhythmias
   e. Paradoxical alkalosis

6. Cyanide produces:
   a. Peripheral and central cyanosis
   b. Profound lactic acidosis
   c. A large difference in arterial versus venous oxygen content
   d. Rotten egg odor
   e. Nongap acidosis

7. Carbon monoxide:
   a. Is associated with a bitter almond odor
   b. Is a metabolite of ethylene chloride spray
   c. Exposure can cause prominent neuropsychiatric sequelae despite recovery from the initial event
   d. Will not bind to myoglobin
   e. Is found in the blood from exogenous sources only

8. Gastrointestinal decontamination should be considered for all of the following hydrocarbons except:
   a. Camphor
   b. Carbon tetrachloride
   c. Mineral seal oil
   d. Heavy metals
   e. Pesticides

9. A 4-year-old ingests an unknown amount of pine oil left in a juice bottle. He is now actively playing in the pediatric area. The most appropriate management includes all of the following except:
   a. Chest radiograph
   b. Pulse oximetry
   c. Serial lung auscultation
   d. Nasogastric lavage
   e. Review the social history

10. All of the following are signs and symptoms of methemoglobinemia toxicity except:
    a. Dark brown arterial blood

b. Central cyanosis
c. Dyspnea
d. Myocardial insufficiency
e. Retinal hyperemia

11. You would most likely expect a patient to appear cyanotic if he or she has which of the following arterial blood gas four-wavelength co-oximetry results?
    a. Oxygen saturation 80%, Hb 12 g/dL
    b. Oxygen saturation 75%, Hb 15 g/dL
    c. Methemoglobinemia 10%, Hb 15 g/dL
    d. Carboxyhemoglobin saturation 25%, Hb 15 g/dL
    e. Methemoglobinemia 15%, Hb 9 g/dL

12. Pulse oximetry in patients with rising methemoglobin levels:
    a. Reads nearly 100% regardless of the methemoglobin level
    b. Approaches 85% regardless of the percentage of deoxyhemoglobin
    c. Correlates appropriately with the percentage oxyhemoglobin
    d. Reads the same as the oxygen saturation performed on routine arterial blood gas without four-wavelength co-oximetry
    e. Approximates the percentage of oxyhemoglobin on four-wavelength co-oximetry

13. All of the following are causes of failure of methylene blue therapy except:
    a. G6PD deficiency
    b. Chlorate toxicity
    c. Hb M disease
    d. NADH reductase deficiency
    e. NADPH reductase deficiency

14. Which of the following is a symptom of lead poisoning?
    a. A whitish line on the fingernail known as a Mees' line
    b. A bluish discoloration along the gingiva known as a Burton's line
    c. A hyperpigmented lesion on the skin that looks like "raindrops on a dusty road"
    d. Pink, painful fingers and an erythematous rash
    e. Multiple crops of clear vesicles on an erythematous base described as "raindrop on a rose."

15. Which of the following completely excludes the diagnosis of lead poisoning?
    a. A normal reticulocyte count
    b. A normal erythrocyte protoporphyrin level
    c. A normal CBC
    d. A normal long bone radiograph
    e. A serum lead level of 7.5 μg/dL

16. All of the following patients have the appropriate chelation therapy plan except:
    a. Encephalopathic child—IV calcium EDTA and oral DMSA
    b. Asymptomatic adult, serum lead level 55 μg/dL—no chelation
    c. Asymptomatic child, serum lead level 55 μg/dL—oral DMSA
    d. Asymptomatic adult, serum lead level 35 μg/dL—no chelation
    e. Asymptomatic child, serum lead level 18 μg/dL—no chelation

Answers

1.b. Intuitively, a substance that is exposed to the entire length of the alimentary canal should produce some injury everywhere. Many studies have demonstrated that this is not the case, and the absence of oropharyngeal burns should not dissuade the clinician from performing endoscopy on a patient with symptoms of esophageal burn. (*Emergency Medicine, Chapter 154, pp 1507–1516*)

2.a. Miniature button batteries produce necrosis by physical, chemical, and electric irritation of the gastrointestinal lining. However, they must be relatively fixed against the mucosa to cause tissue damage, and this is likely to occur in the esophagus. Once past the pylorus, they are generally free floating. Glucagon is least helpful for cervical esophageal impactions of any kind. Emesis of any solid objects increases the risk for aspiration. (*Emergency Medicine, Chapter 154, pp 1507–1516*)

3.d. Cyanide generally does not produce cyanosis, although both are derived from the Greek word for the color blue—*kyanos*. Cyanide and hydrogen sulfide are tissue asphyxiants and produce their toxicity by inhibiting the cytochrome oxidase system. Carbon monoxide produces a falsely normal pulse oximetry reading because the pulse oximeter confuses it with oxyhemoglobin. (*Emergency Medicine, Chapter 154, pp 1507–1516*)

4.e. Chlorine and phosgene require a period of time to dissolve in the respiratory mucus to create their symptoms. Zinc fumes produce metal fume fever—a leukotriene-mediated syndrome with fever and dyspnea. Dermal exposure to low concentrations of hydrofluoric acid is not immediately painful because it is only a weak acid. However, it is acidic enough to be absorbed rapidly in the respiratory tract and produce immediate and often fatal toxicity when inhaled. (*Emergency Medicine, Chapter 154, pp 1507–1516*)

5.e. Hydrofluoric acid complexes calcium and magnesium. This leads to hyperkalemia because cells are unable to maintain electrolyte gradients. The net effect is acidosis and fatal cardiac dysrhythmias. (*Emergency Medicine, Chapter 154, pp 1507–1516*)

6.b. Cyanide poisons the cytochrome oxidase system and prevents oxygen utilization. This leads to poor tissue oxygen extraction and an anion gap acidosis that is accounted for by lactic acid. Approximately half of the population can detect the bitter almond odor of cyanide salts, if present. *(Emergency Medicine, Chapter 154, pp 1507–1516)*

7.c. Carbon monoxide binds to hemoglobin, myoglobin, and cytochromes. It produces no cyanosis. It is also a metabolite of the one carbon molecule, methylene chloride (a paint stripper). Carbon monoxide is produced in the blood as a breakdown product of biliverdin and during heme synthesis, and it can be elevated to nontoxic levels during pregnancy. *(Emergency Medicine, Chapter 154, pp 1507–1516)*

8.c. The primary risk in aliphatic hydrocarbon ingestions such as mineral seal oil is aspiration. This risk is highest in hydrocarbons with low viscosity, low surface tension, and low volatility. Mineral seal oil is a type of hydrocarbon that has poor gastrointestinal absorption and is not associated with other forms of systemic toxicity. Attempts at gastrointestinal decontamination through emesis or lavage may increase this risk of aspiration and turn an asymptomatic ingestion into a serious aspiration. CHAMP is a mnemonic to help remember which hydrocarbons have systemic toxicity potentially needing decontamination: camphor, which produces seizures; halogenated hydrocarbons, such as carbon tetrachloride; aromatics, which can cause CNS depression; metals, with multiple system effects; and pesticides that can cause death by bronchorrhea and weakness of the muscles used in respiration as well as the other systemic effects of organophosphates. *(Emergency Medicine, Chapter 146, pp 1455–1459)*

9.d. Pine oil, like turpentine, is a terpene that presents dual risks of CNS toxicity and aspiration. Formulations often include isopropanol, which can increase CNS depression. Because it has good gastrointestinal absorption, rapid CNS sedation often accompanies toxic ingestion, but these are not demonstrated in this child. Toxicity is unlikely if the patient's sensorium remains normal, there are no signs of respiratory distress, and the chest radiograph is normal. If child abuse is strongly suspected by history or physical examination, the child's social situation should be thoroughly evaluated. *(Emergency Medicine, Chapter 154, pp 1507–1516)*

10.e. Retinal hyperemia is seen in carbon monoxide and cyanide toxicity. Carboxyhemoglobin has a bright red appearance and methemoglobinemia has a brown appearance. This is often detected on an ABG. It becomes especially evident when treatment improves the patient's appearance and a new arterial sample is compared to the pretreatment sample. *(Emergency Medicine, Chapter 149, pp 1470–1475)*

11.c. Cyanosis is visible with 1.5 g/dL of methemoglobin or 5.0 g/dL of deoxyhemoglobin. Thus, anemic patients will require larger percentages of deoxyhemoglobin or methemoglobin to produce a visible cyanosis. Carbon monoxide rarely produces cyanosis because it reflects light in the red spectrum. Carbon monoxide poisoned patients are able to saturate their normal hemoglobin appropriately. *(Emergency Medicine, Chapter 149, pp 1470–1475)*

12.b. The pulse oximeter measures absorbance of light at an infrared and red wavelength at the peak and trough of the pulsatile waveform and then performs a mathematical calculation to report an oxygen saturation. The variable effects of methemoglobin and carboxyhemoglobin on these measurements produce two distinct clinical scenarios. The pulse oximeter errs toward 85% in methemoglobinemia and errs toward 99% in carboxyhemoglobinemia. The effects on the routine blood gas are different because saturation is determined by directly measuring the relationship between oxyhemoglobin and deoxyhemoglobin, which will err toward normal in both situations. A gap between saturation determined by routine blood gas and the pulse oximeter may be a useful clue to toxicity. *(Emergency Medicine, Chapter 149, pp 1470–1475)*

13.d. Because NADH reductase is not necessary for the conversion of methylene blue to leukomethylene blue (the molecule that donates an electron to the Fe^{3+} of methemoglobin to create the normal Fe^{2+} of hemoglobin), NADH-reductase deficiency is never a cause for failure of methylene blue. G6PD deficiency results in poor NADPH production by the hexose monophosphate shunt. NADPH reductase is required to convert methylene blue to leukomethylene blue. Chlorate appears to inactivate G6PD and, when combined with methylene blue, is converted to the more toxic form chlorite. HbM is an abnormal hemoglobin that is permanently in the methemoglobin state because of a stable complex between an abnormal tyrosine substitution and the Fe^{3+}. Patients appear cyanotic but are rarely compromised by this situation except for mild chronic hemolysis. *(Emergency Medicine, Chapter 149, pp 1470–1475)*

14.b. Mees' lines and the hyperpigmented skin lesions are characteristic of arsenic poisoning. The bluish lines on the gingiva are known as Burton's lead lines. Acrodynia (described by answer d) is a characteristic of mercury poisoning in children. Varicella presents with the characteristic lesion in answer e. *(Emergency Medicine, Chapter 148, pp 1465–1469)*

15.e. Screening for lead toxicity used to consist of an erythrocyte protoporphyrin level, but this is an insensitive test of lead toxicity below 25 μg/dL. Since the threshold for toxicity has been reduced to 10 μg/dL, only a serum lead level is a definitive test. Fingerstick lead levels are a useful screen if they are less than 10 μg/dL; if they are higher they may represent skin contamination by lead-containing dirt and debris. *(Emergency Medicine, Chapter 148, pp 1465–1469)*

16.a. Encephalopathic patients are treated optimally with British antilewisite and calcium EDTA. Without British antilewisite, calcium EDTA mobilizes bone stores of lead into the serum and may increase the cerebrospinal fluid lead content. Symptomatic children with lead poisoning but without encephalopathy are also treated with British antilewisite and EDTA at lower doses. Asymptomatic children with lead levels above 45 μg/dl are treated with oral DMSA. The treatment of children with levels of 20 to 45 μg/dl is controversial; many toxicologists will treat with oral DMSA. No chelation therapy is warranted in asymptomatic adults, although levels greater than 50 μg/dl mandate removal of the adult from the environment causing toxicity. ***(Emergency Medicine, Chapter 148, pp 1465–1469, Table 148–2)***

BIBLIOGRAPHY

Brubacher JR: Methemoglobinemia. *In* Howell JM, Altieri M, Jagoda AS, et al (eds): Emergency Medicine. Philadelphia, WB Saunders, 1998, pp 1470–1475.

DeRoos F, Hoffman RS: Lead. *In* Howell JM, Altieri M, Jagoda AS, et al (eds): Emergency Medicine. Philadelphia, WB Saunders, 1998, pp 1465–1469.

Nelson L, Hoffman RS: Physical and chemical irritants and asphyxiants. *In* Howell JM, Altieri M, Jagoda AS, et al (eds): Emergency Medicine. Philadelphia, WB Saunders, 1998, pp 1507–1516.

Papavasiliou J, Kunisaki T: Hydrocarbon ingestions. *In* Howell JM, Altieri M, Jagoda AS, et al (eds): Emergency Medicine. Philadelphia, WB Saunders, 1998, pp 1455–1459.

SECTION EIGHTEEN

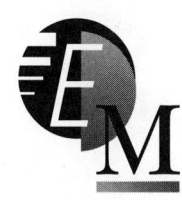

Environmental Emergencies

63 Bites, Stings, and Rabies; Diving Injuries and Illness; and Radiation

JOHN MAHONEY, MD   ERIK HOLT, MD

Bites, Stings, and Rabies

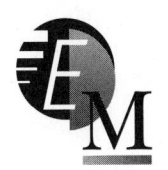

1. Initial treatment of a dog bite includes all of the following except:
   a. Removal of all jewelry from the involved extremity
   b. Administration of an antimicrobial regimen that includes coverage for *Pasteurella multocida*
   c. Assessment of animal health and immunization history
   d. Administration of an antimicrobial regimen that includes coverage for *Eikenella corrodens*
   e. Delayed primary closure for a severely contaminated wound

2. Which of the following is an indication for Td (tetanus-diphtheria) booster after a bite wound?
   a. A patient received a bite wound.
   b. The patient completed initial vaccination series but the last booster was 4 years ago.
   c. The patient is 6 years old with two previous immunizations.
   d. The patient's age is greater than 65 years.
   e. The patient has contaminated wounds and an unclear vaccination history.

3. All of the following are acceptable antimicrobials for human bite prophylaxis except:
   a. Penicillin V
   b. Amoxicillin–clavulanic acid
   c. Erythromycin
   d. Penicillin V and cephalexin
   e. Clindamycin

4. All of the following are associated with an increased likelihood of infection after a dog bite except:
   a. Wounds undergoing initial treatment longer than 2 hours after injury
   b. Hand wounds
   c. Severe crush wounds
   d. Full-thickness wounds
   e. Wounds requiring débridement

5. Initial treatment of a snakebite should include:
   a. Incision and suction
   b. Immobilization of the extremity
   c. Ice to the affected extremity
   d. Elevation of the affected limb
   e. Constricting band tightened to occlude arterial flow

6. A healthy 24-year-old male presents to the ED after being bitten on the hand by a rattlesnake 2 hours ago. He complains of severe pain at the site of the bite and has a temperature of 38.2°C. His treatment should include:
   a. Observation in the ED and local wound care
   b. Local wound care and reexamination in 5 days
   c. Immediate infusion of the appropriate antivenin with reexamination within 24 hours
   d. Diphenhydramine, 50 mg IV, followed by antivenin administration, with one half of the dose given at the wound site and one half given IM
   e. Horse serum skin testing, followed 30 minutes later by antivenin administration if testing is negative

7. A 32-year-old female presents to the ED 25 minutes after being stung on the arm while in the ocean. On initial examination she has a minor wound with minimal surrounding erythema and complains of pain at the wound site. Which of the following does not correctly pair the causative marine organism and appropriate treatment?
   a. Stingray—wound débridement, immersion in hot (45°C) water
   b. Sea sponge—adhesive tape to remove spicules, isopropyl alcohol 40% to 70%, topical steroids
   c. Jellyfish—immersion in 5% acetic acid, shaving the affected area if needed to remove nematocysts
   d. Stonefish—immersion in 5% acetic acid, local wound care, Td booster if needed
   e. Sea urchin—immersion in hot water, local wound care, radiography for retained spines

8. A 26-year-old male presents to the ED after being bitten on the hand by an insect or spider 2 hours prior to arrival. He currently complains of nausea, pain, and a pins-and-needles sensation all over. On his hand there are two red puncture wounds with wheal and surrounding erythema. There are also muscle fasciculations of his forearm. Appropriate treatment is:

339

a. Erythromycin, warm compresses, oral prednisone
b. Appropriate antivenin, calcium gluconate, opioid analgesia
c. Diphenhydramine, stinger removal, antimicrobial
d. Local wound care and admission for observation
e. Excision of wound, antimicrobial, opioid analgesia

9. Which of the following is true regarding rabies infection and treatment after an animal bite?
    a. Human diploid cell vaccine should be administered at the wound site if the animal is known or highly suspected to be rabid.
    b. The full-dose human rabies immune globulin should be administered at the wound site if the animal is known to be or is potentially infected with rabies.
    c. Unprovoked bites by rats, squirrels, and chipmunks pose a particularly high risk for transmission of rabies through the animal's saliva.
    d. Human rabies immune globulin should be given on days 0, 3, 7, 14, and 28.
    e. Human diploid cell vaccine and human rabies immune globulin injections should be given into the deltoid or anterolateral thigh, rather than a gluteal site.

10. Which of the following is true about rabies?
    a. The RNA rabies virus spreads via peripheral nerves to the host's CNS where replication occurs in Negri bodies.
    b. Transmission of rabies is via saliva; a bite wound is the only method of transmission.
    c. Patients with signs of clinical rabies infection can usually be successfully treated with human rabies immune globulin and aggressive supportive care.
    d. Death from rabies infection is the result of progressive muscle spasm resulting from blockade of gamma-aminobutyric acid and glycine at presynaptic nerve terminals.
    e. The severe pain associated with swallowing causes most patients to become hydrophobic.

11. When managing an animal bite, all of the following are true except:
    a. The health department usually requires reporting of both animal bites and rabies.
    b. In most domestic cat and dog bites, other types of infection are more likely than rabies.
    c. Local health officials can provide information on the likelihood of rabies within particular species in a given region.
    d. If an abnormally behaving animal is being killed and examined for evidence of rabies, postexposure prophylaxis should be postponed until the test results are known.
    e. A 10-day quarantine observation of animals that appear healthy can safely exclude rabies infection.

12. The following are true about management of bites and stings except:
    a. Patients who have had an anaphylactic reaction to a bee sting in the past should be immediately treated with subcutaneous epinephrine if they have a subsequent insect sting.
    b. Anaphylaxis is treated with epinephrine, oxygen, IV fluids, antihistamines, steroids, and other supportive measures, whether it is a result of a snake bite, insect sting, or adverse drug reaction.
    c. Hymenoptera, including wasps and yellow jackets, are the insects most often responsible for allergic responses.
    d. IV epinephrine may be required for treatment of severe anaphylaxis with cardiopulmonary collapse.
    e. Signs and symptoms of anaphylaxis may occur after a snakebite or develop during administration of antivenin.

Answers

1.d. Removal of potentially constricting jewelry is important in all cases of extremity trauma. Edema caused by the injury can result in constriction and distal ischemia. *Pasteurella multocida* is responsible for the majority of dog and cat bite infections during the first 24 hours after injury. In contrast, *Eikenella corrodens* is the common early pathogen after human bites. Professional assessment of the responsible animal for signs of rabies is needed if there is any suspicion of rabies infection. **(Emergency Medicine, Chapter 164, pp 1585–1597)**

2.e. In general, the indication for tetanus prophylaxis with Td is if the patient has completed an initial series but has not had a booster within the past 5 years (for dirty wounds) or 10 years for all wounds. All patients with open wounds, including bites, should be considered for tetanus prophylaxis based on their immunization history. An unclear immunization history is also an indication for Td administration. Children up to age 6 years with incomplete initial diphtheria, pertussis, and tetanus vaccinations (less than three doses) should have the series completed with diphtheria, pertussis, and tetanus. For children age 7 and above, Td is recommended instead. Age alone is not an indication for immunization. However, many adult and elderly patients are not adequately immunized. Also note that tetanus immune globulin may be indicated in patients with an unknown status or an incomplete initial series. **(Emergency Medicine, Chapter 164, pp 1585–1597)**

3.e. *Staphylococcus* and *Streptococcus* species found in the human mouth are often beta-lactamase–producing organisms. Cephalexin provides good coverage for most species in the human mouth except *Eikenella corrodens*, which is sensitive to penicillin. Erythromycin may be used if there is severe allergy to penicillin, but it has a higher incidence of treatment failure. *Eikenella* is resistant to clindamycin, metronidazole, and penicillinase-resistant penicillins. Amoxicillin–clavulanic acid is an ideal antimicrobial for prophylaxis of most bites (dog, cat, and human). Established infections are best treated with one or more doses of

IV antimicrobials (depending on co-morbid illnesses and body part involved). *(Emergency Medicine, Chapter 164, pp 1585–1597)*

4.a. Wounds more than 8 hours old are associated with higher infection rates. In addition, advanced age and female sex are associated with an increased incidence of infection. Deep puncture wounds, such as cat bites, are also at high risk. Deeper wounds and punctures may be more likely to develop infection if sutured primarily, so delayed or no closure is a management consideration. Underlying medical conditions that would compromise healing, including vascular disease and immune-compromising diseases, also increase the risk of infection. *(Emergency Medicine, Chapter 164, pp 1585–1597)*

5.b. Immobilization of the extremity and keeping it below the level of the heart are measures to decrease lymphatic spread of venom after snakebite. Elevation of the extremity could increase spread of venom. Constricting bands may decrease lymphatic spread but should not be tight enough to occlude arterial flow. Wound incision, suctioning, and ice have not been shown to be of benefit in envenomations. Identification of the snake can be helpful in determining the most appropriate treatment, but patients should be advised against bringing live snakes to the ED. The attached or decapitated head of a dead snake can still envenomate, so extreme caution is warranted during handling. *(Emergency Medicine, Chapter 164, pp 1585–1597)*

6.e. The envenomation described would be considered moderate, and the patient should receive IV antivenin after skin testing for possible allergy to horse serum. Antivenin is most effective when given within 4 hours of the bite but may be useful up to 24 hours. There is no need for immediate administration of antivenin unless the patient demonstrates symptoms of a severe bite, such as cardiovascular instability. Pit vipers are members of the Crotalidae family, with triangle-shaped heads, elliptical pupils, a heat-sensing pit between the eyes and nose, fangs, and a single row of subcaudal plates at the end of the tail. This is in contrast to nonvenomous snakes, who tend to have rounded heads, round pupils, no fangs, and a double row of caudal plates. Envenomations are graded by the severity of symptoms. Mild bites cause only local and no systemic effects. Moderate bites cause more severe local effects, including severe pain and erythema, and non–life-threatening systemic symptoms (weakness, fever, vomiting, and perioral paresthesias). Severe bites are manifested by more serious systemic symptoms, such as dyspnea, hypotension, tachycardia, and altered consciousness. The most severe bites may result in seizures, shock, and severe laboratory abnormalities (abnormal coagulation parameters and others). Patients with mild bites may be discharged after an extended observation period, but those with more severe bites should be admitted. Diphenhydramine is used as part of the treatment for anaphylaxis, although it is not usually administered directly into a wound. Human rabies immune globulin is given as a divided dose, with half at the wound site and half IM, although snakes do not carry rabies. *(Emergency Medicine, Chapter 164, pp 1585–1597)*

7.d. Stonefish are known to have extremely toxic venom, and use of antivenin is a necessary part of treating envenomations by these animals. When treating wounds from stingrays, sea urchins, starfish, and catfish, remove remaining barb fragments, immerse the wound in hot water (many marine animals have venom that will break down under warm conditions), and obtain a radiograph if foreign body is suspected. In treating jellyfish coelenterate stings, use salt water irrigation to remove loose nematocysts. Avoid fresh water because it may cause remaining nematocysts to discharge. Irrigation with acetic acid or isopropyl alcohol irrigation (or urine if no such solutions are available in the field) is used for primary decontamination followed by gentle shaving to remove any remaining nematocysts. Sea sponges require similar treatment; however, adhesive tape is used to remove embedded spicules. *(Emergency Medicine, Chapter 164, pp 1585–1597)*

8.b. These systemic and local symptoms strongly suggest a black widow spider bite. The black widow venom causes release of norepinephrine and acetylcholine at synapses, causing sustained muscle contractions. This patient's systemic symptoms warrant administration of antivenin, calcium gluconate, and opioids for muscular spasm. These bites may also result in autonomic dysfunction and hypertension, both of which should improve after antivenin but must be treated with general supportive measures if needed. Severe, painful spasm of the abdominal wall musculature can be confused with peritonitis. Erythromycin has been suggested for brown recluse bites. Heat may exacerbate brown recluse bites by potentiating the venom. Spider bites do not typically involve a stinger. *(Emergency Medicine, Chapter 164, pp 1585–1597)*

9.e. Treatment failures have occurred when human diploid cell vaccine has been administered into a gluteal site. The recommendation is to use the deltoid muscle, avoiding the injured side if there is an upper extremity wound. The anterolateral thigh is an alternative in small children. The schedule for human rabies diploid cell vaccination is 1 mL on days 0, 3, 7, 14, and 28. The WHO recommendation includes a later dose at 90 days. Human rabies immune globulin is given only on day 0, in a dose of 20 IU/kg, with half the dose infiltrated at the wound site and the other half in the deltoid muscle, ideally on the injured side. Dogs are the most common carriers of rabies worldwide, but skunks are the most common carriers in the United States. Other common carriers are bats, raccoons, cows, dogs, foxes, and cats. Rodents, lagomorphs (rabbits), reptiles, and birds are not reported to cause rabies in humans. Thorough local wound care and permitting healing via secondary intention are thought to reduce the incidence of rabies infection by up to 90%. *(Emergency Medicine, Chapter 164, pp 1585–1597)*

10.a. Eosinophilic Negri bodies are diagnostic when they are found in animals with rabies, but they are not seen in approximately one quarter of cases. They also occur in humans. Rabies is most commonly transmitted via saliva during a bite by an infected animal, although it has been transmitted through inhalation of infected bat saliva and transplantation of corneal tissue. Universal precautions should be used when exposure to body fluids may occur. Once CNS rabies infection occurs it is almost always fatal, in spite of supportive therapy. Death caused by rabies may follow flaccid or spastic symptoms, with coma, seizures, and apnea as the terminal events. Bulbar, diaphragmatic, and respiratory muscular spasms and seizures that occur with swallowing cause hydrophobia. Progressive muscle spasm resulting from blockade of gamma-aminobutyric acid and glycine at presynaptic nerve terminals is seen in *tetanus*, not rabies. *(Emergency Medicine, Chapter 164, pp 1585–1597)*

11.d. If a biting animal is suspected of being rabid, the routine procedure is for it to be killed and the tissues examined for Negri bodies using fluorescent antibody testing. Because transporting the specimen and performing the tests may take days, the routine procedure is to initiate rabies prophylaxis and discontinue it if the tests are negative. If an animal captured for quarantine is behaving normally at the time of capture, prophylaxis may be postponed and later initiated if any suspicious symptoms develop. Reporting all animal bite wounds to health officials contributes to the effort to maintain surveillance of the incidence of rabies in the region and can facilitate access to information about the prevalence of rabies in a given situation. Different regions in the United States have different patterns of endemic rabies infection. *(Emergency Medicine, Chapter 164, pp 1585–1597)*

12.a. Epinephrine is indicated only after an insect sting from a species similar or identical to the type that caused the previous severe or anaphylactic reaction. At times, patients will self-administer epinephrine when it is not clearly indicated. Physicians are obligated to provide patients with training about the indications for use when prescribing epinephrine injectors. Subcutaneous epinephrine may not be sufficient for more severe cases, and IV epinephrine can be used. Reaction to snakebites may be confounded by reaction to antivenin, which is derived from horses. Thus, performing a horse serum skin sensitivity test can be helpful before administering antivenin, if the patient's condition permits a delay in administering antivenin. Bees and fire ants are also hymenopteran. *(Emergency Medicine, Chapter 164, pp 1585–1597)*

Diving Injuries and Illness

1. A 26-year-old with decompression sickness is to be treated with hyperbaric oxygen therapy. Which of these is a possible initial hyperbaric oxygen regimen?
   a. 100% oxygen at 760 mm Hg for 4 hours
   b. 100% oxygen at 2 to 6 atm absolute (ATA), based on established treatment schedules
   c. 100% oxygen at 14.7 feet of sea water, with gradual decompression according to Naval diver decompression tables
   d. 100% oxygen only; this is not an indication for hyperbaric oxygen
   e. 100% oxygen by high-pressure face mask until symptoms resolve

2. During your first shift at an ED with limited facilities a 26-year-old scuba diver is brought in by paramedics. She complains of severe joint pain and left arm numbness and weakness. You have decided to transport her to a facility with staff specially trained in diving injuries. What studies or therapy may be indicated prior to transfer and how should transport proceed?
   a. 100% oxygen, chest radiograph, CT scan of brain, transport in position most comfortable for the patient
   b. 100% oxygen, CT scan of brain, chest radiograph, ABG, transport in Trendelenburg position
   c. 100% oxygen, ABG, chest radiograph, transport left side down
   d. 100% oxygen, ABG, chest radiograph, transport in Trendelenburg position
   e. 100% oxygen, CT scan of brain, chest radiograph, ABG, transport right side down

3. A 65-year-old scuba diver presents to the ED with fatigue and weakness. The differential diagnosis includes all of the following except:
   a. Stroke
   b. Carbon monoxide poisoning
   c. Upper respiratory infection
   d. Decompression sickness
   e. Dysbaric fatigue syndrome

4. A 30-year-old scuba diver complains of joint pain, rash, and symptoms of vertigo. The most likely diving-related condition is:
   a. Type I decompression sickness
   b. Type II decompression sickness
   c. Inner ear barotrauma
   d. Nitrogen narcosis
   e. Extra-alveolar air syndrome

5. Hyperbaric oxygen therapy can be used to treat all of the following except:
   a. Pneumothorax
   b. Type I decompression sickness
   c. Type II decompression sickness
   d. Air and gas embolism
   e. Barodontalgia

6. The most common cause of death in divers is:
   a. Arterial gas embolism
   b. Decompression sickness
   c. Barotrauma
   d. Drowning
   e. Oxygen toxicity

7. Middle ear barotrauma is manifested by all of the following except:
   a. Tympanic membrane edema
   b. Free blood in the middle ear
   c. Perforation of tympanic membrane
   d. Nystagmus
   e. Tympanic membrane hemorrhage and ear pain

Answers

1.b. 100% oxygen at 2 to 6 ATA is a possible initial regimen. Surface pressure is 1 ATA, 760 mm Hg, 29.9 inches Hg, 14.7 lb/in.^{2} (psi). When diving, the pressure increases 1 ATA for every 33 feet of sea water depth. At a depth of 165 feet of sea water, the pressure is 6 ATA. Scuba divers do not commonly dive below 200 feet. Treatment with 100% oxygen decreases the alveolar concentration of nitrogen, increasing diffusion of nitrogen out of the blood stream into the lungs to be exhaled. Hyperbaric treatment reproduces the pressure effects of a dive. Increasing atmospheric pressure causes a decrease in nitrogen bubble size, therefore increasing tissue perfusion (Boyle's Law). Administration of oxygen at increased pressure also increases dissolved oxygen. This improves delivery to tissues and displacement of nitrogen from gas bubbles. *(Emergency Medicine, Chapter 159, pp 1549–1555)*

2.c. This patient has signs and symptoms consistent with type II decompression sickness. Decompression sickness with neurologic symptoms is an indication for hyperbaric oxygen therapy, and 100% oxygen is an initial therapy that will increase oxygen delivery to tissue and nitrogen gas expulsion. A chest radiograph may reveal evidence of pulmonary barotrauma, such as a pneumothorax, that should be treated prior to transport. Measurement of the ABG may also show evidence of pulmonary embarrassment and the need for more aggressive management. A CT scan of the brain may be performed eventually but is relatively insensitive at detecting abnormalities early in a patient's course and may delay transport. Left lateral decubitus and supine positions allow for air bubbles to be evenly distributed between coronary and cerebral circulation. Sitting upright concentrates air in the cerebral circulation, and the Trendelenburg position increases distribution to the coronary circulation. *(Emergency Medicine, Chapter 159, pp 1549–1555)*

3.e. There is no entity identified as dysbaric fatigue syndrome. The remaining diagnoses are a possibility. Those not specifically caused by the dive could have been exacerbated by diving. Decompression sickness has a variety of presentations from benign to severe and may be missed if a history of diving is not obtained. A detailed history of the dive and surrounding circumstances and a careful physical examination may help to differentiate between a dive injury and other illnesses. For example, divers who refill their own air tanks from an improvised compression source may have an inadvertent carbon monoxide exposure. *(Emergency Medicine, Chapter 159, pp 1549–1555)*

4.b. The symptoms described are of type II decompression sickness. Decompression sickness is thought to be caused by accumulation of nitrogen gas bubbles in tissues and blood. At depth, divers breathe air at increased pressures, increasing the amount of dissolved gas in the blood stream. On return to normal pressure, inert nitrogen and other gases come out of solution and form gas bubbles. Whereas oxygen is metabolized in tissues, nitrogen is an inert gas and accumulates. These bubbles can coalesce in the arterial circulation, causing distal ischemia at a microvascular level and gas embolism if they become large enough. They can also cause direct tissue disruption. Type I "pain only" decompression sickness includes limb or joint pain, rash, and fatigue. Type II decompression sickness includes neurologic symptoms ranging from weakness or vertigo to altered consciousness. Vertigo is a component of inner ear barotrauma, another high-pressure related illness, without systemic involvement. Nitrogen narcosis is intoxication with increasing depth. It resolves on return to the surface. Extra-alveolar air syndromes include gas embolism and pneumothorax and are the second most common cause of death among divers. *(Emergency Medicine, Chapter 159, pp 1549–1555)*

5.a. Untreated pneumothorax is one of the few contraindications for hyperbaric oxygen. The elevated pressure may worsen symptoms. Once a chest tube has been placed, it is safe to proceed with recompression. Hyperbaric oxygen therapy is specific treatment for decompression sickness types I and II. Hyperbaric oxygen compresses gas bubbles after gas embolism, permitting restoration of flow in occluded vessels as the bubbles shrink. Barodontalgia is tooth pain caused by trapped gas that expands during ascent. This mechanism may also manifest in the ear and sinuses. Although barodontalgia can usually be treated symptomatically, severe cases may require hyperbaric treatment. *(Emergency Medicine, Chapter 159, pp 1549–1555)*

6.d. Drowning is the most common cause of death in divers, followed by arterial gas embolism. It is important to also assess survivors of diving accidents as victims of near-drowning and treat accordingly. In gas embolism, nitrogen bubbles concentrate in the left ventricle, forming a large gas bubble. These gas bubbles may then travel through the arterial circulation with catastrophic effects on end organs. The bubbles enter the circulation through ruptured pulmonary veins. Symptoms occur within the first few minutes after surfacing. This may occur in conjunction with a rapid or emergency ascent, so it may be confused with near-drowning after running out of air or an equipment malfunction. (*Emergency Medicine, Chapter 159, pp 1549–1555*)

7.a. Middle ear barotrauma is the most common pressure-related illness associated with diving. It occurs when there is unequal pressure on the tympanic membrane caused by changes in surrounding pressure. Teed classification of middle ear barotrauma includes class 1, erythema of the malleolus and capillary dilatation; class 2, mild tympanic membrane edema; class 3, gross tympanic membrane hemorrhage; class 4, free blood in the middle ear; and class 5, perforation of the tympanic membrane. Middle ear barotrauma can be treated with decongestants, and membrane rupture with antimicrobials. Divers with middle ear barotrauma should be advised to discontinue diving for 3 to 7 days, although those divers with class 1 to 3 barotrauma may continue with slow descent and careful attention to frequently clearing the ears. Nystagmus is associated with inner ear barotrauma and should be referred for evaluation by a specialist. (*Emergency Medicine, Chapter 159, pp 1549–1555*)

Radiation

1. Which is the most effective step in decontaminating patients after typical civilian radiation exposures?
   a. Immediate copious soap and water scrubbing using scrub brushes
   b. Prolonged irrigation at the scene of the incident
   c. Gentle débridement of particles from the skin using nonreactive forceps
   d. Careful removal of contaminated clothing
   e. Early initiation of decorporation therapy

2. Which of the following is equivalent to one roentgen (R)?
   a. 100 rad (radiation-absorbed dose)
   b. 10 rem (roentgen equivalent man)
   c. 1 Gy (Gray)
   d. 1 Sv (Sievert)
   e. 1000 mrem (millirem)

3. Your young female patient's mother is hesitant to permit you to order a diagnostic radiograph. Which of the following is true regarding common radiation exposures?
   a. Typical radiation exposure from watching a color television is only 1 mrem per year.
   b. The human LD50 is 400 millirem.
   c. Patients become measurably radioactive only if exposed to a whole-body dose of greater than 10,000 rem.
   d. After receiving a dose of a radioisotope for a nuclear medicine procedure, all body fluids and secretions pose a serious radiation risk to others for at least 100 days.
   e. An AP chest radiograph results in a dose of 100 mrem.

4. Which of the following is correct regarding the biologic effects of an acute exposure to ionizing radiation?
   a. Survival is unlikely if neurologic symptoms, such as confusion, ataxia, or lethargy, begin within the first few hours after exposure.
   b. Surgical procedures that are needed after a radiation exposure are best postponed until after the first few days, to permit an initial rebound from the radiation insult.
   c. After an ocular exposure, maximal symptoms will develop within 60 days.
   d. Patients with gastrointestinal radiation syndrome have a good chance for survival with early, aggressive supportive care.
   e. Normal peripheral neutrophil counts can be used to predict that a patient has had only a mild exposure.

5. To prepare for incoming patients who may be contaminated with radioactive materials, the ED should:
   a. Maintain a stock of dense shielding materials, such as lead panels and sand bags.
   b. Maintain a stock of specialized radioisotope antidotes, in sufficient quantities to treat the expected number of patients plus the ED staff if necessary.
   c. Maintain a supply of plastic sheeting or paper to prevent contamination of walls and floors, in addition to the usual hazardous materials decontamination supplies.
   d. Evacuate the hospital to prevent other patients from becoming contaminated.
   e. Designate one or two people to do the entire decontamination, to minimize the number of people who may also become exposed.

6. Treatment of radiation-exposed patients includes all of the following except:
   a. Reverse isolation rooms
   b. Tissue biopsy for estimating the radiation dose

c. Human leukocyte antigen typing in preparation for bone marrow transplantation
d. Prophylactic oral antimicrobials for gut sterilization
e. Transfusion of platelets and other blood products

7. During his first day on the job, an industrial radiographer has manually replaced the cesium-137 radioisotope source pellet into its holder several times today when it repeatedly fell out. Which of the following is not true concerning his expected injuries?
   a. The whole-body dose received can be predicted from the severity of the wounds developing on his hands.
   b. Because the exposures were brief, only local injury without systemic sequelae would be expected.
   c. Hand burns from a gamma radiation source are one of the most common types of radiation injuries in the United States.
   d. Bullae and erythema will develop early at the points of skin contact, with very little effect just a few centimeters away.
   e. The low-energy isotopes used for industrial radiography sources are specifically selected because they can safely be handled when needed.

8. An iridium-192 ribbon containing multiple isotope seeds was dislodged from the endotracheal catheter of a patient receiving radiation therapy. After it lay on his neck for 3 hours, the nurse placed it in a basin by the bed. Which of the following is not part of the management of this situation?
   a. Evaluate the patient for local radiation burns on the neck where the ribbon had lain.
   b. Evaluate the nurse for local radiation burns on the hands where she handled the ribbon and initiate monitoring for systemic effects, though unlikely.
   c. Ascertain whether any other patients or workers may have had direct contact or close exposure to the ribbon and therefore require evaluation.
   d. Initiate decontamination of all objects and personnel that the nurse has had contact with since the exposure.
   e. Confirm that all of the isotope seeds have been accounted for.

9. Which of the following treatments are not suggested for management of internal radiation contamination?
   a. Gastric decontamination to limit absorption of ingested radionuclides
   b. Charcoal hemofiltration for removal of unbound circulating radionuclides
   c. Potassium iodide to saturate receptors and block uptake of radioactive iodine
   d. Chelation using dimercaprol for decorporation of radioactive arsenic
   e. Barium sulfate administration to form an insoluble salt for treatment of strontium ingestion

Answers

1.d. Up to 90% of contaminants can be eliminated by removing contaminated clothing. Skin washing, preferably by the patients themselves, improves this up to 98%. Soap and water cleansing is appropriate, but care should be used to avoid abrading the skin and providing a portal of entry for contaminants into the body. Foreign bodies can be removed using conventional techniques and instruments. Decorporation therapy, aimed at treating internal contamination, is a secondary procedure. *(Emergency Medicine, Chapter 155, pp 1517–1524)*

2.e. For most applications, 1 R is equivalent to 1 rad, 1 rem, 1000 mrem, 0.01 Gy, and 0.01 Sv. This is true for beta, gamma, and x radiation. Alpha particles and neutrons have a much more potent biologic effect. Roentgen equivalent man (rem) accounts for these biologic effects. A given rad dose in alpha particles or neutrons will produce up to 20 times more damage than the same dose on gamma rays. This makes the rem and mrem the preferred units of measurement when dealing with biologic systems. *(Emergency Medicine, Chapter 155, pp 1517–1524)*

3.a. Radiation exposure from consumer products including luminous watch dials, television tubes, lantern mantles, and smoke detectors is approximately 2 mrem per year. Natural sources of radiation, including cosmic radiation, radon, and elements naturally found in human tissues, contribute 150 mrem per year. The overall total background radiation dose received in the United States is estimated to be 360 mrem per year. The lethal dose that will result in death to 50% of exposed persons is 400 rem. Patients cannot become radioactive through exposure to ionizing radiation, such as radiographs. If a person becomes contaminated with a radionuclide, then that material may become incorporated into body tissues. Radioisotopes commonly used for nuclear medicine diagnostic procedures have extremely short decay half-lives. Body fluids from these patients are not dangerous, although the low levels of radiation emitted could confound and thus force a delay of subsequent nuclear medicine studies for one or more days after the initial procedure. A diagnostic chest radiograph results in a dose of 10 mrem. *(Emergency Medicine, Chapter 155, pp 1517–1524)*

4.a. Neurovascular symptoms that begin shortly after exposure suggest an acute whole-body dose greater than 30 Gy (3000 rem). In addition to neurologic symptoms, nausea and vomiting will occur early, and skin erythema is expected. Surgical procedures are best performed early, ideally within the first 36 hours, to avoid complication from infection, electrolyte disturbances, and hemorrhage. Cataracts are the most frequent delayed eye injury and typically develop within 3 years. Ocular exposure during diagnostic procedures, such as CT scan of the brain, may accelerate cataract formation in otherwise healthy persons. Tissues that undergo the most rapid cell division are predictably the most radiosensitive. Damage to gastrointestinal mucosa leads to volume depletion and electrolyte disturbances and can permit entry of gastrointestinal pathogens into the vascular system. Patients with this gastrointestinal syndrome also have a very low likelihood of survival even with optimal treatment. The absolute lymphocyte count is used as a biologic dosimeter. A 50% decline in the lymphocyte count within the first 24 hours suggests a severe or possibly lethal exposure. *(Emergency Medicine, Chapter 155, pp 1517–1524)*

5.c. The usual hazardous materials decontamination materials and techniques readily apply to management of radionuclide contaminated patients. Efforts are directed at containment of the substance to as small an area as possible and removal without spread to workers or the facility. In addition to the usual decontamination supplies, an assortment of swabs and plastic bags is helpful to collect specimens from various cavities and wounds for later analysis. Specialized materials, such as protective shielding, are impractical for most facilities and not needed for the majority of situations. Maximizing the distance from the patient and minimizing the time spent by any one worker in the patient's vicinity will reduce the radiation exposure as low as can reasonably be achieved. This may mean rotating staff out of the treatment area frequently. The usual drugs used for decorporation therapy are mostly agents that are used for other purposes, such as chelation after heavy metal ingestion. Certain agents that are less commonly needed can be obtained from designated regional assistance centers if such a need arises. Hospital evacuation is rarely required. Ventilation ducts and access doors should be blocked to prevent spread of contaminants outside of the ED. *(Emergency Medicine, Chapter 155, pp 1517–1524)*

6.b. Reverse isolation, gut sterilization, transfusion of blood products, and other supportive measures used for other immune and bone marrow suppressed patients are indicated for radiation exposure victims. Bone marrow transplantation has improved survival among patients with marrow failure. Invasive procedures are avoided as much as possible because of impaired healing and immune function. Biologic dosimetry indicators include the absolute lymphocyte count and DNA analysis. Various whole-body counting procedures are also used to measure radiation dose. *(Emergency Medicine, Chapter 155, pp 1517–1524)*

7.e. Incidents involving industrial gamma ray radiography units are the most common reported to the nuclear regulating agencies. The radiation source is usually a small cylinder containing an isotope that is deployed from its safety housing along a guide tube. Persons using these instruments should be, but are not always, adequately trained in their safe use. Local effects are most commonly seen, with energy decreasing over distance according to the inverse square law. If particularly severe wounds develop rapidly after exposure, then a larger whole-body exposure would be predicted. Precise determinations of whole-body and local dose are made on the basis of duration of exposure, points of contact, distance from the source, and strength of the source involved. *(Emergency Medicine, Chapter 155, pp 1517–1524)*

8.d. Implanted radioisotope sources are commonly used for local application of radiation to tumors. These are generally safe unless they become dislodged. They typically deliver radiation to tissues within a few centimeters of the source, and the intensity of the radiation decreases with the distance squared. Thus, direct handling or contact with the source can cause local burns, but systemic effects are unlikely. In exposed workers, monitoring for systemic effects is prudent. Other potentially exposed persons should also be examined. The patient and nurse have been irradiated but not contaminated, so there is no indication that decontamination procedures are required. The radiation oncology specialist can assist with determining if all of the radioactive seeds have been retrieved. *(Emergency Medicine, Chapter 155, pp 1517–1524)*

9.b. Nearly all modalities have been attempted as a means to prevent uptake of internal radiation contamination. The best option is always to prevent internal exposure or reduce it before radioisotopes become incorporated into tissues. Gastric decontamination is an option, using gastric lavage preferably over ipecac. Ipecac-induced vomiting can mimic the early symptoms of radiation exposure. Other mechanisms used for treatment of internal contamination include chelation, saturation of receptor sites in tissues, dilution, and precipitation into insoluble salts. Charcoal hemofiltration is not usually used for decorporation of radionuclides. *(Emergency Medicine, Chapter 155, pp 1517–1524)*

BIBLIOGRAPHY

Allison LG, Benitez JG: Diving injuries and illness. In Howell JM, Altieri M, Jagoda AS, et al (eds): Emergency Medicine. Philadelphia, WB Saunders, 1998, pp 1549–1555.

Auerbach PS: Marine envenomations. N Engl J Med 1991; 325:486–493.

Berger ME, Hurtado R, Dunlap J, et al: Accidental radiation injury to the hand: Anatomical and physiological considerations. Health Phys 1997; 72:343–348.

Centers for Disease Control: Rabies Prevention—United States, 1991: Recommendations of the Immunization Practices Advisory Committee (ACIP). MMWR 1991; No. RR-3, pp 1–19.

Dire DJ, Hogan DE, Riggs MW: A prospective evaluation of risk factors for infection from dog bite wounds. Acad Emerg Med 1994; 1:258–266.

Fishbein DB, Robinson LE: Rabies. N Engl J Med 1993; 329:1632–1637.

National Council on Radiation Protection and Measurements Report No. 93: Ionizing radiation exposure of the population of the United States. Bethesda, NCRP, 1987, pp 53–55.

National Council on Radiation Protection and Measurements Report No. 65: Management of persons accidentally contaminated with radionuclides. Bethesda, NCRP, 1980, pp 1–213.

Newman JG: Bites and stings. In Howell JM, Altieri M, Jagoda AS, et al (eds): Emergency Medicine. Philadelphia, WB Saunders, 1998, pp 1585–1597.

Tibbles PM, Edelsburg JS: Hyperbaric-oxygen therapy. N Engl J Med 1996; 334:1642–1648.

Yeskey K: Radiation exposure. In Howell JM, Altieri M, Jagoda AS, et al (eds): Emergency Medicine. Philadelphia, WB Saunders, 1998, pp 1517–1524.

64

Altitude Illness, Heat- and Cold-Related Illness, and Lightning and Electric Injury

LUANNE FREER, MD

Altitude Illness

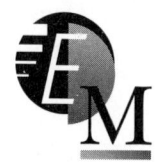

1. All of the following are true about altitude illness except:
   a. It is as common in physically conditioned athletes as in those in poor shape.
   b. The only proven treatment for high-altitude pulmonary edema is descent to lower altitude.
   c. High-altitude cerebral edema is uniformly fatal if untreated.
   d. It is rare below altitudes of 5000 feet.
   e. Medication should be considered only as an adjunct to treatment.

2. All of the following factors contribute to the development of altitude illness except:
   a. Speed of ascent to altitude
   b. Prior history of altitude illness
   c. Altitude reached
   d. Prior medications
   e. Physical conditioning of the individual

3. Treatment of altitude illness may include which of the following?
   a. Descent
   b. Oxygen
   c. Increasing ambient pressure
   d. Rest
   e. All of the above

4. All of the following medications may be used effectively in the treatment of mild altitude illness except:
   a. Anti-inflammatories
   b. Acetaminophen
   c. Acetazolamide
   d. Dexamethasone
   e. Nifedipine

5. Mild to moderate altitude illness is characterized by the development of all of the following signs and symptoms except:
   a. Headache
   b. Insomnia
   c. Anorexia
   d. Altered mental status
   e. Nausea

6. All of the following are true of high-altitude pulmonary edema except:
   a. High pulmonary artery pressures
   b. High cardiac output
   c. Normal to low systemic arterial BP
   d. Low to normal pulmonary capillary wedge pressure
   e. Increased pulmonary vascular resistance

Answers

1.b. High-altitude pulmonary edema is a noncardiogenic pulmonary edema that develops usually on the second day after ascent to altitudes over 2500 m. It can be treated with descent, oxygen, nifedipine, or simulated descent (portable hyperbaric chamber). Studies show that even moderately ill patients with high-altitude pulmonary edema can be managed with oxygen and medication, allowing acclimatization *without* descent. (***Emergency Medicine, Chapter 158, pp 1541–1548***)

2.e. Altitude illness may affect any individual regardless of physical conditioning, depending on individual susceptibility, speed of ascent, height of ascent, prior medications, and history of previous altitude illness. (***Emergency Medicine, Chapter 158, pp 1541–1548***)

3.e. In addition to descent, oxygen, rest, and simulated increase of ambient pressure, medications such as nifedipine, acetazolamide, and furosemide may be considered adjuncts to treatment. (***Emergency Medicine, Chapter 158, pp 1541–1548***)

4.d. Acetazolamide is a carbonic anhydrase inhibitor that causes renal excretion of bicarbonate and therefore acidifies the blood, increasing respiratory drive and PO_2 (especially during sleep). The diuretic effect may also be helpful. Anti-inflammatories and acetaminophen are used to treat the headache associated with acute mountain sickness. Dexamethasone may be used as a last resort for the treatment of high-altitude cerebral edema but has no utility in the treatment or prophylaxis of milder forms of altitude illness. *(Emergency Medicine, Chapter 158, pp 1541–1548)*

5.d. The symptoms of mild to moderate acute mountain sickness are similar to a viral syndrome and may include headache, nausea, dyspnea on exertion, and anorexia. Symptoms usually begin 24 to 48 hours from ascent. Altered sensorium is never present in mild or moderate forms of acute mountain sickness and suggests high-altitude cerebral edema, the most serious form of altitude illness. *(Emergency Medicine, Chapter 158, pp 1541–1548)*

6.b. Only pulmonary artery pressure and pulmonary vascular resistance are elevated in this noncardiogenic pulmonary edema. Cardiac output, mean arterial pressure, and pulmonary capillary wedge pressure usually remain low to normal in high-altitude pulmonary edema. *(Emergency Medicine, Chapter 158, pp 1541–1548)*

Lightning Injuries

1. In the following multiple-patient scenario, all patients were in close proximity to a lightning strike while sitting in bleachers watching a soccer game. Choose the correct triage/treatment priority (in order from first priority to last priority).
   a. iii, i, ii, iv
   b. i, iii, ii, iv
   c. iv, iii, i, ii
   d. iv, i, ii, iii

   i. 36-year-old female 8 months pregnant in labor with abdominal pain and 10% body surface area superficial burns to trunk. Normal vital signs.
   ii. 8-year-old male briefly unconscious and apneic, now with spontaneous breathing and circulation and mildly confused. Normal vital signs.
   iii. 12-year-old female fell from bleachers with angulated deformity of upper extremity without distal pulse. Otherwise normal vital signs.
   iv. 52-year-old male apneic and pulseless with dilated pupils.

2. Which of the following are pathognomonic signs of lightning strike injury?
   a. ii, iv
   b. i, ii
   c. i, iii
   d. i, iv

   i. Lichtenberg figures
   ii. Keraunoparalysis
   iii. Cataracts
   iv. Tympanic membrane rupture

3. Victims of lightning strike are electrically charged and pose a potential threat to rescuers.
   True or False

4. Of the following mechanisms of lightning injury, the most severe injuries are usually seen as a result of:
   a. Sidesplash
   b. Ground current or step voltage
   c. Direct strike
   d. Blast effect
   e. Contact strike

Answers

1.c. In multiple-patient lightning strike incidents, the usual triage prioritization should be reversed for apneic and pulseless patients. Whereas in mass casualties the pulseless are not treated, in lightning injuries, those in cardiopulmonary arrest (patient iv) should be resuscitated first, because a lightning strike generally causes myocardial depolarization, resulting in asystole that may quickly resolve. In addition, CNS respiratory center and diaphragmatic "paralysis" is usually self-limited if the patient has not suffered a substantial anoxic period and respirations are artificially supported. Fixed, dilated pupils may be a transient sign of autonomic dysfunction and not necessarily a bad prognostic sign. Patient iii should be treated next, because realignment and splinting are likely to resolve her circulatory impairment quickly. Patient i needs quick transport to a facility with high-risk obstetric monitoring capabilities; she arguably should be triaged before patient ii because expedient care will be provided to both her and her viable infant. Patient ii may have a minor lightning injury, but the possibility of brain trauma should be ruled out. *(Emergency Medicine, Chapter 160, pp 1556–1562)*

2.b. Lichtenberg figures, superficial ferning on the skin, represent electron showering over the surface of the skin and are pathognomonic for lightning injury. Keraunoparalysis, also specific to lightning injuries, is a lower limb paralysis with vasomotor instability. Although commonly occurring due to electric charge transmission through small vessels of the tympanic membrane or due to direct blast injury in lightning strike, tympanic membrane rupture may result from other causes (e.g., infectious, basilar skull fractures) and is not pathognomonic for lightning injury. Cataracts may form as a result of small tears of the lens capsule from concussive effects of lightning or from vacuole formation replaced by opacities, but they are not pathognomonic signs. *(Emergency Medicine, Chapter 160, pp 1556–1562)*

3. False. Unlike electric injuries caused by alternating current that can be passed on to rescuers if a patient is still in contact with the source, lightning causes a direct current injury and does not leave its victims "charged" or dangerous to rescuers. However, lightning can strike twice, and rescuers should take care to make rescue surroundings as safe as possible for themselves, avoiding tall or isolated trees or buildings, open water, hilltops, and direct contact with metal objects. *(Emergency Medicine, Chapter 160, pp 1556–1562)*

4.c. Although serious injury may result from any type of lightning strike, the most devastating injuries and deaths are a result of direct strike; frequently victims are wearing metal objects on or near their heads (hairpins, umbrellas). The "sidesplash" of current is a result of a direct strike to an object near the victim, who provides a lower-resistance path for the remaining current. When lightning hits the ground, current spreads circumferentially from that strike and may create a circuit between a victim's legs and the ground, resulting in multiple victims of one lightning strike. Blast effect from exploding air may cause injuries from the concussive forces it generates. Contact injuries are a type of direct strike injury in which an individual is in direct contact with an object struck by lightning (e.g., golf club, fishing rod). *(Emergency Medicine, Chapter 160, pp 1556–1562)*

Electric Injuries

1. When resuscitating the victim of electric injury, fluid replacement should follow the "rule of nines."
   True or False

2. Which of the following statements regarding rhabdomyolysis is not true?
   a. Urine containing no RBCs but positive for blood by dipstick is highly suggestive of myoglobinuria.
   b. CK-MB is a reliable indicator of myocardial muscle damage in electric injury.
   c. Mannitol and furosemide are commonly used to maintain urine output.
   d. Alkalinization promotes renal clearance of myoglobin.

3. Of the following paths of electric current injury, which is most likely to result in serious injury?
   a. Hand to foot
   b. Hand to hand
   c. Foot to foot

Answers

1. False. The "rule of nines," which guides fluid replacement for thermal burn injuries by estimating percent body surface area burned, is unreliable in cases of electric injury. This is because the majority of tissue burned in electric accidents is deep soft tissue and bone. In fact, seriously injured victims may appear relatively normal at first glance because most of the burn is under the skin. Intravenous lactated Ringer's is the solution of choice, and urine output is the most reliable indicator of adequate volume replacement; it should be kept at a rate of at least 1 to 1.5 mL/kg per hour. *(Emergency Medicine, Chapter 161, pp 1563–1566)*

2.b. Myoglobinuria may be detected by an orthotolbutamide dipstick test or by the presence of blood by dipstick in the absence of microscopic RBCs. CK-MB fraction, usually a reliable indicator of cardiac muscle infarct, is *not* reliable in cases of electric injury, but the total CK may be a useful prognostic sign for total muscle injury. Adequate fluid resuscitation is the mainstay of treatment for rhabdomyolysis and is guided by urine output (see above); it can be augmented by forced diuresis with mannitol and/or furosemide. Alkalinization of the blood with sodium bicarbonate enhances renal clearance of myoglobin by increasing myoglobin's solubility in urine. *(Emergency Medicine, Chapter 161, pp 1563–1566)*

3.b. The amount of heat generated in electric burn injuries is directly related to the resistance of the tissues; bone, tendon, and fat have higher resistance to flow and suffer the greatest injury, whereas nerves and blood vessels that conduct current more quickly suffer less direct thermal damage. Although serious injuries and cardiac arrhythmias may result from any path of electric current flow, hand-to-hand current is usually the most devastating because of the greater likelihood for current to travel through the heart and spinal column. *(Emergency Medicine, Chapter 161, pp 1563–1566)*

Heat Injuries

1. A patient presents to your ED with a history of syncope while standing outdoors on a hot day. He is now fully oriented and complains of headache and weakness. On examination, his core temperature is 103°F and he appears dehydrated. Your diagnosis is:
   a. Heat syncope
   b. Heat stroke
   c. Heat exhaustion
   d. None of the above

2. All of the following are useful cooling measures for environmental hyperthermia patients except:
   a. Evaporative cooling spray with fans
   b. Cool IV fluids
   c. Salicylates or acetaminophen
   d. Cooling blankets

3. Regarding rehydration in hot environments, which of the following is not correct?
   a. Evaporative fluid losses via sweating may approach 1 to 2 L/hr in hot environments.
   b. For most individuals, relief of thirst is a reliable indicator of adequate fluid replacement.
   c. In general, 500 mL before exertion and 200 to 300 mL every 20 minutes will adequately replace exertional fluid losses.
   d. Fluid losses may be increased in patients who take diuretic medications.

Answers

1.c. Heat illness is a continuum of disease, ranging from heat edema to heat stroke. Heat syncope involves a syncopal episode following prolonged standing in a hot environment and is a diagnosis of exclusion. Other causes of syncope should be excluded, and the patient should have a normal core body temperature. Heat exhaustion typically manifests with symptoms of fatigue, headache, and thirst and clinical signs of dehydration in the setting of elevated core temperature. The patient with heat exhaustion *always* has normal mental status. Patients with altered sensorium following heat exposure have heat stroke until proven otherwise, and other sources of neurologic compromise must be investigated in this setting (e.g., cerebrovascular accident, drug intoxication, hypoglycemia, brain trauma). (*Emergency Medicine, Chapter 162, pp 1567–1573*)

2.c. Active cooling measures should begin as soon as possible in the care of a heat-injured patient. Removing the victim from the source of heat, placing him or her in a cool environment, and initiating IV hydration are the first steps in cooling after addressing basic ABCs. All active cooling measures can induce shivering, which should be avoided. Cooling blankets, tepid water spray with fanning for evaporation, and cool IV fluids are acceptable methods for cooling. However, antipyretics, such as acetaminophen and salicylates, work by resetting the internal thermostat and therefore have no role in environmental hyperthermia and may even be detrimental. Cooling should continue until the core temperature reaches 102.2°F, at which time it should be slowed or stopped to prevent iatrogenic hypothermia. (*Emergency Medicine, Chapter 162, pp 1567–1573*)

3.b. When exposed to heat stress, most individuals will replace only about two thirds of their losses voluntarily, so relief of thirst is not a reliable indicator of adequate hydration. Athletes can acclimatize to hot climates by training for 60 to 90 minutes per day for 1 to 2 weeks, "training" their bodies to sweat more and become more efficient coolers. Many studies recommend beginning with 500 mL of fluid prior to exertion, followed by 200 to 300 mL every 20 minutes during exertion to prevent dehydration. Diuretic use and concurrent illness such as vomiting and diarrhea may increase fluid losses.[1]

Hypothermia and Frostbite

1. The treatment of frostbite includes all of the following except:
   a. Pad and elevate extremities
   b. Begin rewarming as soon as possible in the field to prevent further tissue loss
   c. Leave blisters intact
   d. Rewarm in a water bath at 40°C to 42°C

2. Most hypothermic patients are dehydrated, and the fluid of choice for IV rehydration is lactated Ringer's solution.
   True or False

3. Advanced Cardiac Life Support measures in the hypothermic patient differ from those in the patient without hypothermia in all of the following ways except:

ALTITUDE ILLNESS, HEAT- AND COLD-RELATED ILLNESS, AND LIGHTNING AND ELECTRIC INJURY   351

a. Fixed dilated pupils and lividity are unreliable as signs of death.
b. Lidocaine is the first drug of choice for ventricular fibrillation.
c. Only one round of defibrillation (three attempts) should be made until rewarming is under way.
d. CPR should not be withheld even if it was delayed or interrupted in the field.

4. Chilblains is characterized by all of the following except:
   a. Localized erythema
   b. Nodules
   c. Ulcerations
   d. Response to treatment with nifedipine
   e. Development of gangrene in more severe cases

5. Which of the following is an active external rewarming technique?
   a. Warm water immersion
   b. Aluminum blankets
   c. Heated IV fluids
   d. Airway rewarming

6. Which of the following treatment measures are routinely used to treat frostbite?
   a. i, iii   i. Warm water immersion
   b. i, ii, iii   ii. Narcotic analgesics
   c. ii, iii, iv   iii. Ibuprofen
   d. i, ii, iii, iv   iv. Aloe vera

Answers

1.b. Remove the patient to a safe environment and prevent further heat losses. Rewarming a frozen extremity in the field is rarely practical and may be detrimental if there is *any* chance of refreezing. It is better to leave an extremity frozen than to allow partial rewarming and refreezing because this results in further tissue damage. Blisters should be left intact and the extremity should be splinted, padded, and elevated. The extremity should not be rubbed or stimulated, and wet clothing should be removed. (*Emergency Medicine, Chapter 163, pp 1574–1584*)

2. False. Many hypothermic patients are dehydrated as a result of cold-induced diuresis and third spacing of fluids. Warmed IV fluids (40°C to 42°C) should be introduced early in treatment; microwaving 1 L of IV fluid for 1 to 2 minutes at high power should achieve proper temperature (shake the bag to equalize pockets with higher temperature). Lactated Ringer's solution is not an appropriate rehydration fluid because liver function is diminished in hypothermia and lactate is poorly metabolized; D_5 normal saline is a better choice. Avoid rapid central administration of warmed fluids, which may create arrhythmogenic temperature gradients across an irritable myocardium. (*Emergency Medicine, Chapter 163, pp 1574–1584*)

3.b. In patients with severe hypothermia, lividity, rigor, and fixed pupils may not be reliable indicators of death. However, CPR should not be instituted in a hypothermic patient with a frozen rigid chest, a DNR order, or other lethal injury. CPR should not be withheld even if there were delays or interruptions of CPR in the field; intermittent blood flow will often provide adequate support in severe hypothermia. Bretylium is the only antiarrhythmic drug shown to be effective in hypothermia and is the drug of choice for ventricular fibrillation in the setting of hypothermia. In general, only one round of defibrillation and drugs should be used in the field until definitive rewarming procedures can be instituted, and drug administration should be held to a minimum.[1]

4.e. Chilblains is characterized by development of localized erythema, cyanosis, nodules, and ulcerations on cold-exposed skin. Lesions appear about 12 hours after cold exposure and are associated with burning paresthesias and pruritus. Nifedipine has been used successfully in treatment. Gangrene is not associated with chilblains but may occur with trench foot, which involves neurovascular injury as a result of exposure to wet, cold conditions. Trench foot may result in exquisite cold sensitivity after resolution. (*Emergency Medicine, Chapter 163, pp 1574–1584*)

5.a. Passive external rewarming allows the mildly hypothermic patient to "do the work himself or herself," that is, generate his or her own thermal energy to prevent evaporative or conductive heat loss. Additional clothing, blankets, and aluminum blankets trap patient-generated warmth and allow a hypothermic patient who is shivering to rewarm himself or herself. This is the safest and least invasive rewarming technique. Active external rewarming may be used in mild to moderate hypothermic patients; it involves applying heat directly to the patient's skin by warm water immersion, hot packs, plumbed garments, warming blankets, or radiant heaters. Active core rewarming, used in moderate to severe hypothermia, is more invasive and involves application of heat to the patient's core. Methods used include airway rewarming; heated IV fluids; warm irrigation of gastrointestinal, genitourinary, peritoneal, and chest cavities; diathermy; hemodialysis; and cardiopulmonary bypass. (*Emergency Medicine, Chapter 163, pp 1574–1584*)

6.d. Rapid rewarming is essential in frostbite, and the quickest method for rewarming frozen extremities is warm water immersion at 40°C to 42°C; this should be continued until tissues are soft and pliable. Because rewarming is usually extremely painful, narcotic analgesics are frequently useful. Extremities should be padded and splinted and elevated. Superficial blisters should be aspirated or excised to prevent further tissue contact with prostaglandin $F_{2\alpha}$ and thromboxane A_2. Aloe vera is a thromboxane inhibitor used every 6 hours, and ibuprofen is used to inhibit the arachidonic acid cascade and to promote fibrinolysis. Hydrotherapy and range of motion exercises are useful in the rehabilitation phase. *(Emergency Medicine, Chapter 163, pp 1574–1584)*

REFERENCE

1. Wilderness Medical Society Practice Guidelines, 1995.

BIBLIOGRAPHY

Allison LG, Benitez JG, Dalgleish J: Altitude illness. *In* Howell JM, Altieri M, Jagoda AS, et al (eds): Emergency Medicine. Philadelphia, WB Saunders, 1998, pp 1541–1548.

Auerbach PS: Wilderness Medicine: Management of Wilderness and Environmental Emergencies, 3rd ed. St. Louis, Mosby–Year Book, 1995.

Blum FC, Veach J: Hypothermia and frostbite. *In* Howell JM, Altieri M, Jagoda AS, et al (eds): Emergency Medicine. Philadelphia, WB Saunders, 1998, pp 1574–1584.

Kirkland K: Electric injuries. *In* Howell JM, Altieri M, Jagoda AS, et al (eds): Emergency Medicine. Philadelphia, WB Saunders, 1998, pp 1563–1566.

Manthey DE, Rodgers KG: Heat injuries. *In* Howell JM, Altieri M, Jagoda AS, et al (eds): Emergency Medicine. Philadelphia, WB Saunders, 1998, pp 1567–1573.

Pfaff JA: Lightning injuries. *In* Howell JM, Altieri M, Jagoda AS, et al (eds): Emergency Medicine. Philadelphia, WB Saunders, 1998, pp 1556–1562.

SECTION NINETEEN

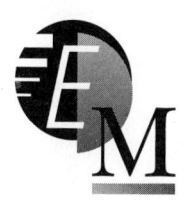

Administration, Emergency Medical Services, and Disaster

65 Pain Management and Sedation

FRED F. TILDEN, MD

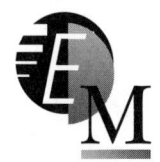

1. Nonpharmacologic interventions for the acute management of pain in the ED include all of the following except:
   a. Immobilization
   b. Elevation
   c. Thermotherapy for arthritis
   d. Cryotherapy for snake bites
   e. Hypnosis

2. Concerning regional anesthetics, all of the following are true except:
   a. Epinephrine prolongs the duration of anesthesia.
   b. Epinephrine should be used for finger lacerations.
   c. Side effects of local or regional anesthetics include tachycardia and hypotension.
   d. To decrease local discomfort, inject anesthetic slowly.
   e. To decrease local discomfort, warm the lidocaine.

3. All of the following statements about regional anesthetics are true except:
   a. Bupivacaine is similar to lidocaine and therefore should not be used in a patient who reports an allergy to lidocaine.
   b. Bupivacaine is an appropriate agent for a complicated finger laceration requiring extensor tendon repair.
   c. Tetracaine is toxic to corneal epithelium and should not be used in the long-term treatment of a corneal abrasion.
   d. Tetracaine, adrenaline, and cocaine (TAC) takes 2 to 5 minutes to induce local anesthesia.
   e. Diphenhydramine is used for local anesthesia.

4. Concerning general analgesics, all of the following are true except:
   a. Naprosyn has efficacy equal to ibuprofen's.
   b. Emergency physicians need not be concerned about opioid addiction when they order a narcotic analgesic to treat acute pain in the ED.
   c. Acetaminophen has anti-inflammatory properties.
   d. Inhaled nitrous oxide should not be used alone for severe pain.
   e. NSAIDs can be effective for severe pain.

5. All of the following are true concerning sedation in the ED except:
   a. Meperidine causes significant euphoria.
   b. Midazolam is the most appropriate benzodiazepine in the ED.
   c. Flumazenil should not be used in the ED.
   d. The pharmacokinetics of chloral hydrate make it an inappropriate agent for use in the ED.
   e. Intranasal benzodiazepines are effective for pediatric sedation.

Answers

1.d. Elevation and immobilization are important interventions for pain management and should begin in the prehospital setting. Chilling tissue decreases pain conduction and is best for burns, tissue swelling, and arthropod envenomations, but not for rheumatologic conditions. Cryotherapy should not be used for snake bites. Thermotherapy is best for rheumatologic conditions, and *after* the acute phase of tissue injury has passed. Hypnosis has been used with good results in some centers. *(Emergency Medicine, Chapter 165, pp 1601–1611)*

2.b. Epinephrine mixed with local anesthetic agents decreases local blood flow and therefore prolongs the duration of anesthesia. It should not be used in an area of terminal vascular supply, i.e., a digit, ear, or penis. Warmed, buffered lidocaine given slowly through a small needle is least painful. *(Emergency Medicine, Chapter 165, pp 1601–1611)*

3.d. Both bupivacaine and lidocaine are amides and therefore are antigenically similar. If a patient reports an allergy to lidocaine, bupivacaine should probably not be used. Most allergic reactions to local anesthetics, however, may in fact be due to the preservative present in the multidose vials. Diphenhydramine can be used if no ester anesthetics are available. Bupivacaine is a longer acting local anesthetic, with duration of action of 200 to 400 minutes. TAC takes 10 to 20 minutes to work (watch for the area to blanch). Tetracaine drops are used to anesthetize the cornea during ED examination but should not be used repeatedly because they may retard corneal healing. *(Emergency Medicine, Chapter 165, pp 1601–1611)*

4.c. Acetaminophen has antipyretic and analgesic effects but is not an anti-inflammatory agent. Emergency physicians must consider the effects of opioids on their patients but should not underdose or withhold opioids from patients with severe pain, because addiction is rare if it did not predate the painful event. Nitrous oxide can augment other medication for severe pain but it is not adequate by itself. Ketorolac has been used effectively for severe pain. Although other NSAIDs have equal analgesic effects in appropriate doses, ketorolac has the advantage of being a parenteral preparation. *(Emergency Medicine, Chapter 165, pp 1601–1611)*

5.c. Midazolam, which can be given by mouth, by rectum, IV, or intranasally, has both a quick onset and short duration of action, making it an excellent sedative for the ED. Chloral hydrate has a slow onset and prolonged duration of action. Flumazenil should always be on hand to reverse benzodiazepines when they are used for conscious sedation. *(Emergency Medicine, Chapter 165, pp 1601–1611)*

BIBLIOGRAPHY

Whiteman C: Pain management and sedation. *In* Howell JM, Altieri M, Jagoda AS, et al (eds): Emergency Medicine. Philadelphia, WB Saunders, 1998, pp 1601–1611.

66 Injury Prevention, Sexual Assault, and Domestic Violence

JANE FEDERMAN, MD

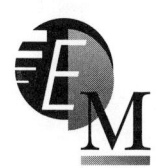

1. All of the following are true statements regarding injuries except:
   a. Injuries result from acute exposure to physical energy.
   b. Most injuries are preventable.
   c. Because they are accidental, injuries should not be thought of as a disease.
   d. Injuries may result from exposure to heat, caustics, and electricity.
   e. Injuries present in predictable patterns in the body.

2. The scope of responsibility for emergency physicians includes all except:
   a. Providing acute care to patients to decrease morbidity and mortality
   b. Performing injury risk factor assessment
   c. Providing injury prevention counseling
   d. Understanding the biomechanics and etiology of an injury
   e. Enforcing mandated legal interventions

3. Haddon's matrix:
   a. Illustrates the causative factors involved in the injury event
   b. Guides EMS providers in their care of injured victims in the prehospital setting
   c. Describes the specific injury findings found in cases of child abuse
   d. Allows for routine screening of all women in EDs to determine the presence of domestic violence
   e. Was determined to be a deterrent in designing strategies to aid in the allocation of resources and identification and development of injury prevention

4. Injury is not categorized by:
   a. Specific risk factors
   b. Demographic distributions
   c. Seasonal variations
   d. A person's hyperactivity
   e. Epidemics

5. Which statistic pertaining to injuries is true?
   a. Approximately three fourths of all injuries are caused by exposure to mechanical or kinetic energy during incidents such as motor vehicle accidents, falls, and discharge of firearms.
   b. Less than one third of all patients treated in EDs seek care owing to an injury.
   c. Only 50% of injured patients seen in EDs are discharged.
   d. More than 1.5 million lives are lost every year to injuries.
   e. Injuries are the leading cause of death in persons older than 45 years.

6. Specific risk factors predisposing persons to injury include all except:
   a. Old age
   b. Drug and alcohol use
   c. Fatigue
   d. Tendency for violent behavior
   e. Proper seat belt use

7. The priority for prehospital care providers is to:
   a. Examine the injury scene and attempt to determine how the injury event occurred
   b. Counsel the less severely injured patients, their families, and their friends to avoid future injuries
   c. Share injury-related information with health and community officials to allow for implementation of prevention strategies
   d. Provide acute care to the injured patient, including assessment, treatment, and transport to a medical facility
   e. Practice primary prevention

8. An important principle of injury control is:
   a. Injury surveillance
   b. Injury may be prevented by modifying the transmission of energy to the individual
   c. Injuries are unavoidable "acts of God"
   d. Performance versus task demands equality
   e. Injuries result from the interaction of three sources of force

9. Findings suggestive of pediatric sexual abuse include all except:
   a. Perihymenal petechiae and edema
   b. Posterior fourchette superficial tears

    c. Posterior hymenal rim width less than 1 mm in knee/chest position
    d. Vaginal foreign body
    e. Thick and redundant hymenal rim

10. Which of the following statements regarding pediatric sexual abuse is true?
    a. Sexual abuse encompasses a wide range of behaviors, including fondling, rape, and commercial exploitation.
    b. The peak age of vulnerability is 7 to 13 years for both boys and girls.
    c. A child's comments about the abuse are important.
    d. Abnormal anal findings are uncommon in abused children.
    e. All of the above are true.

11. When interviewing a child with suspected sexual abuse, all of the following guidelines apply except:
    a. The child should be interviewed alone.
    b. Asking leading questions is preferred because of their young age.
    c. A child interview specialist should be used if possible.
    d. A child should not be forcibly restrained for a genital examination.
    e. Video colposcopy is preferable for the genital examination.

12. Evaluation and treatment in pediatric sexual abuse is directed at all of the following except:
    a. Routine sexually transmitted disease prophylaxis in all children
    b. A pregnancy test and postcoital contraception in those at risk
    c. Crisis intervention and supportive counseling
    d. Performing a forensic examination in pediatric patients presenting as unconscious or intoxicated with unexplained injuries
    e. None of the above

13. Reasonable conclusions that can be made by a physician when there is a lack of physical findings in alleged pediatric sexual abuse include all except:
    a. There was a delay in seeking care.
    b. There was rapid and complete tissue healing.
    c. The child is attention-seeking.
    d. Rape can occur without ejaculation or tissue damage.
    e. All of the above can be concluded.

14. Behavioral tactics used against abused women include:
    a. Economic abuse
    b. Verbal abuse
    c. Intimidation and coercion
    d. Isolation
    e. All of the above

15. Physician responsibilities when dealing with victims of abuse (male or female) include:
    a. Empowering the victim of abuse
    b. Providing support services and referrals in actual or suspected abuse
    c. Assessing an abuse victim's safety level if she is being discharged
    d. Maintaining awareness of abuse in a medical evaluation of all female patients
    e. All of the above

16. A true statement regarding adult abuse is:
    a. Women are less likely to be battered while pregnant.
    b. Few women are killed by their abusive partners.
    c. A domestic violence social history should not be solicited unless there is evidence of injury.
    d. Mandatory reporting laws have been shown to deter domestic violence.
    e. None of the above are true.

17. Adult victims of abuse display which of the following symptoms or behavior?
    a. Eating disorders
    b. Sexual dysfunction
    c. Sleeping disorders
    d. Suicide attempts
    e. All of the above

18. Common findings in victims of abuse include all except:
    a. Fear and shame
    b. Avoiding eye contact
    c. Continuous and unrelenting abuse
    d. Overly solicitous and protective partners
    e. A sense that they are responsible for the abuse

19. Which of the following statements regarding sexual assault is true?
    a. Although acts of sexual violence are defined legally, when dealing with the victim of a sexual assault, it is not the job of the emergency physician to determine the legal issues.
    b. Sexual assault victims are triaged according to their reported injuries; thus, patients without significant injuries should wait their appropriate turn in line.
    c. Based on the theory of implied consent, it is unnecessary to obtain formal consent for the collection of evidence during an examination after sexual assault.
    d. Once collection of evidence is performed in the ED, the patient is obligated to press charges should the offender be caught.
    e. Rape survivors rarely present to a private physician's office, so it is unnecessary in that setting to include routine screening for current or past victimization in the history of a patient who presents with innocuous complaints.

20. Important information to be elicited during the history of a sexual assault victim includes all but which of the following?
    a. A description of any and all acts perpetrated
    b. Use of birth control devices
    c. Any injuries sustained and how they occurred
    d. Report of all sexual history, such as number of recent sex partners and last intercourse, even if it occurred more than 72 hours earlier
    e. Pertinent past medical history, including last menstrual period, perineal and/or anal injuries, procedures, or medical treatments

21. Routine evaluation of a sexual assault victim includes all except:
    a. Photographs in the ED with the assistance of law enforcement
    b. Scanning the body with a Wood's lamp
    c. Colposcopy
    d. Anoscopy or proctoscopy
    e. Wet mount slides to check for sperm

22. A victim of a sexual assault presents to your ED. Appropriate treatment includes all of the following except:
    a. Prophylaxis of sexually transmitted diseases
    b. Postcoital estrogens to women of childbearing age who present within 72 hours of assault
    c. Counseling regarding support services and community agency referrals
    d. Routine psychiatric evaluation
    e. HIV testing or referral for HIV testing

23. True statements regarding rape include all except:
    a. There has been a significant rise in the awareness of sexual assault of women and children.
    b. Victims will often meet the criteria for post-traumatic stress disorder, which over the long term is characterized by psychic numbing, flashbacks, avoidance of associated stimuli, and intense distress.
    c. Adolescents and young adult women are most at risk for acquaintance and date rape.
    d. Sexual assault of males often goes unreported.
    e. Most rapists are sadistic and are sexually excited by the infliction of pain on the victim.

Answers

1.c. Injury may be defined as any damage to the human body that results from excess exposure to a source of energy or from deprivation of essential entities such as heat and oxygen. Although blunt and penetrating trauma account for many injuries, injury is a broader term that includes exposure to thermal, electrical, radiant, and chemical energy. Energy transmission follows the laws of physics; thus, injuries present in predictable patterns in the body. The emergency physician must have the ability to predict or suspect injuries based on the mechanism of injury. Although injuries had been conceived of as accidental and thus unavoidable, they are preventable. Injury is a disease that behaves similar to any classic infectious disease, with measurable risk factors, demographics, and temporal variations. *(Emergency Medicine, Chapter 166, pp 1612–1617)*

2.e. It is clear that the emergency physician provides acute patient care with the intention of decreasing morbidity and mortality. An understanding of the biomechanics and etiology of injury is necessary to perform a complete and accurate patient assessment by predicting the possible injuries and then to guide interventions accordingly. Emphasis has long been placed on treating victims of injuries, with the aspects of injury control and prevention ignored. It is critical that emergency physicians perform an injury risk factor assessment for each patient, and then counsel and educate them in ways to prevent future injury. This includes appropriate referrals for drug and alcohol rehabilitation, social services, and other community resources. Exacting compliance of legal interventions is the responsibility of law enforcement agencies and the judicial system, not the emergency physician. *(Emergency Medicine, Chapter 166, pp 1612–1617)*

3.a. Haddon's matrix is an epidemiologic tool that illustrates the causative factors involved in the various phases of an injury: preinjury, injury, and postinjury. It may aid in the allocation of resources and identification and development of injury prevention strategies. Within each phase of injury, there are host (e.g., alcohol use, osteoporosis), vehicle (e.g., worn-out tires), and environmental (e.g., visibility, access to EMS, drunk-driving laws) factors that contribute to the outcome of an event. Most injuries are the product of a large number of causal factors and are not just random occurrences. *(Emergency Medicine, Chapter 166, pp 1612–1617)*

4.d. Injury can be regarded as a disease. There are identifiable demographic distributions, seasonal variations, and epidemics. To illustrate, the introduction of in-line skating has led to an epidemic of specific injuries sustained during the sport. Water sport–related injuries tend to increase in number during the warm weather months when people flock to pools and beaches. There are specific risk factors that increase the chances of a person's sustaining an injury. For example, patients in different age groups are at different risks for specific sports injuries because of changes in the body's ability to resist a specific injury with age. Contrary to belief, injury is not usually a result of a behavioral problem of the victim. However, certain behaviors are associated with increased risk, such as alcoholism and violent tendency. *(Emergency Medicine, Chapter 166, pp 1612–1617)*

5.a. Approximately three fourths of all injuries are caused by exposure to mechanical or kinetic energy during incidents such as motor vehicle accidents, falls, and gunfire. Over one third of all patients treated in EDs seek care owing to an injury. Each year, injuries claim the lives of more than 150,000 people and account for 2.3 million hospitalizations. Of the 23 million annual ED visits, about 90% of the injured patients seen are discharged. Injury is the leading cause of death in individuals up to 44 years old, surpassing even cancer and heart disease as the leading cause of years of potential life lost before the age of 65. The total cost of injury is estimated to be more than $200 billion annually. *(Emergency Medicine, Chapter 166, pp 1612–1617)*

6.e. Subgroups of the population possess specific risk factors that predispose them to injury. Those at the extremes of age are known to be at risk because of their physical attributes as well as their social situation. The use of alcohol or drugs causes impairment in thinking and judgment and affects reaction times during critical moments. Fatigue can also compromise a person by diminishing the ability to react in a given situation. Those persons with a tendency toward violent behavior put themselves in situations where there is a greater chance for injury, such as frequenting establishments where there is a possibility of becoming involved in a fight. Other risk factors, to name just a few, include poor vision, inexperience, failure to use seat belts, using seat belts incorrectly, inadequate maintenance of a vehicle, inclement weather conditions, and poor lighting. *(Emergency Medicine, Chapter 166, pp 1612–1617)*

7.d. Although acute care of the injured victim is the priority in the prehospital setting, the prehospital care provider is in a unique position to evaluate the circumstances surrounding injuries. Documentation of information regarding the demographics, location, mechanism of injury, and associated risk factors is important in identifying problem injuries and designing and implementing prevention strategies. Information should be relayed to ED personnel for consideration in the assessment and treatment of the injured victim. Prehospital care providers should practice primary prevention as they interact directly with the injured and their families and friends. Counseling on how injuries can be prevented in the future should be addressed so that patients can return to a safer environment. In addition, EMS personnel may be the first to notice an increase in a particular type of injury. A mechanism should be in place to share this information with appropriate officials. *(Emergency Medicine, Chapter 166, pp 1612–1617)*

8.b. The most important principle of injury control is that injury is a disease that is subject to prevention by modifying transmission of energy to the individual. Some of the factors involved may be amenable to prevention strategies or interventions designed to reduce the incidence or severity of injury. Interventions may be educational, legal, or biomechanical or engineering related. Educational programs may encourage seat belt use or carbon monoxide detector placement for increased safety. Laws against drunk driving or for mandatory helmet use by motorcyclists are aimed to change behaviors. Modifications in engineering and design such as air bags, softer dashboards, and improved road design may be effective in reducing the incidence and severity of injury. *(Emergency Medicine, Chapter 166, pp 1612–1617)*

9.e. Digital trauma may produce petechiae and edema involving the perihymenal tissue and clitoris. Labial intercourse may produce erythema and edema of the perihymenal tissue and superficial tears of the posterior fourchette without causing much discomfort. Although there is controversy about the hymenal findings (dependent on factors such as age, pubertal development, positioning, relaxation state), a posterior rim width less than 1 mm in the knee/chest position is abnormal and considered suspicious for abuse. The emergency physician should be familiar with variations of normal genital findings and nonspecific changes such as hymenal tags and urethral dilation. The hymenal rim may appear thick and redundant in the first few years of life and at the beginning of puberty. Girls with a vaginal foreign body should be evaluated for sexual abuse and screened for sexually transmitted disease if a discharge is present. *(Emergency Medicine, Chapter 167, pp 1619–1625; Chapter 168, pp 1626–1637)*

10.e. Sexual abuse encompasses numerous behaviors, including fondling; exhibitionism; oral, anal, or vaginal intercourse; forcible rape; and commercial exploitation. The peak age of vulnerability is 7 to 13 years for both sexes, but physical signs of sexual abuse are found even in infants. Sexual abuse experts agree that the child's comments about the abuse are the most useful part of the sexual abuse evaluation. Abnormal anal findings are not common in abused children. Acute signs of anal trauma such as bruising, edema, and lacerations can disappear within 1 week. Anal findings mimicking abuse may be caused by Crohn's disease, hemolytic-uremic syndrome, chronic constipation with anal fissures, and rectal prolapse. *(Emergency Medicine, Chapter 167, pp 1619–1625; Chapter 168, pp 1626–1637)*

11.b. Taking the child's history and documenting it appropriately are critical to the medical record and for evidence in court. If possible, the child should be interviewed alone, preferably by a child interview specialist. Repeated interviewing may result in further trauma to the child and may increase the child's suggestibility as a witness. The interviewer should not ask leading questions and should avoid suggesting answers, being judgmental, or displaying emotions. The majority of children requiring evaluation are not frightened and do not perceive the examination as a reenactment of the abuse. Under no circumstances should a child be forcibly restrained for a genital examination. For the uncooperative child, the examination can be rescheduled if there is no likelihood of reexposure to the alleged perpetrator, or facilitated using conscious sedation or general anesthesia. The use of a video colposcope is ideal for the genital examination because it allows for better visualization, provides a clear permanent record, and often helps relax the child by demystifying the examination procedure. *(Emergency Medicine, Chapter 167, pp 1619–1625; Chapter 168, pp 1626–1637)*

12.a. Any unconscious or intoxicated child with unexplained injuries should be considered for a forensic examination. Any patient at risk for pregnancy should receive a pregnancy test and postcoital contraception. Prophylaxis of sexually transmitted diseases is not recommended in prepubertal children because of low prevalence. The exception is for those children assaulted by a perpetrator known to have a sexually transmitted disease. The discovery of sexual abuse is a psychosocial emergency. The most important aspect of treatment is crisis intervention and supportive counseling. Referral for psychologic treatment services should be a priority, and at least one medical follow-up visit should be scheduled for between 2 and 6 weeks.

(Emergency Medicine, Chapter 167, pp 1619–1625; Chapter 168, pp 1626–1637)

13.c. There are many reasons for a lack of physical findings in pediatric sexual abuse, including a delay in seeking care, rapid and complete tissue healing, and tissue elasticity. In addition, hormonal effects on tissues may obscure changes. Rape can occur without ejaculation or tissue damage. Evidence of seminal fluid is found only infrequently. The anal sphincter can accommodate stool larger than the penile diameter, and vaginal penetration is in fact uncommon in child sexual abuse. Child sexual abuse often consists of fondling, rubbing, or oral-genital contacts that are unlikely to produce evidence of injury. It is dangerous for the emergency physician to assume that a child with a normal examination is merely attention-seeking. A complete evaluation with the involvement of all necessary agencies and services is indicated whenever there is such an allegation. *(Emergency Medicine, Chapter 167, pp 1619–1625; Chapter 168, pp 1626–1637)*

14.e. Adult abuse involves primarily spousal violence and elder abuse. Domestic violence most often is an issue of power and control of men over women. It is characterized by a pattern of coercive behavior that may include repeated battering, emotional abuse, sexual assault, progressive social isolation, deprivation, and intimidation. The abuser may also use economic means, such as preventing a woman from taking a job or having access to family income, as a way to control her. The abuser uses a variety of methods of power and control to keep the victim within the confines of the relationship. Abusers believe they have the right and duty to control the other partner, and they justify their violence by blaming the victim's behavior. *(Emergency Medicine, Chapter 167, pp 1619–1625; Chapter 168, pp 1626–1637)*

15.e. The emergency physician must do several things when dealing with abuse victims. Essential is maintaining an awareness of abuse in the medical evaluation of all patients. Although the most graphic, trauma is not the only manifestation of abuse. Violence must be asked about when taking the social history of patients. Positive intervention by the physician validates the victim's fears and acknowledges the abuse. The victim must be empowered so that over time he or she feels a growing sense of worth as a person, with an ability to make decisions and ultimately consider the risk of leaving the abusive relationship. Decisions regarding the patient's care should be respected and accepted. Provision of literature and referrals to community support services should be made discretely. Prior to discharge, the patient's safety upon return home or to a relationship must be ascertained. He or she should be educated in developing a safety plan for the patient and children should a hasty departure be needed. Admission is appropriate if it is the only sanctuary available to the victim. *(Emergency Medicine, Chapter 167, pp 1619–1625; Chapter 168, pp 1626–1637)*

16.e. As part of a routine medical evaluation, a physician should elicit, by direct questioning, answers regarding the possibility of sexual and physical abuse. It is incumbent on the examiner to create an atmosphere supportive of such disclosure, especially in light of the fact that domestic violence is life-threatening. Approximately 40% to 50% of women murdered in the United States are the victim of an abusive partner. Pregnancy is an especially dangerous time for women because they are less able to avoid blows and escape attacks, thus putting themselves and their fetuses at risk. Some states have adopted mandatory reporting laws, but frequently these have resulted in increased danger to victims because abusers will often attempt retaliation when they can regain access to their victims. Legal remedies have been in a constant state of change. A physician should be aware of the applicable state laws and the services available in the community. *(Emergency Medicine, Chapter 167, pp 1619–1625; Chapter 168, pp 1626–1637)*

17.e. Victims of abuse do not suffer only from the direct physical trauma. Sometimes a victim may present with multiple somatic complaints, including sexual dysfunction, musculoskeletal disorders, anxiety, depression, and eating or sleeping disorders. An extreme response is seen in victims who present after a suicide attempt. After the initial feelings of shock, anger, and hurt, they become confused and fearful, and they lose their self-esteem. Finally, they develop emotional numbness, passivity, and helplessness. Victims are known to suffer from post-traumatic stress syndrome. *(Emergency Medicine, Chapter 167, pp 1619–1625; Chapter 168, pp 1626–1637)*

18.c. An insightful and effective examiner will be aware of patient cues during an interview. Victims of abuse are often fearful and ashamed and can display low self-esteem by avoiding eye contact. Because victims lose their perspective with chronic abuse, they begin to believe that they are responsible for the abuse events. Abuse tends to be cyclic. There is a tension-building phase of variable length that can be initiated by various factors, often unrelated to the victim. This is followed by the battering episode. Subsequently, the abuser enters the "honeymoon" phase of kindness and remorse. The victim craves this kind of attention from this partner she wants in her life, resulting in "traumatic bonding"; she doesn't want the relationship to end, she only wants the battering to stop. Observing a partner to be overly solicitous, protective, and hypervigilant of the patient is a strong clue to an abusive relationship. Partners who insist on answering questions not posed to them or refuse to leave the patient's side should further heighten suspicion. *(Emergency Medicine, Chapter 167, pp 1619–1625; Chapter 168, pp 1626–1637)*

19.a. Although the history is clear in the individual who presents shortly after an attack and acknowledges a rape, many rape survivors present to an ED or to a private physician's office with a variety of nonspecific symptoms without ever revealing that an assault took place. Therefore, it is important that all physicians include routine screening for current or past victimization in the history, including intimate physical and sexual assault. All sexual assault victims must be triaged as a priority, with the individual's privacy protected by placing the individual in a quiet area. It is best if a friend, relative, or patient advocate stays with the victim for the duration of the victim's stay in the ED. A consent should be obtained early to collect evidence, but it must be explained to the victim that the collection of evidence does not commit the victim to reporting the assault or pressing charges later. To reduce the mental and physical trauma while maximizing the collection of useful forensic evidence, a thorough history and physical examination must be completed with clear and objective documentation of the findings. However, based on the evidence obtained through law enforcement and medical channels, the acts of sexual violence are ultimately defined by the legal system. Physicians do not determine the legal issues. *(Emergency Medicine, Chapter 132, pp 1367–1371)*

20.d. Specific information about the alleged assault for the record includes the person providing the history; the date, time, and location of the assault; any and all acts perpetrated (penetration, objects used); whether ejaculation occurred; any birth control devices used; injuries sustained; and how injuries occurred (weapons used, restraints, coercion). It is also important to note if the victim has urinated, defecated, or wiped or washed the assaulted area. Finally, a review of the victim's past medical history is necessary, including the last menstrual period and recent perineal or anal injuries, procedures, operations, or medical treatments. The only sexual history that must be ascertained is if there was consenting sexual intercourse within the previous 72 hours; any other sexual history is irrelevant. *(Emergency Medicine, Chapter 132, pp 1367–1371)*

21.e. Evidence should be collected in the ED on any patient who sustained an assault less than 72 hours before arrival. Photographs should be taken with the assistance of a law enforcement officer to document clearly any signs of trauma, skin marks, or bruises. In addition to a thorough general physical examination, a careful genital-anal examination must be conducted. The entire body should be scanned with a Wood's lamp in a darkened room to look for dried or moist secretions, and samples should be taken from these sites with a moistened swab as well as from a control site free of secretions. Colposcopy will allow for better visualization of subtle signs of trauma that could be missed with the naked eye. If rectal injury is suspected by history, it is appropriate to perform anoscopy or proctoscopy for a more careful evaluation. Wet mount slides for the physician to look for sperm are no longer recommended. *(Emergency Medicine, Chapter 132, pp 1367–1371)*

22.d. Prophylactic antibiotic therapy for sexually transmitted diseases should be geared toward the most likely pathogens (*Chlamydia trachomatis, Trichomonas vaginalis, Neisseria gonorrhea,* and syphilis), with patient referrals for sexually transmitted disease screens at 2 and 12 weeks after presentation. It is also appropriate to address the hepatitis B status of a victim if indicated. Women of childbearing age should be offered postcoital estrogens if they present within 72 hours of the assault. Information must be provided regarding support services, counseling, and other community agencies that can be of assistance to the victim. Victims should be offered the option of being tested for HIV while in the ED if that service is available, or they can be referred to an anonymous alternative testing site. If injuries or medical concerns do not pose a threat to the victim's safety, then the individual can be discharged. Psychiatric evaluation is indicated if a rape survivor expresses suicidal thoughts, for which inpatient psychiatric hospitalization may be necessary. At times, a safe house may be in order for victims of spousal or other similar kinds of abuse. *(Emergency Medicine, Chapter 132, pp 1367–1371)*

23.e. Survivors of rape experience long-term effects, including persistent fears, avoidance of situations that trigger memories of the violation, profound feelings of shame, and difficulty reestablishing intimate relationships. They often meet criteria for post-traumatic stress disorder. Adolescents and young adult women are most at risk for acquaintance and date rape and at least risk from someone unknown to them. Sexual assault of males is rarely reported despite the increased awareness of sexual assault in women and children. There may be an underlying notion that the criminal justice system will not be sympathetic to the male victim or that male victims are not "real men." Perpetrators of sexual assault are motivated by power and anger. The most common profile of a rapist is that of a power rapist (55%) who wants to theoretically possess the victim sexually to compensate for feelings of inadequacy or to actively express his concept of virility. Anger rapists (40%) consider rape the ultimate offense they can commit against another person. Sadistic rapists (5%) are sexually excited by the infliction of pain on the victim and usually plan a rape of a stranger. Gang rapes are associated with male camaraderie. Last, there are rapists who have a sense of entitlement, such as in the case of father-daughter incest. *(Emergency Medicine, Chapter 132, pp 1367–1371)*

BIBLIOGRAPHY

Linder J: Sexual assault. *In* Howell JM, Altieri M, Jagoda AS, et al (eds): Emergency Medicine. Philadelphia, WB Saunders, 1998, pp 1367–1371.

Olson K: Pediatric sexual assault. *In* Howell JM, Altieri M, Jagoda AS, et al (eds): Emergency Medicine. Philadelphia, WB Saunders, 1998, pp 1619–1625.

Ortega C, Olson K: Family violence and abuse. *In* Howell JM, Altieri M, Jagoda AS, et al (eds): Emergency Medicine. Philadelphia, WB Saunders, 1998, pp 1626–1637.

Williams JM: Injury control and emergency medicine. *In* Howell JM, Altieri M, Jagoda AS, et al (eds): Emergency Medicine. Philadelphia, WB Saunders, 1998, pp 1612–1617.

67 Approach to a Disaster, EMS Systems Organization and Operation, Patient Transfer, and Air Medical Transport

NEILL S. OSTER, MD

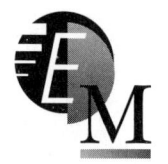

Approach to a Disaster

1. During a disaster, triage tags are used to categorize victims. Which color is associated with "walking wounded"?
   a. Red
   b. Yellow
   c. Yellow' (prime)
   d. Green
   e. Gold

2. The Joint Commission on Accreditation of Hospital Organizations (JCAHO) requires a hospital's disaster plan to be activated how many times per year?
   a. One
   b. Two
   c. Three
   d. Four
   e. Five

3. Using the American College of Emergency Physicians (ACEP) definition of a medical disaster, which of the following would constitute a disaster?
   a. An airplane fire at an urban airport with 200 victims transported to area hospitals for treatment of smoke inhalation
   b. A six car pile-up, with 2 dead and 18 transported to two local trauma centers
   c. An overturned schoolbus with 40 children injured and transported to a rural community hospital
   d. A two-train collision, with 150 "walking wounded," 25 yellow tags, and 30 red tags in a busy city

4. While critiquing disasters and disaster drills, which of the following is constantly identified as a major problem?
   a. Preparedness
   b. Communications
   c. Personnel
   d. Triage
   e. Hazardous material management

5. Triage:
   a. Requires doing everything possible for all victims
   b. Uses all available resources to treat as many patients as possible
   c. Is a dynamic process requiring reevaluation and reassessment
   d. Happens only at the disaster site
   e. Allows the "walking wounded" to help the more critically injured patients

6. All of the following are sections under the National Disaster Medical System (NDMS) except:
   a. Department of Health and Human Resources
   b. Department of Defense
   c. Disaster Medical Assistance Teams
   d. Emergency Medical Services
   e. Federal Emergency Management Agency

7. Regarding the Incident Command System (ICS), all are true except:
   a. It is part of the implementation phase.
   b. It has a command staff.
   c. It collects and evaluates information obtained to predict future needs.
   d. It sets up a clear chain of command for support services.
   e. It oversees the financial section.

Answers

1.d.
- Red: Urgent, unstable, hospitalization, and intervention necessary
- Yellow: Stable, requires transport to prevent decompensation
- Yellow': Unstable, death imminent, treat and transport only after Red and Yellow patients. May not receive treatment. "Greatest good for greatest number of people"
- Green: Stable. Minor injuries. "Walking wounded"
- Gold: Not used

(Emergency Medicine, Chapter 171, pp 1657–1663)

2.b. JCAHO requires activation of the disaster plan twice a year. Hospitals should exercise at least one internal

364 ADMINISTRATION, EMERGENCY MEDICAL SERVICES, AND DISASTER

and one external disaster scenario. *(Emergency Medicine, Chapter 171, pp 1657–1663)*

3.c. ACEP defines a medical disaster as "when the destructive effects of natural or man made forces overwhelm the ability of a given area or community to meet the demand for healthcare." As written, the scenarios in answers a, b, and d would be considered mass casualty incidents, all occurring in areas capable of handling medical health care needs. In the scenario in answer c, 40 children being taken to a rural community hospital with assorted injuries would likely overwhelm the staff and their ability to deliver health care. *(Emergency Medicine, Chapter 171, pp 1657–1663)*

4.b. Communications is the most commonly encountered problem. Many reasons have been identified: poor organization, equipment failure, human error, multiple and incompatible radio frequencies, lack of backup power, lack of standard communication protocol, and varied agency jargon. *(Emergency Medicine, Chapter 171, pp 1657–1663)*

5.c. The tenet of triage is to do the greatest amount of good for the greatest amount of victims. Physicians may have a difficult time with this concept because it is extremely difficult to watch a critical patient die who under normal conditions would have been afforded all available resources and may have survived. Triage is a dynamic process in which reevaluation may save additional lives and may avoid missing decompensating patients. "Walking wounded" should be sent to a separate collection point to avoid congestion and overcrowding of the triage site. *(Emergency Medicine, Chapter 171, pp 1657–1663)*

6.d. EMS is a section of the National Highway Traffic Safety Administration (NHTSA) within the Department of Transportation (DOT). The other organizations listed, as well as the Department of Veterans Affairs, comprise NDMS. The goal of NDMS is to provide assistance at the disaster site, with evaluation, triage, treatment, and stabilization of injured individuals. *(Emergency Medicine, Chapter 171, pp 1657–1663)*

7.a. The disaster response is divided into three phases: activation, implementation, and recovery. The ICS is part of the activation phase responsible for rapid formation of management and logistical units, setting up a command post, and controlling all phases of disaster response. The implementation phase ensures safety and security of the site and coordinates appropriate team interventions. The recovery phase assesses what happened and how the team responded. This phase is critical to the long-term functioning of the disaster team. Critical incident stress management is an integral part of the recovery phase. *(Emergency Medicine, Chapter 171, pp 1657–1663)*

EMS Systems Organization and Operation, Patient Transfer

1. Public Law 93-154, the EMS Systems Act of 1973, included all of the following elements except:
   a. Training
   b. Communications
   c. Financial support
   d. Public safety agencies
   e. Disaster management

2. The 1994 EMT-Basic Curriculum allows EMT-Bs to do all except:
   a. Assist patients with taking medications
   b. Perform automatic defibrillation
   c. Control open hemorrhage
   d. Administer IV fluids
   e. Initiate closed chest compression

3. Under the Emergency Medical Transport and Active Labor Act (EMTALA), all of the following are true except:
   a. An appropriate medical screening examination must be provided to any patient requesting treatment.
   b. Patients identified as having an emergency medical condition or in active labor must be treated and stabilized within the capabilities of the hospital.
   c. Preferential transfer of patients with comprehensive insurance is desirable.
   d. A consent for transfer, stating the reasons for transfer and summarizing the risks/benefits of transfer, must be signed by the patient.
   e. On transfer, a copy of the medical record, including the results of any laboratory tests, must be sent with the patient.

4. The Consolidated Omnibus Budget Reconciliation Act (COBRA) states all of the following regarding patient transfers except:
   a. The patient or legal guardian must agree to the transfer.

b. The receiving hospital must have a bed for the patient.
c. The referring physician and the receiving physician must agree upon the mode of transport and care to be delivered during transport.
d. The patient must be stabilized as much as possible prior to transport.
e. Women in active labor should be transferred immediately.

5. EMS quality assurance programs include time criteria, protocol compliance, skill success rates, and patient outcomes. Which aspect of quality assurance may incorporate all of these elements?
    a. Prospective evaluation
    b. Concurrent evaluation
    c. Retrospective evaluation
    d. Continuous quality assurance
    e. None of the above

Answers

1.c. In 1973 Congress passed Public Law 93-154 with the goal of improving EMS on a national scale. In order to receive funding, 15 elements had to be included. Financial support is not one of these elements. States use discretionary federal highway safety funds and trauma funds to support EMS development. *(Emergency Medicine, Chapter 172, pp 1664–1676)*

2.d. EMT-Basic certified medics may perform all the above-mentioned functions except administration of medications and IV fluids. Under certain circumstances, they may perform endotracheal intubation. *(Emergency Medicine, Chapter 172, pp 1664–1676)*

3.c. EMTALA impacts directly upon emergency physicians and EMS. This legislation, also known as COBRA, was intended to protect patients against inappropriate transfers, improve access to appropriate health care, and deter patient transfers based purely on economic criteria. EMTALA is an amendment to the Social Security Act with responsibility for enforcement delegated to the Health Care Financing Administration (HCFA). It impacts both on the sending hospital, which must comply with the provisions of the law, and on the receiving hospital, which has a responsibility to accept appropriate patients and to report inappropriate transfers to HCFA. *(Emergency Medicine, Chapter 170, pp 1645–1653)*

4.e. COBRA was enacted by Congress in 1986. COBRA violations are subject to fines of up to $50,000 for physicians and potential termination of the hospital from the Medicare reimbursement program. It was instituted to prevent transfer of financially undesirable patients. Women in active labor who risk delivery during transport should not be transferred unless there is a clear medical necessity. A physician who refuses a medically appropriate transfer without good cause is also subject to investigation. Recently, HICFA has determined that hospitals that fail to report such inappropriate transfers are also subject to investigation and penalties. *(Emergency Medicine, Chapter 172, pp 1664–1676)*

5.c. Concurrent quality assurance provides real-time evaluation and immediate information. Prospective evaluation includes training, ensuring appropriate protocols, and system design. Retrospective evaluation is the easiest but may not provide an accurate picture of the performance of the complete patient care system. *(Emergency Medicine, Chapter 172, pp 1664–1676)*

Air Medical Transport

1. Factors that may contribute to hypoxemia and hypoperfusion during air medical transport include all of the following except:
    a. Anemia
    b. History of carbon monoxide poisoning
    c. Flying altitude of 2500 feet
    d. History of cyanide poisoning
    e. Acute blood loss

2. According to Boyle's law, the volume of a confined gas will expand with increases in altitude. This effect is important in all the following patients except:
    a. Those receiving 100% O_2 by face mask
    b. Those with IV solutions in bottles
    c. Those wearing military antishock trousers
    d. Those with pneumothorax
    e. Those who are intubated

3. The etiology of high-altitude pulmonary edema is:
    a. i, ii, iii
    b. i, iii
    c. ii, iv
    d. iv
    e. i, ii, iii, iv

    i. Cardiomegaly and pulmonary hypertension
    ii. Pulmonary vascular constriction and arteriolar hypertension
    iii. Expansion of confined gases
    iv. Alveolar capillary leakage and release of inflammatory cell mediators

Answers

1. c. Because PaO_2 is a function of barometric pressure, as the aircraft ascends, the decreasing atmospheric pressure causes a decreasing PaO_2. The PaO_2 at sea level is 100 mm Hg; 4000 feet, 80 mm Hg; and 8000 feet, 60 mm Hg. Therefore, flying at 2500 feet should not significantly contribute to worsening hypoxia. *(Emergency Medicine, Chapter 173, pp 1677–1682)*

2. a. Because increases in altitude cause expansion of the volume of gas, as surrounding atmosphere pressure falls, IV solutions should be in plastic bags. Endotracheal cuffs and military antishock trousers pressures must be closely observed during altitude changes, and patients with a pneumothorax should have a tube thoracostomy before flights, whenever possible. Oxygen delivery by face mask is not in a confined system and therefore not subject to Boyle's law. *(Emergency Medicine, Chapter 173, pp 1677–1682)*

3. c. Hypoxia leads to pulmonary arteriolar constriction, which may result in pulmonary hypertension if extensive. The heart is usually of a normal size. *(Emergency Medicine, Chapter 173, pp 1677–1682)*

BIBLIOGRAPHY

Benson NH, Brown LH, Bunn BD: Emergency medical services: Systems organization and operation. *In* Howell JM, Altieri M, Jagoda AS, et al (eds): Emergency Medicine. Philadelphia, WB Saunders, 1998, pp 1664–1676.

March JA, Prasad NH, Gough JE: Approach to a disaster. *In* Howell JM, Altieri M, Jagoda AS, et al (eds): Emergency Medicine. Philadelphia, WB Saunders, 1998, pp 1657–1663.

Rose WD: Air medical transport. *In* Howell JM, Altieri M, Jagoda AS, et al (eds): Emergency Medicine. Philadelphia, WB Saunders, 1998, pp 1677–1682.

Smith LB: Patient transfers. *In* Howell JM, Altieri M, Jagoda AS, et al (eds): Emergency Medicine. Philadelphia, WB Saunders, 1998, pp 1645–1653.

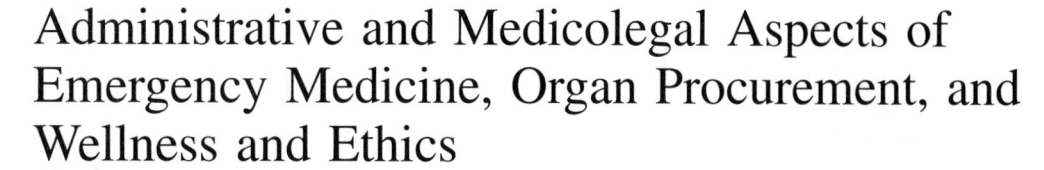

68 Administrative and Medicolegal Aspects of Emergency Medicine, Organ Procurement, and Wellness and Ethics

DONALD BARTON, MD   NEILL S. OSTER, MD

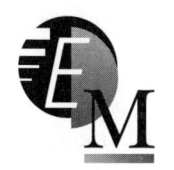

Administrative and Medicolegal Aspects of Emergency Medicine, and Organ Procurement

DONALD BARTON, MD

1. Administration brings to your attention a complaint from a patient who had waited in the ED for several hours for what appears to have been an unnecessary radiographic study. After investigation you find that the radiologist on call was delayed because he was at a party. The best initial strategy for handling this complaint would be to:
   a. Indicate to administration that the delay occurred because the radiologist was at a party
   b. Initiate a quality assurance (QA) project to monitor ED waiting times for radiographic studies
   c. Speak to the ED attending involved and determine his rationale for ordering the study
   d. Have the ED attending involved prepare a talk for the department on the indications for the study that he had ordered
   e. Take responsibility for the delay by informing administration that the study was not indicated

2. Which of the following is not considered to be an essential activity of an ED?
   a. Deliver high-quality, cost-effective, compassionate care
   b. Establish appropriate QA/continuous quality improvement (CQI) projects to collect data for presentation to the Joint Commission
   c. Provide adequate staffing
   d. Maintain effective lines of communication both within and outside the department
   e. All are essential activities

3. Scheduling:
   a. Can contribute to burnout if improperly done
   b. Should always be individualized to meet the needs of the staff
   c. Should be as predictable and stable as possible
   d. Should be fair
   e. All of the above

4. Which of the following is not a likely source of conflict with hospital administration?
   a. The perceived cost of ED care
   b. The importance of providing adequate patient care
   c. The provision of adequate staffing
   d. The recognition of the stress resulting from shift work and managing highly acute patients on a continuous basis
   e. All are sources of conflict

5. All the following are true regarding hospital committees except:
   a. They should be seen as an essential "tool of the trade."
   b. They provide an opportunity to improve relations with physicians outside the department of emergency medicine.
   c. Involvement should be active, with opinions given on all issues brought before the committee.
   d. Timing often conflicts with the staffing requirements of the department.
   e. All of the above are true.

6. Which of the following statements concerning similarities between Emergency Departments and Departments of Emergency Medicine is incorrect?
   a. Both require proper administrative support.
   b. The principal goal of each is to render superior patient care.
   c. Both engage in educational activities.
   d. Analysis of clinical data is essential for both.
   e. All of the above are correct.

7. Which statement about information in the National Practitioner Data Bank is true?
   a. The National Practitioner Data Bank includes reports of all medical malpractice awards
   b. The National Practitioner Data Bank includes reports of all adverse licensure actions
   c. The National Practitioner Data Bank includes reports of all adverse professional review and professional society membership actions

d. Information is available to the individual physician but unavailable to private individuals, medical malpractice insurance payers, and plaintiffs' attorneys
e. Although voluntary resignations do not have to be reported if privileges are surrendered before formal investigation begins, resignations must be reported if they are in exchange for aborting an investigation.

8. All are true of peer review except:
   a. It is a process of internal evaluation that seeks to improve patient care and delivery of health care services.
   b. It encompasses the process of credentialing.
   c. A decision made during peer review may lead to restriction, suspension, or revocation of a physician's clinical privileges.
   d. It is protected by the Health Care Quality Improvement Act.
   e. The process is considered confidential and is therefore unavailable to review by the courts and outside agencies.

9. All of the following statements are true regarding proving of medical malpractice in a court of law except:
   a. It must be proved that the physician had a duty to treat, and there was a breach in that duty.
   b. It must be proved that failure to provide adequate care resulted in an injury.
   c. It must be proved that some damage occurred as a result of the injury.
   d. Malpractice must be proved beyond a shadow of a doubt.
   e. Malpractice can be instituted against a physician who acts as a "good samaritan."

10. Which statement concerning signing a patient out against medical advice is false?
    a. It requires meticulous documentation that the patient understands, and preferably vocalizes, the risks of leaving, including disability or even death.
    b. It protects the physician against liability because of patient negligence.
    c. It should not be permitted if the patient is thought to be incompetent or incapacitated.
    d. It is generally considered worthless by the courts.
    e. It should be followed by providing appropriate follow-up care, including prescriptions.

11. A 27-year-old male is brought to the ED by EMS on a backboard with a cervical collar in place after a traffic accident. The patient sustained a 6-inch laceration involving the face and scalp. He is generally uncooperative with the evaluation process. A nurse tells you that while performing vital signs she detected the odor of alcohol on his breath. The patient becomes increasingly agitated after the arrival of a police officer, who intends to investigate the accident, and the patient announces that he wants to sign out against medical advice. Which of the following statements is true?
    a. Because alcohol is noted on his breath, you can restrain the patient until an ethyl alcohol level is obtained.
    b. If the patient suddenly jumps off the backboard, knocks down a nurse, and runs for the exit during the evaluation process it is your responsibility to stop and restrain him.
    c. If the patient eventually consents to treatment, the police officer can be given a blood specimen for ethyl alcohol level determination.
    d. If the patient's insurance carrier requests a copy of the medical record, the patient's ethyl alcohol level can be included with the record.
    e. If you permit the patient to leave against medical advice, he cannot leave the ED until he signs the against medical advice form.

12. Continuous Process Improvement (CPI) was introduced as an alternative to traditional QA. Problems associated with traditional QA methodology include all the following except:
    a. Indicator thresholds are artificially set and often limit the potential for improvement.
    b. QA methodology ignores the performance of nearly 90% of the workforce.
    c. QA methodology is outcome based.
    d. Most quality problems are not under worker control.
    e. All of the above are true.

13. Using traditional QA methods, all of the following would be useful indicators for study in the ED except:
    a. Rate of return to the ED within 24 hours
    b. Rate of difference between radiograph reading by the ED and by radiology
    c. Rate at which patients walk out of the ED without being seen
    d. Rate at which RhoGAM is not given to Rh-negative patients who miscarry
    e. Rate that nursing deviates from the ED policy on vital sign monitoring

14. All of the following statements about CPI are true except:
    a. It is predicated on the premise that most quality problems are the result of the system, not people.
    b. It can be successful only if employees are empowered to make changes to the system.
    c. Management has no role in the process.
    d. It is iterative.
    e. It must have a strong consumer focus.

15. When a patient dies in the ED, the one true statement is:
    a. When faced with the situation of informing the family of the death of a family member, the ED physician should always be completely truthful.
    b. A problem faced by the ED physician in informing the family of a patient's death is that most often there has been no opportunity to establish a trusting relationship with them.
    c. In order to preserve the patient-physician relationship, it is important that the ED physician maintain as much distance as possible when talking to the family members of a deceased patient.
    d. Because of the possibility of severe psychological trauma, children in the family usually should be told

as little as possible about the patient's death while in the ED.
   e. Expressions of sincere sympathy to the family, such as saying "I'm sorry," help let the family know that the ED physician cared.

16. Although grief is a normal response to the death of a family member, it is important that the ED physician look for signs of pathologic grief. All of the following are true of pathologic grief except:
   a. The determination of what is pathologic grief is often influenced by the family's cultural and social background.
   b. Pathologic grief is characterized by grief of abnormally prolonged duration or intensity.
   c. Expressions of guilt by the survivor suggest the need for further intervention.
   d. Certain situations surrounding the patient's death especially predispose to pathologic grief.
   e. The use of sedating medication for severely agitated survivors may actually prolong the grieving process.

17. Which of the following statements about organ donation is true?
   a. If a deceased patient has a properly filled out donor card, his or her organs can be harvested whether or not the next of kin agrees.
   b. Cardiorespiratory death 2 hours prior to being brought to the hospital precludes the need to inquire about organ donation.
   c. Because of the time required to harvest organs, organ donation inevitably delays the funeral arrangements of the deceased.
   d. Although 90% of the public approves of the idea of organ donation and 70% to 80% of patients' families approached about organ donation agree to it, less than 20% of potential organs are in fact donated.
   e. Although a desirable goal, requests for organ donation are at the discretion of the physician.

Answers

1.c. When confronted with a complaint or quality issue it is extremely important that all information about the incident be collected before any formal response is made. Discussing the rationale for ordering the test with the physician involved is the most appropriate first step, both to determine if there were any management issues not apparent from the documentation and also to determine the physician's understanding of what information he or she expected the test to provide. If, after investigation, it appears that the physician involved had a knowledge deficit about the test that was ordered, one solution is to have the physician prepare a talk for the department. The response to administration should depend on the results of your investigation. Although it would be easy to blame the radiologist, unless the test was clearly indicated, the possible adverse effect on the relationship between emergency medicine and radiology should be considered. If, in fact, the study was not indicated, it would be reasonable to take responsibility for the delay and indicate what corrective plan you had implemented. Although a QA project to determine radiology waiting times might be an appropriate approach to a chronic problem (e.g., this was not just a single incident), the time commitment required and the likelihood of successful completion of such a project should be considered before attempting implementation. *(Emergency Medicine, Chapter 175, pp 1691–1696)*

2.b. As in any branch of medicine, the primary mission of the ED is to provide high-quality, compassionate patient care. With the ongoing changes in the health care system, consideration of the cost of the care being delivered has become an issue, although, after eliminating obvious waste, it often seems unclear where costs can be trimmed without compromising patient care. One area where administration can cut costs is personnel; however, because adequate staffing is essential to maintain quality care, the staffing needs of the department must be carefully determined and clearly presented to hospital administration. By maintaining lines of communication within the department, information can be effectively transferred, both from the bottom up and from the top down. Mechanisms should be in place for keeping departmental administration informed of the problems that the physicians, nurses, and clerical staff face on a daily basis and, in turn, to disseminate solutions to those personnel. By maintaining effective lines of communication with other departments, problems can be openly discussed, common goals identified, and common solutions developed. Maintaining effective lines of communication with hospital administration keeps them informed of the particular needs of and problems faced by the ED and allows for feedback to the department of what administration expects of it. QA is a mechanism to assess performance of the department and to identify any systematic problems, whereas CQI projects are attempts to identify the components of the total system that have an impact on an identified problem and to develop and test solutions to correct it. Although the Joint Commission will often ask about departmental QA and CQI projects, the purpose of QA and CQI projects is to meet departmental needs and not simply to satisfy the Joint Commission. *(Emergency Medicine, Chapter 175, pp 1691–1696)*

3.e. One of the more important job assignments in the ED is scheduling. Schedules must be written to meet the needs not only of the department but also of the staff, whom it directly affects. Although schedules inevitably vary month to month, predictable work patterns should be maintained as much as possible. Changes to the schedule should be made as little as possible once the schedule is distributed. The schedule should be fair, with undesirable shifts, weekends, and nights evenly distributed. Failure to do so will result in dissatisfaction and, inevitably, burnout. Although staff requests must be acknowledged and met where possible, the needs of the department, that is, maintaining adequate staff to provide safe patient care, must always come first. This must be recognized by the staff and to some extent anticipated by departmental administration, whose job it is to see that an adequate number of staff are available. *(Emergency Medicine, Chapter 175, pp 1691–1696)*

4.b. A successful hospital administration is one that can simultaneously meet the needs of the hospital's sponsoring corporate entity, its medical departments, and the community it serves. This is accomplished by providing quality medical care within the budget of the hospital. Medical departments and administration usually disagree over what resources it takes to maintain this level of care, not the goal of quality care. The care provided in the ED is perceived as expensive by administration because it is one of the few areas of the hospital that is always open and requires near full staffing 24 hours a day. Unless the staffing needs are clearly understood by hospital administration, the administration will attempt to reduce staffing because personnel costs are a recurring, high-overhead cost. The ED is also seen as the place where expensive, often futile, stabilizing maneuvers are performed. It is important that administration understands how effective, timely, and adequate ED stabilization decreases the overall cost of hospitalization. Finally, the ED is often the place where patient evaluations are initiated, and although the costs of these evaluations are often attributed to the ED, administration should understand that they are components of both inpatient and outpatient care, and, if properly done, save time and money. It is unlikely that physicians who do not work in the ED, let alone administration, will ever understand the stressful nature of the work done in the ED. *(Emergency Medicine, Chapter 175, pp 1691–1696)*

5.c. Although committees usually meet on a regular basis, ED schedules frequently change in response to vacation and personal requests by various members of the department. Because regular participation in a committee is necessary to become established as an effective member, ED schedules must often be carefully tailored to allow committee attendance. Participation in hospital-wide committees provides an opportunity to work with physicians from other departments and a chance to establish alliances based on common needs. Participation in these committees by representatives of the ED is essential, because the needs of the department may not be recognized by physicians outside of the department and, even if recognized, will often conflict with their own department's requirements. Although emergency physicians can often provide unique insights into many problems, it is important that opinions not be expressed on every issue brought before a committee. Choosing the appropriate battles to fight is an important skill in committee work. *(Emergency Medicine, Chapter 175, pp 1691–1696)*

6.e. With the exception of an academic mission, Emergency Departments and Departments of Emergency Medicine provide essentially the same service. Although Departments of Emergency Medicine will often have more resources, both attempt to provide quality patient care, both engage in community-oriented educational activities, both engage in data analysis to help improve patient care, and both require adequate administrative support. *(Emergency Medicine, Chapter 175, pp 1691–1696)*

7.d. The National Practitioners Data Bank was created by the Health Care Improvement Act to restrict the ability of incompetent practitioners to avoid discovery by moving to other states. It is a repository for all malpractice awards, adverse licensure actions, adverse professional reviews, and professional society membership actions. During screening of an applicant for staff appointments or granting clinical privileges, hospitals must query the database. Although individual practitioners can review their own records, these records are unavailable to private individuals and medical malpractice payers. Although in general malpractice attorneys do not have access to the database, if a physician is named in an action against a hospital and the attorney can provide evidence demonstrating that the hospital failed to submit a mandatory query of the database, the attorney can obtain a data bank report. *(Emergency Medicine, Chapter 178, pp 1708–1716)*

8.e. Peer review is an ongoing process of internal evaluation of physician competence and conduct by other physicians. It begins when a physician first applies for hospital privileges and continues throughout the entire period a physician is associated with the hospital. Peer review is done both on a case-by-case basis and during periodic re-credentialing. The Health Care Improvement Act was passed by Congress to encourage peer review participation. The act requires that hospitals query the National Practitioners Data Bank at the time of initial credentialing to determine if a pattern of adverse actions against the physician exists. It also provides conditional immunity from lawsuits based on antitrust, interference of business, and libel and slander, provided that the hospital acts in good faith at the time of the review. Confidentiality of peer review records is granted by individual states, provided that the peer review process remains confidential. If evidence can be provided that the discussion of confidential peer review matters occurred in public or outside the peer review process, the protection of confidentiality may be lost. Moreover it is advisable that a physician involved in a peer review action not be present while the case is discussed, because although the records of the peer review process may be protected, the physician can be questioned regarding his or her recollection of the discussion. In addition, peer review records are not protected during investigation by various state agencies, such as the Department of Health. *(Emergency Medicine, Chapter 178, pp 1708–1716)*

9.d. To win a medical malpractice suit, a plaintiff must prove four separate elements: the physician must have had a duty to treat the patient; there must have been a breach of this duty by failing to provide reasonable care; the failure to provide reasonable care must be shown to have caused an injury; and the injury must have resulted in either physical or psychological damage. Proof must be at the level of more-likely-than-not, with the preponderance of evidence, that is, just over 50%, supporting physician liability. Emergency physicians obviously have a duty to treat patients who present to the ED. What constitutes reasonable care is determined by a jury after consideration of both national standards and the testimony of expert witnesses. Medicine does not guarantee a correct diagnosis or successful treatment, and physicians are not liable for pursuing one of several acceptable courses of therapy, so long as an acceptable standard of care is met. Damages are awarded on the basis of quantifiable economic or noneconomic losses. All states have laws that provide immunity from civil liability when emergency aid is rendered at the scene of an accident, provided no remuneration is sought and the care is provided in a non-negligent manner. *(Emergency Medicine, Chapter 178, pp 1708–1716)*

10.b. Although physicians often consider having a patient sign out against medical advice as a means of transferring patient care responsibility from themselves back to the patient, in fact it is uncommon for health care providers to escape liability because of patient negligence in this context. Against medical advice forms are considered by the courts as contracts of adhesion, that is, nothing was negotiated or agreed upon, and they are therefore worthless. The disparity of knowledge and skill between a physician and a patient places a duty on the physician to protect patients from harm, even from themselves. Before allowing a patient to sign out against medical advice, a physician must be able to ascertain that a patient has the capacity to make an informed decision. The patient must not have an impaired sensorium or be incapacitated by drugs or alcohol, and the patient must be able to understand the risks of leaving and the arrangements made at discharge for treatment and follow-up. This process must be carefully documented. *(Emergency Medicine, Chapter 178, pp 1708–1716)*

11.d. Although alcohol is noted on his breath, this does not constitute intoxication. Unless the patient is properly evaluated and shown to be incapacitated, restraining the patient against his will may constitute false imprisonment. It is not the responsibility of a treating physician to place himself or herself in harm's way, and after the patient absconds from the hospital the proper authorities should be informed. If the providers release a sample of blood to the police without specific permission, they run the risk of being charged with a violation of the patient's civil rights. This may expose the providers to charges of assault and battery. Although wanting to leave the hospital, a patient may still refuse to sign an against medical advice form. Under these circumstances the physician should still attempt to give discharge instructions and proper follow-up, documenting this and the patient's refusal to sign the against medical advice form in the chart. Since the insurance carrier was informed of the accident, for the purpose of reimbursement of medical expenses, it has a right to the medical record, which may include the patient's alcohol level. *(Emergency Medicine, Chapter 178, pp 1708–1716)*

12.c. The traditional QA process attempts to improve quality by monitoring performance. Indicators are selected, measured, and trended. Indicators can be structural-based (do all the defibrillators work properly?), process-based (what is radiography turnaround time?), or outcome-based (what is the number of unexpected returns to the ED within 48 hours?). Thresholds are selected for each indicator. If performance remains within the predetermined threshold, then quality is considered adequate with regard to that indicator. If the threshold is exceeded, then management attempts to identify the problems that caused the high failure rate and attempts to correct them. Often the problem identified is that of individual performance. One problem with this approach is that there are often no "standards" to help set an indicator threshold (is a 5% return rate acceptable or should it be 2%?), and because no action is taken if the threshold is met, opportunities to further improve performance can be missed. A second problem is that most workers (up to 90%) are never involved in situations that result in outliers and therefore never have an opportunity to have their performance evaluated or improved. Perhaps the greatest shortcoming of the traditional QA approach is that most quality problems are, in fact, the result of problems with the overall system, which if corrected would avoid situations that give the worker an opportunity to make an error in the first place. *(Emergency Medicine, Chapter 176, pp 1697–1701)*

13.d. To be useful, QA indicators should monitor high-risk, high-volume, or problem-prone areas. Data are collected on the total number of cases that meet inclusion criteria (e.g., number of radiographs read by ED staff) and the number of cases that fail the screen (e.g., number of discrepant readings between the ED and radiology), and a ratio is calculated and trended. In most EDs, it is unlikely, in the case of a miscarrying woman who did not receive RhoGAM, that either the denominator (Rh-negative miscarriage patients) or the numerator (Rh-negative miscarriage patients who do not receive RhoGAM) will be sufficiently large to calculate ratios that can be validly trended. A better approach to evaluate this type of problem would be to use sentinel event screening, another traditional QA approach, which involves careful analysis of the index case to determine specifically what went wrong. *(Emergency Medicine, Chapter 176, pp 1697–1701)*

14.c. The underlying premise of CPI is that 85% of quality problems result from problems in the system and only 15% from worker performance. Improvement comes about when the workers themselves are empowered to analyze the system and modify it. A strong consumer focus is required because success must ultimately be measured against "consumer satisfaction" with the product or service delivered. The plan-do-check-act model of CPI is an iterative process in which ideas for improvement are suggested, tested, introduced, and evaluated. Management's role in the process is both that of a coach and that of a servant, providing workers with the resources they need to improve their work environment. *(Emergency Medicine, Chapter 176, pp 1697–1701)*

15.b. By the nature of the practice of emergency medicine, ED physicians usually have little opportunity to establish a relationship with either the dying patient or the surviving family. To some extent this can be ameliorated by involving the family early, for example, by taking the time to obtain a history from them, keeping them informed of changes in the patient's status, and, under certain circumstances, even allowing a family member to be present during the resuscitation effort. Although it is best to be truthful when dealing with any patient, there are certain circumstances, especially in the situation of informing family of the death of a loved one, in which being completely truthful may in fact be detrimental. Examples of this would include a telephone call to the family for them to come to the hospital, in which it is recommended to tell them that the patient had a serious accident or is very ill; reassurance, unless obviously untrue, that the deceased felt no pain; or reassurance that the outcome would have been the same regardless of any earlier intervention they might have made. A compassionate approach to the family, including a caring touch and sitting down when discussing the patient's death, projects a sense that the ED physician cares and can prevent a feeling of dissatisfaction with the care given in the ED. Although it is acceptable to express sympathy, it is preferred to state that "you have my utmost sympathy," because "I'm sorry" may be misconstrued as an expression that the care that was delivered may not have been adequate. Surviving children are especially problematic because they are often not prepared intellectually or emotionally to deal with the death of a loved one, but nonetheless will be aware of their loss. It is recommended that the ED physician advise parents to use simple, direct terms when relating the death to a child and, if requested by family, allow the child to view the body. Excluding children from the mourning process deprives them of the opportunity to work through their feelings and isolates them from the rest of the family. *(Emergency Medicine, Chapter 169, pp 1639–1644)*

16.c. Pathologic grief is the result of an incomplete or unresolved grieving process. It is characterized by grief of abnormally prolonged duration or intensity, often is remitting and exacerbating, and frequently results in personal disability. Guilt is a common reaction to the death of a loved one, because family members often blame themselves for not having recognized the seriousness of the patient's problem or not forcing the patient to seek medical attention sooner. In general, guilt should be discouraged by reassuring the family that they had done all that could have been done under the circumstances. Cultural and social traditions often determine a family member's immediate grief response. Knowledge of these traditions will help the ED physician understand the response and recognize deviations from normal. The death of a child or a spouse of many years, death by suicide or homicide, or death in which the survivor may have been contributory all predispose to an abnormal grieving reaction. Although the judicious, short-term use of sedating medication may be indicated under certain circumstances, in general these medications only postpone and prolong the grieving process. *(Emergency Medicine, Chapter 169, pp 1639–1644)*

17.d. The Uniform Anatomical Gift Act provides a national standard by which adult patients can provide for donation of their organs after cardiorespiratory or brain death. Although a properly filled out donor card technically allows for organ donation regardless of the wishes of the next of kin, in practice, transplant coordinators require their permission. Current legislation requires that the physician make a request for organ donation. In fact, failure to recognize the wishes of the deceased to donate organs or to make a request for organ donation of the next of kin may place the physician at risk for a lawsuit. Even if death occurred several hours earlier, tissue grafts (such as skin, bone, heart valves, and corneas) can still be obtained. Although time is required for the transplant team to arrive at the hospital and obtain the organs, families can be reassured that funeral arrangements will not be altered and that there will be no visible disfigurement to the body of the donor. *(Emergency Medicine, Chapter 169, pp 1639–1644)*

Wellness and Ethics

NEILL S. OSTER, MD   DONALD BARTON, MD

1. All of the following are true regarding night shift work except:
   a. It is associated with increased injuries during the commute to and from work.
   b. Working long blocks of night shifts has fewer deleterious effects on sleep patterns.
   c. Sleeping as soon as possible after a night shift is desirable.
   d. Eating high-protein meals before a night shift and high-carbohydrate meals toward the end of a shift is recommended.
   e. Recovery time from a single night shift generally takes 1 to 2 days.

2. Regarding stress and women in emergency medicine, all are true except:
   a. Patients expect more time and nurturing from female physicians.
   b. Family issues and career demands conflict with traditional home roles.
   c. Nurses expect female physicians to share gender-related tasks (i.e., bladder catheterization of female patients).
   d. The rate of depression is equal to that for males in emergency medicine residencies.
   e. The length of medical training is a constant reminder of the "biological clock" and childbearing.

3. Which of the following is not a symptom of burnout among emergency physicians?
   a. Thinking that everyone who complains of pain is seeking drugs
   b. Compulsive behavior
   c. Acceptance of abuses
   d. Hostility to patients with seemingly minor complaints
   e. Emotional withdrawal

4. Potential deleterious effects on emergency physician wellness include all of the following except:
   a. Dealing with pain, suffering, and death
   b. Negative interactions with other services
   c. Shift work
   d. Emergency department noise
   e. Participation in follow-up of cases

5. Effective stress management includes all except:
   a. Exercise
   b. Healthy diet: low fat, high fiber, and high carbohydrates
   c. Attention to family and friends
   d. Putting the job first
   e. Networking to share problems and blow off steam

6. A 34-year-old man is brought to the ED after being discovered unresponsive in his room. The patient is accompanied by his friend, who had called EMS and who indicates that he needs to talk to you. A rapid assessment reveals vital signs: heart rate 100, RR 14, oxygen saturation 98%. The patient is sleepy, but responsive to verbal stimuli. After ordering an IV and continuous monitoring, you go out to speak to his friend. His friend, who had lived with him for 3 years, indicates that while both he and his roommate use heroin, they were otherwise in good health. You are struck by how upset he is about his roommate's condition. When questioned why, he explains that his roommate does not like going to doctors, so much so that the roommate had been made to promise that he would never call an ambulance if the patient ever got sick and certainly never allow him to be resuscitated if he ever were to have an arrest, saying he didn't want to become a "vegetable." While still talking to his friend, the nurse comes out of the room and states that the patient's RR and oxygen saturation are dropping. As you enter the room, the patient seizes and subsequently suffers full cardiopulmonary arrest. Ethically, you should:
   a. Not resuscitate based on the principle of beneficence
   b. Give Narcan but do not resuscitate based on what the patient's surrogate had told you
   c. Resuscitate because the patient's friend is a drug addict and therefore unreliable
   d. Resuscitate because a written advance directive is not available
   e. Resuscitate because the patient is otherwise well and likely to survive the arrest

7. Problems faced by the ED physician when approaching ethical issues during patient management include:
   a. Documentation
   b. Lack of time
   c. Determination of decision-making capacity
   d. Conflict between what the physician believes is needed for the patient and what the patient wants provided
   e. All of the above

8. Examples of ethical values include all the following except:
   a. Compassion
   b. Distributive justice
   c. Technical competence
   d. Freedom from financial burdens
   e. Freedom from pain

Answers

1.b. When working night shifts in long blocks, emergency physicians state that they seem to perform better while at work but have greater sleep difficulties and use more caffeine and sedatives compared to when they work isolated night shifts. Other problems reported are difficulty initiating day sleep, inadequate time with family, inadequate total sleep time, interference with daytime duties, decreased ability to socialize, and disruption of exercise regimens. *(Emergency Medicine, Chapter 174, pp 1685–1690)*

2.d. Among emergency medicine residents, the rate of depression for female residents is significantly higher than for males, and sexual harassment of female residents occurs at least three times the rate for male residents. The other statements are all true. *(Emergency Medicine, Chapter 174, pp 1685–1690)*

3.b. Burnout among emergency physicians results from a combination of factors, including varying shift work that includes night call, excessive patient loads, emotional response to unavoidable but poor patient outcomes, and continuous demands placed on them by patients, other ED and hospital staff, and hospital administration. Other services often view the ED team as creating work for them, resulting in hostility that is frequently reflected in abusive behavior toward the ED staff. Burnout is often reflected by a change, either abrupt or gradual, in a physician's attitude toward patients and other staff members. Compulsive behavior per se is not necessarily a sign of burnout, because increased attention to the details of history, evaluation, management, and improved documentation are, in fact, desirable in today's medical environment and may represent an attempt at an appropriate adaptive change. Although often little can be done about the abusive patient, when the ED physician becomes the target of abusive behavior from other physicians in the hospital, the appropriate response should be to properly document the specific abusive event and submit this information to ED administration so that the behavior of the abusive physician can be modified. *(Emergency Medicine, Chapter 174, pp 1685–1690)*

4.e. Emergency physicians must feel supported by their colleagues and their directors. To strengthen the support and increase job satisfaction, active recording of case successes should be done. Active follow-up on patients admitted through the ED will strengthen the ED physician's sense of appreciation. For example, emergency physicians can justifiably ask how and why personnel in the ED should be expected to decide in a few hours what it took days for the inpatient service to figure out. *(Emergency Medicine, Chapter 174, pp 1685–1690)*

5.d. Attention to personal needs is an important component of stress management. It has been recommended to adopt a strategy of "my family is the most important thing to me." Work-related decisions can then be made with a clear thought process. Exercise, diet, and networking all contribute to healthy stress management. *(Emergency Medicine, Chapter 174, pp 1685–1690)*

6.e. From the conversation with the patient's roommate it is apparent that the patient had clear wishes not to be resuscitated. Although a written advance directive to this effect is not available, ethically management should be based on the patient's wishes. Given the patient's current lack of capacity, a surrogate decision maker must be found for him. The patient's roommate meets all the tests of an appropriate surrogate: he knows the patient, has frequent contact with him, and has a very clear idea of the patient's treatment preference. The fact that the friend uses heroin does not invalidate the wishes of the patient. The principle of beneficence concerns the duty of the physician to act in the patient's best interest. Although the patient had expressed to his roommate a wish not to be resuscitated, it is nonetheless in the patient's best interest to resuscitate him. Other than drug use, the patient is in good health and has had a witnessed respiratory arrest, with a very low probability of a bad outcome ("becoming a vegetable") if resuscitation is initiated rapidly. It should be noted that in some states, even if an advance directive is available, given the circumstances of the arrest and the fact that the patient is otherwise well, the legally as well as ethically appropriate management would be to resuscitate. *(Emergency Medicine, Chapter 177, pp 1702–1707)*

7.e. Whether consciously aware of it or not, ethical considerations regularly influence the ED physician's decision-making process. Because of time constraints, most busy, experienced physicians have developed a set of rules to deal with common situations faced in the ED, based on ethical principles and their own, as well as on an expectation of the patient's values. Problems occur when rules conflict or do not exist for a particular situation. At these times, it is important that the physician take time to consider the ethical situation that confronts him or her. The physician should discuss with the patient (or surrogate) the problem, giving the patient and the physician the chance to exchange information on the ethical problem and the relative importance of the values in each of their value structures. During this process, the physician must assess the decision-making capacity of the patient (or surrogate), because if the patient (or surrogate) does not have this capacity, the physician, by default, must make decisions for the patient, based on what the physician considers to be a course that a reasonable adult would want to follow under similar circumstances. This process should be documented on the chart. *(Emergency Medicine, Chapter 177, pp 1702–1707)*

8.b. Distributive justice (the obligation to allocate resources fairly within the population) is an ethical principle, not a value. Ethical principles, which are derived from our religious and philosophical traditions as well as social norms, are the basis for all ethical decision making. In addition to justice, they include beneficence (the duty of the physician to act in the patient's best interest), autonomy (the right of the patient to control his or her own destiny), and the sanctity of human life. Values are derived from the application of ethical principles in the real world, reflecting what is of practical importance to the individual. Because each individual's life experience is different, the relative importance of any value in any individual's value structure is likely to differ from another's. Although problems are occasionally encountered when ethical principles conflict, e.g., the right of a patient to refuse treatment (autonomy) may result in the patient's death (sanctity of human life), problems are more likely to result from unrecognized differences in the physician's and the patient's values. As the relative priority of values differs among individuals, there is often no one correct solution to a problem, only better or best solutions. It is important that physicians appreciate these differences and make an attempt to determine their patients' values while explaining their own, because poor communication, lack of time, misunderstanding, or conflict in the importance of values can result in patient dissatisfaction despite appropriate medical management. *(Emergency Medicine, Chapter 177, pp 1702–1707)*

BIBLIOGRAPHY

Allison LG: Ethics. *In* Howell JM, Altieri M, Jagoda AS, et al (eds): Emergency Medicine. Philadelphia, WB Saunders, 1998, pp 1702–1707.

Burkland CD: Quality assurance and continuous process improvement. *In* Howell JM, Altieri M, Jagoda AS, et al (eds): Emergency Medicine. Philadelphia, WB Saunders, 1998, pp 1697–1701.

McNamara R: Wellness. *In* Howell JM, Altieri M, Jagoda AS, et al (eds): Emergency Medicine. Philadelphia, WB Saunders, 1998, pp 1685–1690.

Paulson D: Organ procurement and delivering bad news. *In* Howell JM, Altieri M, Jagoda AS, et al (eds): Emergency Medicine. Philadelphia, WB Saunders, 1998, pp 1639–1644.

Prescott JE: Departmental administration. *In* Howell JM, Altieri M, Jagoda AS, et al (eds): Emergency Medicine. Philadelphia, WB Saunders, 1998, pp 1691–1696.

Smith LB: Medicological aspects of emergency medicine. *In* Howell JM, Altieri M, Jagoda AS, et al (eds): Emergency Medicine. Philadelphia, WB Saunders, 1998, pp 1708–1716.

SECTION TWENTY

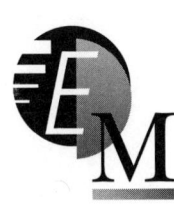

Procedures

69 Emergency Department Thoracotomy and Tube Thoracostomy

SIMON ROY, MD

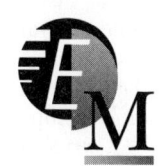

1. The highest survival rates are obtained when ED thoracotomy is performed for:
   a. Open cardiac compression
   b. Aortic cross clamping to redistribute blood flow
   c. Relief of pericardial tamponade
   d. Control of great vessel hemorrhage
   e. Intracardiac volume/medication administration

2. Appropriate technical maneuvers to be performed on entering the chest include all of the following except:
   a. Pericardiotomy
   b. Aortic cross clamping
   c. Local hemorrhage control
   d. Open cardiac compression
   e. Direct cannulation of great veins for venous access

3. All of the following are true statements regarding the technique of ED thoracotomy except:
   a. Incision is made from sternum to midaxillary line along the left fourth or fifth intercostal space.
   b. The entire incision from skin to pleura should be made with a No. 10 blade scalpel.
   c. An intercostal retractor maintains exposure once the incision is made.
   d. Pericardiotomy should be performed longitudinally and anterior to the phrenic nerve.
   e. An acceptable substitute to cross clamping the descending aorta (when technically difficult) is aortic compression.

4. All of the following are complications or pitfalls to be avoided when performing ED thoracotomy except:
   a. Laceration of the internal mammary artery with uncontrollable bleeding
   b. Incomplete medial and lateral wound extension resulting in inadequate exposure
   c. Inadequate elevation of the pericardium off the epicardium prior to pericardiotomy, resulting in cardiac laceration
   d. Esophageal perforation while attempting aortic cross clamping
   e. Pulmonary laceration due to lung hyperinflation on entering the chest cavity

5. Important technical principles in chest tube placement include all of the following except:
   a. In general, the fifth intercostal space in the midaxillary line is an appropriate position.
   b. The skin and chest wall incisions should be enlarged as needed if exposure is limited.
   c. A 36F tube should be placed for most adult trauma patients.
   d. Pleural adhesions and diaphragmatic hernia are potential obstacles to uneventful placement.
   e. Tube placement should be performed along the superior aspect of the intercostal space.

6. Which of the following is not an appropriate indication for chest tube placement?
   a. Tension pneumothorax
   b. Massive hemothorax
   c. Emphysema-related blebs
   d. Residual pneumothorax after chest tube placement
   e. Development of large pleural effusion after pancreatic trauma

7. During tube placement and after careful blunt finger dissection, a well-defined pleural space cannot be defined because of dense pleural adhesions. The next appropriate step is to:
   a. Use more aggressive blunt dissection
   b. Begin sharp dissection
   c. Move the insertion site to a different location
   d. Reconsider the need for the tube
   e. Proceed directly to the OR

8. During difficult chest tube placement, a sudden jet of pulsatile arterial blood appears from the chest wound. The patient is otherwise stable. The next course of action should be:
   a. Place a pressure dressing and abort tube placement.
   b. Prepare the patient for the OR.
   c. Continue with placement through the same incision.
   d. Locally explore the wound for presumed iatrogenic intercostal vessel damage, with local ligation.
   e. Infiltrate the area with lidocaine/epinephrine solution.

9. A patient sustains extensive blunt chest trauma. Chest radiograph demonstrates a 25% pneumothorax on the right side. While the operator is preparing for chest tube placement, the patient becomes hypotensive and hypoxemic. The most appropriate next step is:
   a. Needle decompression of the right chest
   b. Expedited chest tube placement
   c. Intubation
   d. Transfusion with packed RBCs
   e. Transfer to the OR

Answers

1. c. Pericardial tamponade relief has been found to be the most survivable indication for ED thoracotomy. This probably relates to the technical ease of opening the pericardium as compared to the more demanding other intrathoracic maneuvers and also to the usually preserved blood volume of tamponade patients. Penetrating etiologies of tamponade are more survivable than their blunt counterparts, and stab wounds are more survivable than gunshot wounds.[1] *(Emergency Medicine, Chapter 100, pp 1027–1039)*

2. e. Cannulation of great veins is technically difficult from the usual left anterolateral thoracotomy approach and can result in tearing. All the other maneuvers are standard. *(Emergency Medicine, Chapter 12, pp 99–105)*

3. b. Performing the entire incision with a scalpel increases the chances of iatrogenic injury to both the lung and heart. It is easier, safer, and faster to use Mayo scissors to make the final pleural level of dissection. The left fourth or fifth intercostal space yields excellent access to the vital intrathoracic structures. Pericardiotomy should be well anterior and longitudinal to the phrenic nerve to avoid damage. Aortic occlusion can be easily performed by using a fist, sponge-tipped clamp, or custom-made "aortic occluder" to compress the vessel against the vertebral column. *(Emergency Medicine, Chapter 12, pp 99–105)*

4. a. The internal mammary artery is commonly transected when adequately extending the medial aspect of the dissection. This is easily controllable and rarely causes significant bleeding. Incomplete medial and lateral wound extension is a far greater problem, severely limiting exposure. The pericardium should be elevated with forceps (if not already distended away from the heart by blood) prior to pericardiotomy. Unless the aorta can be completely encircled by blunt dissection prior to cross clamping, it is safer to use compression/occlusion techniques to avoid esophageal injury. Right main stem intubation and transient hypoventilation are methods to decrease lung volume while incising the pleura.[1] *(Emergency Medicine, Chapter 12, pp 99–105)*

5. e. The intercostal neurovascular bundle is located along the inferior aspect of the ribs. Therefore, the chest tube should be placed directly above the lower rib, through the inferior aspect of the intercostal space to avoid bundle damage. The fifth space usually avoids both subclavian vascular and peridiaphragmatic abdominal structures. One of the most common mistakes in placement is not performing a large enough chest wall incision to provide adequate exposure. A large incision can always be closed with additional simple sutures. A 36F tube allows both air and blood evacuation in the adult patient. Any previous pleural insult can lead to local adhesion formation. Possible pleural adhesions, combined with a high index of clinical suspicion for diaphragmatic hernia, mandate careful digital exploration of the pleural space prior to tube insertion. *(Emergency Medicine, Chapter 12, pp 99–105)*

6. c. Blebs related to COPD are something to beware of when looking at a radiograph with a possible pneumothorax. One must always be sure that a pneumothorax is present and that the tube is not directed into the bleb cavity (to avoid creation of massive bronchopleural fistula). Pancreatic pleural effusion is an appropriate indication for chest tube placement.

7. c. It is dangerous to proceed further at the same site, especially in an aggressive or sharp fashion. Lung laceration with bleeding and air leak may ensue. The need for the tube should have been determined before technical problems began. Transport to the OR would be appropriate only if the patient had an operative indication, and most instances in which chest tubes are used are not operative situations. Attempting tube placement at a site away from the adhesions is the best course of action. *(Emergency Medicine, Chapter 12, pp 99–105)*

8. d. Difficult tube placement can often result in laceration of intercostal vessels. If bleeding is accompanied by stable vital signs, it is unlikely that the source is a deep viscus. Figure-of-eight sutures can easily control the bleeding. Pressure and lidocaine with vasoconstrictors are unlikely to control arterial bleeding. Intercostal vessel injury rarely requires transfer to the OR. *(Emergency Medicine, Chapter 12, pp 99–105)*

9. a. Tension pneumothorax is most likely and can most rapidly be alleviated by needle decompression. A rushed chest tube placement will most likely result in iatrogenic injury. Transport to the OR will only result in delay in resolution of an easily correctable situation. Blood transfusion is not indicated. Intubation may be harmful because tension may be worsened by positive pressure ventilation. *(Emergency Medicine, Chapter 10, pp 85–92)*

REFERENCE

1. Read RA, Moore EE, Moore JB: Emergency department thoracotomy. *In* Mattox KL, Moore EE, Feliciano DV (eds): Trauma. Norwalk, CT, Appleton & Lange, 1996, pp 193–206.

BIBLIOGRAPHY

Hauda WE II: Tube and needle thoracostomy. *In* Howell JM, Altieri M, Jagoda AS, et al (eds): Emergency Medicine. Philadelphia, WB Saunders, 1998, pp 85–92.

Morgan JA, King JA: Emergency department resuscitative thoracotomy. *In* Howell JM, Altieri M, Jagoda AS, et al (eds): Emergency Medicine. Philadelphia, WB Saunders, 1998, pp 99–105.

Rothenhaus TC, Ulrich AS: Chest trauma. *In* Howell JM, Altieri M, Jagoda AS, et al (eds): Emergency Medicine. Philadelphia, WB Saunders, 1998, pp 1027–1039.

70

Cricothyroidotomy and Percutaneous Transtracheal Ventilation and Peritoneal Lavage

JUDD E. HOLLANDER, MD   ADAM J. SINGER, MD

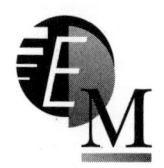

1. Cricothyroidotomy may be considered in all of the following situations except:
   a. A 21-year-old female trauma patient with a LeFort grade 3 midface fracture and blood in the airway
   b. A 32-year-old male paralyzed from the neck down due to a diving injury
   c. A 2-year-old who has upper airway obstruction from a coin
   d. A 19-year-old hemophiliac in a car accident with blood in the oropharynx in whom attempts at nasal and orotracheal intubation have failed

2. Proper performance of a cricothyroidotomy requires attention to all of the following details except:
   a. When possible, the patient should be preoxygenated.
   b. When time allows, the patient should receive local anesthesia prior to incision.
   c. After the skin incision is made, bleeding should be controlled with silver nitrate cautery.
   d. The skin incision should be made in the vertical direction.
   e. The tracheostomy tube cuff should be inflated after placement in the airway.

3. Percutaneous translaryngeal ventilation should not be performed in which of the following circumstances?
   a. A child with angioedema precluding visualization of the vocal cords
   b. An adult who has a foreign body in her upper airway
   c. An adult with a gunshot wound to the neck and a large amount of blood in the oropharynx
   d. An adult patient with a coagulopathy

4. Absolute contraindications to peritoneal lavage include:
   a. Prior surgery
   b. Pregnancy
   c. Eviscerated bowel
   d. Obesity
   e. All of the above

5. All of the following indicate a positive peritoneal lavage except:
   a. Aspiration of 10 mL of gross blood
   b. Greater than 100,000 RBC/mL
   c. Greater than 500 WBC/mL
   d. Aspiration of bile or food particles
   e. An amylase level greater than 100 units/mL

6. All of the following are indications for peritoneal lavage except:
   a. Treatment of hypothermia
   b. Unexplained hypotension in a patient with multiple trauma
   c. A multiple-trauma patient with an altered mental status
   d. A multiple-trauma patient with free air below the diaphragm on chest radiograph
   e. Penetrating lower thoracic wound

7. The following fluid is indicated for peritoneal lavage in a 15-kg child:
   a. 1000 mL lactated Ringer's solution
   b. 150 mL 5% glucose in water
   c. 150 mL lactated Ringer's solution
   d. 700 mL lactated Ringer's solution
   e. 500 mL normal saline

8. A supraumbilical approach to peritoneal lavage is indicated in all of the following situations except:
   a. Obesity
   b. Children
   c. Pregnant patient
   d. Lower intra-abdominal masses
   e. After open cholecystectomy

Answers

1.c. Cricothyroidotomy may be indicated in patients with maxillofacial trauma, distorted anatomy, and bleeding precluding visualization of the vocal cords; cervical spine injury precluding movement of the neck; upper airway obstruction; or failure of oral or nasal intubation. Relative contraindications include known or suspected laryngeal disease, age less than 10 years, distortion of anatomy, and a coagulopathy. Children with upper airway obstruction should have percutaneous translaryngeal jet ventilation with tracheostomy shortly thereafter. Although a coagulopathy is a relative contraindication, if it is the only available option, cricothyroidotomy needs to be performed. *(Emergency Medicine, Chapter 9, pp 79–84)*

2.c. While the physician is preparing to perform a cricothyroidotomy, patients should be preoxygenated, adequate lighting should be available, and the appropriate equipment should be secured. When time allows, the patient should receive local anesthesia with an epinephrine-containing solution to minimize bleeding after the incision. The skin incision should be made in the vertical direction to avoid the vessels that lie adjacent to the trachea. There should be no attempt to control the bleeding. It is essential to establish the airway as rapidly as possible. Once the airway is established, the tracheostomy tube is placed. The cuff should be inflated and the tube secured. *(Emergency Medicine, Chapter 9, pp 79–84)*

3.b. Percutaneous translaryngeal ventilation can be used to establish a temporary airway. The insertion of a needle in the cricothyroid membrane may allow adequate ventilation for 3 to 45 minutes until a more definitive airway can be established. The indications are essentially the same as for cricothyroidotomy, but percutaneous translaryngeal ventilation is preferred over cricothyroidotomy in children younger than 10 years old. The one absolute contraindication is in patients with upper airway obstruction, because the air inserted under high pressure cannot escape through the small lumen of the needle, which in turn leads to severe barotrauma. *(Emergency Medicine, Chapter 9, pp 79–84)*

4.c. The only *absolute* contraindication to peritoneal lavage is a clear-cut indication for laparotomy, such as an eviscerated bowel. Relative contraindications include pregnancy, prior pelvic or abdominal surgery, or inability to insert a Foley catheter or nasogastric tube to decompress the bladder or stomach, respectively. *(Emergency Medicine, Chapter 8, pp 73–78)*

5.e. Peritoneal lavage is considered positive if there is greater than 5 to 10 mL of gross blood on aspiration, greater than 100,000 RBC/mL or greater than 500 WBC/mL, or bile or food particles present. In patients with penetrating trauma to the lower chest or upper abdomen, some consider greater than 5000 RBC/mL positive. An amylase level of greater than 100 units/mL is not considered positive. *(Emergency Medicine, Chapter 8, pp 73–78)*

6.d. Peritoneal lavage is particularly helpful in trauma patients with an unreliable physical examination, such as with intoxication, an altered mental status, or lower rib injuries. It is also indicated in multiple-trauma patients with unexplained hypotension. Peritoneal lavage may also be used to infuse warm fluid in hypothermic patients. The presence of free intraperitoneal air indicates bowel perforation, which requires laparotomy and is therefore an absolute contraindication to peritoneal lavage. *(Emergency Medicine, Chapter 8, pp 73–78)*

7.c. In children, 10 to 20 mL/kg of solution should be infused intraperitoneally. In adults, 1000 mL should be infused. Both normal saline and lactated Ringer's solution may be used. *(Emergency Medicine, Chapter 8, pp 73–78)*

8.e. In most healthy adults, an infraumbilical approach is preferred. In children, obese patients, pregnant patients, and patients with lower abdominal masses, a supraumbilical approach is recommended. *(Emergency Medicine, Chapter 8, pp 73–78)*

BIBLIOGRAPHY

Anderson DM: Cricothyroidotomy and percutaneous transtracheal ventilation. *In* Howell JM, Altieri M, Jagoda AS, et al (eds): Emergency Medicine. Philadelphia, WB Saunders, 1998, pp 79–84.

Coleridge ST: Peritoneal lavage. *In* Howell JM, Altieri M, Jagoda AS, et al (eds): Emergency Medicine. Philadelphia, WB Saunders, 1998, pp 73–78.

71 Lumbar Puncture and Gastrostomy Tubes

JUDD E. HOLLANDER, MD   ADAM J. SINGER, MD

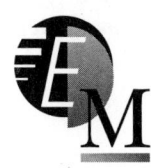

1. Lumbar puncture can be safely performed in all of the following patients except:
    a. A 32-year-old female with sudden onset of the worst headache of her life who has had a normal CT scan
    b. A previously healthy 29-year-old male with severe headache, fever to 104°F, and a normal neurologic and fundoscopic examination
    c. A 25-year-old HIV-positive male with low-grade fever, stiff neck, and a headache
    d. A 26-year-old female with a history of pseudotumor cerebri who has a nonfocal neurologic examination, papilledema, and a normal head CT

2. Which of the following can decrease the likelihood of a postdural headache following lumbar puncture?
    a. Using a small-diameter spinal needle
    b. Using a shorter spinal needle
    c. Performing the procedure in left lateral recumbent position
    d. Having another person support the patient during the procedure

3. Treatment of postdural headache may include:
    a. Aminophylline
    b. A blood patch
    c. Angiography and embolization
    d. Placing the patient in Trendelenburg position for 2 hours

4. Complications with reinsertion of gastrostomy tubes are not associated with which of the following?
    a. Size of the gastrostomy tube
    b. Duration of time since the initial tract was created
    c. Size of the internal balloon
    d. Failure to obtain a plain abdominal radiograph after reinsertion

5. All of the following suggest a problem with a gastrostomy tube placed 2 weeks ago except:
    a. Protracted nausea and vomiting
    b. Free air under the diaphragm in an abdominal radiograph
    c. Aspiration pneumonia
    d. Fluid leakage around the tube

Answers

1.c. Patients with an increased likelihood of increased intracranial pressure should undergo CT before spinal puncture. This group of patients includes patients with malignancy likely to metastasize to the CNS and patients with HIV. Patients with pseudotumor cerebri are often treated with lumbar puncture for removal of cerebrospinal fluid. In this setting, papilledema is not a contraindication to the procedure. CT alone does not exclude subarachnoid hemorrhage. Lumbar puncture will detect patients with subarachnoid bleeds not detected by CT scan. In patients not at risk for elevated intracranial pressure, it is reasonable to proceed to lumbar puncture without CT. On the other hand, empiric treatment with antimicrobials followed by CT and then lumbar puncture is also reasonable. (*Emergency Medicine, Chapter 7, pp 69–71*)

2.a. Postdural headaches follow one third of all spinal taps. They generally develop within 48 hours of the procedure and can last up to 2 weeks. At times they can be more severe than the headache that led to the procedure. The risks of postdural headache can be minimized by the use of small-diameter spinal needles. Some additional techniques that may reduce the likelihood of postdural headache include having the patient lie flat or even prone following the procedure and ensuring that the patient remains hydrated. (*Emergency Medicine, Chapter 7, pp 69–71*)

3.b. Usually hydration and analgesia are sufficient for management of postdural headaches. In more severe cases, IV caffeine can be used; however, it is contraindicated in patients with elevated aminophylline levels, cardiac dysrhythmias, and potential subarachnoid hemorrhage. Blood patches are useful for persistent leaks and are usually efficacious in relieving headaches. (*Emergency Medicine, Chapter 7, pp 69–71*)

4.d. Fistulous tracts created within the past 1 to 2 weeks can be disrupted by percutaneous replacement of feeding tubes. Great care must be taken with patients whose tubes become dislodged within this time period. Reinsertion of gastrostomy tubes should be accomplished in a timely manner because the tracts may close within as little as 1 to 2 hours. When the exact tube size is unknown, it is helpful to know that the size used for the average adult is 18F to 20F. Reinsertion of replacement tubes that are smaller than the original tube may result in peristomal leak or reduction in the size of the fistulous tract. Longer tubes may be associated with more stress at the skin surface, and this increased pivoting may result in a larger stoma with more peristomal leak. The choice of balloon size can be critical in infants, in whom the balloon may occupy a large portion of the stomach, reducing the amount of nutrition that the child receives. Reinsertion of gastrostomy tubes into tracts created within the past several months should be followed by contrast radiography to confirm placement in the gastrointestinal tract. Plain radiography will not be sufficient. *(Emergency Medicine, Chapter 13, pp 106–112)*

5.b. Protracted nausea and vomiting or leakage around the tube suggests problems with the gastrostomy tube. In patients with signs of upper intestinal obstruction, the balloon is one possible culprit. After confirming balloon position, the balloon should be deflated and repositioned. Fluid leakage around the tube can occur from gastric outlet obstruction, using a tube that is so long that it causes pressure on the skin with widening of the stomal opening, or obstruction of the tube itself. Aspiration pneumonia can occur from feeding volumes that are too large or tube positioning in the esophagus. Free air can be detected under the diaphragm for several weeks after gastrostomy tube placement. *(Emergency Medicine, Chapter 13, pp 106–112)*

BIBLIOGRAPHY

Kenders K: Gastric tube management. *In* Howell JM, Altieri M, Jagoda AS, et al (eds): Emergency Medicine. Philadelphia, WB Saunders, 1998, pp 106–112.

Salik RM: Lumbar puncture. *In* Howell JM, Altieri M, Jagoda AS, et al (eds): Emergency Medicine. Philadelphia, WB Saunders, 1998, pp 69–71.

72 Percutaneous Central Venous Catheterization and Pericardiocentesis

ADAM J. SINGER, MD   JUDD E. HOLLANDER, MD

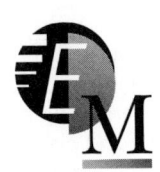

1. Which of the following concerning the mechanics of flow through intravenous catheters is true?
    a. The larger the catheter diameter, the faster the flow.
    b. The longer the catheter, the slower the flow.
    c. The higher the viscosity of the infused fluid, the lower the flow.
    d. Catheter diameter is the critical dimension concerning flow.
    e. All of the above are true.

2. Select the best approach for central venous cannulation in the following case presentations.
    i. Subclavian vein approach
    ii. Internal jugular vein approach
    iii. Femoral vein approach

    a. A young cardiac arrest patient who was intubated by EMS prior to ED arrival who presents with ongoing CPR and inability to cannulate peripheral veins.
    b. An awake patient with an isolated midcervical spine fracture who might need to have endotracheal intubation to support respirations in the near future.
    c. A victim of major upper torso trauma who simultaneously requires intubation and bilateral tube thoracostomy.
    d. A 32-year-old female with primary pulmonary hypertension on chronic warfarin therapy in whom peripheral access cannot be established.

3. Which of the following signs is considered most pathognomonic of a pericardial tamponade?
    a. Hypotension
    b. Muffled heart sounds
    c. Elevated central venous pressure
    d. Electrical alternans
    e. Pulses alternans

4. All of the following are causes of cardiac tamponade except:
    a. Trauma
    b. Malignancy
    c. Tuberculosis
    d. Renal failure
    e. Myocarditis

5. Which of the following pairs of approaches and positions for pericardiocentesis is most appropriate?
    a. Subxiphoid approach—supine
    b. Parasternal approach—sitting up 45 degrees
    c. Subxiphoid approach—sitting up 45 degrees
    d. Apical approach—in left lateral decubitus position
    e. Apical approach—supine

6. Complications of pericardiocentesis include all of the following except:
    a. Pneumothorax
    b. Laceration of a coronary artery
    c. Perforation of the stomach
    d. Cardiac tamponade
    e. All are complications

7. Considering pericardiocentesis, which statement is most correct?
    a. Endocardial contact is recognized by ST and/or PR segment elevation on the V lead of the ECG.
    b. Aspiration of clotting blood usually originates from the right ventricle.
    c. Aspiration of nonclotting blood is nondiagnostic.
    d. Pericardiocentesis is absolutely contraindicated in all patients with coagulopathy.
    e. The Seldinger technique is not recommended for insertion of a soft catheter.

Answers

1.e. Flow through a tube is expressed using Poiseuille's law.

$$\text{Flow} = \frac{\text{Pi (radius)}^4 \times \text{(pressure gradient across the device)}}{8 \text{ (viscosity)} \times \text{(length)}}$$

The largest determinant of the speed of flow is the radius of the catheter. Flow is directly related to the catheter radius, whereas it is inversely related to the viscosity and length of the catheter. As a result, short, large-bore catheters are ideal when large volumes of fluid need to be rapidly administered. Conversely, long, narrow-lumen catheters, like some triple lumen catheters, are poorly suited for rapid fluid administration. *(Emergency Medicine, Chapter 6, pp 61–68)*

2.a. ii; b. i; c. iii; d. iii. The internal jugular vein can usually be cannulated while CPR is in progress. The internal jugular approach is preferred over subclavian vein catheterization while CPR is being performed because it has a lower complication rate and a higher success rate. Theoretical advantages over the femoral route are the delivery of high doses of cardioactive medications directly into the heart. In patients requiring active airway management, the subclavian approach would be preferred because rotation and positioning of the neck with the internal jugular approach make intubation and cervical spine immobilization more difficult. The femoral approach provides successful access to the central circulation when the patient may require many upper torso and airway procedures at the same time. In addition, it is the only compressible central vein, making it the route of choice in patients with coagulation disorders. *(Emergency Medicine, Chapter 6, pp 61–68)*

3.d. The classic findings of cardiac tamponade were first described by Beck and include hypotension, distended neck veins, and muffled heart sounds. However, only one third of patients with traumatic tamponade present with this triad. Additional findings include pulsus paradoxus and an enlarged cardiac silhouette on chest radiograph. Although uncommon, electrical alternans of the P wave, QRS complex, and T wave is virtually pathognomonic of cardiac tamponade. *(Emergency Medicine, Chapter 11, pp 93–98)*

4.e. The three most common causes of cardiac tamponade are neoplastic disease, idiopathic pericarditis, and uremia. Other causes include trauma, open heart surgery, and coagulopathies. Myocarditis is not a cause of cardiac tamponade. *(Emergency Medicine, Chapter 11, pp 93–98)*

5.c. Although there are several approaches to pericardiocentesis, the safest route is the subxiphoid approach because it avoids the pleura, coronary arteries, and internal mammary artery. By sitting the patient at an angle of 45 degrees, the heart is brought closer to the anterior chest wall. *(Emergency Medicine, Chapter 11, pp 93–98)*

6.e. Pericardiocentesis is not a benign procedure and has many potential complications, including puncture of the heart with hemopericardium, pneumothorax, injury to surrounding organs such as the stomach and colon, and laceration of a coronary or internal mammary artery. As with any invasive procedure, there is also a risk of introducing infection. *(Emergency Medicine, Chapter 11, pp 93–98)*

7.b. When performing pericardiocentesis, the metal hub of the needle should be attached to an alligator clip and the V lead of an ECG. Epicardial contact is recognized by the presence of ST and/or PR segment elevation or ectopic beats. Blood in the pericardium does not usually clot because it has undergone fibrinolysis, whereas blood from the right ventricular chamber usually clots. Coagulopathy is a *relative* contraindication to pericardiocentesis. In the hemodynamically compromised patient, this procedure may be lifesaving. *(Emergency Medicine, Chapter 11, pp 93–98)*

BIBLIOGRAPHY

Rodriguez M: Pericardiocentesis. *In* Howell JM, Altieri M, Jagoda AS, et al (eds): Emergency Medicine. Philadelphia, WB Saunders, 1998, pp 93–98.

Younger JG, Dronen SC: Percutaneous central venous catheterization. *In* Howell JM, Altieri M, Jagoda AS, et al (eds): Emergency Medicine. Philadelphia, WB Saunders, 1998, pp 61–68.

73. Joint Aspiration, Major Joint Reduction, and Intraosseous Infusion

ADAM J. SINGER, MD   JUDD E. HOLLANDER, MD

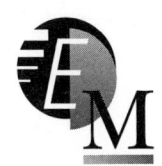

1. Which of the following conditions is an absolute contraindication to arthrocentesis?
   a. Bleeding diathesis
   b. Infection overlying the joint
   c. Oral anticoagulation
   d. Oral antimicrobials
   e. Allergy to local anesthetics

2. Which of the following pairs describes the preferred positioning for specific joint aspirations?
   a. Shoulder—internally rotated
   b. Knee—flexed at 90 degrees
   c. Elbow—flexed at 90 degrees
   d. Ankle—foot in dorsal flexion
   e. Wrist—hand in 60 to 90 degrees of dorsal flexion

3. The knee joint may be aspirated from which of the following approaches?
   a. The medial aspect of the inferior patella border
   b. The lateral aspect of the patella
   c. The infrapatellar ligament
   d. The medial aspect of the midportion of the patella
   e. All of the above

4. Which of the following positions of the extremities are common in major joint dislocations?
   a. Abduction and external rotation of the shoulder with anterior dislocation
   b. Internal rotation and adduction of the shoulder with anterior dislocation
   c. Flexion of the elbow with anterior dislocation
   d. Shortening and external rotation of the leg with posterior hip dislocation
   e. Medial displacement of the patella with patellar dislocation

5. In which of the following situations should the joint be reduced immediately, prior to obtaining radiographic confirmation?
   a. Recurrent anterior dislocation of the shoulder
   b. Lateral dislocation of the patella
   c. Posterior dislocation of the hip
   d. Elbow dislocation associated with a supracondylar fracture
   e. Ankle dislocation with a cool foot and no palpable foot pulse

6. Which of the following methods is not recommended for reduction of an anterior dislocation of the shoulder?
   a. Stimson's technique
   b. Scapular manipulation
   c. Hippocratic technique
   d. Traction-countertraction
   e. All of the above methods are appropriate

7. All of the following are true about IO line placement in the proximal tibia except:
   a. It usually requires less than 5 minutes to perform.
   b. It is done over the anteromedial surface, 1 to 3 cm below the tibial tuberosity.
   c. It can be done in a 10-year-old male in cardiac arrest.
   d. It should not be performed on the side of a femur fracture.
   e. Bone marrow aspiration is not necessary to confirm placement.

8. All of the following are reported complications of IO infusions except:
   a. Osteomyelitis
   b. Mediastinitis
   c. Subcutaneous extravasation of fluids
   d. Local infection
   e. Fat embolism

Answers

1.b. Although bleeding disorders and oral anticoagulation are relative contraindications to arthrocentesis, only an overlying infection is an absolute contraindication to joint aspiration because of the risk of introducing an infection. *(Emergency Medicine, Chapter 15, pp 117–119)*

2.c. In order to facilitate joint aspiration, the elbow should be held at 90 degrees of flexion. The shoulder should be held in the neutral position and the knee should be fully extended or only slightly flexed. For ankle joint aspiration, the foot should be held in plantar flexion. Wrist joint aspiration is performed with the wrist held in 20 to 30 degrees of flexion. *(Emergency Medicine, Chapter 15, pp 117–119)*

3.e. Although the preferred approach to the knee joint is through the medial aspect of the joint, the joint may be aspirated from the medial, the lateral, or the inferior aspect. *(Emergency Medicine, Chapter 15, pp 117–119)*

4.a. The most common major joint dislocation is an anterior dislocation of the shoulder in which the arm is usually held in abduction and external rotation. Posterior dislocation of the shoulder, in which the arm is usually adducted and internally rotated, is rare. The elbow is usually dislocated posteriorly with flexion at an angle of 90 degrees. Most hip dislocations are posterior and the leg is internally rotated and shortened. *(Emergency Medicine, Chapter 16, pp 120–125)*

5.e. Many dislocations of major joints may be associated with fractures. Therefore, radiographic confirmation should be obtained in all cases before attempting reduction except where there is vascular compromise such as with an ankle dislocation with a cool and pulseless foot. In this case, the joint must be reduced prior to radiography. *(Emergency Medicine, Chapter 16, pp 120–125)*

6.c. Anterior dislocation of the shoulder is the most common major joint dislocation. It may be reduced by many methods such as placing the patient prone and attaching a 10-pound weight to the wrist, medial rotation of the scapular tip with the patient sitting or prone, and traction-countertraction with traction of the affected arm while an assistant applies countertraction with a sheet wrapped around the chest. The Hippocratic method, in which the physician's foot is placed in the patient's axilla, is not recommended because it is associated with neurovascular complications. *(Emergency Medicine, Chapter 16, pp 120–125)*

7.c. Intraosseous infusion is indicated when immediate IV access is necessary and there is inability to obtain peripheral IV access. The proximal tibia is the most commonly used site and can be used in children until 6 years of age. After 6 years of age the tibia becomes significantly less vascular and should not be used. Once the stylet is removed, bone marrow usually can be aspirated. In cases where marrow cannot be aspirated but saline is easily flushed through, placement is usually correct. *(Emergency Medicine, Chapter 14, pp 113–116)*

8.e. The most common complication of IO infusion is local infection (3.7%). Osteomyelitis occurs at a rate of 0.7%. This usually occurs when there is prolonged infusion or when placement is done in a bacteremic patient. Sternal IO infusions can be done in adults although it is not recommended in children. Posterior sternal puncture may cause mediastinitis. Extravasation of fluid can occur anywhere there is a break in the cortex of the bone, at holes from previous unsuccessful attempts, or fracture sites. Compartment syndromes have been reported from significant extravasation of fluid. Fat embolism without any clinical significance has been reported in dogs. There have been no reported cases in humans. *(Emergency Medicine, Chapter 14, pp 113–116)*

BIBLIOGRAPHY

Druckenbrod GG, Bishow RM: Major joint reduction. *In* Howell JM, Altieri M, Jagoda AS, et al (eds): Emergency Medicine. Philadelphia, WB Saunders, 1998, pp 120–125.

Eljaiek LF Jr: Arthrocentesis. *In* Howell JM, Altieri M, Jagoda AS, et al (eds): Emergency Medicine. Philadelphia, WB Saunders, 1998, pp 117–119.

Ross PA: Intraosseous infusion. *In* Howell JM, Altieri M, Jagoda AS, et al (eds): Emergency Medicine. Philadelphia, WB Saunders, 1998, pp 113–116.

INDEX

Note: Page numbers in *italics* refer to illustrations.

AAA (abdominal aortic aneurysm), 46, 48
Abdomen, pain in, transmission of, 75, 76
  radiographic findings in, 75, 76
  trauma to, 261–265
Abdominal aortic aneurysm (AAA), 46, 48
Abortion, 302–303, 304
Abrasions, corneal, 145, 148
Abruptio placentae, 301, 305
  signs of, 273, 274
Abscess(es), alveolar, 163, 167
  anorectal, 89, 91
  hepatic, 79, 80
  perianal, treatment of, 89, 91
  periapical, 163, 164, 167
  perinephric, 212, 215
  peritonsillar, 158, 161
  pharyngeal, 157, 159
  renal, 212, 215
  retropharyngeal, 158, 160, 161
  tubo-ovarian, 310
Absence seizures, 204, 206
Abuse, child, historical/radiographic findings in, 293, 295–296
  injuries prompting investigation for, 272, 273
  pediatric rheumatologic disease confused with, 118, 121
  sexual, 357–358, 360–361
  elder, 361
  sexual. See *Sexual abuse/assault.*
  spousal, 361
  substance, 238–240
Acetaminophen, for altitude illness, 347
  hepatotoxicity of, 318, 319
  overdose of, 79, 80, 317–318, 318, 319
Acetazolamide, for altitude illness, 347
Acetic acid, compresses with, for *Pseudomonas* folliculitis, 228, 229
  for cerumen removal, 152, 154
Acidosis, in painful sickle cell crises, 180, 181
  metabolic, in asthma, 67, 68
  in diabetic ketoacidosis, 135, 138
  respiratory, COPD management and, 64, 65, 66
  in asthma, 67, 68
Acne, 223, 225
Acoustic neuromas, 154
Acquired immunodeficiency syndrome (AIDS), 99–101
Acyclovir, for Ramsay Hunt syndrome, 152, 154
Adenosine, for pediatric SVT, 7, 9
  for ventricular tachycardia, 35, 39
  interactions with, 32, 37
Adenovirus infection, 161
Administrative aspects, of emergency medicine, 367, 369
Adrenal crisis, 135, 136, 138, 139
Adrenal insufficiency, 135, 136, 138–139
Adrenaline, in topical anesthetic, 277, 278

Adrenalitis, autoimmune, primary adrenal insufficiency from, 135, 138
Adriamycin, cardiotoxicity from, 173, 176
Afterload, medications reducing, 28, 30
Agitated patient, 234–235, 236
AIDS (acquired immunodeficiency syndrome), 99–101
Air, cold, asthma and, 67, 68
Air embolism, hyperbaric oxygen therapy for, 343
  pulmonary, 62, 63
Air medical transport, 365–366
Airway, esophageal gastric tube, 15, 16–17
  esophageal obturator, 15, 16–17
  hyperactivity of, in bronchopulmonary dysplasia, 69, 70
  injury to, 254, 255
  management of, 15–18
  obstruction of, in anaphylaxis, 123, 124
    with mandibular fracture, jaw thrust maneuver in, 15, 16
  oropharyngeal, size of, 15, 16
  pediatric, 6, 7–8, 271, 272
    vs. adult, 159, 162
  pharyngotracheal lumen, contraindications to, 15, 17
  suctioning of, 15, 16
  upper, obstruction of, in generalized tonic-clonic seizures, 159, 162
  sudden, 157, 160
Albuterol sulfate, in emergency asthma management, 67, 68
Alcohol, abuse of, 238–240
  frequent intake of, gastrointestinal bleeding and, 83, 85
  intoxication with, precipitating sickle cell crisis, 180, 182
  withdrawal of, seizures from, 203, 205
Alcoholic ketoacidosis, 137, 141
Allergic conjunctivitis, 146, 149
Allergic reactions, 123–125
  to IV contrast agents, 218, 219
Allergy, procaine, medications safe in, 277, 278
Allopurinol, for tumor lysis syndrome, 174, 177
Alpha$_1$-protease deficiency, COPD and, 64, 65
Altitude illness, 347–348
Aluminum hydroxide antacids, for tumor lysis syndrome, 174, 177
Alveolar abscess, 163, 167
Alveolar bone, tooth impacted into, 165, 168
Alveolar osteitis, 164, 167
Alveolar ridge, to midtrachea, distance calculation of, for pediatric patient, 15, 17
Alzheimer's disease, psychosis in, 233, 235
Amatoxin, liver failure and, 329, 330–331
Amaurosis fugax, 197, 198
Amniotic fluid, pulmonary embolism and, 62, 63
Amoxicillin, bacteria resistant to, otitis media from, 151–152, 154

Amoxicillin-clavulanic acid, for human bite prophylaxis, 339, 340
Amphotericin B, for mucormycosis, 151, 153
Ampicillin, *Clostridium difficile* overgrowth from, 75, 77
  for perforated appendix, 84, 86
Amputated finger, replantation of, 286, 288
Amylase, serum, in pancreatitis, 79, 81
Amyloidosis, complicating multiple myeloma, 173, 175–176
Anal fissure, 82, 84
  chronic, 89, 91
Analgesics, general, 355, 356
Anaphylactoid reaction, to radiocontrast media, 123, 124
Anaphylaxis, 123–125
Anemia, sickle cell, 181, 182
Anesthesia, regional, 355–356
Anesthetic, local, for laceration repair, 277–278
  topical, for laceration repair, 277, 278
Aneurysm, aortic, 46, 47–48
  coronary artery, complicating Kawasaki's disease, 228, 229
Anger rapist, 362
Angina, Ludwig's, presentation of, 157, 160, 161
  management of, 164, 167
  Prinzmetal's, conditions associated with, 21, 23
    ECG changes in, 22, 24–25
  stable, unstable angina vs., 21, 23
  unstable, characteristics of, 21, 23
  variant, conditions associated with, 21, 23
    ECG changes in, 22, 24–25
  Vincent's, complications of, 161
    presentation of, 160, 164, 168
Angiodysplasias, gastrointestinal bleeding in, 82, 84
Angiography, cerebral, in third cranial nerve palsy, 198, 199
  in pelvic trauma, 266, 268
  pulmonary, 62, 63
Angioplasty, emergency, indications for, 28, 29–30
Ankle, injuries of, 290–291, 292
Anorectal abscess, 89, 91
Anorexia, in altitude illness, 347, 348
Antacids, aluminum hydroxide, for tumor lysis syndrome, 174, 177
Anterior cord syndrome, 244, 246
Anticholinergic toxidrome, vs. sympathomimetic toxidrome, 329, 330
Anticholinergics, in emergency asthma management, 67, 68
  toxicity of, 321, 322
Anticonvulsants, 325, 326, 327–328
Antidepressants, toxicologic effects of, 321, 322–323
  tricyclic, overdose of, *34*, 35, 38

391

Antidiuretic hormone, inappropriate, syndrome of, 174, 176
  from vincristine, 130, 133
Anti-inflammatories, for altitude illness, 347
  nonsteroidal. See *Nonsteroidal anti-inflammatory drugs (NSAIDs)*.
Antimalarials, in systemic lupus erythematosus, 117, 119
Antimicrobials, allergic reactions to, 123, 124
  for febrile neutropenic patient, 174, 176
  for Lyme disease, 110
  for sepsis, 102, 103
  for sexual assault victim, 359, 362
  for systemic lupus erythematosus, 117, 119
  in pregnancy, 273, 274, 309, 312
  prophylactic, for human bite, 339, 340–341
  for oral lacerations, 163, 166
Antipsychotics, 233–234, 235–236
Antitrypsin deficiency, COPD and, 64, 65
Anxiety, in thyroid storm, 136, 139
  in thyrotoxicosis, 136, 139
Anxiety disorders, 234, 236
Aorta, aneurysm of, 46, 47–48
  dissection of, hypertension with, drug regimen for, 39, 40
  prehospital management of, 46, 47
  therapy for, 22, 24
  stenosis of, symptoms/physical findings in, 22, 23–24
Aortic arch tear, 258, 259
Aortic outflow tract syncope, 41, 42
Aortocaval compression, in pregnancy, 304, 305
Apgar score, 301, 302
Apical capping, mediastinal widening with, 257, 259
Apnea, in infant, 11–12
Apoplexy, 135, 138
Appendicitis, 75, 76, 83–84, 86–87
  pregnancy and, 309, 312
Arrhythmias, 32–39
  cocaine-induced, drugs for, 34, 37
  complicating myocardial infarction, 35, 39
  cyclic antidepressant-induced, 321, 323
  from thrombolytic therapy, 32, *33,* 37
  in digoxin toxicity, 35, 38
  in Lyme disease, treatment of, 35, 38
  pediatric, 7, 9
  syncope from, 41, 42
Arsenic poisoning, 334
Arterial blood gases (ABGs), in adult respiratory failure, 13–14
Arterial catheters, febrile illness and, 96, 98
Arterial embolus, therapy for, 45, 47
Arteriography, in penetrating neck trauma, 254, 255
Arteritis, giant cell, ophthalmic manifestations of, 117, 119
  temporal, 146, 149, 205, 207
Artery(ies). See also specific artery, e.g., *Aorta*.
  cerebral, right anterior, infarct of, 197, 198
  embolism in, 45, 47
  ophthalmic, infarct of, 197, 198
  retinal, central, occlusion of, 146–147, 149
Arthritis, gonococcal, 294, 297
  Lyme, 110
  monoarticular, acute, 294, 297
  rheumatoid, 117, 119
    ophthalmic manifestations of, 117, 120
  viral infections and, 294, 297
Arthrocentesis, 389
Aspiration, joint, 389–390
Aspirin, odontophagia from, 78, 80
Asthma, 67–69
  adenosine and, 32, 37
  in pregnancy, 309, 312

Asystole, therapy for, 3, 5
Atacurium, histamine release from, 17
  metabolism of, by plasma enzymes, 15–16, 17
Atelectasis, aspirated foreign body and, 157, 160
Atenolol, pediatric ingestion of, 322, 323
Atrial fibrillation, admission criteria for, 32, 36
  complicating myocardial infarction, 35, 39
  conditions associated with, 34, 38
  in digoxin poisoning, 322, 323
  new-onset, management of, 34, 37–38
    medications for, 34, 38
  treatment of, 35, 39
  with preexcitation pattern, treatment of, 35, *36,* 39
Atrioventricular (AV) block, 32, *33,* 37
Atropine, in resuscitation, 3–4, 5
Auditory canal, external, foreign bodies in, 152, 154
Aura, 204, 206
Autoimmune adrenalitis, primary adrenal insufficiency from, 135, 138
Autoimmune disorders, 117–122
Auto-PEEP, in mechanically ventilated patient, 13, 14
Autotransfusion, in thoracic trauma, 258, 260
AV (atrioventricular) block, 32, *33,* 37
Avulsion fractures, site of, 266, 267

Babinski's sign, in right-sided hemispheric lesion, 191, 193
Back pain, 295, 297, 298
  in adrenal insufficiency, 135, 138
Bacteremia, complicating acute bacterial prostatitis, 212, 214–215
Bacterial keratitis, topical corticosteroids and, 146, 148
Bacterial prostatitis, acute, 212, 214–215
Bacterial sinusitis, 151, 153
Bacterial vaginosis, 308, 311
Bacteriuria, relapse of, 212, 215
Bacteroides melaninogenicus, pneumonia with cavitation from, 69, 70
Baker's cyst, in rheumatoid arthritis, 117, 119
Barodontalgia, hyperbaric oxygen therapy for, 343
Barotrauma, COPD management and, 64, 65
  middle ear, 343, 344
Barrel chest, in COPD, 64, 65
Basilar skull fracture, 248, 250
Battered spouse, 358, 361
Battery, button, ingestion of, 332, 333
Behavioral disorders, 231–240
Behçet's disease, 118, 120
Benadryl, for scombroid, 76, 77
Benzathine penicillin G, for syphilis, 114
Benzodiazepines, for cocaine intoxication, 329, 330
  in pregnancy, 273, 274
  overdose of, 325, 326, 327
Beta-agonist therapy, hypokalemia from, 130, 132
Beta-agonist toxicity, 322, 323–324
Bicarbonate, sodium, in cardiac arrest, 3, 4
Bicycle handlebar injury, pediatric, 261–262, 264
Biliary colic, 78, 80
Bipolar illness, psychosis in, 233, 235
Bite(s), dog, 339, 340
  human, prophylaxis for, 339, 340–341
  insect, allergic reactions to, 123–124
  management of, 340, 342
  snake, 339, 341
  spider, 339–340, 341
Black widow spider bite, 339–340, 341

Bladder, decompression of, 217, 218
  trauma to, 262, 263, 265
Blalock-Taussig shunt, classic, 56, 58
Blast injuries, 281–282
Bleeding. See *Hemorrhage*.
Blindness, cortical, 197, 198
Blood, loss of, in multiple trauma, 243, 245
  transfusions of, complications of, 82, 84
Blood gases, arterial, in adult respiratory failure, 13–14
  in hypoxemia from hypoventilation, 4, 5
Blood pressure, lowering of, in hypertensive encephalopathy, goals for, 40
Blood vessels, compromised, in extremity trauma, 269
  in neck trauma, 253, 254, 255
  injuries to, in blunt extremity trauma, 269, 270
  in supracondylar fracture, 285–286, 287–288
Blumberg's sign, in appendicitis, 75, 76
Boerhaave's syndrome, 24
Bone, alveolar, tooth impacted into, 165, 168
Bone marrow transplantation, for sickle cell disease, 180, 182
Borchardt's triad, in gastric volvulus, 88, 89
Borderline personality disorder, 234, 236
Borrelia burgdorferi infection, dysrhythmia from, treatment of, 35, 38
  Lyme disease from, 109, 110
Botulism, 75–76, 77, 200, 201
Boutonnière deformity, in rheumatoid arthritis, 117, 119
Boyle's law, 365, 366
Bradycardia, post-MI, asymptomatic, therapy for, 35, 39
  sinus, complicating myocardial infarction, 35, 39
  therapy for, 3, 5
Brain. See also *Cerebral* entries.
  herniation of, uncal, 247, 249
Brain stem, infarct of, 197, 198
  lesion of, 191
"Breakbone" fever, 112, 113
Breast, cancer of, diagnosis of, 313, 314
  metastatic, hypercalcemia from, 137, 141
  disorders of, 313–314
  postpartum engorgement of, 313, 314
  trauma to, 313–314
Breathing, pursed-lip, in COPD, 64, 65
Bronchiolitis, respiratory syncytial virus, apnea in infants and, 11
Bronchopulmonary dysplasia, 69, 70–71
Bronchospasm, pulmonary embolism from, death in, 62, 64
Brown-Séard syndrome, 295, 298
Brugada criteria, in VT vs. SVT, 32, 36–37
Bulla, 223, 224–225
Bullous pemphigoid, 224, 225
Bundle branch block, left, in acute myocardial infarction, 26, 27
Burnout, in emergency physicians, 373, 374
Burns, 279–281
  palatal, 164, 167
Bursitis, olecranon, traumatic, 286, 288
Burton's line, in lead poisoning, 333, 334
Button battery, ingestion of, 332, 333

Cafe coronary, 157, 160
Calcitonin, for hypercalcemia, 138, 141
  of malignancy, 173, 176
Calcium channel blockers, for hypertension, 135, 138

Calcium chloride, for tumor lysis syndrome, 174, 177
Calcium gluconate, for hyperkalemia, 130, 132
Calculi, salivary, 158, 161–162
Caloric reflex, 191
Camphor, gastrointestinal decontamination for, 332, 334
Cancer, breast, diagnosis of, 313, 314
　　metastatic, hypercalcemia from, 137, 141
　emergencies related to, 173, 177
　hematologic, cause of death in, 174, 176
　lung, superior vena cava syndrome in, 173, 174–175, 176
　metabolic abnormalities in, 174, 177
　metastatic. See *Metastasis(es)*.
　prostate, epidural spinal cord compression in, 173, 175
Candidiasis, oral, 157, 159, 161
Canine space infection, 165, 168
Cannabis abuse, 238, 240
Capillary refill, in dehydration, 129, 130
Carbamazepine, adenosine and, 32, 37
　for trigeminal neuralgia, 198
　toxicity of, 326, 327
Carbamide peroxide, for cerumen removal, 152, 154
Carbon dioxide detectors, colorimetric, disposable end-tidal, 16, 17
　readings from, 16, 18
Carbon monoxide, poisoning by, 279–281, 332, 334
　scuba diving and, 342, 343
Carbon tetrachloride, gastrointestinal decontamination for, 332, 334
Carboxyhemoglobin level, signs/symptoms associated with, 279–281
Cardiac. See also *Heart*.
Cardiac arrest, pediatric, 6–7, 8
　predicting survival in, 3, 4
Cardiac tamponade, 51, 53, 387, 388
　presentation of, 54
Cardiogenic shock, acute transmural MI with, emergency angioplasty for, 28, 29–30
　after myocardial infarction, risk factors for, 29, 31
　dobutamine in, 25, 26
　hemodynamic profile in, 28, 30
　rapid-sequence intubation in, 28, 30
　signs of, 28, 30
Cardiogenic syncope, 1-year mortality for, 41–42
Cardiomyopathy, dilated, from acute myocarditis, 51, 53
　hypertrophic, 21, 23
Cardiovascular system, in Kawasaki syndrome, 23, 25
Cardioversion, 56, 57
Carpal bone fractures, 287, 289
Cataracts, from topical corticosteroids, 146, 148
　in lightning injuries, 348
Catheter(s), arterial, febrile illness and, 96, 98
　central venous, febrile illness and, 96, 98
　percutaneous, 387–388
　dialysis, 211, 213–214
　　Foley, contraindications to, 262, 264
Caustic ingestions, 332, 333
Cavernous sinus thrombosis, 159
Cavitation, pneumonia with, organisms causing, 69, 70
Cefaclor, *Clostridium difficile* overgrowth from, 75, 77
　for cystitis, 212, 214
Cefazolin, allergic reactions and, 123, 124
Ceftazidime, allergic reactions and, 123, 124
Ceftriaxone, for perforated appendix, 84, 86
　for Rocky Mountain spotted fever, 108, 109

Cellulitis, orbital, 146, 149
　periorbital, 147–148, 150
Central cord syndrome, 244, 246
Central nervous system (CNS), dysfunction of, in thyrotoxicosis, 136, 139
　infections of, 105–106. See also *Meningitis*.
　lesions in, HIV infection and, 100, 101
Central pontine myelinolysis, 130, 133
Central retinal artery occlusion, 146–147, 149
Central venous catheter(s), febrile illness and, 96, 98
Central venous catheterization, percutaneous, 387–388
Cephalexin, for human bite prophylaxis, 339, 340
Cerebral angiography, in third cranial nerve palsy diagnosis, 198, 199
Cerebral artery, right anterior, infarct of, 197, 198
Cerebral demyelination, 130, 133
Cerebral metastases, intracranial pressure elevation from, 173, 175
Cerebral palsy, fever from, 95, 97
Cerebrospinal fluid (CSF), values for, in newborn, 105, 106
Cerebrovascular accident, in HgbSS disease, 180, 182
Cerebrovascular emergencies, 197, 198–199
Cerumen removal, 152, 154
Cervical spine, fracture of, 257, 259
　immobilization of, 243, 245
　pseudosubluxation of, 293, 295
　trauma to, 244, 246
Chagas' disease, 112, 113
Chance fracture, thoracolumbar, 244, 246
Chancre, in syphilis, 113, 114
Chancroid, 311
Charcoal, activated, 322, 323
　N-acetylcysteine and, 318, 319
Chelation therapy, 333, 334–335
Chemoprophylaxis, against meningitis, 105, 106
Chemotherapeutic agents, cardiotoxicity from, 173, 176
Chest, barrel, in COPD, 64, 65
　flail, 257, 259
　pain in, 21–25. See also *Myocardial infarction (MI); Myocardial ischemia*.
　　cocaine-associated, 21, 23
　　deep inspiration and, 22, 24
　　ECG in, 22, 24–25
　　esophageal etiology and, 78, 79
　　in children, causes of, 22–23, 25
　　in cocaine use, 329, 330
　　in Dressler's syndrome, therapy for, 22, 24
　　in esophageal reflux disease, 22, 24
　　in sickle cell disease, 23, 25
　　noncardiac, differential diagnosis of, 22, 24
　trauma to, 257–260
　　blunt, tension pneumothorax in, 380
Chest tube placement, 379–380
CHF (congestive heart failure), 28–31. See also *Congestive heart failure (CHF)*.
Chilblains, 351
Child abuse, historical/radiographic findings in, 293, 295–296
　injuries prompting investigation for, 272, 273
　rheumatologic disease confused with, 118, 121
　sexual, 357–358, 360–361
Chlamydia, 308, 311–312
Chlamydial conjunctivitis, 146, 149
Chlorine gas, toxicity of, 332, 333
Chlorpropamide overdose, hypoglycemia from, 137, 141
Cholangitis, acute, Reynold's pentad in, 78, 80
Cholecystitis, acute, diagnosis of, 78, 80

Cholecystitis *(Continued)*
　in elderly, 75, 76
Cholelithiasis, 24
Cholesteatoma, 152, 154
Cholesterol gallstones, 78, 80
Christmas disease, gastrointestinal bleeding in, 194, 196
Chronic obstructive pulmonary disease (COPD), 64–66
Cigarette smoking, COPD and, 64, 65
Ciguatera, 76, 77
Cimetidine, for anaphylactoid reactions to radiocontrast media, 123, 124
Ciprofloxacin, for cystitis, 212, 214
　for *Shigella* and *Salmonella*, 75, 77
Clavicle, fracture of, 285, 287
Clindamycin, *Clostridium difficile* overgrowth from, 75, 77
　for perforated appendix, 84, 86
Clonidine, toxicity of, in child, 322, 323
Closed-fist injuries, 277, 278
Clostridium difficile overgrowth, 75, 77
Clozapine (Clozaril), 233, 235–236
Clozaril (clozapine), 233, 235–236
Clubbing, of fingers, in COPD, 64, 65
Cluster headaches, 204–205, 207, 208
Coagulation, disseminated intravascular, 184, 185, 186, 187
　from autotransfusion, 260
Coagulation pathways, measures of, 185, 187
COBRA (Consolidated Omnibus Budget Reconciliation Act), 364–365
Cocaine, abuse of, 238, 239, 240
　arrhythmias induced by, drugs for, 34, 37
　chest pain associated with, 21, 23
　hypertension induced by, drugs for, 34, 37
　in topical anesthetic, 277, 278
　intoxication with, 329, 330
Coccyx, avulsion fractures of, 266, 267
Cold air, asthma and, 67, 68
Cold intolerance, in myxedema, 136, 139
Colic, biliary, 78, 80
　renal, 217, 218, 219
Coma, cyclical, from carbamazepine, 326, 327
　hyperosmolar nonketotic, 136, 140
　myxedema, 135, 139
　pediatric causes of, 191–192, 193
Coma cocktail, 238–239, 240
Community-acquired pneumonias, 161
Compartment syndrome(s), complicating IO infusions, 389, 390
　posterior, 269, 270
Complex partial seizures, 204, 206
Computed tomography (CT), of nasal-orbital-ethmoid fracture, 251, 253
Concussion, dental, 164, 167
Condylar fracture, 251, 252
Condylomata lata, 312
　in syphilis, 113, 114
Congenital heart disease, 56–58
Congestive heart failure (CHF), 28–31
　cause of, 4, 5
　conditions precipitating, 29, 31
　descriptive terms for, 29, 31
　dobutamine in, 28, 30
　endotracheal intubation in, 28, 29
　initial therapy for, 28, 29
　mortality from, 29, 31
　pediatric, causes of, 29, 31
　　findings in, 29, 31
　respiratory failure in, treatment of, 28, 30
Conjunctival lacerations, 146, 148
Conjunctivitis, herpes simplex, 147, 150
　types and features of, 146, 149
Consolidated Omnibus Budget Reconciliation Act (COBRA), 364–365

Constipation, in cancer-related hypercalcemia, 174, 177
  pediatric, 88, 90
Continence, normal, 217, 218
Continuous positive airway pressure (CPAP), conditions benefited by, 16, 18
Continuous Process Improvement (CPI), 368, 371–372
Contraceptives, "morning after," 307, 310
Contrast media, IV, allergic reactions to, 218, 219
Contusion, myocardial, 257, 258–259
  pulmonary, 258, 259
Coprine, disulfiram-like reactions to, 329, 331
Cornea, abrasions of, 145, 148
  foreign bodies in, 146, 148–149
Coronary artery aneurysm, complicating Kawasaki's disease, 228, 229
Cortical blindness, 197, 198
Corticosteroids, for adrenal crisis, 135, 138
  for sickle cell disease, 180, 182
  in emergency asthma management, 67, 68
  ocular, topical, adverse effects of, 146, 148
Cortinarius, 329, 330
Corynebacterium minutissimum, erythrasma from, 227, 228
Cough, inhaled foreign body causing, 157, 159
"Count of Monte Cristo" syndrome, 191, 193
Coxsackievirus, 157, 158, 159, 160–161
CPAP (continuous positive airway pressure), conditions benefited by, 16, 18
Cranial nerve disorders, 197–198, 199
CREST syndrome, 227, 228–229
Cricothyroidotomy, 383–384
Croup, 158, 161
Cryoprecipitate, for thrombotic thrombocytopenic purpura, 184, 185
Cryptococcal meningitis, AIDS and, 99, 100, 101
CT (computed tomography), of nasal-orbital-ethmoid fracture, 251, 253
Cushing's syndrome, 136–137, 140
Cyanide, toxicity of, 332, 333–334
Cyanosis, in COPD, 64, 65
  in neonate, 56, 57
  methemoglobinemia and, 333, 334
Cyclic antidepressants, toxicologic effects of, 321, 323
Cyclical coma, from carbamazepine, 326, 327
Cyst(s), Baker's, in rheumatoid arthritis, 117, 119
  epidermal, 224, 225
  pilonidal, treatment of, 89, 91
Cystic fibrosis, COPD and, 64, 65
Cystitis, 212, 214
Cytomegalovirus retinitis, 99, 100

Dacryoadenitis, 147, 150
Death, 368–369, 372
  from hematologic malignancies, cause of, 174, 176
DeBakey classification system, for thoracic aortic dissections, 46, 48
Decompression sickness, 342, 343
Deep tendon reflexes, in myxedema, 136, 139
Deep venous thrombosis (DVT), lower-extremity, evaluation of, 45, 47
  pulmonary embolism and, 61, 62
  risk factors for, 45, 47
  therapy for, 45, 47
Defibrillation, 3, 4
Defibrillators, automatic external, 4, 5
Dehydration, hyponatremic, 129, 130–132
  in child, 76, 77

Dehydration *(Continued)*
  rehydration solution for, 129, 130
  rehydration for, 75, 76
Delirium, causes of, 235, 237
  dementia vs., 233, 235
Delivery, normal, 301–302
Demyelination, cerebral, 130, 133
Dementia, delirium vs., 233, 235
Dengue fever, 112, 113
Dengue shock syndrome, 112, 113
Dental. See also *Tooth (teeth)*.
Dental emergencies, 163–169
Dental injuries, 251, 252
Departments of Emergency Medicine, Emergency Departments and, 367, 370
Depression, in emergency personnel, 373, 374
Dermatitis, 223, 224, 225
Dermatologic disorder(s), 221–229
  rashes as, 223, 225. See also *Rash*.
  skin cancer as, 227, 228
Dermatomyositis, 117, 119, 120
  juvenile, fever in, 118, 120
Dexamethasone, for adrenal insufficiency, 135, 138–139
Diabetes insipidus, central, hypernatremic dehydration in infant from, 129, 130
Diabetes mellitus, cranial nerve disorders in, 198
  hypoglycemia in, 137, 141
  Kussmaul's respirations in, 137, 140
  malignant otitis externa and, 152, 154
  mucormycosis complicating, 151, 153
  pediatric, vomiting and dehydration in, 129, 130
Diabetic ketoacidosis, abdominal pain from, 75, 76
  abnormalities associated with, 135, 138
  hypokalemia from, 130, 132
  sodium correction in, 137, 140–141
  therapeutic goals in, 135, 138
Dialysis, catheters for, 211, 213–214
  indications for, 317, 319
Diaphragm, ipsilateral flattening of, aspirated foreign body and, 157, 160
  trauma to, 258, 259–260
Diarrhea, 75, 76–77
  diet and, 130, 132
  in thyrotoxicosis, 136, 139
  infectious, HIV and, 100, 101
Diazepam, for cocaine-induced hypertension and arrhythmias, 34, 37
DIC (disseminated intravascular coagulation), 184, 185, 186, 187
  from autotransfusion, 260
Diet, diarrhea and, 130, 132
Digital rectal examination, contraindications to, 266, 267
Digoxin toxicity, 35, 38, 322, 323
Dilated cardiomyopathy, from acute myocarditis, 51, 53
Diltiazem, for Wolff-Parkinson-White syndrome, 35, 39
Diphenhydramine, for anaphylactoid reactions to radiocontrast media, 123, 124
  for scombroid, 76, 77
Diphtheria, 157, 159, 160
Dipyridamole, adenosine and, 32, 37
Disaster plan/approach, 363–364
Discitis, infectious, 295, 298
Dislocation(s), anterior shoulder, reduction of, 285, 287
  facet, cervical spine, 244, 246
  glenohumeral, 285, 287
  hip, 294, 297
  humeral head, 285, 287
  joint, reduction of, 389, 390

Dislocation(s) *(Continued)*
  knee, 290, 291
  mandibular condyle, 164–165, 168
  temporomandibular joint, 251, 252
Disseminated intravascular coagulation (DIC), 184, 185, 186, 187
  from autotransfusion, 260
Dissociation, electromechanical, causes of, 3, 4
Distributive justice, 373, 374–375
Distributive shock, in infant, 129, 130
Diuresis, for hypercalcemia, in Paget's disease, 137–138, 141
Diuretics, hypokalemia from, 130, 132
  loop, for hypercalcemia of malignancy, 173, 176
Diving injuries/illness, 342–344
Dizziness, 192, 194
Dobutamine, in cardiogenic shock, 25, 26
  in congestive heart failure, 28, 30
Dog bite, 339, 340
Dopamine, for hypotension, 102, 103
Down's syndrome, congenital heart disease and, 56, 58
Doxorubicin, cardiotoxicity from, 173, 176
Doxycycline, odontophagia from, 78, 80
Dressler's syndrome, 54
  chest pain in, therapy for, 22, 24
Drowning, 343–344
Drug(s). See also named drug or drug group.
  abuse of, 238–240
  for cocaine-induced hypertension and arrhythmias, 34, 37
  in pregnancy, 273, 274
  phototoxic reactions from, 227, 229
  reactions to, 227, 228
Drug fever, 98
Dry socket, 164, 167
Duct(s), nasolacrimal, obstruction of, 140, 147
  Stensen's, 165, 168
  Wharton's, 165, 168
Duodenal injury, 261–262, 264
Dust, asthma and, 67, 68
Dysarthria, 191
Dysequilibrium, 192, 194
Dysfunctional uterine bleeding, 307, 308, 310, 311
Dysphasia, 191
Dysplasia, bronchopulmonary, 69, 70–71
Dyspnea, inhaled foreign body causing, 157, 159
Dysrhythmias. See *Arrhythmias*.
Dystonia, 330, 331

Eating disorders, in adult abuse victims, 358, 361
ECG (electrocardiogram). See *Electrocardiogram (ECG)*.
Eclampsia, 304, 305
  treatment of, 40
Ectopic pregnancy, 83, 86, 302, 303, 304
  ruptured, 304–305, 308, 311
Eczema herpeticum, 223, 225
Edema, pulmonary, high-altitude, 347, 348
  etiology of, 365, 366
  in bronchopulmonary dysplasia, 69, 70
Edrophonium chloride, diagnostic uses of, 201, 202
EGTA (esophageal gastric tube airway), 15, 16–17
Ehrlichiosis, 108–109
Elbow, nursemaid's, 293–294, 296
Elderly, abuse of, 361
  gastric ulcer in, endoscopic diagnosis of, 82, 84–85

Elderly *(Continued)*
    gastrointestinal bleeding in, risk factor for, 83, 85
Electric injuries, 349
Electrocardiogram (ECG), in acute myocardial infarction, 25–26, 27
    in acute pericarditis, 22, 24
    in chest pain, 22, 24–25
    in digoxin poisoning, 322, 323
    in pericarditis, 51, 53
    prehospital, 25, 26
Electrolyte abnormalities, in end-stage renal disease, 211, 213
Electromechanical dissociation, causes of, 3, 4
ELISA, positive, in Lyme disease, 110, 111
Embolus(i), arterial, 45, 47
    with absent distal pulses, therapy for, 45, 47
    pulmonary. See *Pulmonary embolism.*
Emergency Departments, Departments of Emergency Medicine and, 367, 370
Emergency Medical Transport and Active Labor Act (EMTALA), 364, 365
Emotional stress, precipitating sickle cell crisis, 180, 182
Empyema, 69–71
EMS system, 364–365
EMTALA (Emergency Medical Transport and Active Labor Act), 364, 365
Encephalopathy, hypertensive, goals of lowering blood pressure in, 40
Endocardial cushion defect, in Down's syndrome, 56, 58
Endocarditis, 52–53, 54
Endocrine disorder(s), 135–141
    adrenal crisis as, 135, 138
    adrenal insufficiency as, 135, 138–139
    diabetes mellitus as, 137, 140–141
    diabetic ketoacidosis as, 135, 138
    myxedema coma as, 135, 139
    pheochromocytoma as, 135, 138
    pituitary necrosis as, 135, 138
    thyroid storm as, 135–136, 139
Endotracheal intubation, in congestive heart failure, 28, 29
    rapid-sequence, in cardiogenic shock, 28, 30
    thiopental and, 15, 17
Endotracheal tube, drugs given by, 271, 272
    pediatric, size of, 6, 8, 15, 17
    uncuffed, 16, 17
Enterocolitis, necrotizing, gastrointestinal bleeding from, 82, 84
Environmental emergencies, 337–352
Enzymes, plasma, nondepolarizing agents metabolized by, 15–16, 17
EOA (esophageal obturator airway), 15, 16–17
Epidermal cysts, 224, 225
Epididymitis, complicating acute bacterial prostatitis, 212, 214–215
Epidural hematomas, 247, 249
Epidural spinal cord compression, in prostate cancer, 173, 175
Epinephrine, for allergic reactions, 124
    in local anesthesia, 277–278
Epiphysis, humeral, separation of, 285, 287
    slipped capital femoral, 294, 295, 296–297
Episiotomy, 301, 302
Epistaxis, 151, 152–153
Erysipelas, 228, 229
Erythema marginatum, 227, 228
Erythema migrans, in Lyme disease, 109, 110
Erythema multiforme, 224, 225, 226
Erythema nodosum, 224, 225–226
    in systemic lupus erythematosus, 117, 119
Erythema toxicum neonatorum, 224, 226
Erythrasma, 227, 228, 311

Erythrocyte(s), sickled, in painful sickle cell crises, 180, 181
Erythrocyte sedimentation rate (ESR), elevated, in Lyme disease, 110
Erythromycin, *Clostridium difficile* overgrowth from, 75, 77
    for chlamydia in pregnancy, 308, 311–312
    for human bite prophylaxis, 339, 340
    for Rocky Mountain spotted fever, 108, 109
    hearing loss from, 152, 154
    uses of, 309, 312
Escherichia coli, infantile infections from, 95, 97
Esophageal gastric tube airway (EGTA), 15, 16–17
Esophageal obturator airway (EOA), 15, 16–17
Esophageal reflux, 78, 79
Esophageal reflux disease, chest pain in, 22, 24
Esophagus, chest pain related to, 78, 79
    food impaction in, 158–159, 162
    foreign bodies in, 78, 79
    injuries to, 254–255
    Mallory-Weiss tear of, 82, 84
    perforation of, 78, 79–80
ESR (erythrocyte sedimentation rate), elevated, in Lyme disease, 110
Estrogens, postcoital, for sexual assault victim, 359, 362
Ethambutol, for tuberculosis, 107
Ethanol, cafe coronary and, 157, 160
    metabolism of, 325
Ethics, 373–375
Ethylene glycol toxicity, 325, 326–327
Etidronate disodium, for hypercalcemia, 138, 141
Exercise, asthma and, 67, 68
    hypoglycemia from, 137, 141
Extensor tendon, lacerations of, 286, 288
Extraction, dental, complications of, 164, 167
Extremity(ies), lower, trauma to, 290–292
    trauma to, 269–270
    upper, trauma to, 285–288
Eye(s), disorders of, 145–150
    chemical injuries as, 145, 148
    traumatic injuries as, 145, 148
    strain of, headache from, 205, 207–208
Eyelids, margins of, lacerations of, 146, 148
    pathology of, 147, 149

Face, trauma to, 243, 245
Facet dislocation, of cervical spine, 244, 246
Factor IX deficiency, 194, 196
Familial hemiplegic migraine, 205, 208
Fatigue, in myxedema, 136, 139
    respiratory muscle, in asthma, 67, 68
Febrile child, 95–98
Febrile seizure, 203, 205
Femoral epiphysis, slipped capital, 294, 295, 296–297
Femoral line, percutaneous, for pediatric patients, 7, 9
Femur, fracture of, 290, 291
    trochanteric, 295, 297
Fetal loss, in systemic lupus erythematosus, 117, 119
Fetus, risks to, from maternal trauma, 274, 275
Fever, drug, 98
    harmful level of, 95, 97
    in acute cholangitis, 78, 80
    in adrenal insufficiency, 135, 138
    in pediatric rheumatologic diseases, 118, 120
    in thyroid storm, 136, 139
    in thyrotoxicosis, 136, 139
    measurement of, in children, 95, 97

Fever *(Continued)*
    noninfectious causes of, 95, 97
Fibrillation, atrial. See *Atrial fibrillation.*
    ventricular, arrest from, intervention for, 4, 5
Fibrotic lung disease, COPD and, 64, 65
Finger(s), amputated, replantation of, 286, 288
    clubbing of, in COPD, 64, 65
Fitz-Hugh-Curtis syndrome, 307, 308, 310, 311
Flail chest, 257, 259
Flank pain, in adrenal insufficiency, 135, 138
Flash burns, 281, 282
Fluid(s), for hypercalcemia of malignancy, 173, 176
    IV, for hypotension from septic shock, 102, 103
Fluid and electrolyte management, 129–133
Flumazenil, 326, 327
Foley catheter, contraindications to, 262, 264
Folliculitis, *Pseudomonas,* 228, 229
Fomepizole, 325, 327
Foot injuries, 290, 292
Foreign body(ies), aspirated, 157, 160
    corneal, 146, 148–149
    esophageal, 78, 79
    external auditory canal, 152, 154
    in children, febrile illness and, 96, 98
    ingestion of, 158, 162
    inhalation of, 157, 159–160
    nasal, 151, 153
    pulmonary embolism and, 62, 63–64
    rectal, 89, 90–91
    vaginal, in child, 307, 310
Fracture(s), ankle, 290–291, 292
    avulsion, sites of, 266, 267
    basilar skull, 248, 250
    carpal bone, 287, 289
    cervical spinal, 244, 246
    cervical spine, 257, 259
    clavicular, 285, 287
    condylar, of mandible, 251, 252
    femoral, 290, 291
        trochanteric, 295, 297
    foot, 290, 292
    Galeazzi, 288
    hamate, 287, 289
    hangman's, 244, 245–246
    hip, 294–295, 297
    humeral, 285, 287
    LeFort, 251, 253
    mandibular, 251, 252
        jaw thrust maneuver and, 15, 16
    maxillofacial, 251, 252
    metatarsal, 290, 291–292
    Monteggia, 288
    nasal-orbital-ethmoid, CT scan of, 251, 253
    orbital rim, 251, 252
    pediatric, 293, 296
    pelvic, major, 266, 268
    penile, 262, 265
    rib, 257, 259
    sternal, 258, 260
    supracondylar, 285–286, 287
    thoracolumbar Chance, 244, 246
    tooth, 164, 167
        classification and management of, 166, 169
    triquetrum, 287, 289
    ulnar, midshaft, 286, 287–288
    zygoma, 251, 252
Frontal sinus, 151, 153
Frostbite, 350–352
Fungal keratitis, topical corticosteroids and, 146, 148
Furosemide, hearing loss from, 152, 154

Galeazzi fracture, 288

Gallstones, cholesterol, 78, 80
Gardnerella vaginalis, bacterial vaginosis from, 308, 311
Gas embolism, hyperbaric oxygen therapy for, 343
Gastric volvulus, 88, 89
Gastritis, hemorrhagic, management of, 82, 84
Gastrointestinal tract, anticholinergic poisoning and, 321, 322
  bleeding in, 82–83, 84–85
  disorders of, 73–92
  obstruction of, 88–92
Gastrostomy tubes, 385–386
Genital lesions, 308, 311
Genital warts, 312
Genitourinary injuries, pediatric, 263, 265
Gentamicin, for febrile neutropenic patient, 174, 176
  for perforated appendix, 84, 86
Giant cell arteritis, ophthalmic manifestations of, 117, 119
Glasgow Coma Scale, 243, 245
  in intracranial injury evaluation, 247, 249–250
Glaucoma, acute angle-closure, signs and symptoms of, 146, 147, 149, 150
  complicating hyphema, in sickle cell anemia, 181, 182
Glenohumeral dislocation, 285, 287
Globe, lacerations of, 145, 148
Glucocorticoids, in systemic lupus erythematosus, 117, 119
Glucose, endogenous sources of, in starvation, 137, 141
Gonococcal arthritis, 294, 297
Gonococcal conjunctivitis, 146, 149
Granuloma, noncaseating, in sarcoidosis, 117, 119
Granulomatosis, Wegener's, in rheumatoid arthritis, 117, 119
Grief, 369, 372
Guillain-Barré syndrome, 200, 201, 202
Gunshot wound, 261, 263
  of thigh, 269–270
Gyrometrin, seizures and, 329, 330–331

Haddon's matrix, 357, 359
Haemophilus influenzae, infections from, HgbSS disease and, 180, 182
  pediatric, 96, 98
  otitis media from, 154
  pneumonia from, 69, 70
Haldol (haloperidol), indications for and contraindications to, 233, 235
Hallpike maneuver, 154
Hallucinations, 233, 235
Haloperidol (Haldol), indications for and contraindications to, 233, 235
Hamate fractures, 287, 289
Hand injuries, 286, 288
  closed-fist, 277, 278
Hangman's fracture, 244, 245–246
Head trauma, assessment of, 243, 245
  pediatric, 272
Headache(s), cluster, 204–205, 207, 208
  in altitude illness, 347, 348
  in pheochromocytoma, 135, 138
  in pituitary necrosis, 135, 138
  in Rocky Mountain spotted fever, 108, 109
  in subarachnoid hemorrhage, 204, 207
  migraine, 204, 205, 207, 208
  pain mechanism in, 205, 208
  postdural, after lumbar puncture, 385
Hearing loss, 151–152, 153–154
Heart. See also *Cardiac; Cardio-* entries.

Heart *(Continued)*
  arrhythmias of, 32–39. See also *Arrhythmias.*
  damage to, from doxorubicin, 173, 176
  disease of, congenital, 56–58
  failure of, acute left-sided, clinical findings in, 28, 30
    complicating COPD, 64, 65
    congestive, 28–31. See also *Congestive heart failure (CHF).*
    high-output, 28, 30
  ischemia of, silent, predisposing factors for, 21, 23
  Lyme disease and, 110
  pain in, altered perception of, predisposing factors for, 21, 23
  wide complex pulseless rhythms of, 3, 4
Heart block, 35, 38
Heart valve, mitral, prosthetic, febrile illness and, 96, 98
Heat injuries, 350
Heavy metals, gastrointestinal decontamination for, 332, 334
Heliotrope rash, in dermatomyositis, 117, 119
Hemarthrosis, in hemophilia A, 186, 194
Hematochezia, 82–83, 84
Hematologic malignancies, cause of death in, 174, 176
Hematoma(s), epidural, 247, 249
  retroplacental, 274, 275
Hematuria, 262, 264
  causes of, 211, 214
Hemi-cord syndrome, 295, 298
Hemiplegic migraine, 205, 208
Hemispheric lesion, right-sided, 191, 193
Hemoglobinopathies, 180–183
Hemolytic uremic syndrome, 185, 187
Hemophilia, 184, 185, 186
Hemorrhage, extremity, control of, 269
  gastrointestinal, 82–83, 84–85
  in pelvic trauma, management of, 265, 266
  intracranial, in hemophilia, 184–185, 186
    altered mental status and, 203, 205
  postpartum, 305, 306
  retrobulbar, 145–146, 148
    in orbital rim fracture, 251, 252
  subarachnoid, 197, 198
    headache in, 204, 207
  uterine, dysfunctional, 307, 308, 310, 311
  vaginal, third trimester, 304, 305
  variceal, management of, 82, 84
  ventral pons, 191, 193
  vitreous, 146, 149
Hemorrhagic gastritis, management of, 82, 84
Hemorrhagic shock, pediatric, 271, 272
Hemorrhoid(s), 89, 90
  treatment of, 89, 91
Hemostasis, disorders of, 184–187
Hemothorax, traumatic, 257, 259
Henoch-Schönlein purpura, child abuse confused with, 118, 121
  renal complications of, 118, 120
Hepatitis, acute, 79, 80
Herniation, uncal brain, 247, 249
Herpes simplex, conjunctivitis from, 147, 150
  treatment of, 307–308, 310–311
Herpes zoster, abdominal pain from, 75, 76
HgbSS disease, 180, 181
Hill-Sachs deformity, 285, 287
Hip, dislocation of, 294, 297
  fractures of, 294–295, 297
Hirschsprung's disease, 88, 90
Histamine, in allergic reactions, 124, 125
  release of, drugs causing, 15, 17
Histrionic personality disorder, 234, 236
HIV (human immunodeficiency virus) infection, 99–101

Hordeolum, 147, 149
Horner's syndrome, 197, 199
  ipsilateral, 191
"Hot tub," 228, 229
Human bite prophylaxis, 339, 340–341
Human immunodeficiency virus (HIV) infection, 99–101
Humeral epiphysis separation, 285, 287
Humeral head, dislocation of, 285, 287
Humerus, fractures of, 285, 287
Hutchinson's sign, 227, 228
Hydration, for hypercalcemia, in Paget's disease, 137–138, 141
Hydrocarbons, gastrointestinal decontamination for, 332, 334
Hydroceles, 217, 219
Hydrofluoric acid, toxicity of, 332, 333
Hydrogen peroxide, for cerumen removal, 152, 154
Hydroxyurea, for sickle cell disease, 180, 182
Hyperactivity, airway, in bronchopulmonary dysplasia, 69, 70
Hyperbaric oxygen therapy, 342, 343
  for carbon monoxide poisoning, 279
Hyperbilirubinemia, in neonate, 79, 80–81
Hypercalcemia, cancer-related, symptoms/signs of, 174, 177
  treatment of, 173, 176
  causes of, 137, 141
  in Paget's disease, 137–138, 141
  therapy for, 138, 141
Hypercapnia, in asthma, 67, 68
Hypercortisolism, 136–137, 140
Hyperdefecation, in thyrotoxicosis, 136, 139
Hyperemesis gravidarum, 303, 304
Hyperkalemia, from hydrofluoric acid, 332, 333
  in adrenal insufficiency, 136, 139
  in diabetic ketoacidosis, 135, 138
  in renal failure, 130, 132
Hyperleukocytic syndrome, 173, 175
Hypermagnesemia, 211, 213
Hypernatremia, therapy for, 130, 133
Hypernatremic dehydration, pediatric, 129, 130–132
Hyperosmolar nonketotic coma, 136, 140
Hyperparathyroidism, hypercalcemia from, 137, 141
Hyperpigmentation, in adrenal insufficiency, 136, 139–140
Hyperpyrexia, in Rocky Mountain spotted fever, 108, 109
Hyperreflexia on left, in right-sided hemispheric lesion, 191, 193
Hypersensitivity, 123–125
Hypertension, 39–41
  cocaine-induced, drugs for, 34, 37
  from phenelzine, treatment of, 34, 37
  in cranial nerve disorders, 198
  in pheochromocytoma, 135, 138
  with aortic dissection, drugs for, 39, 40
Hypertensive crisis, treatment of, 40, 41
Hypertensive emergency, in chronic renal failure, 211, 213
  treatment plan for, 40–41
Hypertensive encephalopathy, lowering blood pressure in, 40
Hypertensive urgency, treatment of, 39–40
Hyperthermia, 350
  in sepsis, 102, 103
Hypertrophic cardiomyopathy, 21, 23
Hyperviscosity syndrome, 173–174, 176
  complicating COPD, 64, 65
  complicating multiple myeloma, 173, 175–176
Hyphema, 146, 148
  in sickle cell anemia, 181, 182

Hypocalcemia, from thyroidectomy, 137, 140
  signs/symptoms of, 130, 132
Hypocapnia, in sepsis, 102, 103
Hypoglycemia, causes of, 137, 141
  from chlorpropamide overdose, 137, 141
  in adrenal insufficiency, 136, 139
  postictal altered mental status and, 203, 205
Hypokalemia, causes of, 130, 132
Hyponatremia, 129–130, 130, 131–132, 133
  in adrenal insufficiency, 136, 139
  in diabetic ketoacidosis, 135, 138
  in infant, 129, 130
  treatment of, central pontine myelinolysis from, 130, 133
Hypoparathyroidism, from thyroidectomy, 137, 140
Hypoperfusion, in air medical transport, 365–366
Hypotension, from septic shock, 102, 103
  in anaphylaxis, 123, 124
  in septic shock, 102, 103
  in tuberculosis patient, 107, 108
  myocarditis with, 51, 53
  orthostatic, diagnosis of, 192, 194
Hypothermia, 350–351
  complicating multiple blood transfusions, 82, 84
  in infant, 95, 97
Hypoventilation, hypoxemia from, 4, 5
Hypovolemic shock, in pediatric patient, 129, 130
Hypoxemia, COPD management and, 64, 65
  from hypoventilation, 4, 5
  in air medical transport, 365–366
Hypoxia, in painful sickle cell crises, 180, 181

Ibuprofen, hearing loss from, 152, 154
ICS (Incident Command System), 363, 364
Ileal obstruction, 88, 89
Iliopsoas test, in appendicitis, 75, 76
Immune disorders, 115–125
Immunization, tetanus, 277, 278
Immunofluorescence testing, for diphtheria, 157, 159
Impetigo, 228, 229
Impingement syndromes, 285, 287
Incident Command System (ICS), 363, 364
Infant(s), apnea in, 11–12
  CSF values in, 105, 106
  full-term, resuscitation of, 7, 8
  heart failure in, 29, 31
  hypernatremic dehydration in, 129, 130–132
  otitis media in, 152, 154–155
  pathogens in, 105, 106
  premature, hypothermia in, 6, 7
  sepsis in, 95, 97
Infarction, brain stem, 197, 198
  myocardial. See *Myocardial infarction (MI)*.
  non–Q-wave, 21, 23
  ophthalmic artery, 197, 198
  posterior fossa, 197, 199
  right anterior cerebral, 197, 198
  subendocardial, 21, 23
  ventral pons, 191, 193
Infection(s), 93–114. See also specific infection, e.g., *Pneumonia*.
  breast, 313, 314
  canine space, 165, 168
  central nervous system, 105–106. See also *Meningitis*.
  complicating IO infusions, 389, 390
  dog bite and, 339, 341
  genitourinary tract, localization of, 212–213, 215
  in end-stage renal disease, 211, 213

Infection(s) *(Continued)*
  masticator space, 164, 167–168
  mycoplasma, extrapulmonary manifestations of, 69, 70
  organisms causing, 95, 97
  parvovirus, sickle cell anemia and, 181, 182
  plantar puncture, 290, 291
  precipitating sickle cell crisis, 180, 182
  sinus, asthma and, 67, 68
  tendon sheath, purulent, 286, 288
  urinary tract, 96, 98, 212–213, 214, 215
  uvular edema from, 158, 162
  viral, arthritis and, 294, 297
Infectious discitis, 295, 298
Infectious mononucleosis, 161
Infusion, intraosseous, 389, 390
Inhalation, foreign body, 157, 159–160
Injection injury, 286, 288
Injury(ies). See *Trauma*.
Insect, in external auditory canal, 152, 154
Insect bites, allergic reactions to, 123–124
Insomnia, in altitude illness, 347, 348
Insulin overdose, hypoglycemia from, 137, 141
Intermittent mandatory ventilation, 16, 17–18
Intestines, small, obstruction of, 88, 89–90
Intoxication, alcohol, 238, 240
  precipitating sickle cell crisis, 180, 182
  cocaine, 329, 330
  drug, 238, 240
Intracranial hemorrhage, in hemophilia, 184–185, 186
  postictal altered mental status and, 203, 205
Intracranial injury, 247–250
Intracranial mass, in AIDS patient, 100, 101
Intracranial pressure, elevated, cerebral metastases and, 173, 175
Intraocular pressure, elevated, from topical corticosteroids, 146, 148
Intraosseous (IO) access, in children, 271, 272
Intraosseous (IO) infusion, 389, 390
Intraosseous (IO) lines, for pediatric patients, 7, 9
Intubation, endotracheal. See *Endotracheal intubation*.
  in anaphylaxis, 123, 124
  in septic shock, 102, 103
  nasotracheal, blind, contraindications to, 16, 17
  tracheal, in COPD exacerbations, 64, 65
  inadvertent, 15, 16–17
Intussusception, diagnosis of, 83, 86
  gastrointestinal bleeding from, 82, 84
  in Henoch-Schönlein purpura, 118, 122
  management of, 174, 177
  presenting symptoms/findings of, 88, 90
Ionizing radiation, 344, 345
Iron pill, odontophagia from, 78, 80
Iron poisoning, 318, 319–320
Irritability, paradoxical, 96, 97
Irritable mood, causes of, 234, 236
Ischemia, cardiac, predisposing factors for, 21, 23
Isoniazid, for tuberculosis, 107
  pericarditis and, 51, 53

Jaundice, in acute cholangitis, 78, 80
Jaw thrust maneuver, mandibular fracture and, 15, 16
Jellyfish sting treatment, 339, 341
Joint(s). See also named joint, e.g., *Hip*.
  aspiration of, 389–390
  metacarpophalangeal, lacerations over, 286, 288
  reduction of, 389, 390

Joint(s) *(Continued)*
  temporomandibular, dislocation of, 251, 252
Jugular venous thrombosis, 159
Justice, distributive, 373, 374–375
Juvenile dermatomyositis, fever in, 118, 120
Juvenile rheumatoid arthritis, 118, 120, 121–122
  fever in, 118, 120

Kanavel's four cardinal signs, of purulent tendon sheath infection, 286, 288
Kaposi's varicelliform eruption, 223, 225
Kawasaki syndrome, cardiovascular complications of, 23, 25
Kawasaki's disease, coronary artery aneurysm complicating, 228, 229
  history/physical examination in, 56, 57–58
Kehr's sign, 75, 76
Keratitis, topical corticosteroids and, 146, 148
Keraunoparalysis, in lightning injuries, 348
Ketoacidosis, alcoholic, 137, 141
  diabetic. See *Diabetic ketoacidosis*.
Kidney(s), abscess of, 212, 215
  contusion of, 212, 214
  disease of, end-stage, 211, 213
  failure of, acute, caused by acute tubular necrosis, 211, 213
    determining cause of, 211, 213
    treatment plan for, 40–41
  chronic, 211, 213
  hyperkalemia in, 130, 132
  orellanine and, 329, 330–331
  pericarditis in, 52, 54
  infarction of, in polyarteritis nodosa, 118, 122
  injury to, risk factors for, 262, 265
  methotrexate and, 173, 176
  pediatric rheumatologic conditions involving, complications of, 118, 120
  surgical exploration of, 262, 265
  visual imaging of, 263, 265
Kiesselbach's plexus, in anterior epistaxis, 153
Klebsiella pneumoniae, pneumonia with cavitation from, 69, 70
Knee, injuries to, 290, 291
Kocher method, for anterior shoulder dislocation reduction, 285, 287
Kussmaul's respirations, in diabetes mellitus, 137, 140

Labetalol, for hypertension and aortic dissection, 39, 40
Labor, normal, 301–302
  premature, 304–305
Labyrinthitis, suppurative, 154
Lacerations, extensor tendon, 286, 288
  facial, 252, 253
  oral, 163, 166
  over metacarpophalangeal joint, 286, 288
  repair of, topical anesthetic for, 277, 278
Lambert-Eaton syndrome, 200, 201, 202
Laparoscopy, diagnostic, 261, 263
  in abdominal trauma, 261, 264
Laparotomy, in abdominal trauma, 261, 263–264
Laryngitis, 160
Laryngospasm, in hypocalcemia, 130, 132
Laryngotracheobronchitis, 158, 161
Lasix, for hypercalcemia, 138, 141
Lavage, peritoneal, 383, 384
  diagnostic, 261, 262, 263, 264, 266, 267
Laxatives, hypokalemia from, 130, 132
LBBB (left bundle branch block), in acute myocardial infarction, 26, 27
Lead poisoning, 333, 334

LeFort fractures, 251, 253
Left bundle branch block (LBBB), in acute myocardial infarction, 26, 27
Legg-Calvé-Perthes disease, 294, 296
Legionella pneumonia, 69, 70
Leptospirosis, 113–114
Lethargy, in cancer-related hypercalcemia, 174, 177
Leukemia, acute myelogenous, hyperleukocytic syndrome in, 173, 175
　fever from, 95, 97
　neutropenic, typhlitis in, 174, 177
　vincristine for, hyponatremia from, 130, 133
Leukocytosis, in sepsis, 102, 103
Leukostasis syndrome, 173, 175
Lice, in eyelashes, sexual abuse and, 227, 228
Lichen planus, 224, 226
Lichtenberg figures, in lightning injuries, 348
Lidocaine, for cocaine-induced hypertension and arrhythmias, 34, 37
　for ventricular tachycardia, 35, 39
　in acute myocardial infarction, 26, 27
　in local anesthesia, 277–278
Ligaments, ankle, 291, 292
Lightheadedness, 192, 194
Lightning injuries, 348–349
Liquefaction necrosis, in external auditory canal, 152, 154
Listeria monocytogenes, infantile infections from, 95, 97
Listeria sepsis, pediatric fever from, 96, 98
Lithium, for thyrotoxicosis, 136, 139
　toxicologic effects of, 321
Liver, abscess of, 79, 80
　acetaminophen toxicity and, 318, 319
　blunt trauma to, 261, 264
　failure of, amatoxin and, 329, 330–331
　　fulminant, 78–79, 80
"Locked-in syndrome," 191, 193
Loop diuretics, for hypercalcemia of malignancy, 173, 176
Lorazepam, for status epilepticus, 203–204, 206
LSD, 329, 331
Ludwig's angina, management of, 164, 167
　presentation of, 157, 160, 161
Lugol's solution, for thyrotoxicosis, 136, 139
Lumbar puncture, 385
　contraindications to, 105, 106
Lung(s). See also *Pulmonary; Respiratory* entries.
　blast, 281–282
　cancer of, superior vena cava syndrome in, 173, 174–175, 176
　contusion of, 258, 259
　disease of, 59–72
　　chronic obstructive, 64–66
　　fibrotic, 64, 65
　edema of, high-altitude, 347, 348
　　etiology of, 365, 366
　in bronchopulmonary dysplasia, 69, 70
　hyperexpansion of, aspirated foreign body and, 157, 160
Lupus erythematosus, systemic, 117, 119
　pediatric, pseudotumor cerebri in, 118, 122
Lyme disease, 109–111, 227, 228
　dysrhythmia in, treatment of, 35, 38
Lymph node syndrome, mucocutaneous, 56, 57–58
　cardiovascular complications of, 23, 25
Lymphadenopathy, parotid gland, in Lyme disease, 110
Lymphogranuloma venereum, 311
Lymphoma, non-Hodgkin's, pericardial tamponade in, 174, 177

Malabsorption syndrome, 185, 187

Malaria, 112, 113
Malignancy(ies). See also *Cancer.*
　hypercalcemia of, treatment of, 173, 176
Malignant otitis externa, 152, 154
Mallory-Weiss tear, 82, 84
Malpractice suit, 368, 370–371
Mandible, fracture of, 251, 252
　jaw thrust maneuver and, 15, 16
Mandibular condyles, dislocation of, 164–165, 168
　fracture of, 251, 252
MANTRELS score, 83, 86
Marijuana abuse, 238, 240
Masticator space infection, 164, 167–168
Mastitis, postpartum, 313, 314
Mastoiditis, complicating otitis media, 152, 154
Maxillary sinus, 151, 153
Maxillofacial fracture, 251, 252
Maxillofacial trauma, 163, 166, 251–253
McCarthy Infant Observation Scale, 95–96, 97
Measles, vs. Rocky Mountain spotted fever, 108, 109
Measles-mumps-rubella vaccination, 96, 98
Mechanical outflow obstruction, pulmonary embolism from, 62, 64
Mechanical ventilation, for asthma, 67, 68
　in respiratory distress, 13, 14
Meconium, resuscitation of newborn with, 6, 8
Mediastinal shift, contralateral, aspirated foreign body and, 157, 160
Mediastinal widening, evaluation of, 257, 259
Mediastinitis, complicating IO infusions, 389, 390
Medical advice, signing out against, 368, 371
Medical malpractice suit, 368, 370–371
Medical transport, air, 365–366
Medicolegal aspects, of emergency medicine, 368, 370–371
Mees' lines, 333, 334
Melanoma, 227, 228
Melena, investigation of, 82, 84
Meniere's disease, 152, 154
Meningitis, 96, 98, 105–106
　complicating otitis media, 152, 154
　cryptococcal, AIDS and, 99, 100, 101
　in infants, 95, 97
Meningococcemia, petechial rash from, 224, 225
　vs. Rocky Mountain spotted fever, 108, 109
Menstruation, precipitating sickle cell crisis, 180, 182
Mental status, altered, 191–192, 193–194
　in acute cholangitis, 78, 80
　pediatric causes of, 191–192, 193
Metabolic acidosis, in asthma, 67, 68
　in diabetic ketoacidosis, 135, 138
Metacarpophalangeal joint, lacerations over, 286, 288
Metastasis(es), cerebral, intracranial pressure elevation from, 173, 175
　from breast cancer, hypercalcemia from, 137, 141
　spinal cord compression in, 174, 177
Metatarsal fractures, 290, 291–292
Methanol toxicity, 325, 326–327
Methemoglobinemia toxicity, 332–333, 334
Methotrexate, adverse effects of, 173, 176
Methyldopa, pericarditis and, 51, 53
Methylene blue therapy, failure of, 333, 334
Methylxanthines, adenosine and, 32, 37
Metronidazole, for *Clostridium difficile*–induced colitis, 75, 77
　for perforated appendix, 84, 86
Micturition, normal, 217, 218
Middle ear barotrauma, 343, 344
Midface trauma, 243, 245

Migraine headache, 204, 205, 207, 208
　hemiplegic, 205, 208
Milch method, for anterior shoulder dislocation reduction, 285, 287
Military antishock trousers, 243, 245
Mineral oil, cerumen removal with, 152, 154
Mini-mental status examination, impaired, 235, 237
Miosis, 197, 198
　causes of, 191
Mithramycin, for hypercalcemia, 138, 141
Mitral valve prosthesis, febrile illness and, 96, 98
Moban (molindone), 233, 235–236
Mobitz AV block, 32, *33,* 37
Molar pregnancy, 303, 304
Molindone (Moban), 233, 235–236
Mondor's disease, 313, 314
Moniliasis, 158, 161
Monoamine oxidase inhibitor–tyramine interaction, 321
Monoarticular arthritis, acute, 294, 297
Mononucleosis, 157, 159
　infectious, 161
Monteggia fracture, 288
Mood, irritable, causes of, 234, 236
Moraxella catarrhalis, otitis media from, 154
　pneumonia from, 69, 70
Morbilliform reaction, 227, 228
Morison's pouch, fluid in, 305
"Morning after" pills, 307, 310
Morphine, for nephrolithiasis, in hemophilia, 194, 196
Motor neuron disease, 200, 201
Mucocutaneous lymph node syndrome, 56, 57–58
　cardiovascular complications of, 23, 25
Mucormycosis, 151, 153
Mucosa, dry, anterior epistaxis from, 151, 153
Mucositis, from methotrexate, 173, 176
Mucus plugging, COPD management and, 64, 66
Multiple myeloma, complications of, 173, 175–176
Muscarinic symptoms, of organophosphate poisoning, 330, 331
Muscle(s), relaxants of, for pediatric near-drowning victim, 7, 9
　respiratory, fatigue of, in asthma, 67, 68
　weakness of, in cancer-related hypercalcemia, 174, 177
　in hypocalcemia, 130, 132
Musculoskeletal injuries, 283–298
Mushrooms, paraquat and, 329, 330
Myasthenia gravis, 200, 201
Mycobacterial disease, 107–108
Mycobacterium tuberculosis, pneumonia with cavitation from, 69, 70
Mycoplasma, infection from, extrapulmonary manifestations of, 69, 70
　sinusitis from, 151, 153
Mydriasis, 197, 198
Myelinolysis, central pontine, 130, 133
Myelogenous leukemia, acute, hyperleukocytic syndrome in, 173, 175
Myocardial contusion, 257, 258–259
Myocardial infarction (MI), abdominal pain from, 75, 76
　acute, adjunctive therapies for, 26, 27
　characteristics of, 21, 23
　ECG in, 25–26, 27
　inferolateral, management of, 25, 26–27
　left bundle branch block in, 26, 27
　management of, 26, 27
　risk factors for, 21, 23

Myocardial infarction (MI) *(Continued)*
   serum markers for, 26, 27
   transmural, emergency angioplasty for, 28, 29–30
   asymptomatic bradycardia after, therapy for, 35, 39
   cardiogenic shock after, risk factors for, 29, 31
   chest pain in, therapy for, 22, 24
   dysrhythmias complicating, 35, 39
   ventricular ectopy after, 34, 37
Myocardial ischemia, 25–27
   presenting complaint in, 22, 24
Myocarditis, presenting symptoms of, 52, 54
   with hypotension and respiratory distress, management of, 51, 53
Myxedema, ECG in, 51, 53
Myxedema coma, 135, 139

N-acetylcysteine (NAC), for acetaminophen overdose, 317–318, 319
Nalozone, in opioid overdose, 329, 330
Narcissistic personality disorder, 234, 236
Nasal disorders, 151, 152–153
Nasal-orbital-ethmoid fracture, CT scan of, 251, 253
Nasolacrimal duct obstruction, 147, 150
Nasotracheal intubation, blind, contraindications to, 16, 17
Nasotracheal tube, size of, 15, 17
National Disaster Medical System (NDMS), 363, 364
National Practitioner Data Bank, 367–368, 370
Nausea, in adrenal insufficiency, 135, 138
   in altitude illness, 347, 348
NDMS (National Disaster Medical System), 363, 364
Near drowning, pediatric, 7, 9
Near-syncope, 192, 194
Neck trauma, 253–255
Necrotizing enterocolitis, gastrointestinal bleeding from, 82, 84
Neisseria meningitidis, pediatric infections from, 96, 98
Nephrolithiasis, 218, 219
   in hemophilia, 194, 196
Nervous system, disorders of, 189–208
Neuralgia, trigeminal, 198
Neuritis, retrobulbar, 107
Neuroleptic malignant syndrome, 330, 331
Neurologic disorder(s), 189–208
   altered mental status as, 191–192, 193–194
   cerebrovascular emergencies as, 197, 198–199
   coma as, 191–192, 193. See also *Coma.*
   cranial nerve disorders as, 197–198, 199
   dizziness as, 192, 194
   from penetrating neck trauma, 254, 255
   headaches as, 204–205, 207–208. See also *Headache(s).*
   in supracondylar fractures, 285–286, 287–288
   neuromuscular, 200–202
   seizures as, 203–204, 205–207. See also *Seizures.*
   urinary retention in, 217, 219
   vertigo as, 192–195
Neuromas, acoustic, 154
Neuromuscular disorders, 200–202
Neurovascular symptoms, from ionizing radiation exposure, 344, 345–346
Neutropenia, febrile patient with, antimicrobials for, 174, 176
   from methotrexate, 173, 176
Neutropenic leukemia, typhlitis in, 174, 177
Nifedipine, for altitude illness, 347
   for hypertensive urgencies, 39–40

Night shift work, 373–374
Nitrites, organisms producing, 212, 214
Nitroglycerin, for cocaine-induced hypertension and arrhythmias, 34, 37
   sublingual, adverse effects of, 28, 29
Nitroprusside, for cocaine-induced hypertension and arrhythmias, 34, 37
Nodules, subcutaneous, in rheumatoid arthritis, 117, 119
Nonconvulsive status, 203, 205
Nondepolarizing agents, metabolized by plasma enzymes, 15–16, 17
Non-Hodgkin's lymphoma, pericardial tamponade in, 174, 177
Non–Q-wave infarction, 21, 23
Nonsteroidal anti-inflammatory drugs (NSAIDs), for pericarditis, 52, 54
   for Ramsay Hunt syndrome, 152, 154
   in pregnancy, 273, 274
   in systemic lupus erythematosus, 117, 119
   toxicity of, 317, 319
Norepinephrine, for hypotension from septic shock, 102, 103
Nosebleed, 151, 152–153
NSAIDs (nonsteroidal anti-inflammatory drugs), for pericarditis, 52, 54
   for Ramsay Hunt syndrome, 152, 154
   in pregnancy, 273, 274
   in systemic lupus erythematosus, 117, 119
   toxicity of, 317, 319
Nursemaid's elbow, 293–294, 296
Nystagmus, 192, 194–195

Obesity, abdominal injury patterns and, 262, 264
Obstetric disorders, 301–306
Obstructive uropathy, complicating multiple myeloma, 173, 175–176
Obturator test, in appendicitis, 75, 76
Occult blood, in stool, 83, 85
Ocular disorders, 145–150
Ocular palsy, in pituitary necrosis, 135, 138
Oculovestibular reflex, 191
Odontophagia, medications causing, 78, 80
Olanzapine (Zyprexa), 233, 235–236
Olecranon bursitis, traumatic, 286, 288
Oncologic emergencies, 173–177
Ophthalmic artery infarct, 197, 198
Opioid overdose, 329, 330
Orbital cellulitis, 146, 149
Orbital rim fractures, 251, 252
Orellanine, renal failure and, 329, 330–331
Organ donation, 369, 372
Organophosphate poisoning, 330, 331
Oropharyngeal airway, size of, 15, 16
Orthopedic emergencies, pediatric, 293–298
Orthostasis, diagnosis of, 192, 194
Osteitis, alveolar, 164, 167
Osteomyelitis, complicating IO infusions, 389, 390
Osteonecrosis, in sickle cell anemia, 181, 182
Osteoporosis, sternal fracture and, 260
Otitis externa, malignant, 152, 154
Otitis media, 151–152, 154–155
Otohematoma, 152, 154
Ottawa ankle rules, 290, 291, 292
Oximetry, pulse, 332, 333, 334
Oxygen dependence, in bronchopulmonary dysplasia, 69, 70
Oxygen therapy, hyperbaric, 342, 343
   in emergency asthma management, 67, 68
Oxygenation, assessment of, in pulmonary embolism, 61, 62–63

Pacemaker, 32, 37
Paget's disease, hypercalcemia from, 137–138, 141
Pain, abdominal, transmission of, 75, 76
   back, 295, 297, 298
   in adrenal insufficiency, 135, 138
   cardiac, altered perception of, predisposing factors for, 21, 23
   chest. See *Chest, pain in.*
   flank, in adrenal insufficiency, 135, 138
   in pericarditis, 22, 24
   management of, 355–356
Palate, burns of, 164, 167
Palpitations, in pheochromocytoma, 135, 138
Pamidronate, for hypercalcemia of malignancy, 173, 176
Pancreatic pseudocyst, 79, 81
Pancreatitis, acute, 79, 81
Pancuronium, histamine release from, 15, 17
Paradoxical irritability, 96, 97
Paralysis, 200–202
Parasitic diseases, 112–113
Parkinson's disease, psychosis in, 233, 235
Parotid glands, lymphadenopathy around, in Lyme disease, 110
Paroxysmal supraventricular tachycardia recurrence, 4, 5
Parvovirus infection, sickle cell anemia and, 181, 182
Patella injuries, 290, 291
Patient transfers, 363–364
Pediatric patient. See also *Infant(s).*
   abdominal trauma in, 262, 264
   airway of, 6, 7–8
   altered mental status/coma in, 191–192, 193
   alveolar ridge to midtrachea distance in, 15, 17
   ankle injuries in, 291, 292
   appendicitis, 83, 86
   arrhythmias in, 7, 9
   asthma in, differential diagnosis of, 67–68, 68–69
   atenolol ingestion by, 322, 323
   bicycle handlebar injury in, 261–262, 264
   cardiac arrest in, 6–7, 8
   chest pain in, causes of, 22–23, 25
   clonidine toxicity in, 322, 323
   dehydration in, 76, 77
   rehydration solution for, 129, 130
   distributive shock in, 129, 130
   endotracheal tube for, size of, 6, 8, 15, 17
   uncuffed, 16, 17
   febrile, 95–98
   fluid and electrolyte disorders in, 129–131
   foreign body ingestion by, 158, 162
   genitourinary injuries in, 263, 265
   head trauma in, 247, 249
   heart failure in, causes of, 29, 31
   near drowning in, 7, 9
   orthopedic emergencies in, 293–298
   pneumonia in, pathogens causing, 69, 70
   resuscitation of, 6–10
   rheumatologic conditions in, 118, 120
   sexual abuse in, 357–358, 360–361. See also *Child abuse.*
   sickle cell disease in, chest pain and, 23, 25
   trauma in, 271–273
   tuberculosis in, 107, 108
   vaginal foreign bodies in, 307, 310
   vascular access for, 7, 9–10
Pediculosis capitis, 227, 228
PEEP (positive end-expiratory pressure), 16, 18
Peer review, 368, 370
Pelvic inflammatory disease, 307, 308, 309, 310, 311, 312

Pelvic inflammatory disease *(Continued)*
  appendicitis differentiated from, 83, 86
Pelvic ring disruption, Young classification of, 266, 267–268
Pelvis, fractures of, 266, 268
  trauma to, 265–268
Pemphigoid, bullous, 224, 225
Pemphigus vulgaris, 224, 225
Penicillin, allergic reactions and, 123, 124
  for oral lacerations, 163, 166
  for syphilis, 114
  pericarditis and, 51, 53
Penicillin V, for human bite prophylaxis, 339, 340
Penis, fracture of, 262, 265
Percutaneous central venous catheterization, 387–388
Percutaneous femoral line, for pediatric patients, 7, 9
Percutaneous transtracheal ventilation, 383, 384
Perianal abscess, treatment of, 89, 91
Periapical abscess, 163, 164, 167
Pericardial effusion/tamponade, in chronic renal failure, 211, 213
Pericardial friction rub, 52, 53–54
Pericardial knock, 54
Pericardial tamponade, ED thoracotomy for, 379, 380
  electrical alternans in, 387, 388
  in non-Hodgkin's lymphoma, 174, 177
Pericardiocentesis, 387, 388
Pericarditis, acute, ECG findings in, 22, 24
  constrictive, 54
  ECG in, 51, 53
  etiology and features of, 51, 53
  in systemic lupus erythematosus, 117, 119
  juvenile rheumatoid arthritis and, 118, 122
  malignant, 54
  management of, 51–52, 53, 54
  pain in, 22, 24
Pericoronitis, 163, 167
Perihepatitis, 307, 310
Perinephric abscess, 212, 215
Periodic paralysis, 200, 201–202
Periorbital cellulitis, 147–148, 150
Peritoneal lavage, 383, 384
  diagnostic, 261, 262, 263, 264, 266, 267
Peritonitis, 310
Peritonsillar abscess, 158, 161
Personality disorders, 234, 236
Pesticides, gastrointestinal decontamination for, 332, 334
Petechiae, in endocarditis, 53, 54
Petechial rash, from meningococcemia, 224, 225
Pharyngeal abscess, 157, 159
Pharyngitis, streptococcal, abdominal pain from, 75, 76
  viral, 161
Pharyngotracheal lumen airway, contraindications to, 15, 17
Phencyclidine, toxicity of, 329–330, 331
Phenelzine, interactions with, 34, 37
Phenobarbital, elimination of, 326, 328
Phentolamine, for hypertension from phenelzine, 34, 37
  for hypertension in pheochromocytoma, 135, 138
Phenylephrine, for hypotension from septic shock, 102, 103
  rhinitis medicamentosa from, 151, 153
Phenytoin, pericarditis and, 51, 53
  uses of, 325, 326
Pheochromocytoma, 135, 136, 138, 139, 140
Phlegmasia cerulea dolens, characteristics of, 45–46, 47

Phosgene, toxicity of, 332, 333
Photophobia, in pituitary necrosis, 135, 138
Phototoxic drug reactions, 227, 229
Physicians, emergency, burnout in, 373, 374
Physostigmine, 321, 322
Pilonidal cyst, treatment of, 89, 91
Pine oil ingestion, 332, 334
Pituitary gland, necrosis in, 135, 138
  tumor of, 129, 130
Placenta previa, 301, 305
Plantar puncture, 290, 291
Plantar reflex, in right-sided hemispheric lesion, 191, 193
Plasma, fresh frozen, for Christmas disease, 194, 196
  for thrombotic thrombocytopenic purpura, 184, 185
  indications for, 185, 187
Plasma enzymes, nondepolarizing agents metabolized by, 15–16, 17
Plasma exchange, for thrombotic thrombocytopenic purpura, 184, 185–186
Platelet transfusion, for thrombotic thrombocytopenic purpura, 184, 185
Pleurisy, 69–71
Pneumocystis carinii pneumonia, 99, 100–101
Pneumonia, 69–71
  AIDS-related, 99, 101
  community-acquired, 161
  complicating COPD, 64, 65
  Pneumocystis carinii, 99, 100–101
Pneumothorax, 258, 259, 260
  complicating COPD, 64, 65
  tension, in blunt chest trauma, 380
Poiseuille's law, 387–388
Poisoning, anticholinergic, 321, 322
  arsenic, 334
  carbon monoxide, 279–281
    scuba diving and, 342, 343
  cyanide, 332, 333–334
  digoxin, 35, 38, 322, 323
  ethylene glycol, 325, 326–327
  iron, 318, 319–320
  lead, 333, 334
  organophosphate, 330, 331
  salicylate, 317, 319
  superwarfarin rodenticide, 330, 331
Poliomyelitis, 200, 201
Pollen, asthma and, 67, 68
Polyarteritis nodosa, pediatric, fever in, 118, 121
  renal complications of, 118, 120
  renal infarction in, 118, 122
Polymorphic ventricular tachycardia, 42
Polyps, gastrointestinal bleeding from, 82, 84
Polyvalent pneumococcal vaccines, 69, 70
Pons, ventral, hemorrhage/infarction of, 191, 193
Positive end-expiratory pressure (PEEP), 16, 18
Postdural headache, after lumbar puncture, 385
Posterior compartment syndrome, 269, 270
Posterior fossa infarctions, 197, 199
Post-myocardial infarction syndrome, chest pain in, therapy for, 22, 24
Postpartum hemorrhage, 305, 306
Post-traumatic stress disorder, 234, 236
Potassium, depletion of, in diabetic ketoacidosis, 135, 138
  supplemental, odontophagia from, 78, 80
Power rapist, 362
Prazosin, for hypertension in pheochromocytoma, 135, 138
Prednisone, Cushing's syndrome and, 136–137, 140
  for Ramsay Hunt syndrome, 152, 154
Preeclampsia, 40, 304, 305
Pregnancy, antimicrobials in, 273, 274, 309, 312

Pregnancy *(Continued)*
  appendicitis in, 83, 86, 309, 312
  asthma in, 309, 312
  chlamydia in, 308, 311–312
  early, complications of, 302–304
  eclampsia in, treatment of, 40
  ectopic, 83, 86, 302, 303, 304
    ruptured, 304–305, 308, 311
  late, complications of, 304–306
  medications in, 273, 274
  molar, 303, 304
  normal physiologic changes in, 273, 274
  pelvic trauma in, 265, 266–267
  perforated appendix in, antimicrobials for, 84, 86
  physiologic changes in, 305, 306
  pruritic urticarial papules and plaques of, 224, 226
  tests for, 302, 303
  trauma in, 273–275
Preload, medications reducing, 28, 30
Premature infant, hypothermia in, 6, 7
Premature labor, 304–305
Premature ventricular beats, management of, 36, 39
Priapism, 217, 219
Prinzmetal's angina, conditions associated with, 21, 23
  ECG changes in, 22, 24–25
Procainamide, for atrial fibrillation with preexcitation pattern, 35, 39
  in resuscitation, 3, 4
Procaine allergy, medications safe in, 277, 278
Prochlorperazine, for migraine headache, 205, 208
Propoxyphene, toxicity of, 329, 330
Propylthiouracil, for thyrotoxicosis, 136, 139
Prostaglandin E, for cyanotic newborn, 56, 57
Prostate gland, cancer of, epidural spinal cord compression in, 173, 175
  hypertrophy of, benign, 217, 219
Prostatitis, 212, 214–215
Prosthesis, mitral valve, febrile illness and, 96, 98
Pruritic urticarial papules and plaques, of pregnancy, 224, 226
Pruritus, vulvovaginal, 307, 309
Pseudocyst, pancreatic, 79, 81
Pseudoephedrine, interaction with phenelzine, 34, 37
Pseudomonas aeruginosa, malignant otitis externa from, 152, 154
Pseudomonas folliculitis, 228, 229
Pseudosubluxation, cervical spine, pediatric, 293, 295
Pseudotumor cerebri, in systemic lupus erythematosus, 118, 122
Psychogenic seizures, 204, 207
Psychosis, 233–237
  in systemic lupus erythematosus, 117, 119
Ptosis, 197–198, 199
Public Law 93–154, 363, 364
Pulmonary angiography, 62, 63
Pulmonary edema, high-altitude, 347, 348
  etiology of, 365, 366
  in bronchopulmonary dysplasia, 69, 70
Pulmonary embolism, A-a gradient in, 62, 63
  clinical diagnosis of, 62, 63
  clinical signs of, 61, 62
  death from, conditions associated with, 62, 64
  deep venous thrombosis and, 61, 62
  demographics of, 62, 63
  oxygenation assessment in, 61, 62–63
  risk factors for, 61, 62
  therapy for, 62, 63

Pulmonary embolism *(Continued)*
  thrombolytic therapy and, 22, 24
Pulmonary vasoconstriction, 62, 64
Pulse oximetry, 332, 333, 334
Pulse pressure, in thyrotoxicosis, 136, 139
Pulsus paradoxus, in COPD, 64, 65
Pupils, asymmetry of, 192, 194
Purpura, acute immune thrombocytopenic, 184, 186
  differential diagnosis of, 223, 225
  Henoch-Schönlein, child abuse confused with, 118, 121
    renal complications of, 118, 120
  thrombotic thrombocytopenic, 184, 185–186, 187, 227, 228
Pursed-lip breathing, in COPD, 64, 65
Pyelogram, intravenous, "one-shot," 262, 265
Pyelonephritis, 212, 214
  complicating bacterial prostatitis, 212, 214–215
  xanthogranulomatous, 212, 214
Pyloric stenosis, 88, 90
Pyrethrin toxicity, 330, 331

Quality assurance (QA) programs, EMS, 364, 368, 371
Quinolones, for *Shigella* and *Salmonella*, 75, 77

Rabies, 340, 341–342
Radiation, 344–346
Radioactive contamination, 344, 346
Radiocontrast media (RCM), anaphylactoid reaction to, 123, 124
Rales, in thyroid storm, 136, 139
Ramsay Hunt syndrome, 152, 154
Rape. See *Sexual abuse/assault.*
Rash, from methotrexate, 173, 176
  heliotrope, in dermatomyositis, 117, 119
  in childhood rheumatologic disorders, 118, 121
  in Lyme disease, 109, 110
  in Rocky Mountain spotted fever, 108–109
Rattlesnake bite, 339, 341
Raynaud's phenomenon, 118, 121
  in scleroderma, 117, 119
RCM (radiocontrast media), anaphylactoid reaction to, 123, 124
Rectum, digital examination of, contraindications to, 266, 267
  for temperature measurement, in children, 95, 97
  foreign bodies in, 89, 90–91
  prolapse of, 89, 91–92
Reflex(es), caloric, 191
  deep tendon, in myxedema, 136, 139
  oculovestibular, 191
Regional anesthesia, 355–356
Reiter's syndrome, 117, 118
Renal colic, 217, 218, 219. See also *Kidney(s).*
Respirations, Kussmaul's, in diabetes mellitus, 137, 140
Respiratory acidosis, COPD management and, 64, 65, 66
  in asthma, 67, 68
Respiratory depression, from opioid overdose, 329, 330
Respiratory distress, myocarditis with, 51, 53
Respiratory failure, adult, 13–14
  impending, warning signs of, 67
  in congestive heart failure, treatment of, 28, 30
Respiratory muscle fatigue, in asthma, 67, 68

Respiratory syncytial virus bronchiolitis, infant apnea and, 11
Respiratory syncytial virus pneumonia, 69, 70
Resuscitation, adult, 3–5
  pediatric, 6–10
Retinal artery, central, occlusion of, 146–147, 149
Retinal detachment, 145, 148
Retinitis, AIDS, 99, 101
  cytomegalovirus, 99, 100
Retrobulbar hemorrhage, 145–146, 148
  in orbital rim fracture, 251, 252
Retrobulbar neuritis, from ethambutol, 107
Retrobulbar pressure, increased, 146, 149
Retrograde urography, indications for, 266, 267
Retropharyngeal abscess, 158, 160, 161
Retroplacental hematoma, 274, 275
Rewarming techniques, external, 351
Reye's syndrome, 192, 193–194
Reynold's pentad, in acute cholangitis, 78, 80
Rhabdomyolysis, 349
Rheumatic fever, erythema marginatum in, 227, 228
Rheumatoid arthritis, 117, 119
  juvenile, 118, 120, 121–122
  ophthalmic manifestations of, 117, 120
Rhinitis medicamentosa, 151, 153
Rhonchi, in COPD, 64, 65
Rhythms, cardiac, wide complex pulseless, 3, 4
Rib fractures, 257, 259
Rickettsia rickettsii, Rocky Mountain spotted fever from, 108, 109
Rifampin, for tuberculosis, 107
Rinne test, 151, 153–154
Risperidone (Risperal), 233, 235–236
Rocky Mountain spotted fever, 108–111
Rovsing's sign, in appendicitis, 75, 76
Rule of nines, 279, *280,* 281

Sadistic rapist, 362
Salicylate toxicity, 317, 319
Saline, for hypernatremia, 130, 133
  for hypovolemic shock, 129, 130
Salivary calculi, 158, 161–162
Salmonella, antimicrobial agents for, 75, 77
  infection from, HgbSS disease and, 180, 182
Salter-Harris injury classification, 293, 296
Saphenous vein cutdown, for pediatric patients, 7, 9
Sarcoidosis, 117, 119
  hypercalcemia from, 137, 141
  ophthalmic manifestations of, 117, 120
Scheduling, 367, 369–370
Schizoid disorder, vs. schizophrenia, 234, 236
Schizophrenia, 233, 235
Schizotypal disorder, vs. schizophrenia, 234, 236
Scleritis, 147, 150
Scleroderma, 117, 119
  chest radiograph in, 118, 122
  renal complications of, 118, 120
Scombroid, 76, 77
Sea sponge wound, 339, 341
Sea urchin wound, 339, 341
Seat belt syndrome, 244, 246
Seborrheic dermatitis, 223, 225
Sedation, 355, 356
  for pediatric near-drowning victim, 7, 9
Seizures, 203–204, 205–207
  absence, 204, 206
  complex partial, 204, 206
  cyclic antidepressant–induced, 321, 323
  from carbamazepine, 326, 327
  from isoniazid, 107

Seizures *(Continued)*
  generalized tonic-clonic, altered mental status in, 203, 205
    febrile, 203, 205
    upper airway obstruction in, 159, 162
  gyrometrin and, 329, 330–331
  in hypernatremic dehydration, 129, 131
  in pregnancy, treatment of, 273, 274
  psychogenic, 204, 207
  tonic, 204, 206
Sepsis, 102–104
  from abdominal trauma, 261–262, 264
  in hematologic malignancies, 174, 176
  in newborn, 95, 97
  in systemic lupus erythematosus, 117, 119
  Listeria, pediatric fever from, 96, 98
  Rocky Mountain spotted fever differentiated from, 108, 109
  viral, pediatric fever from, 96, 98
Septic shock, hypotension from, drugs for, 102, 103
  in acute cholangitis, 78, 80
Serotonin receptors, in headache pain, 205, 208
Serotonin-reuptake inhibitors, toxicologic effects of, 321
Serum amylase, in pancreatitis, 79, 81
Serum markers, for acute myocardial infarction, 26, 27
Serum sickness, fever from, 95, 97
Sexual abuse/assault, evaluation of, 359, 362
  history taking in, 358, 362
  lice in eyelashes and, 227, 228
  pediatric, 357–358, 360–361. See also *Child abuse.*
  treatment of, 359, 362
Sexual dysfunction, in adult abuse victims, 358, 361
Sexually transmitted disease, prophylaxis for, in sexual abuse victims, 359, 362
Shaken baby syndrome, 247, 248–249
Shigella, antimicrobial agents for, 75, 77
Shock, cardiogenic. See *Cardiogenic shock.*
  distributive, in infant, 129, 130
  hypovolemic, in pediatric patient, 129, 130
  pediatric, 271, 272
  septic, hypotension from, drugs for, 102, 103
    in acute cholangitis, 78, 80
  spinal, 244, 246
Shoulder dislocation, anterior, reduction of, 285, 287, 389, 390
Shunt, Blalock-Taussig, classic, 56, 58
  central nervous system, *Staphylococcus epidermidis* causing infection of, 105, 106
  ventriculoperitoneal, febrile illness and, 96, 98
Sialoadenitis, 161
Sialolithiasis, 158, 161–162
Sickle cell disease, 180–182
  in children, chest pain in, 23, 25
Sigmoid volvulus, 88, 90
Silent cardiac ischemia, predisposing factors for, 21, 23
Sinus(es), age of aeration of, 151, 153
  infection of, asthma and, 67, 68
Sinus bradycardia, complicating myocardial infarction, 35, 39
Sinus tachycardia, treatment of, 35–36, 39
Sinusitis, 151, 153
Sjögren's syndrome, ophthalmic manifestations of, 117, 120
Skew deviation, 191
Skin, disorders of, 221–229
  in endocarditis, 53, 54
  in myxedema, 136, 139
Skull fracture, basilar, 248, 250
Sleeping disorders, in adult abuse victims, 358, 361

Slipped capital femoral epiphysis, 294, 295, 296–297
Small bowel obstruction, 88, 89–90
Smoking, COPD and, 64, 65
Snakebite, 339, 341
Sodium, diabetic ketoacidosis and, 137, 140–141
Sodium bicarbonate, for cyclic antidepressant–induced cardiac dysrhythmias, 321, 323
 for tumor lysis syndrome, 174, 177
 in cardiac arrest, 3, 4
Sodium nitroprusside, for hypertension, and aortic dissection, 39, 40
 in pheochromocytoma, 135, 138
Sphenoid sinus, 151, 153
Spider bite, 339–340, 341
Spinal cord, compression of, complicating multiple myeloma, 173, 175–176
 in metastatic cancer, 174, 177
 epidural, compression of, in prostate cancer, 173, 175
 injury to, pediatric, 293, 295
Spinal shock, 244, 246
Spine, cervical. See Cervical spine.
 thoracic, compression of, 174, 177
 trauma to, 243, 244, 245–246
 pediatric, 272–273
Spleen, trauma to, blunt, 261, 264
 in children, 262, 264
Spousal violence, 361
Stanford classification system, for thoracic aortic dissections, 46, 48
Staphylococcal conjunctivitis, 146, 149
Staphylococcus aureus, pneumonia from, 69, 70
 with cavitation, 69, 70
 toxic shock syndrome from, 309, 312
Staphylococcus epidermidis, CNS shunt infection from, 105, 106
Starvation, endogenous glucose source in, 137, 141
 hypoglycemia from, 137, 141
Status epilepticus, 203–204, 206
Stensen's duct, 165, 168
Sternal fracture, 258, 260
Steroids, Cushing's syndrome and, 136–137, 140
 gastrointestinal bleeding and, 83, 85
Stevens-Johnson syndrome, 224, 225
 trimethoprim-sulfamethoxazole and, 123, 124
Stimson method, for anterior shoulder dislocation reduction, 285, 287
Sting(s), jellyfish, treatment of, 339, 341
 management of, 340, 342
Stingray wound treatment, 339, 341
Stomach ulcer, endoscopic diagnosis of, 82, 84–85
Stool guaiac test, positive, 83, 85
Strep throat, 157, 159
Streptococcal pharyngitis, abdominal pain from, 75, 76
Streptococcus, group A beta-hemolytic, 157, 159
 group B, infantile infections from, 95, 97
Streptococcus pneumoniae, infection from, HgbSS disease and, 180, 182
 infantile, 95, 97
 pediatric, 96, 98
 otitis media from, 154
 pneumonia from, 69, 70
Streptokinase, hypersensitivity to, 123, 124
Streptomycin, for Rocky Mountain spotted fever, 108, 109
 for tuberculosis, 107
Stress, disorders from, 234, 236
 emergency personnel and, 373, 374
 emotional, precipitating sickle cell crisis, 180, 182

Stress *(Continued)*
 heat, 350
 management of, 373, 374
 seizure disorders and, 203, 205
Stridor, in anaphylaxis, 123, 124
 inhaled foreign body causing, 157, 159
Stroke, 197, 198–199
 in HgbSS disease, 180, 182
Subarachnoid hemorrhage, 197, 198
 headache in, 204, 207
Subendocardial infarction, 21, 23
Substance abuse, 238–240
Succinylcholine, metabolism of, 15, 17
Suicide, 234, 236
 attempted, in adult abuse victims, 358, 361
Sulfonamides, phototoxic reaction from, 227, 229
Superficial thrombophlebitis, therapy for, 45, 47
Superior vena cava syndrome, 173, 174–175, 176
Superwarfarin rodenticide poisoning, 330, 331
Suppurative jugular venous thrombosis, 159
Suppurative labyrinthitis, 154
Supracondylar fracture, 285–286, 287
Supraglottitis, 158, 160, 161
Supranuclear pathway lesion, 191
Supraventricular tachycardia (SVT), in children, treatment of, 7, 9
 paroxysmal, recurrence of, 4, 5
 ventricular tachycardia differentiated from, 34, 38
 Brugada criteria for, 32, 36–37
Sutures, materials for, 277, 278
 removal of, 277, 278
SVT (supraventricular tachycardia). See *Supraventricular tachycardia (SVT).*
Sweating, in pheochromocytoma, 135, 138
Sympathomimetic agents, interaction of, with phenelzine, 34, 37
Sympathomimetic toxidrome, vs. anticholinergic toxidrome, 329, 330
Sympathomimetics, rhinitis medicamentosa from, 151, 153
Syncope, 41–42
Syndrome of inappropriate antidiuretic hormone (SIADH), 174, 176
 from vincristine, 130, 133
Synovitis, transient, 294, 296
Syphilis, 113, 114, 311
 congenital, pediatric fever from, 96, 98
Syrup of ipecac, 317, 318
Systemic lupus erythematosus, 117, 119
 pediatric, fever in, 118, 120
 pseudotumor cerebri in, 118, 122
 renal complications of, 118, 120

Tachy-brady syndrome, 38
Tachycardia, from carbamazepine, 326, 327
 in neonate, 56, 57
 in sepsis, 102, 103
 in thyroid storm, 136, 139
 reentrant, in Wolff-Parkinson-White syndrome, treatment of, 35, 39
 sinus, treatment of, 35–36, 39
 supraventricular, paroxysmal, recurrence of, 4, 5
 ventricular, unsustained, lidocaine for, 26, 27
 wide complex, regular, 34, 38
Tachypnea, in sepsis, 102, 103
Td (tetanus-diphtheria) booster, after bite wound, 339, 340
Temperature, afebrile, reported as fever, 96, 98
 measurement of, in children, 95, 97
Temporal arteritis, 146, 149, 205, 207

Temporal lobe, uncal herniation of, 247, 249
Temporomandibular joint dislocation, 165, 168, 251, 252
Tendon(s), lacerations of, 286, 288
Tendon sheath infection, purulent, 286, 288
Tensilon test, 201, 202
Tension pneumothorax, 380
Testicular torsion, 217, 219
Testicular trauma, 263, 265
Tetanus immunization, 277, 278
Tetanus-diphtheria (Td) booster, after bite wound, 339, 340
Tetany, in hypocalcemia, 130, 132
Tetracaine, in topical anesthetic, 277, 278
Tetracycline, for acne, side effects of, 223, 225
 for cystitis, 212, 214
Tetralogy of Fallot, 56, 57
Thalassemia, 181, 182–183
Theophylline, adenosine and, 32, 37
 toxicity of, 322, 323–324
Thiopental, endotracheal intubation and, 15, 17
Third cranial nerve palsy, 197, 198, 199
Thoracic aortic aneurysm, 46, 47–48
Thoracic duct, ruptured, 258, 259
Thoracic spine, compression of, 174, 177
Thoracolumbar Chance fracture, 244, 246
Thoracostomy, tube, ED, 379–380
Thoracotomy, ED, 379, 380
Thorax, trauma to, autotransfusion in, 258, 260
Thrombocytopenia, 184, 186
Thrombocytopenic purpura, acute immune, 184, 186
 thrombotic, 184, 185–186, 187, 227, 228
Thrombolytics, arrhythmias from, 32, 33, 36
 for myocardial ischemia, 25, 26
 hypersensitivity to, 123, 124
 risks of, 22, 24
Thrombophlebitis, superficial, therapy for, 45, 47
Thrombosed hemorrhoids, acute external, treatment of, 89, 91
Thrombosis, cavernous sinus, 159
 deep venous, 45, 47
 jugular venous, suppurative, 159
Thrombotic thrombocytopenic purpura, 184, 185–186, 187, 227, 228
Thrush, 161
Thyroid storm, 135–136, 139
Thyroidectomy, complications of, 137, 140
Thyrotoxicosis, 135–136, 139
 fever from, 95, 97
Tick-borne disease(s), 108–111
 ehrlichiosis as, 108–109
 Lyme disease as, 109–111
 Rocky Mountain spotted fever as, 108–109
Tidal volume, in ventilated patient, 16, 18
Tissue plasminogen activator (TPA), indications for, 45, 47
Toad venom, ingestion of, 322, 323
Tobramycin, hearing loss from, 152, 154
Tocolysis, contraindications to, 305, 306
Tonic seizures, 204, 206
Tonic-clonic seizure, generalized, altered mental status in, 203, 205
 febrile, 203, 205
Tonsillitis, 160
Tooth (teeth), avulsed, transport media for, 165, 168
 concussion of, 164, 167
 eruption of, 164, 167
 extraction of, 166, 169
 complications of, 164, 167
 fractures of, 164, 167
 classification and management of, 166, 169
 identification of, 165, 168
 impacted into alveolar bone, 165, 168

Tooth (teeth) *(Continued)*
  injuries to, 251, 252
    management of, 166, 168–169
      permanent, avulsed, emergency, 164, 165–166, 167, 168
      reimplantation of, 163, 166–167
    primary, avulsed, 165, 168
Topical anesthetic, for laceration repair, 277, 278
Torsades de pointes, 42
Toxic epidermal necrolysis, 224, 225
Toxic shock syndrome, 309, 312
Toxicologic emergencies, 315–335. See also *Poisoning.*
Toxidrome, sympathomimetic, vs. anticholinergic toxidrome, 329, 330
TPA (tissue plasminogen activator), indications for, 45, 47
Trachea, intubation of, inadvertent, 15, 16–17
  middle of, to alveolar ridge, calculation of, for pediatric patient, 15, 17
Tracheal intubation, in COPD exacerbations, 64, 65
Tracheostomy, in neck trauma, 253, 254
Transfers, patient, 363–364
Transfusion(s), blood, complications of, 82, 84
  in sickle cell disease, 180, 181
  platelet, for thrombotic thrombocytopenic purpura, 184, 185
Transient ischemic attacks, 145, 148
  in HgbSS disease, 180, 182
Transient synovitis, 294, 296
Transplantation, bone marrow, for sickle cell disease, 180, 182
Transtracheal ventilation, percutaneous, 383, 384
Trauma, 241–282, 357, 359–360
  abdominal, 261–265
  anterior epistaxis from, 151, 153
  breast, 313–314
  chest, 257–260
    blunt, 380
  dental, 251, 252
    management of, 165, 168
    prehospital care for, 163, 166
  diaphragmatic, 258, 259–260
  esophageal, 254–255
  extremity, 269–270
  head, 247–250
    assessment of, 243, 245
    pediatric, 272
  in pregnant patient, 273–275
  lower extremity, 290–292
  maxillofacial, 163, 166, 251–253
  multiple, 243–246
  neck, 253–255
  pediatric, 271–273
  pelvic, 265–268
  spinal, 243–246
    pediatric, 272–273
  thoracic, autotransfusion in, 258, 260
  upper extremity, 285–288
  urogenital, 262, 264
Traumatic hemothorax, 257, 259
Traumatic olecranon bursitis, 286, 288
Tremors, in thyrotoxicosis, 136, 139
Trench mouth, complications of, 158, 161
Treponema pallidum, 113, 114. See also *Syphilis.*
Triage, 363, 364
Trichomonas vaginalis, 308, 312
Tricyclic antidepressant, overdose of, *34*, 35, 38
Trigeminal neuralgia, 198
Trimethoprim, for cystitis, 212, 214
Trimethoprim-sulfamethoxazole, allergic reactions to, 123, 124
Triquetrum fractures, 287, 289
Trousseau's sign, in hypocalcemia, 130, 132

Trypanosomiasis, 112, 113
Tube(s), chest, placement of, 379–380
  endotracheal, pediatric, size of, 6, 8, 15, 17
  uncuffed, 16, 17
  gastrostomy, 385–386
Tube thoracostomy, ED, 379–380
Tuberculosis, 107–108
Tubo-ovarian abscess, 310
Tubular necrosis, acute, acute renal failure caused by, 211, 213
Tumor(s). See also *Cancer;* specific neoplasm.
  anterior epistaxis from, 151, 153
  pituitary, hypernatremic dehydration in infant from, 129, 130
Tumor lysis syndrome, treatment of, 174, 177
Tympanic membrane, perforation of, 152, 154
  in lightning injuries, 348
Typhlitis, 174, 177

Ulcer, gastric, endoscopic diagnosis of, 82, 84–85
Ulna, fracture of, midshaft, 286, 287–288
Ultrasound, in abdominal trauma, 261, 263
  in acute cholecystitis, 78, 80
  in early pregnancy, 302, 303
  in pyloric stenosis, 88, 90
Uncal brain herniation, 247, 249
Uncal herniation, 191, 193
Uniform Anatomical Gift Act, 369, 372
Uremic syndrome, hemolytic, 185, 187
Ureteral obstruction, 217, 218, 219
Ureterolithiasis, 218, 219
Urethra, injuries to, 262, 263, 265
Urethrography, retrograde, indications for, 266, 267
Urinalysis, 212, 214
Urinary bladder. See *Bladder.*
Urinary extravasation, 218, 219
Urinary retention, 217, 218, 219
Urinary tract, chronic outlet obstruction of, 217, 218
  infections of, 96, 98, 212–213, 214, 215
Urine culture, indications for, 212, 214
Urine dipstick, false-positive, 212, 214
Urogenital trauma, 262, 264
Uropathy, obstructive, complicating multiple myeloma, 173, 175–176
Urticaria, 223–224, 225, 226
Uterus, bleeding from, dysfunctional, 307, 308, 310, 311
Uvular edema, 158, 162

Vaccine, measles-mumps-rubella, fever from, 96, 98
  polyvalent pneumococcal, 69, 70
Vagina, bleeding from, third trimester, 304, 305
  foreign body in, 307, 310
  itching in, 308, 311
Vaginosis, bacterial, 308, 311
Variant angina, conditions associated with, 21, 23
  ECG changes in, 22, 24–25
Variceal bleed, management of, 82, 84
Varicose veins, therapy for, 45, 47
Vascular access, pediatric, 7, 9–10
Vasoconstriction, pulmonary, 62, 64
Vasopressors, for adrenal crisis, 135, 138
Vein(s), femoral, percutaneous line in, for pediatric patients, 7, 9
  saphenous, cutdown of, for pediatric patients, 7, 9
  varicose, therapy for, 45, 47

Venom, toad, ingestion of, 322, 323
Venous thrombosis, deep, risk factors for, 45, 47
  therapy for, 45, 47
Ventilation, intermittent mandatory, 16, 17–18
  mechanical, for asthma, 67, 68
  in respiratory distress, 13, 14
  tidal volume and, 16, 18
  percutaneous transtracheal, 383, 384
Ventricular ectopy, post-MI, 34, 37
Ventricular fibrillation arrest, intervention for, 4, 5
Ventricular septal defect (VSD), clinical findings in, 56–57, 58
  in Down's syndrome, 56, 58
Ventricular tachycardia (VT), complicating myocardial infarction, 35, 39
  drugs for, 35, 39
  indications of, 4, 5
  polymorphic, 42
  supraventricular tachycardia vs., 34, 38
    Brugada criteria for, 32, 36–37
  unsustained, lidocaine for, 26, 27
Ventriculoperitoneal shunt, in children, febrile illness and, 96, 98
Vertebrobasilar insufficiency, 197, 198
Vertigo, 193–195
Vincent's angina, complications of, 161
  presentation, 160, 164, 168
Vincristine, hyponatremia from, 130, 133
Violence. See also *Abuse.*
  management of, 234–235, 236
  potential, 234, 236
  spousal, 358, 361
Viral conjunctivitis, 146, 149
Viral keratitis, topical corticosteroids and, 146, 148
Viral pharyngitis, 161
Virus(es), human immunodeficiency, 99–101
  infections from, arthritis and, 294, 297
  fever and, 96, 98
    Rocky Mountain spotted fever vs., 108, 109
  pediatric fever from, 96, 98
  respiratory syncytial, bronchiolitis from, infant apnea in, 11
  pediatric pneumonia from, 69, 70
Visual field defects, in pituitary necrosis, 135, 138
Vitreous detachment, posterior, 145, 148
Vitreous hemorrhage, 146, 149
Volume deficits, in sepsis, 103, 104
Volvulus, gastric, 88, 89
  gastrointestinal bleeding from, 82, 84
  sigmoid, 88, 90
Vomiting, in adrenal insufficiency, 135, 138
  in pituitary necrosis, 135, 138
von Willebrand's disease, 184, 185, 186
V/Q scanning, 61–62, 63
VT (ventricular tachycardia). See *Ventricular tachycardia (VT).*
Vulvovaginal pruritus, 307, 309

Waldenström's macroglobulinemia, hyperviscosity syndrome from, 173–174, 176
Warfarin therapy, complications of, 185, 187
Warts, genital, 312
Weakness, in adrenal insufficiency, 135, 138
  in cancer-related hypercalcemia, 174, 177
  in myxedema, 136, 139
Weber test, 151, 153
Wegener's granulomatosis, in rheumatoid arthritis, 117, 119
Wellness, 373–375
Wharton's duct, 165, 168

Wheezing, in COPD, 64, 65
  inhaled foreign body causing, 157, 159
Withdrawal, alcohol/substance abuse, 238, 239, 240
  benzodiazepine, 326, 327
Wolff-Parkinson-White syndrome, 32, *33,* 37, 38
  atrial fibrillation with preexcitation pattern in, treatment of, 35, *36,* 39
  reentrant tachycardia in, treatment of, 35, 39
Wound management, 277–278

Wrist trauma, 286–287, 288–289

Xanthogranulomatous pyelonephritis, 212, 214
X-rays, in pediatric orthopedic emergencies, 295, 297

Yale Infant Observation Scale, 95–96, 97

Young classification system, of pelvic ring disruption, 266, 267–268

Zinc fumes, toxicity of, 332, 333
Zygoma fracture, 251, 252
Zyprexa (olanzapine), 233, 235–236